Pediatric Urology

Mario Lima • Gianantonio Manzoni
Editors

Pediatric Urology

Contemporary Strategies from Fetal Life to Adolescence

Foreword by Göran Läckgren

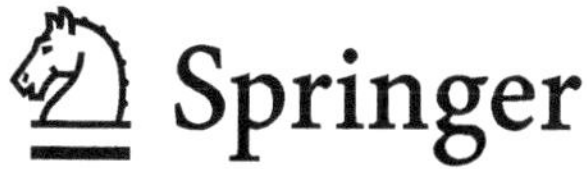

Editors
Mario Lima
Pediatric Surgery
S. Orsola-Malpighi University Hospital
Bologna
Italy

Gianantonio Manzoni
Pediatric Urology
Fondazione IRCCS Ca' Granda –
Ospedale Maggiore Policlinico
Milano
Italy

ISBN 978-88-470-5692-3 ISBN 978-88-470-5693-0 (eBook)
DOI 10.1007/978-88-470-5693-0
Springer Milan Heidelberg New York Dordrecht London

Library of Congress Control Number: 2014951711

Printed on acid-free paper

Springer is part of Springer Science+Business Media (www.springer.com)

Foreword

In Europe, Pediatric Urology is a subspecialty to either urology or pediatric surgery, and has developed quickly over the last decades. The need for a separate specialty to handle congenital anomalies and diseases in the urogenital tract in children is a natural consequence of the big differences in physiology, anatomy and disease panorama presentation between children and adults. The development of our specialty has been parallel to the progress in neonatology, antenatal diagnostics and radiology. New imaging techniques, molecular biology, genetics, and minimal invasive surgery have contributed to earlier diagnosis, better and safer approaches to the treatment and surgery of congenital urogenital malformations. Pediatric Urology is basically reconstructive urology of congenital malformations, but also deals with functional disturbances in the urogenital tract, tumors, stones etc. Many of our patients carry "their problems" into adulthood and need continuous and sometimes life-long follow-up with doctors that have good knowledge of the primary anomalies and their treatment.

The European Society for Pediatric Urology (ESPU) was founded for these reasons as a scientific society in 1990. One of the most important activities has been to arrange educational courses for the young urologists/surgeons and also to encourage and support other institutions to arrange courses and training in pediatric urology.

This book is based on the state-of-the-art lectures presented at the *Menarini Symposium* on Pediatric Urology in Bologna, June 2013. The Editors have managed to assemble some of the leading international experts in pediatric urology, and this book is based on current knowledge and the clinical experience of the authors. For ESPU it is very important that we can encourage organizers of courses to publish and spread the current state of the art in Pediatric Urology, and this book may serve as a reference source for pediatric urologists as well as urologists, pediatricians and surgeons dealing with patients with congenital abnormalities in the urogenital tract.

Göran Läckgren

Preface

Pediatric Urology is defined as the subspecialty of both Urology and Pediatric Surgery concerned with clinical recognition, prevention, treatment (surgical and non-surgical) and the rehabilitation of congenital and acquired diseases, malformations and functional problems of the genitor-urinary system in children and adolescents.

Over the years Pediatric Urology has unofficially developed, expanded, matured and established its diverse body of knowledge and proficiency. Some procedures performed today are so demanding that they should only be performed in centres where this sub-specialist knowledge and skill has been accumulated and well developed.

Last year, a very successful symposium held in Bologna on "Innovative Strategies in Pediatric Urology" represented the starting point for this new book. The subsequent idea to be able to incorporate into a dynamic and modern way the opinions of some of the best world's leading experts in this field has become a reality! The *European Society for Paediatric Urology (ESPU)* acknowledged the extraordinary opportunity to include this course as a 2013 ESPU event, and we are indeed honoured of the further privilege of a very prestigious Foreword from its President, Prof. Goran Lackgren.

As Editors, we are extremely pleased and thankful to all the Authors for their outstanding contribution, and we hope that all the potential readers will thoroughly enjoy this book as we did.

Mario Lima
Gianantonio Manzoni

Contents

Part III Bladder

Part IV Urethra

Part V Genitalia

Contributors

Annalisa Amaduzzi Department of General Surgery and Transplantation, S. Orsola-Malpighi University Hospital, Bologna, Italy

Claudio Antonellini Department of Pediatric Surgery, S. Orsola-Malpighi University Hospital, Bologna, Italy

Simonetta Baroncini Department for Mother and Child Health, S. Orsola-Malpighi University Hospital, Bologna, Italy

Federico Baronio Department of Pediatrics, S. Orsola-Malpighi University Hospital, Bologna, Italy

Alfredo Berrettini Pediatric Urology Unit, Fondazione IRCCS Ca' Granda – Ospedale Maggiore Policlinico, Milan, Italy

Marco Busutti Pediatric Nephrology and Dialysis Unit, Department of Pediatrics, S. Orsola-Malpighi University Hospital, Bologna, Italy

Paolo Caione Department of Nephrology-Urology, Children's Hospital Bambino Gesù, Rome, Italy

Noemi Cantone Department of Pediatric Surgery, S. Orsola-Malpighi University Hospital, Bologna, Italy

Irene Capelli Dialysis, Nephrology and Transplantation Unit, Department of Experimental, Diagnostic and Specialty Medicine, S. Orsola-Malpighi University Hospital, Bologna, Italy

Maria Luisa Capitanucci Department Nephrology–Urology, Robotic Surgery and Urodynamic Division, Children's Hospital Bambino Gesù, Rome, Italy

Filomena Carfagnini Department of Pediatric Radiology, S. Orsola-Malpighi University Hospital, Bologna, Italy

Marco Castagnetti Urology Unit, Section of Pediatric Urology, University Hospital of Padua, Padua, Italy

Francesco Corazza Department of Pediatrics, S. Orsola-Malpighi University Hospital, Bologna, Italy

Mario De Gennaro Department Nephrology–Urology, Robotic Surgery and Urodynamic Division, Children's Hospital Bambino Gesù, Rome, Italy

Delphine Demède Department of Pediatric Urology, HFME Mother and Child Hospital, Lyon, France

Francesca Destro Department of Pediatric Surgery, S. Orsola-Malpighi University Hospital, Bologna, Italy

Alaa El Ghoneimi Department of Pediatric Urology, University Children Hospital Robert Debré, APHP, University of Paris Diderot, Paris Cedex, France

Monica Fae Department for Mother and Child Health, S. Orsola-Malpighi University Hospital, Bologna, Italy

Giorgio Feliciangeli Dialysis, Nephrology and Transplantation Unit, Department of Experimental, Diagnostic and Specialty Medicine, S. Orsola-Malpighi University Hospital, Bologna, Italy

Andrea Gentili Department for Mother and Child Health, S. Orsola-Malpighi University Hospital, Bologna, Italy

Michele Guidotti Department of Nephrology-Urology, Children's Hospital Bambino Gesù, Rome, Italy

Claudia Guiducci Pediatric Nephrology and Dialysis Unit, Department of Pediatrics, S. Orsola-Malpighi University Hospital, Bologna, Italy

Gaetano La Manna Dialysis, Nephrology and Transplantation Unit, Department of Experimental, Diagnostic and Specialty Medicine, S. Orsola-Malpighi University Hospital, Bologna, Italy

Claudio La Scola Pediatric Nephrology and Dialysis Unit, Department of Pediatrics, S. Orsola-Malpighi University Hospital, Bologna, Italy

Mario Lima Department of Pediatric Surgery, S. Orsola-Malpighi University Hospital, Bologna, Italy

Gianantonio Manzoni Pediatric Urology Unit, Fondazione IRCCS Ca' Granda – Ospedale Maggiore Policlinico, Milan, Italy

Riccardo Masetti Department of Pediatrics – Pediatric Hematology and Oncology "Lalla Seràgnoli", S. Orsola-Malpighi University Hospital, Bologna, Italy

Fraia Melchionda Department of Pediatrics, S. Orsola-Malpighi University Hospital, Bologna, Italy

Francesca Mencarelli Pediatric Nephrology and Dialysis Unit, Department of Pediatrics, S. Orsola-Malpighi University Hospital, Bologna, Italy

Emilio Merlini Division of Pediatric Urology, Regina Margherita Children's Hospital, Citta' Della Salute e Della Scienza Di Torino, Torino, Italy

Michela Maffi Department of Pediatric Surgery, S. Orsola-Malpighi University Hospital, Bologna, Italy

Dario G. Minoli Pediatric Urology Unit, IRCCS Ca' Granda – Ospedale Maggiore Policlinico, Milan, Italy

Cristina Mondardini Department for Mother and Child Health, S. Orsola-Malpighi University Hospital, Bologna, Italy

Giovanni Montini Pediatric Nephrology and Dialysis Unit, Department of Pediatrics, S. Orsola-Malpighi University Hospital, Bologna, Italy

Giovanni Mosiello Department Nephrology–Urology, Robotic Surgery and Urodynamic Division, Children's Hospital Bambino Gesù, Rome, Italy

Pierre Mouriquand Department of Pediatric Urology, HFME Mother and Child Hospital, Lyon, France

Flavia Neri Department of General Surgery and Transplantation, S. Orsola-Malpighi University Hospital, Bologna, Italy

Andrea Pession Department of Pediatrics, S. Orsola-Malpighi University Hospital, Bologna, Italy

Craig A. Peters Surgical Innovation, Technology and Translation, The Sheikh Zayed Institute for Pediatric Surgical Innovation, Children's National Health System, Washington DC, USA

Matthieu Peycelon Department of Pediatric Urology, University Children Hospital Robert Debré, APHP, University of Paris Diderot, Paris Cedex 19, France

Gianluigi Pilu Department of Medicine and Surgery, Chair of Obstetrics and Gynecology, University of Bologna, Bologna, Italy

Antonio Daniele Pinna Department of General Surgery and Transplantation, S. Orsola-Malpighi University Hospital, Bologna, Italy

Arcangelo Prete Department of Pediatrics – Pediatric Hematology and Oncology "Lalla Seràgnoli", S. Orsola-Malpighi University Hospital, Bologna, Italy

Philip Ransley Division of Pediatric Urology, Civil Hospital, Sindh Institute of Urology and Transplantation, Karachi, Pakistan

Matteo Ravaioli Department of General Surgery and Transplantation, S. Orsola-Malpighi University Hospital, Bologna, Italy

Waifro Rigamonti Pediatric Surgery and Urology Unit, Burlo Garofalo Hospital, Trieste, Italy

Richard C. Rink Department of Pediatric Urology, Riley Hospital for Children, Indiana University School of Medicine, Indianapolis, USA

Giovanni Ruggeri Department of Pediatric Surgery, S. Orsola-Malpighi University Hospital, Bologna, Italy

Federico Scottoni Department of Nephrology-Urology, Children's Hospital Bambino Gesù, Rome, Italy

Sajid Sultan Department of Pediatric Urology, Sindh Institute of Urology and Transplantation, Karachi, Pakistan

Konrad M. Szymanski Department of Pediatric Urology, Riley Hospital for Children, Indiana University School of Medicine, Indianapolis, USA

Giovanni Tani Department of Pediatric Radiology, S. Orsola-Malpighi University Hospital, Bologna, Italy

Serdar Tekgul Division of Pediatric Urology, Department of Urology, Hacettepe University, Ankara, Turkey

Marco Togni Department of Pediatrics – Pediatric Hematology and Oncology "Lalla Seràgnoli", S. Orsola-Malpighi University Hospital, Bologna, Italy

Santiago Vallasciani Pediatric Urology Unit, IRCCS Ca' Granda – Ospedale Maggiore Policlinico, Milan, Italy

Francesca Vendemini Department of Pediatrics – Pediatric Hematology and Oncology "Lalla Seràgnoli", S. Orsola-Malpighi University Hospital, Bologna, Italy

Christopher R.J. Woodhouse Emeritus Professor of Adolescent Urology, Department of Urology, University College, London, UK

Daniele Zama Department of Pediatrics – Pediatric Hematology and Oncology "Lalla Seràgnoli", S. Orsola-Malpighi University Hospital, Bologna, Italy

Part I

General Aspects

Prenatal Diagnosis or Urological Abnormalities

1

Gianluigi Pilu

Anomalies of the genitourinary tract are among the most common malformations, with an overall prevalence in the range of 2–6 cases per 1,000 births. Most likely, this figure is an underestimation of the true incidence because in many cases the diagnosis of a urological problem is only made after the first months or years of life.

In Europe ultrasound examinations are performed in virtually all pregnancies. Patients with an increased risk of a fetal anomaly, usually because of a familial history, are referred to tertiary care centers for detailed sonograms. But even patients without specific risk factors undergo screening ultrasound examinations, usually between 11 and 13 weeks' gestation and 20 weeks' gestation. A direct consequence of this policy is the detection of abnormal fetal urinary tract findings in a tangible number of cases. Some of these findings are clear cut and allow the diagnosis of a specific malformation. In other cases, they only arise the suspicion of an abnormality. The sensitivity and specificity of universal ultrasound screening for fetal anomalies in pregnancy has been investigated in many large surveys, with variable results [1–4]. It is clear that both false negatives and positives are frequent. Indeed, the value of universal screening for anatomic malformations is debated [2–4].

After the identification of abnormal or suspicious fetal sonographic findings, pediatric specialists are frequently consulted to discuss the management strategy in the perinatal period and the prognosis. Such consultations have a particular relevance when the diagnosis is made in early gestation and the couples are considering the option of a pregnancy termination. It seems important to stress that caution is necessary when discussing the implications of antenatal diagnosis. The accuracy of sonography is limited, and anomalies identified in utero tend to have a different outcome than those that are identified after birth. Ancillary methods are now available for prenatal diagnosis in selected cases, including genetic testing and magnetic resonance, and multidisciplinary discussion is certainly indicated [5, 6].

In the following pages, we will briefly review the state of the art of prenatal diagnosis of urinary tract anomalies, focusing upon the information that seem relevant for the pediatric urologist and nephrologist who work in close contact with obstetric departments.

1.1 Standard Sonographic Examination of the Fetal Urinary Tract

In most countries, ultrasound examination is performed at 11–13 weeks' gestation with the aim to recognize multiple pregnancies, assess fetal

G. Pilu
Department of Medicine and Surgery,
Chair of Obstetrics and Gynecology,
University of Bologna, Via Massarenti 13,
Bologna 40138, Italy
e-mail: gianluigi.pilu@unibo.it

M. Lima, G. Manzoni (eds.), *Pediatric Urology: Contemporary Strategies from Fetal Life to Adolescence*,
DOI 10.1007/978-88-470-5693-0_1, © Springer-Verlag Italia 2015

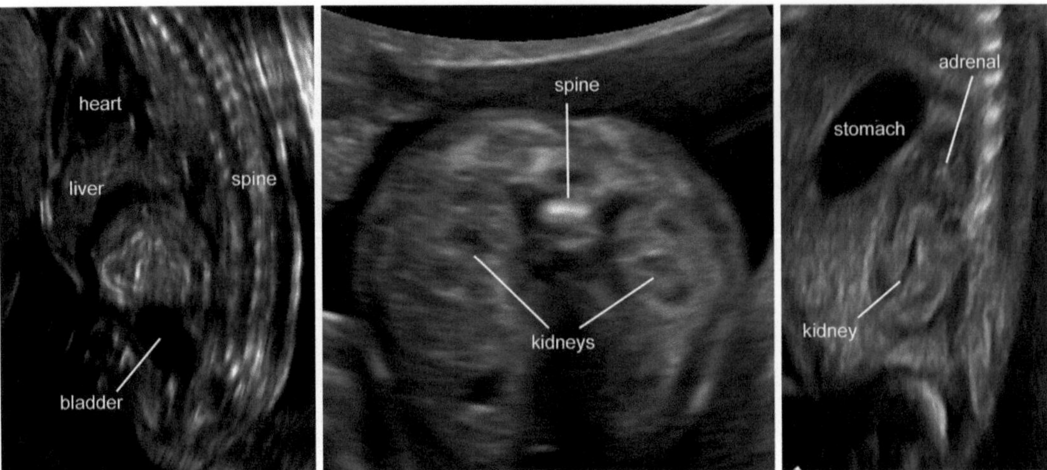

Fig. 1.1 Normal appearance of the fetal urinary tract at 20 weeks' gestation

viability, and screen for aneuploidies. At this time in gestation, the fetus is too small to allow a detailed examination of fetal anatomy. However, the bladder can be seen frequently, and gross dilatation (megacystis), due to urethral obstruction or more complex anomalies, can be identified [7–9]. Most efforts to diagnose anomalies are however made at around 20 weeks' gestation. At this time, there is a general consensus that the kidneys and bladder should always be identified (Fig. 1.1) [4]. An important clue of the integrity of the urinary tract is also the presence of a normal amount of amniotic fluid. Starting from about 16 weeks' gestation, the amniotic fluid is almost exclusively formed by fetal urine. Oliguria results in oligohydramnios and alerts to the possible presence of a urinary abnormality.

1.2 Renal Agenesis

Bilateral renal agenesis is found in 1 per 5,000 births; unilateral agenesis is found in 1 per 2,000 births. Renal agenesis is usually an isolated sporadic abnormality, but in a few cases, it may be secondary to a chromosomal abnormality or part of a genetic syndrome (such as Fraser syndrome) or a developmental defect (such as VACTERL association).

Bilateral renal agenesis is rarely missed at 20 weeks' gestation. The predominant findings at this time include severe oligohydramnios and failure to visualize the fetal bladder. However, severe oligohydramnios may be encountered also with premature rupture of the membranes or severe uteroplacental insufficiency. A specific diagnosis requires the demonstration of the absence of the kidneys, and this may be difficult at times. Examination of the renal areas is often hampered by the absence of amniotic fluid and the "crumpled" position adopted by these fetuses. Vaginal sonography with high-frequency high-resolution probes is useful in these cases. Useful clues in these cases is the almost constant presence of hypertrophic cardiomyopathy as well as the abnormal position of the adrenal glands that extend inferiorly to the renal fossae ("lying down" adrenals) (Fig. 1.2) [10]. Bilateral renal agenesis is a lethal condition. The presence of amniotic fluid is necessary for the normal development of the lungs up to 22–24 weeks. Early severe oligohydramnios results in a disruptive sequence commonly referred to as Potter syndrome, featured by pulmonary hypoplasia and limb mechanical deformations. Infants usually die in the neonatal period of respiratory insufficiency [11, 12].

Prenatal diagnosis of unilateral renal agenesis is generally difficult because in these cases the sonographic findings are subtle (Fig. 1.2) [13]. Amniotic fluid and bladder volume are normal. At midgestation the renal capsule is thin and the renal parenchyma difficult to differentiate from the

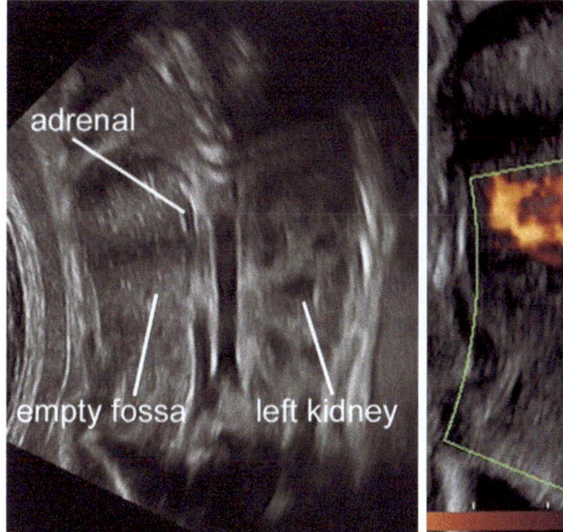

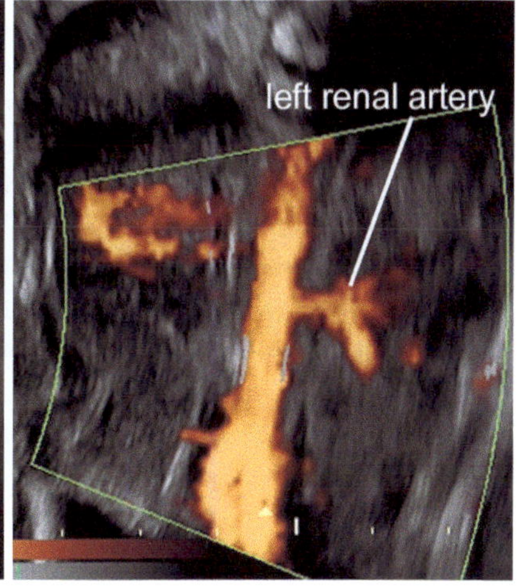

Fig. 1.2 Unilateral renal agenesis in fetus at midgestation; while the left kidney is well demonstrated, the right renal fossa appears empty; the diagnosis is supported by the observation of a vertical direction of the adrenal gland and by the failure to demonstrate the right renal artery with color Doppler ultrasound

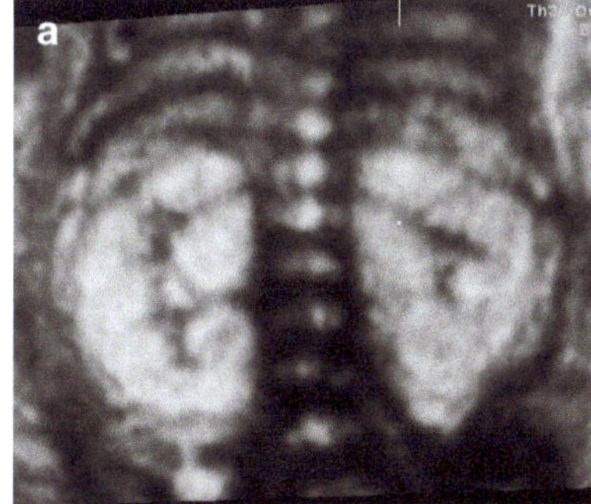

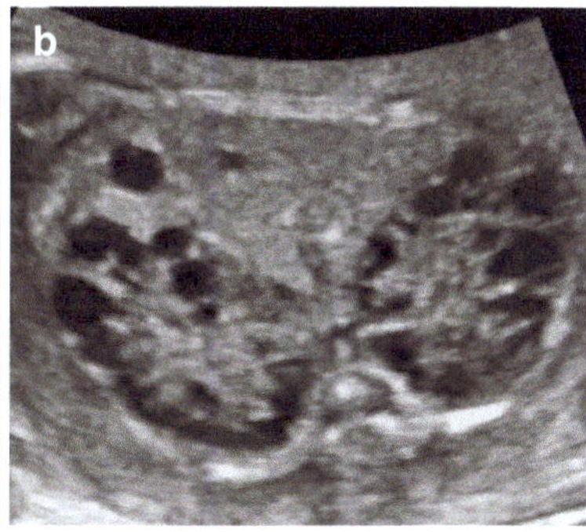

Fig. 1.3 Variable sonographic appearance of fetal bilateral renal dysplasia; (**a**) the kidneys are enlarged and contain multiple microcysts that are not individually demonstrated by sonography but result in increased echogenicity of the renal parenchyma; (**b**) the kidneys are enlarged and contain multiple macroscopic cysts

surrounding abdominal organs, and being positive about the absence of one kidney may be hard. The possibility of renal ectopia should also be considered in these cases. Progressive intrauterine development is also possible. At least in some cases, absence or severe hypoplasia of one kidney may not be a failure of embryogenesis but rather a disruption secondary to vascular of infectious causes. In such cases, the kidneys may have an unremarkable appearance at midgestation. The prognosis of unilateral agenesis is usually good, but significant associated anomalies occur in 30 % of cases. In particular, contralateral vesico-urinary reflux is present in about 20 % of cases [14].

1.3 Cystic Dysplastic Kidneys

Cystic dysplastic kidneys are a heterogeneous group of conditions with variable etiology, pathology, and clinical course. Sonographically, kidneys may present with either recognizable cystic collections or present increased echogenicity due to intraparenchymal disseminated microcysts (Fig. 1.3) [5, 6, 15–17]. Usually, early diagnosis of the specific type is impossible but for three different conditions: multicystic kidney, Meckel-Gruber syndrome, and renal dysplasia associated with early and severe obstructive uropathy.

Multicystic kidneys are usually unilateral and appear as a cluster of multiple irregular cysts of variable size with little intervening hyperechogenic stroma [6, 17, 18]. In the majority of cases, this is a sporadic abnormality but chromosomal abnormalities (mainly trisomy 18), genetic syndromes, and other defects (mainly cardiac) are present in about 50 % of the cases. The affected kidney may be large or small, and variations of the size can be encountered throughout gestation, either as the consequence of progressive atrophy or enlargement of the cysts. Large kidneys have been reported to cause polyhydramnios, but this is rare. In most cases vaginal delivery at term is possible. Isolated multicystic kidneys have a good prognosis, but the main factor influencing the outcome is a high prevalence of abnormalities (up to 40 % of cases) of the contralateral kidney, including vesicoureteral reflux, renal agenesis, and ureteral obstruction, that frequently require surgery and may result in progressive deterioration of renal function [18].

Meckel-Gruber syndrome is featured by the combination of cystic dysplasia, polydactyly, and cerebral malformations including cephalocele, posterior fossa cystic abnormalities, and anencephaly. It is a lethal condition transmitted as an autosomal recessive trait. A confident diagnosis can be made when the typical combination of digital, renal, and cerebral finding is encountered. The condition should also be suspected when there is bilateral macrocystic dysplasia of the kidneys prior to midgestation [9].

Early and persistent obstruction of the lower urinary tract is associated with *secondary cystic dysplasia* of the kidneys that appear hyperechogenic, increased in size, and small cysts spread in the parenchyma. In these cases the diagnosis is favored by the simultaneous demonstration of obstructive uropathy (distended bladder and ureters, pyelectasia, oligohydramnios). The prognosis is poor, and renal insufficiency is virtually always observed [6, 19].

Autosomal recessive cystic kidneys (also referred to as infantile polycystic kidneys) are characterized by markedly enlarged kidneys with cystic dilatation of the renal tubules, often with associated hepatic fibrosis. Sonographically, the kidneys appear enlarged on both sides and hyperechogenic. These sonographic appearances may however be manifest only in late gestation. The prognosis is variable. Cases appearing early in gestation are associated with oligohydramnios since the second trimester and are usually lethal due to a combination of renal failure and pulmonary hypoplasia. In most cases however the onset of the disease occurs later on in gestation or after birth, and there is a variable progression towards renal failure [5, 6, 16, 20].

Autosomal dominant cystic kidneys, one of the most common genetic diseases, is usually asymptomatic until the third or fourth decade of life. Sonography will not demonstrate abnormalities prior to the second or third decade. In a handful of cases, however, affected fetuses have demonstrated findings similar to the autosomal recessive variety: enlarged and echogenic kidneys. The experience with prenatal diagnosis is limited. It would not seem however that intrauterine presentation is not necessarily associated with a poor prognosis [6, 15, 16].

Cystic kidney is also found with many other genetic and nongenetic disorders such as tuberous sclerosis, Jeune syndrome, Sturge-Weber syndrome, Zellweger syndrome, and Laurence-Moon-Biedl syndrome [5, 6].

One major problem is differentiating early manifestation of autosomal recessive cystic kidneys from other types of dysplasias, such as autosomal dominant cystic kidney that has a much more favorable prognosis. Particularly in early gestation, when large echogenic kidneys are found with signs of normal renal function (normal amniotic fluid and bladder volume), a precise diagnosis may be impossible [16].

1.4 Enlargement of the Urinary Tract

Enlargement of the urinary tract is one of the most common abnormal findings that are identified with antenatal ultrasound.

Mild hydronephrosis or pyelectasia is by far the entity most frequently encountered. Although this is not universally agreed, this is defined by an anteroposterior diameter of the pelvis of >4 mm at midgestation weeks and >10 mm in the third trimester [21–25]. Most infants with a prenatal diagnosis of mild hydronephrosis will be found to have no urinary tract abnormality at birth. It has been suggested that distention of the renal pelves may be due to relaxation of smooth muscle of the urinary tract by the high levels of circulating maternal hormones or maternal-fetal overhydration. When the pelvis measured in the anteroposterior diameter is less than 10 mm and there is no calyceal dilatation, over 90 % of neonates will be normal. When the measurement is 10–15 mm and

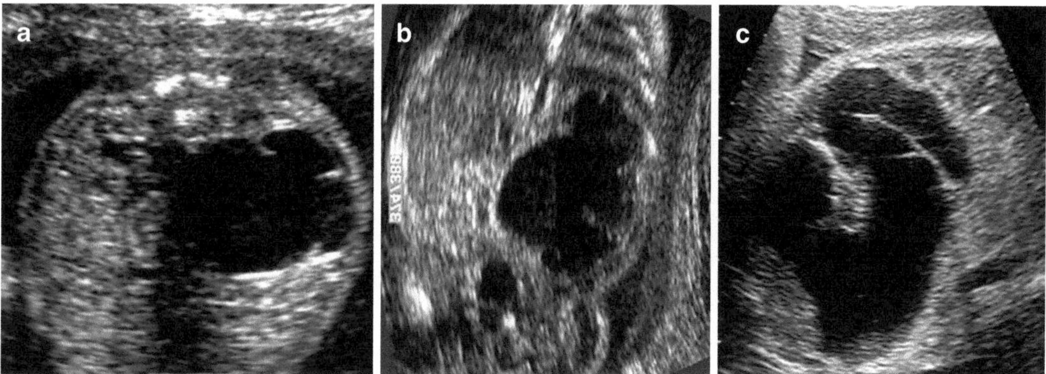

Fig. 1.4 Upper urinary tract enlargement: (**a**, **b**) hydronephrosis; (**c**) megaureter

there is no obvious calyceal dilatation, roughly 40 % of infants will require medical or surgical intervention. When the measurements are more than 15 mm and/or there is calyceal enlargement, most fetuses will require surgery (Fig. 1.4) [21–26]. Sonographically, it may be difficult at times to distinguish severe hydronephrosis with significant calyceal enlargement from multicystic kidney [17]. Hydronephrosis is usually the consequence of either ureteropelvic junction obstruction or vesicoureteric reflux. These are sporadic conditions, and although in some cases there is an anatomic cause, in most instances, the underlying cause is thought to be functional. In 80 % of cases, the condition is unilateral. Very rarely associated anomalies are found, albeit a slightly increased risk of chromosomal aberrations has been suggested for infants with mild dilatation. Independently from the degree or progression of hydronephrosis, the prognosis is generally good. The presence of a normal amount of amniotic fluid is reassuring with regard to renal function, and no modification of standard obstetric care is required. Vaginal delivery can occur at term.

Hydroureteronephrosis in the presence of a normal bladder may result from either ureterovesical reflux or ureterovesical junction obstruction (Fig. 1.4). Under normal condition, the small ureter cannot be visualized with antenatal ultrasound. The dilated ureter appears as a tortuous fluid-filled tubular structure interposed between the renal pelvis, which is variably dilated, and the bladder. Very rarely, a primary megaureter will be present, with a normal renal pelvis [20–22, 24–26]. The outcome and management principles are similar to the ones outlined for hydronephrosis.

Renal duplication can be associated with hydronephrosis and megaureter. A specific diagnosis is possible when two distinct renal pelves can be seen within one kidney (Fig. 1.5). Typically, there is some degree of dilatation of the upper renal pole [27, 28].

Megacystis is defined as a gross enlargement of the urinary bladder and is most frequently the consequence of urethral obstruction (Fig. 1.6). Typically, it is seen in the early midtrimester and has been visualized as early as 11 weeks' gestation [7, 8, 11, 12, 21]. The bladder is usually greatly enlarged, occupying most of the abdomen and distending it. Urethral obstruction can be caused by urethral agenesis, persistence of the cloaca, urethral stricture, or posterior urethral valves. Posterior urethral valves occur only in males and are the commonest cause of bladder outlet obstruction. The condition is sporadic and is found in about 1 in 3,000 male fetuses. With posterior urethral valves, there is usually incomplete or intermittent obstruction of the urethra, resulting in an enlarged and hypertrophied bladder with varying degrees of hydroureters, hydronephrosis, a spectrum of renal hypoplasia and dysplasia, oligohydramnios, and pulmonary hypoplasia. In some cases, there is associated urinary ascites from rupture of the bladder or transudation of urine into the peritoneal cavity.

When megacystis is found in association with either normal or increased amount of amniotic fluid, the possibility of megacystis-microcolon-intestinal

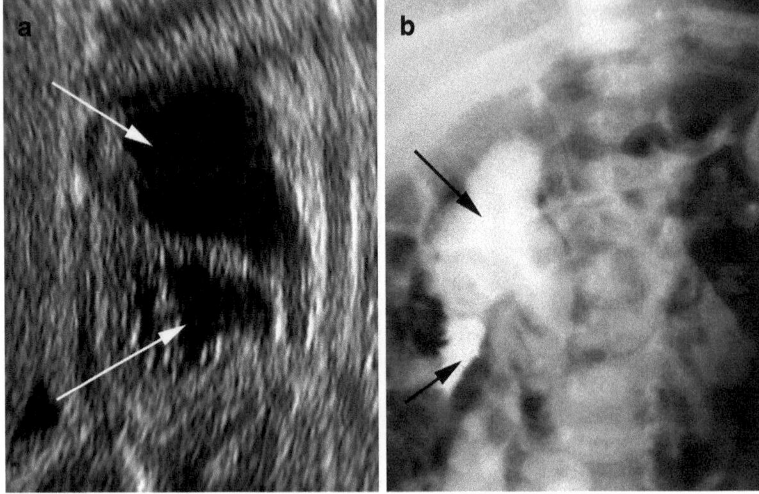

Fig. 1.5 Renal duplication (*arrows*) demonstrated by prenatal sonography (**a**) and postnatal urography (**b**)

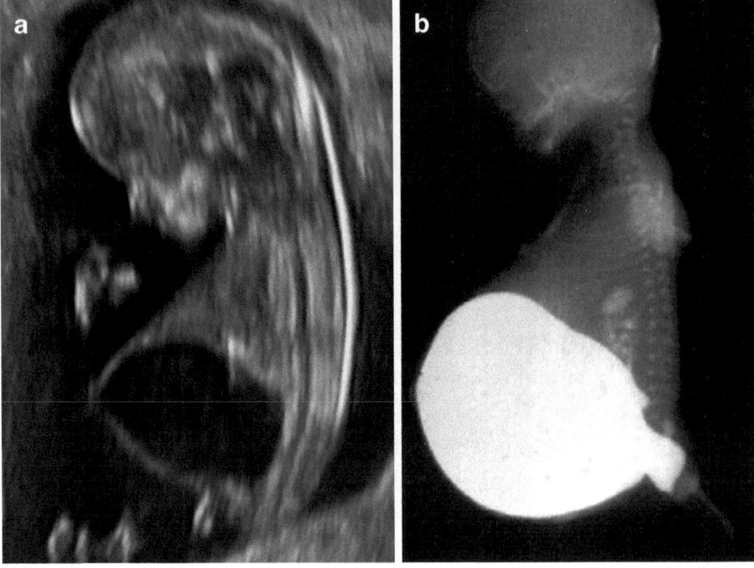

Fig. 1.6 Fetal megacystis demonstrated by antenatal sonography (**a**) and postnatal urography (**b**)

hypoperistalsis syndrome (MMIHS) should be considered [29]. This is a sporadic abnormality characterized by a massively dilated bladder and hydronephrosis in the presence of normal or increased amniotic fluid; the fetuses are usually female. There is associated shortening and dilatation of the proximal small bowel and microcolon with absent or ineffective peristalsis. The condition is usually lethal due to bowel and renal dysfunction (Fig. 1.7).

The outcome of urethral obstruction depends upon how severe and early this occurs. Complete persistent obstruction occurring in the early midtrimester (e.g., urethral atresia, early posterior urethral valves) results in massive distension of the bladder and abdominal wall (prune-belly abdomen), severe oligohydramnios, dysplastic kidneys, and pulmonary hypoplasia. Obstruction occurring in late gestation may be associated with oligohydramnios and hydronephrosis, but

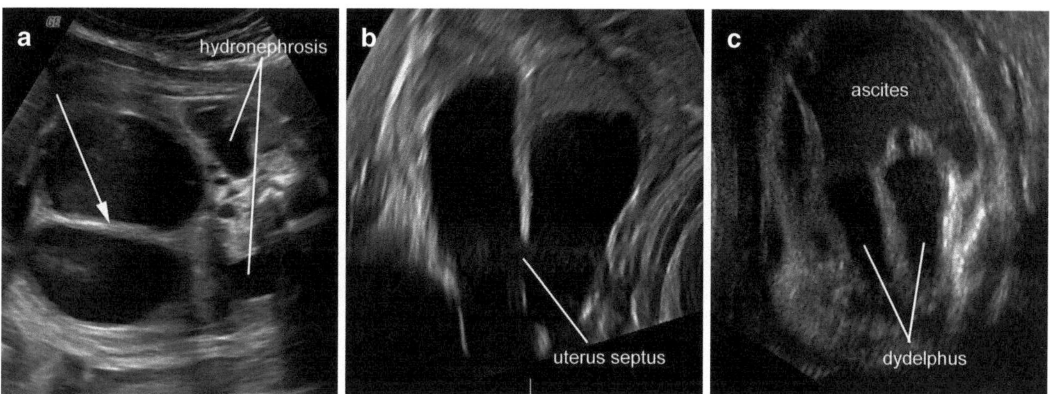

Fig. 1.7 Hydrometrocolpos; (**a**, **b**) the presence of an incomplete median septum (*arrow*) within a large midline abdominal cyst in a fetus with concomitant bilateral hydronephrosis suggests the presence of a uterus septus; a urogenital tract malformation was identified at birth; (**c**) in a fetus with ascites, ultrasound demonstrates a midline cystic structure suggestive of uterus didelphys; common cloaca was demonstrated after birth

does not result in pulmonary hypoplasia and dysplastic kidneys. Management of early-appearing megacystis is debated. Shunting the fetal bladder is feasible, although there is no conclusive evidence that such intervention improves renal or pulmonary function beyond what can be achieved by postnatal surgery [20, 30]. Antenatal evaluation renal function relies on a combination of ultrasonographic findings and analysis of fetal urine obtained by puncture of the bladder or renal pelvis. An attempt to assess the severity of renal compromise should however be done before embarking fetal therapy. Poor prognostic signs are (a) the presence of bilateral multicystic or severely hydronephrotic kidneys with echogenic kidneys, suggestive of renal dysplasia; (b) anhydramnios implying complete urethral obstruction; and (c) high urinary sodium, calcium, and ß2-microglobulin levels. In these cases, there are little chances of the infant surviving [20].

1.5 Bladder Exstrophy and Cloacal Exstrophy

Exstrophic anomalies are a group of disorders derived by a maldevelopment of the caudal fold of the anterior abdominal wall. In bladder exstrophy there is defect in the lower abdominal wall and the bladder is exposed and everted. Cloacal exstrophy is a more radical anomaly involving a large defect of the lower abdomen and perineum, separation of the pelvic bones, and eversion of the bladder and colon. Associated anomalies are rarely seen with bladder exstrophy but are found in most cloacal exstrophies and include neural tube defects, renal malformations, omphalocele, and congenital heart disease.

Exstrophy of the bladder is difficult to recognize antenatally, and the main finding is the persistent failure to visualize the bladder in the presence of a normal amount of amniotic fluid and normal kidneys [31]. The index of suspicion is increased by the presence of an irregularity in the lower abdominal wall caudad to the umbilical cord insertion. Exstrophy of the cloaca results in the presence of a complex mass arising from the lower abdomen, with no evidence of a urinary bladder.

1.6 Hydrometrocolpos

Hydrometrocolpos is a distention of the uterus and vagina caused by an obstruction to the drainage of genital secretions. This may arise from imperforate hymen, an abnormal transverse membrane, or agenesis of vagina or cervix. In most cases the condition is only manifest in adolescence. Rarely, gross distension resulting in a pelvic mass has been seen antenatally, usually in association with urogenital sinus or cloacal malformations. The sonographic appearance is a cystic pelvic mass, often with low-level echoes or a debris level, posterior to the bladder and extending into the abdomen [32]. A specific diagnosis from other intra-abdominal masses may be impossible, but for cases presenting with a septate or didelphys uterus that result in a very typical image on sonography.

Conclusion

Although the exact sensitivity and specificity of the prediction of fetal malformations by ultrasound examinations remains unclear, these examinations will frequently reveal abnormal findings indicating the presence of a urinary tract anomaly. This will trigger a multidisciplinary discussion on the relevance of the finding. Mild enlargement of the urinary tract, the most common entity, is a normal variant in many cases. The probability of an anomaly depends upon the degree of enlargement, but the outcome remains difficult to predict. Although in general a specific diagnosis of fetal renal anomalies is difficult, some entities have a clear-cut appearance in early gestation. Such list includes mostly bilateral renal agenesis, severe urethral obstruction, Meckel syndrome, multicystic kidney, and bladder and cloacal exstrophy.

References

1. Crane JP, LeFevre ML, Winborn RC, Evans JK, Ewigman BG, Bain RP, Frigoletto FD, McNellis D (1994) A randomized trial of prenatal ultrasonographic screening: impact on the detection, management, and outcome of anomalous fetuses. The RADIUS Study Group. Am J Obstet Gynecol 171(2):392–399. PubMed PMID: 8059817
2. Ewigman BG, Crane JP, Frigoletto FD, LeFevre ML, Bain RP, McNellis D (1993) Effect of prenatal ultrasound screening on perinatal outcome. RADIUS Study Group. N Engl J Med 329(12):821–827. PubMed PMID: 8355740
3. Grandjean H, Larroque D, Levi S (1999) The performance of routine ultrasonographic screening of pregnancies in the Eurofetus Study. Am J Obstet Gynecol 181(2):446–454. PubMed PMID: 10454699
4. Salomon LJ, Alfirevic Z, Berghella V, Bilardo C, Hernandez-Andrade E, Johnsen SL, Kalache K, Leung KY, Malinger G, Munoz H, Prefumo F, Toi A, Lee W, Committee ICS (2011) Practice guidelines for performance of the routine mid-trimester fetal ultrasound scan. Ultrasound Obstet Gynecol 37(1):116–126. PubMed PMID: 20842655
5. Roume J, Ville Y (2004) Prenatal diagnosis of genetic renal diseases: breaking the code. Ultrasound Obstet Gynecol 24(1):10–18. PubMed PMID: 15229910
6. Zerres K, Volpel MC, Weiss H (1984) Cystic kidneys. Genetics, pathologic anatomy, clinical picture, and prenatal diagnosis. Hum Genet 68(2):104–135
7. Kagan KO, Staboulidou I, Syngelaki A, Cruz J, Nicolaides KH (2010) The 11–13-week scan: diagnosis and outcome of holoprosencephaly, exomphalos and megacystis. Ultrasound Obstet Gynecol 36(1):10–14. PubMed PMID: 20564304
8. Sebire NJ, Von Kaisenberg C, Rubio C, Snijders RJ, Nicolaides KH (1996) Fetal megacystis at 10–14 weeks of gestation. Ultrasound Obstet Gynecol 8(6):387–390. PubMed PMID: 9014277
9. Ickowicz V, Eurin D, Maugey-Laulom B, Didier F, Garel C, Gubler MC, Laquerriere A, Avni EF (2006) Meckel-Gruber syndrome: sonography and pathology. Ultrasound Obstet Gynecol 27(3):296–300. PubMed PMID: 16450359
10. Hoffman CK, Filly RA, Callen PW (1992) The "lying down" adrenal sign: a sonographic indicator of renal agenesis or ectopia in fetuses and neonates. J Ultrasound Med 11(10):533–536. PubMed PMID: 1404583
11. Anumba DO, Scott JE, Plant ND, Robson SC (2005) Diagnosis and outcome of fetal lower urinary tract obstruction in the northern region of England. Prenat Diagn 25(1):7–13. PubMed PMID: 15662711
12. Robyr R, Benachi A, Daikha-Dahmane F, Martinovich J, Dumez Y, Ville Y (2005) Correlation between ultrasound and anatomical findings in fetuses with lower urinary tract obstruction in the first half of pregnancy. Ultrasound Obstet Gynecol 25(5):478–482. PubMed PMID: 15816021
13. Jeanty P, Romero R, Kepple D, Stoney D, Coggins T, Fleischer AC (1990) Prenatal diagnoses in unilateral empty renal fossa. J Ultrasound Med 9(11):651–654. PubMed PMID: 2258997
14. Westland R, Schreuder MF, Ket JC, van Wijk JA (2013) Unilateral renal agenesis: a systematic review on associated anomalies and renal injury. Nephrol Dial Transplant 28(7):1844–1855. Epub 2013 Feb 28
15. Brun M, Maugey-Laulom B, Eurin D, Didier F, Avni EF (2004) Prenatal sonographic patterns in autosomal dominant polycystic kidney disease: a multicenter study. Ultrasound Obstet Gynecol 24(1):55–61, PubMed PMID: 15229917
16. Chaumoitre K, Brun M, Cassart M, Maugey-Laulom B, Eurin D, Didier F, Avni EF (2006) Differential diagnosis of fetal hyperechogenic cystic kidneys unrelated to renal tract anomalies: a multicenter study. Ultrasound Obstet Gynecol 28(7):911–917. PubMed PMID: 17094077

17. Rizzo N, Gabrielli S, Pilu G, Perolo A, Cacciari A, Domini R, Bovicelli L (1987) Prenatal diagnosis and obstetrical management of multicystic dysplastic kidney disease. Prenat Diagn 7(2):109–118. PubMed PMID: 3554210
18. van Eijk L, Cohen-Overbeek TE, den Hollander NS, Nijman JM, Wladimiroff JW (2002) Unilateral multicystic dysplastic kidney: a combined pre- and postnatal assessment. Ultrasound Obstet Gynecol 19(2):180–183. PubMed PMID: 11876812
19. Johnson MP, Bukowski TP, Reitleman C, Isada NB, Pryde PG, Evans MI (1994) In utero surgical treatment of fetal obstructive uropathy: a new comprehensive approach to identify appropriate candidates for vesicoamniotic shunt therapy. Am J Obstet Gynecol 170(6):1770–1776. PubMed PMID: 8203438. discussion 1776–9
20. Johnson CE, Elder JS, Judge NE, Adeeb FN, Grisoni ER, Fattlar DC (1992) The accuracy of antenatal ultrasonography in identifying renal abnormalities. Am J Dis Child 146(10):1181–1184. PubMed PMID: 1415046
21. Grignon A, Filion R, Filiatrault D, Robitaille P, Homsy Y, Boutin H, Leblond R (1986) Urinary tract dilatation in utero: classification and clinical applications. Radiology 160(3):645–647. PubMed PMID: 3526402
22. Nguyen HT, Kogan BA (1998) Upper urinary tract obstruction: experimental and clinical aspects. Br J Urol 81(Suppl 2):13–21. PubMed PMID: 9602791
23. Orzechowski KM, Berghella V (2013) Isolated fetal pyelectasis and the risk of Down syndrome: a meta-analysis. Ultrasound Obstet Gynecol 42(6):615–621. PubMed PMID: 23712390
24. Podevin G, Mandelbrot L, Vuillard E, Oury JF, Aigrain Y (1996) Outcome of urological abnormalities prenatally diagnosed by ultrasound. Fetal Diagn Ther 11(3):181–190. PubMed PMID: 8739585
25. Sairam S, Al-Habib A, Sasson S, Thilaganathan B (2001) Natural history of fetal hydronephrosis diagnosed on mid-trimester ultrasound. Ultrasound Obstet Gynecol 17(3):191–196. PubMed PMID: 11309166
26. Lepercq J, Beaudoin S, Bargy F (1998) Outcome of 116 moderate renal pelvis dilatations at prenatal ultrasonography. Fetal Diagn Ther 13(2):79–81. PubMed PMID: 9650651
27. Abuhamad AZ, Horton CE Jr, Horton SH, Evans AT (1996) Renal duplication anomalies in the fetus: clues for prenatal diagnosis. Ultrasound Obstet Gynecol 7(3):174–177. PubMed PMID: 8705408
28. Whitten SM, McHoney M, Wilcox DT, New S, Chitty LS (2003) Accuracy of antenatal fetal ultrasound in the diagnosis of duplex kidneys. Ultrasound Obstet Gynecol 21(4):342–346. PubMed PMID: 12704741
29. White SM, Chamberlain P, Hitchcock R, Sullivan PB, Boyd PA (2000) Megacystis-microcolon-intestinal hypoperistalsis syndrome: the difficulties with antenatal diagnosis. Case report and review of the literature. Prenat Diagn 20(9):697–700. PubMed PMID: 11015695
30. Morris RK, Malin GL, Khan KS, Kilby MD (2010) Systematic review of the effectiveness of antenatal intervention for the treatment of congenital lower urinary tract obstruction. BJOG 117(4):382–390. PubMed PMID: 20374578
31. Cacciari A, Pilu GL, Mordenti M, Ceccarelli PL, Ruggeri G (1999) Prenatal diagnosis of bladder exstrophy: what counseling? J Urol 161(1):259–261. discussion 62. PubMed PMID: 10037419
32. Davis GH, Wapner RJ, Kurtz AB, Chhibber G, FitzSimmons J, Blocklinger AJ (1984) Antenatal diagnosis of hydrometrocolpos by ultrasound examination. J Ultrasound Med 3(8):371–374. PubMed PMID: 6384541

2 Antenatal and Perinatal Management of Urinary Malformations

Francesca Destro, Noemi Cantone, Michela Maffi, and Mario Lima

2.1 Introduction

Maternal US was introduced in the 1970s and it has increased in frequency and popularity, until the 1980s when it became a routine practice. Nowadays all pregnancies have a detailed US anomaly scan. The urinary tract anomalies (UTAs) are the commonest anomalies found in utero, not only for their high incidence but also because these abnormalities result in alterations easily recognizable on ultrasound as hydronephrosis or variations of parenchymal echogenicity [1]. The sensitivity and specificity of US are operator dependent [2, 3]. These abnormalities are detected at 16–20 weeks of gestation, with an incident of 1 in 50–100 pregnancies, depending on the US criteria. Most of these findings will resolve spontaneously before birth [2, 4]. About 70 % of UTAs are diagnosed by 20 weeks of gestation, while the other 30 % are found either on a third trimester scan or more commonly as a consequence of an obstetric complication.

It is fundamental to have a pre- and postnatal collaboration with obstetrics and other colleagues in order to produce the best data, statistics, and counseling [1, 4]. In fact the prenatal diagnosis of UTA may cause a huge amount of anxiety for the family that may be related to a poor counseling, misunderstanding, and insufficient collaboration. The difficult interaction between specialists may be related to the lack of standardized parameters used for pre- and postnatal US measurements [5, 6].

The goal of the prenatal diagnosis is not only to obtain a differential diagnosis but also to achieve a definition of the prognosis, foreseeing the natural history of these anomalies. The biggest challenge in the prenatal assessment is to identify the population at risk in which an early diagnosis and treatment can prevent urinary tract or systemic complications. In fact, only a small part (<5 %) of neonates with a prenatal diagnosis of UTA develops a renal insufficiency or requires renal transplantation, whereas the remaining part of them leads a normal life.

For this reason we should consider different parameters to discriminate the fetuses that require follow-up and intervention from those who do not [7–9].

The elements identified during prenatal evaluation are specific or nonspecific. Specific abnormalities represent 20 % of prenatal US findings, and they include duplex kidney with or without ureterocele and multicystic kidney for which there is a well-accepted treatment. The main problem with prenatal diagnoses is that more than 80 % of US findings are nonspecific (variations of renal echogenicity, cystic disease, variations of renal dimensions, oligohydramnios, hydronephrosis, etc.). All these findings

F. Destro • N. Cantone • M. Maffi • M. Lima (✉)
Department of Pediatric Surgery,
S. Orsola-Malpighi University Hospital,
Via Massarenti 11, Bologna 40138, Italy
e-mail: francesca_destro@hotmail.com;
noemicantone@hotymail.com; michela.maffi@libero.it;
mario.lima@unibo.it

M. Lima, G. Manzoni (eds.), *Pediatric Urology: Contemporary Strategies from Fetal Life to Adolescence*,
DOI 10.1007/978-88-470-5693-0_2, © Springer-Verlag Italia 2015

end up with a huge variety of possible diagnoses. In these cases explaining the differential diagnoses to parents could be impossible for the obstetrician.

The most frequent abnormalities suspected with pregnancy scans are ureteropelvic junction obstruction (44–65 %), vesicoureteral reflux (15 %), multicystic kidney (10 %), ureteroceles (10 %), megaureter (9 %), and posterior urethral valves (4 %) [4]. The aim of prenatal investigation and postnatal evaluation is to detect asymptomatic patients that will develop symptoms or severe renal function alterations, in other words, to identify patients at risk. The key to do that is to know the natural history of prenatal abnormalities. It is also fundamental to use a limited number and types of postnatal investigations selecting only those that are likely to influence the clinical outcome.

Patients' evaluation always starts with prenatal history that should include detailed parameters (detailed measures and not unspecific terminology). Prenatal history permits to decide if the prenatal abnormality is the end result of a utero event (e.g., multicystic kidney, transient urethral obstruction) and if it is clinically significant or not [1, 9].

2.2 Hydronephrosis

Hydronephrosis is the most common (and unfortunately nonspecific) finding during prenatal ultrasounds [4]. It consists of a dilated renal pelvis and calices with or without ureter and bladder dilatation. Its interpretation is not always easy and requires a thorough process of differential diagnosis. In fact, the causes of prenatal hydronephrosis can vary from self-limiting conditions to others associated with a high risk of renal failure in the postnatal period. The most common pathologies presenting with prenatal hydronephrosis are summarized in Table 2.1 [4, 9, 10].

The parameter used to define hydronephrosis is the anteroposterior diameter (ADP) of the pelvis in the transverse plane of the kidney at the hilum [4, 9, 10]. On these bases, hydronephrosis is commonly evaluated as follows (Fig. 2.1) [11]:

Grade 1 – pelvic APD of 1 cm and no caliectasis

Grade 2 – pelvic APD of 1–1.5 cm and no caliectasis

Grade 3 – pelvic APD is greater than 1.5 cm and slight caliectasis

Grade 4 – pelvic APD is greater than 1.5 cm and moderate caliectasis

Grade 5 – pelvic APD is greater than 1.5 cm and severe caliectasis and cortical atrophy (cortex <2 mm thick)

Hydronephrosis may be defined as mild (<15 mm), moderate (15–20 mm), and severe (>20 mm), on the base of prenatal renal pelvis dilatation at third trimester US. In each case the presence or absence of calyceal dilatation should be evaluated [12].

Anyway prenatal ultrasounds should give a lot of other information such as longitudinal diameter of the kidney (which include up and low pole calices), transverse diameter (which include the mid pole), parenchymal echogenicity, ureteral dilatation, thickness of the bladder wall, bladder content (Fig. 2.2), and amniotic fluid volume [1, 4].

Recently the Society for Fetal Urology has proposed a grading system for postnatal hydronephrosis on US [13, 14]:

Grade 0: intact central renal complex + normal parenchyma

Grade 1: slight central renal complex splitting + normal parenchyma

Grade 2: central renal complex splitting confined within renal border + normal parenchyma

Grade 3: wide splitting of central renal complex + pelvis dilated outside renal border + calices dilated with normal parenchyma

Table 2.1 Causes of prenatal hydronephrosis

Causes of prenatal hydronephrosis
Ureteropelvic junction obstruction
Vesicoureteral reflux
Primary nonrefluxing megaureter
Ureterocele
Ureterovesical junction obstruction
Ureteral ectopia
Posterior urethral valves
Megacystic megaureter
Physiologic dilatation
Multicystic dysplastic kidney
Autosomal recessive polycystic kidney disease
Exstrophy
Prune belly syndrome

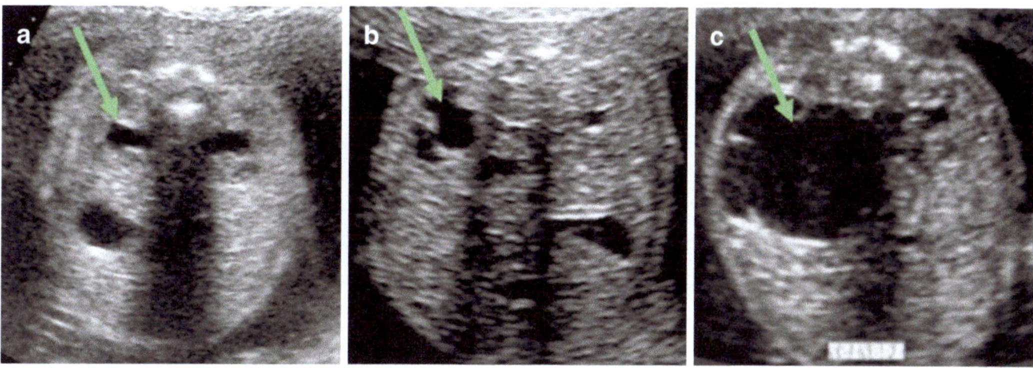

Fig. 2.1 Prenatal hydronephrosis on US: grade I with renal pelvis dilatation (*green arrow* in **a**), grade II with renal pelvis and calyceal dilatation (*green arrow* in **b**), and grade III with severe dilatation of both pelvis and calyces (*green arrow* in **c**) and cortical atrophy (**c**)

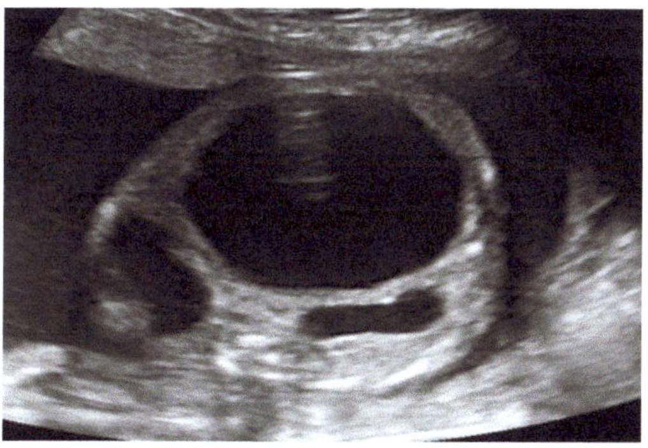

Fig. 2.2 US evaluation, at 20 weeks of gestational age, is completed with examination of the lower urinary tract. The abdominopelvic transversal scan shows the presence of a distended bladder

Grade 4: large dilated calices + further dilation of renal pelvis + thinning of parenchyma (less than half that of the contralateral of <4 mm if bilateral)

All these data, combined with the fetal well-being, the age of detection of the anomaly, and the unilaterality versus the bilaterality, should be considered for a correct management. The problem is still the lack of accurate prognostic factors and the fact that prenatal hydronephrosis may be caused by various etiologies (obstructive and nonobstructive). Different prenatal prognostic elements have been investigated [15–17]. The presence of oligohydramnios and increased renal echogenicity seem to be related to obstruction, thus identifying patients that may require fetal intervention (e.g., vesicoamniotic shunt) [9, 16]. Isotonic urine is thought to be related to poor outcome, whereas selective reabsorption of sodium and chloride by normal kidneys makes the urine hypotonic. In particular biochemical parameters identified as predictors of poor functional outcome include: fetal urinary sodium of >100 mEq/L, elevated urinary calcium (>1.2 mmol/L), and increased β2 microglobulin [17]. Predictors of good function seem to be normal moderately decreased amniotic fluid, normal sonographic appearance, and urine outcome >2 mL/min [15–17].

Unfortunately the postnatal management of these children remains controversial (in terms of timing and types of interventions). Investigations performed immediately after birth may be altered by perinatal dehydration and lower glomerular filtration. We recommend to wait at least 3–7 days (for unilateral dilatations with normal contralateral kidney also 10–14 days) to perform a sonogram once oligohydramnios, urethral obstruction, multicystic renal dysplasia, and bilateral severe hydronephrosis have been excluded. In fact prompt postnatal US in the first day of life is essential for fetuses with suspected lower urinary tract obstruction or pathologies that put at risk the kidneys [4, 18].

The role of the micturating cystourethrogram (MCU) has not been completely established, especially in children with prenatal hydronephrosis and normal postnatal US. MCU is used in case of abnormal bladder (suspicion of outflow obstruction), bilateral upper tract dilatation, ureter dilatation, and duplex kidneys to detect vesicoureteral reflux, ectopic ureteroceles, and posterior urethral valves [1, 4, 9].

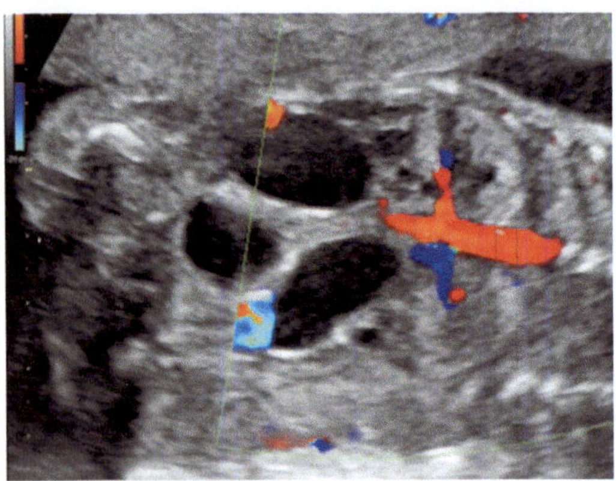

Fig. 2.3 US abdominopelvic coronal scan showing severe dilated ureter

Vesicoureteral reflux (*VUR*) causes nonspecific prenatal hydronephrosis. VUR cannot be diagnosed prenatally except for bilateral cases. Bilateral hydronephrosis, bilateral VUR, and distended bladder represent megacystis and megaureter. Postnatal surgery (Deflux or ureteroneocystostomy) is required on the base of laterality and grade [4, 10, 19].

An *ureterocele* is a cystic dilatation of the distal ureter in a solitary or duplicated collecting system (usually the upper pole). It causes obstruction and subsequent dilatation of the upper urinary tract. After birth, it is managed by endoscopic decompression (with or without heminephrectomy) when intravesical. Extravesical forms should be treated conservatively [4, 10].

A dilated ureter (Fig. 2.3) and renal pelvis with MCU negative for VUR may indicate the presence of aperistalsis in the distal ureter (*nonrefluxing megaureter*). This condition tends to reduce spontaneously [4, 10].

Babies with prenatal unilateral mild hydronephrosis (prenatally pelvic dilatation <15 mm, stable in the first 6 months of life) and normal echogenicity and without ureteric-calyceal dilatation should be managed by pediatricians with US. The population described is the one with no clinical significance. They do not need either VCUG or antibiotic prophylaxis (Table 2.2 resumes the need for antibiotics in newborns with prenatally detected uropathies) [1].

Table 2.2 Antibiotic prophylaxis

No
Mild isolated renal dilatation <15 mm and normal calyces
Multicystic kidney with normal contralateral kidney
Ectopic kidney without dilatation
Yes: all other cases
Trimethoprim 2 mg/kg/day, single dose

US evaluation should be completed with MAG3 renogram when ureteral dilatation has been ruled out and an *ureteropelvic junction* (*UPJ*) *obstruction* is suspected [4].

UPJ obstruction is the most common cause of severe hydronephrosis without dilatation of ureter and bladder. The cause of obstruction may be intrinsic or extrinsic (e.g., accessory vessels).

Obstruction makes the half-life ($t½$) on MAG3 greater than 20 min (normal is between 0 and 10 min) [4, 20].

The postnatal treatment of patients with hydronephrosis is still debated [1, 10]. In fact the majority of patients with a dilatation <20 mm have a good renal function and do not require any intervention. Among them there are two populations at risk that include patients with intrarenal hydronephrosis and patients with increasing dilatation. Intrarenal hydronephrosis might be a sign of UPJ obstruction. The obstruction is responsible for massive calyceal dilatation that represents a threat for the renal parenchyma. At MAG3 the parenchyma appears stretched and thinned. Many intrarenal hydronephroses are detected prenatally as multicystic kidneys because all those calices look like cysts. However, the renal function is still present, differently from the multicystic kidneys, and the US shows a central cystic structure with multiple dilated and uniform-sized lateral calyces communicating with the central cystic structure. It is important to differentiate severe hydronephrosis and multicystic kidneys because intrarenal hydronephrosis requires prompt surgical correction.

The second group at risk is the one with increasing dilatation that seems to be related to 15–20 mm dilatation (moderate) with calyceal involvement. If a moderate dilatation with calyceal involvement is identified, it is useful

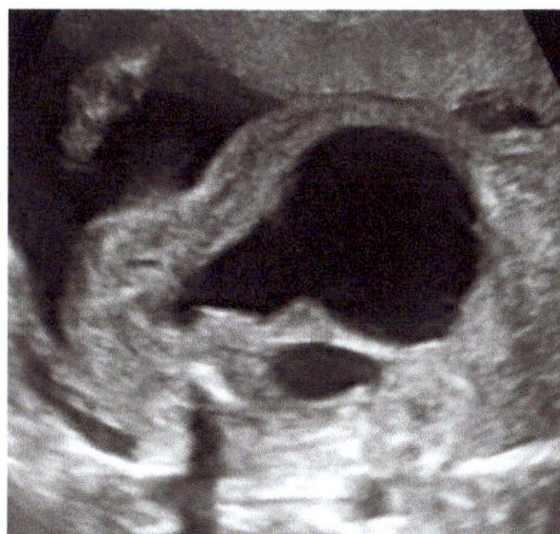
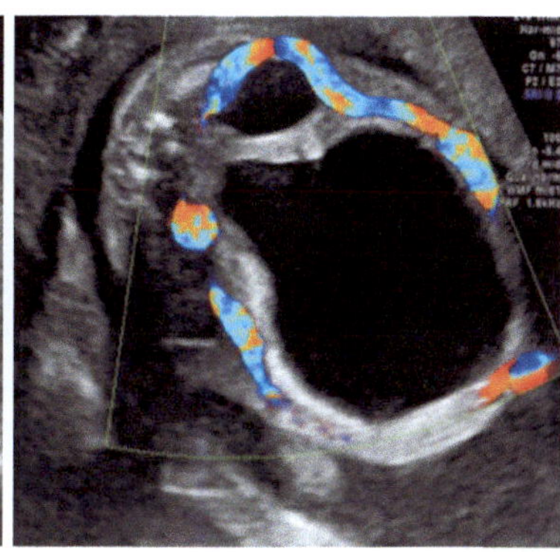

Fig. 2.4 Dilated bladder with keyhole sign that indicates a low urinary tract obstruction

to perform a baseline MAG3 and to start a US follow-up. Surgery is required in case of changes at US follow-up.

Prompt evaluation with diuretic renogram is necessary in case of grade 3 or 4 hydronephrosis (severe dilatation >20 mm) and suspected bilateral ureteropelvic obstruction, to assess renal function.

Among patients with severe hydronephrosis, there are some that will benefit a prophylactic pyeloplasty. A dilatation of 30 mm seems associated with deterioration in all cases and it represents a clinical significant population that requires surgery. In all other cases, surgery is required when the dilatation increases, the function drops under 40 %, and symptoms (urinary tract infections, pain, etc.) occur [1, 4, 10, 18].

Prenatal US hydronephrosis with oligohydramnios may indicate the presence of *posterior urethral valves* (*PUV*). PUVs are mucosal flaps that cause bladder outlet obstruction. US findings also include dilated urinary bladder and posterior urethra (keyhole sign) and subcortical renal cyst formation (Fig. 2.4) [4, 10, 21].

Increased postnatal mortality is predicted by severe bilateral upper tract dilatation (renal AP diam. >10 mm), renal parenchymal changes, and severe oligohydramnios or anhydramnios. After birth patients are evaluated with US and MCU. The bladder should be voided with a small feeding tube and surgery performed early (transurethral valve ablation with Bugbee, cutaneous pyelostomy/ureterostomy/vesicostomy). Positive prognostic factors are serum creatinine level <0.8–1.0 mg/dL 1 month after surgery and the presence of a pop-off valve mechanism that protects high systems.

Urethral obstruction might also be transient. *Transient urethral obstruction* is the end result of an in utero event. In these cases prenatal US shows a distended bladder, bilateral hydronephrosis, dilated ureters, and normal/reduced amniotic fluid. The condition is transient and by 25 weeks there is a spontaneous resolution with the bladder emptying, the fluid restored, and the hydronephrosis improved. The cause is often a syringocele that derives from the Cowper's duct and it is in the anterior urethra. MCU shows a pattern similar to those of resected PUV. MCU should be performed via suprapubic in order to leave the urethra virgin. In fact, syringoceles are very flimsy and easy to rupture. These children usually have an abnormal bladder, dilated posterior urethra, and prominent bladder neck [4, 22]. Another rare form of functional lower tract obstruction is the *congenital megalourethra*. It is caused by abnormal development or hypoplasia of the penile erectile tissue, secondary to distal urethral obstruction. When the amniotic fluid volume is normal, survival is possible. However, all liveborn infants have voiding, renal, and sexual dysfunction. Megalourethra should be considered in all male fetuses with megacystis and elongated and/or distended phallic structure (Fig. 2.5) [23].

2.3 Cystic Renal Disease

Cystic renal disease is another good example of the end result of an in utero event. The *multicystic dysplastic kidney* (*MCDK*) appears on prenatal

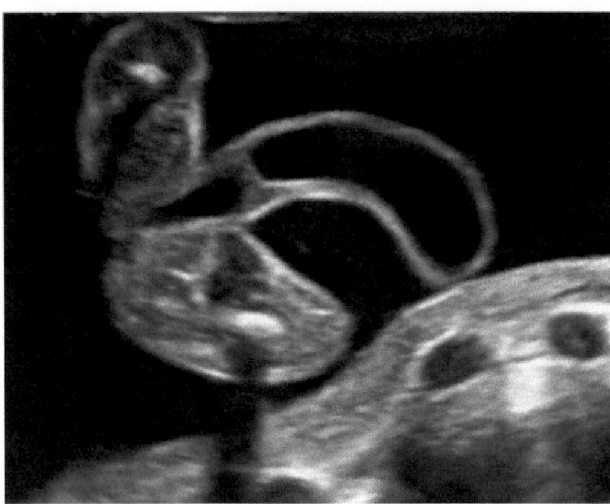

Fig. 2.5 Megacystis and distended phallic structure on prenatal 20-week US scan

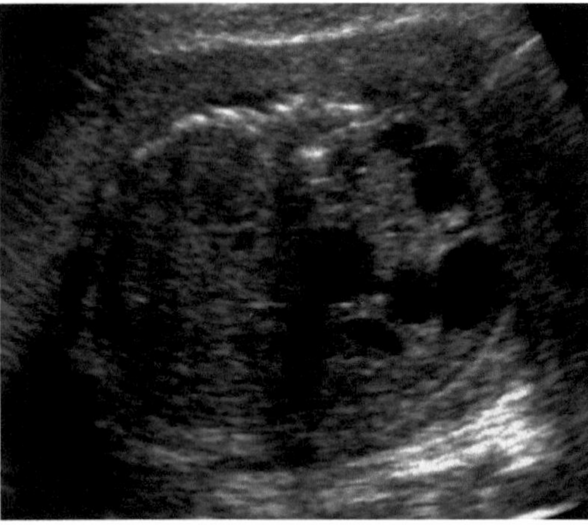

Fig. 2.6 Monolateral multicystic kidney: many non-communicating cysts appear in the renal parenchyma

US as a group of multiple, variable-sized, non-communicating cysts and minimal parenchyma (specific diagnoses) (Fig. 2.6).

Before the advent of prenatal US, MCDK were almost always diagnosed as a mass in the abdomen. Nowadays 80 % of patients with MCDK are asymptomatic. The MCDK may involute (45 % prenatally and 25 % within 14 months, 50 % by 5 years of age) or may represent a threat because of its mass effect over surrounding structures. Dimensions are used as a parameter for involution. In particular kidneys >7 cm do not involute. The smaller they are, the more and the sooner they shrink away. Small kidneys can be followed conservatively with routine US to monitor renal involution, malignancy development, and blood pressure measurements (risk of hypertension). The diagnosis is confirmed by renal scan that does not demonstrate function. MCU is useful to exclude VUR. It is a described associated anomaly of the contralateral kidney that is the clinically significant kidney (the one that we have to follow). In case of VUR patients are followed conservatively since resolution occurs in 68 % of cases.

Cystic diseases can also involve just segments of the kidney (*segmental cystic dysplasia*). In these cases the DMSA scan shows a function reduction that is related to cystic involution and not to an ongoing parenchymal damage.

A lethal cystic renal disease is the *autosomal recessive polycystic disease* (*ARPKD*). Kidneys are large, uniform, and echogenic, with no visible cysts. The condition is associated with pulmonary failure and Potter's syndrome [24, 25].

2.4 Prenatal Management and Fetal Intervention

The outcome of prenatally detected severe obstructive pathologies is influenced by active intervention during pregnancy. Active intervention has been proposed to treat conditions with high probability of intrauterine death or early postnatal demise (e.g., bilateral renal agenesis, bilateral multicystic kidneys). In case of PUV, preterm delivery has been suggested as an alternative but it is not universally accepted.

Fetal intervention includes: diagnostic procedure (karyotype to evaluate chromosomal abnormalities), termination of pregnancy (often chosen in case of cloacal and classic bladder exstrophy), and therapeutic intervention, usually vesicoamniotic shunting.

Fetal intervention is indicated in case of oligohydramnios with bladder outlet obstruction, normal karyotype, and singleton pregnancy. Vesicoamniotic shunt provides for the insertion of a double pigtail shunt into the fetal bladder under US surveillance in order to obtain decompression of the upper urinary tract. Unfortunately the results have been disappointing (high mortality rate, premature labor, renal insufficiency). These data might be influenced by the fact that patients selected for shunting procedures are at the severer end of the obstructed spectrum [2, 26].

References

1. Dillon HK (2008) Prenatal diagnosis. In: Thomas DFM, Duffy PG, Rickwood AMK (eds) Essential of pediatric urology, 2nd edn. Informa Healthcare, London, pp 133–142
2. Carr MC, Kim SS (2010) Prenatal management of urogenital disorders. Urol Clin North Am 37(2):149–158
3. Fugelseth D, Lindemann R, Sande HA, Refsum S, Nordshus T (1994) Prenatal diagnosis of urinary tract anomalies. The value of two ultrasound examinations. Acta Obstet Gynecol Scand 73(4):290–3
4. Hubert KC, Palmer JS (2007) Current diagnosis and management of fetal genitourinary abnormalities. Urol Clin North Am 34(1):89–101. Review
5. Johnson CE, Elder JS, Judge NE, Adeeb FN, Grisoni ER, Fattlar DC (1992) The accuracy of antenatal ultrasonography in identifying renal abnormalities. Am J Dis Child 146(10):1181–1184
6. Morin L, Cendron M, Crombleholme TM, Garmel SH, Klauber GT, D'Alton ME (1996) Minimal hydronephrosis in the fetus: clinical significance and implications for management. J Urol 155(6):2047–2049
7. Thomas DF, Madden NP, Irving HC, Arthur RJ, Smith SE (1994) Mild dilatation of the fetal kidney: a follow-up study. Br J Urol 74(2):236–239
8. Mandell J, Blyth BR, Peters CA, Retik AB, Estroff JA, Benacerraf BR (1991) Structural genitourinary defects detected in utero. Radiology 178(1):193–196
9. Elder JS (2006) Management of prenatal hydronephrosis. In: Puri P, Höllwarth M (eds) Pediatric surgery. Springer, Berlin, pp 825–838
10. Rao PK, Palmer JS (2009) Prenatal and postnatal management of hydronephrosis. Sci World J 9:606–614. doi:10.1100/tsw.2009.85. Review
11. Grignon A, Filion R, Filiatrault D, Robitaille P, Homsy Y, Boutin H, Leblond R (1986) Urinary tract dilatation in utero: classification and clinical applications. Radiology 160(3):645–647
12. Lee RS, Cendron M, Kinnamon DD, Nguyen HT (2006) Antenatal hydronephrosis as a predictor of postnatal outcome: a meta-analysis. Pediatrics 118(2):586–593
13. Fernbach SK, Maizels M, Conway JJ (1993) Ultrasound grading of hydronephrosis: introduction to the system used by the Society for Fetal Urology. Pediatr Radiol 23(6):478–480
14. Maizels M, Reisman ME, Flom LS, Nelson J, Fernbach S, Firlit CF, Conway JJ (1992) Grading nephroureteral dilatation detected in the first year of life: correlation with obstruction. J Urol 148(2 Pt 2):609–614. discussion 615–616
15. Glick PL, Harrison MR, Golbus MS, Adzick NS, Filly RA, Callen PW, Mahony BS, Anderson RL, deLorimier AA (1985) Management of the fetus with congenital hydronephrosis II: prognostic criteria and selection for treatment. J Pediatr Surg 20(4):376–387
16. Fefer S, Ellsworth P (2006) Prenatal hydronephrosis. Pediatr Clin North Am 53(3):429–447. vii. Review
17. Crombleholme TM, Harrison MR, Golbus MS, Longaker MT, Langer JC, Callen PW, Anderson RL, Goldstein RB, Filly RA (1990) Fetal intervention in obstructive uropathy: prognostic indicators and efficacy of intervention. Am J Obstet Gynecol 162(5): 1239–1244
18. Wiener JS, O'Hara SM (2002) Optimal timing of initial postnatal ultrasonography in newborns with prenatal hydronephrosis. J Urol 168(4 Pt 2):1826–1829. discussion 1829
19. Elder JS, Peters CA, Arant BS Jr, Ewalt DH, Hawtrey CE, Hurwitz RS, Parrott TS, Snyder HM 3rd, Weiss RA, Woolf SH, Hasselblad V (1997) Pediatric vesicoureteral reflux guidelines panel summary report on the management of primary vesicoureteral reflux in children. J Urol 157(5):1846–1851
20. Palmer LS, Maizels M, Cartwright PC, Fernbach SK, Conway JJ (1998) Surgery versus observation for managing obstructive grade 3 to 4 unilateral hydronephrosis: a report from the Society for Fetal Urology. J Urol 159(1):222–228
21. Krishnan A, de Souza A, Konijeti R, Baskin LS (2006) The anatomy and embryology of posterior urethral valves. J Urol 175(4):1214–1220. Review
22. Avni EF, Schulman CC (1996) The origin of vesicoureteric reflux in male newborns: further evidence in favour of a transient fetal urethral obstruction. Br J Urol 78(3):454–459
23. Promsonthi P, Viseshsindh W (2010) Case report and review: prenatal diagnosis of congenital megalourethra. Fetal Diagn Ther 28(2):123–128. Epub 2010 Jul 31. Review
24. Al Naimi A, Baumüller JE, Spahn S, Bahlmann F (2013) Prenatal diagnosis of multicystic dysplastic kidney disease in the second trimester screening. Prenat Diagn 33(8):726–731. Epub 2013 Jun 3
25. Bearman SB, Hine PL, Sanders RC (1976) Multicystic kidney: a sonographic pattern. Radiology 118(3): 685–688
26. Harrison MR, Nakayama DK, Noall R, de Lorimier AA (1982) Correction of congenital hydronephrosis in utero II. Decompression reverses the effects of obstruction on the fetal lung and urinary tract. J Pediatr Surg 17(6):965–974

Urinary Tract Imaging

3

Filomena Carfagnini and Giovanni Tani

The radiologic studies for the evaluation of the urinary tract in children are those most frequently performed in daily practice; the number of children studied was also significantly increased in recent years, in proportion to the spread on the territory and the practice of routine prenatal ultrasound.

Many diagnostic techniques are available, such as ultrasound further which was refined in the last decade, while others have become obsolete in the different diagnostic algorithms, replaced by new techniques that are recently introduced, and in either case, knowledge of these advances is essential for a modern diagnostic approach in terms of accuracy, efficiency, and radiation protection [1].

3.1 Ultrasonography (US)

US is definitely the most widely used imaging technique for the study of the urinary tract in children. Already identified in the past as a technique of approach and guidance for the evaluation of the urinary tract, it is now universally recognized as the investigation of choice, allowing accurate diagnosis of many pathological conditions, significantly reducing the need for further radiological examinations.

The ultrasound examination remains real-time operator dependent and requires, particularly in light of the new applications, skilled and experienced operators in whose hands often becomes the only exam required for diagnosis to be able to direct the next diagnostic algorithm [2–5].

Ultrasound examinations for the study of the urinary tract in children require high-resolution multi-frequency transducers, convex or linear (3–18 MHz).

The use of these probes allows a thorough examination, which must include the meticulous study of the kidneys including its location, size, and parenchymal structure and a detailed assessment of the bladder, perivesical space, as well as ureteral and pelvicalyceal dilatation.

It requires, when possible, a well-hydrated child with adequate bladder filling and post-void assessment.

It is essential that the examiner is familiar with the age-dependent US changes of the pediatric urogenital tract. Knowledge of these variations is critical to capture all the possible renal parenchymal changes, which may orient quickly to the presence of specific diseases.

In the neonatal period the kidneys retain the characteristic fetal lobulation presenting typical notches and wave profile (Fig. 3.1). The renal cortex is initially hyperechoic relative to the liver, especially in premature infants small for gestational age with the exaltation of the normal corticomedul-

F. Carfagnini (✉) • G. Tani
Department of Pediatric Radiology,
S. Orsola-Malpighi University Hospital,
Via Albertoni 15, Bologna, 40138, Italy
e-mail: filomena.carfagnini@aosp.bo.it;
gianni.tani@libero.it

M. Lima, G. Manzoni (eds.), *Pediatric Urology: Contemporary Strategies from Fetal Life to Adolescence*,
DOI 10.1007/978-88-470-5693-0_3, © Springer-Verlag Italia 2015

lary differentiation. After the neonatal period, cortical echogenicity progressively decreased to become similar to that of the liver between the fourth and sixth months of life. The medullary pyramids are hypoechoic compared to the cortex, so less and less evident with increasing age. The excretory cavity, only visible when extended, is anechoic (Fig. 3.2). The renal sinus is not represented by the absence or scarcity of fat. The bladder should be considered including its morphology and size and wall thickness and any endoluminal formation should be evaluated and identified.

In addition to the usual applications, there are other recently introduced applications which have great importance in the study of the urinary tract in children [5–7].

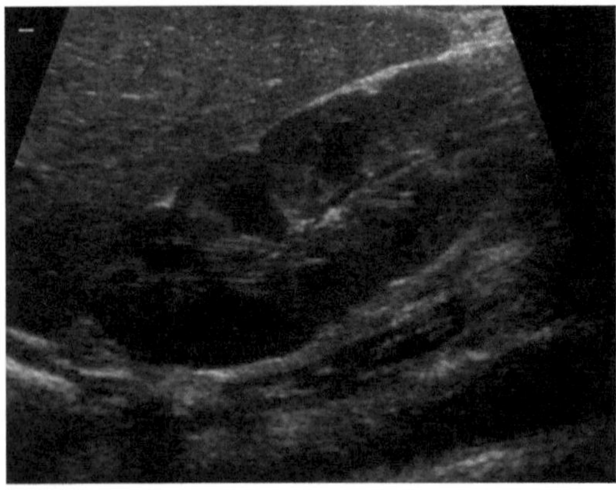

Fig. 3.1 US study: neonatal kidney with the typical fetal lobulation and clear corticomedullary differentiation

- *Motion-mode* (M-mode) helps evaluate the movement and, therefore, is able to provide a semiquantitative evaluation and documentation of the ureteral peristalsis.
- *Harmonic imaging (HI)* is a new US technique based not on the reflection of the fundamental frequency of the ultrasound beam but on the harmonic response generated by the tissue or, when used, by the contrast medium. It provides a better definition of the profiles, particularly of the fluid structure systems, such as dilated collectors; reduces artifacts; and improves the representation of the contrast medium.
- *Panoramic US* uses consecutive US images acquired during a steady shift of the transducer; these are added after shift vector analysis to reconstruct a larger field of view. The technique is extremely useful to demonstrate large pathologies or for measuring very large structures, too large for the normal range of conventional transducers.
- Transperineal US with high-frequency linear probes allows optimal visualization of the urethra, vagina, and surrounding structures.
- Three-dimensional US (3D US) is a relatively new technique that provides a multiaxial demonstration of the entire kidney and bladder. It is applicable to neonates and children even at the bedside. It improves renal parenchymal volume calculation, particularly in irregularly shaped kidneys or in hydronephrosis, as the dilated collecting system can be deducted

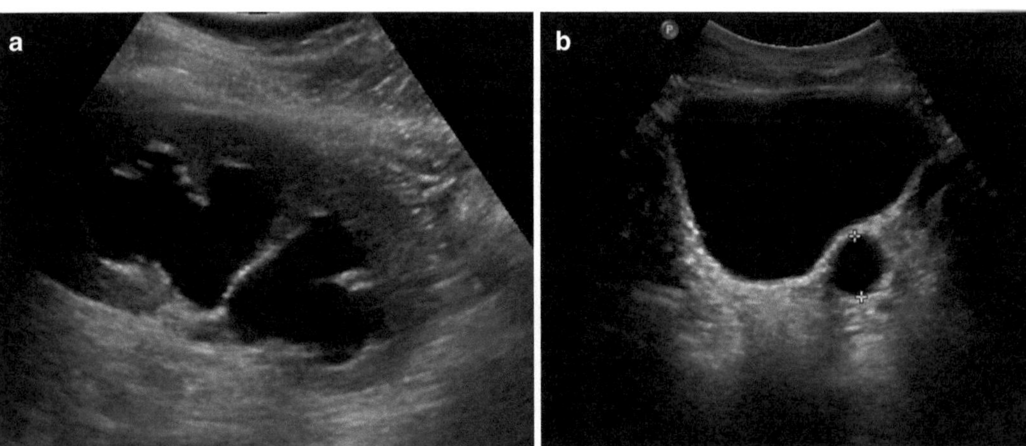

Fig. 3.2 (**a**, **b**) US study: left hydroureteronephrosis

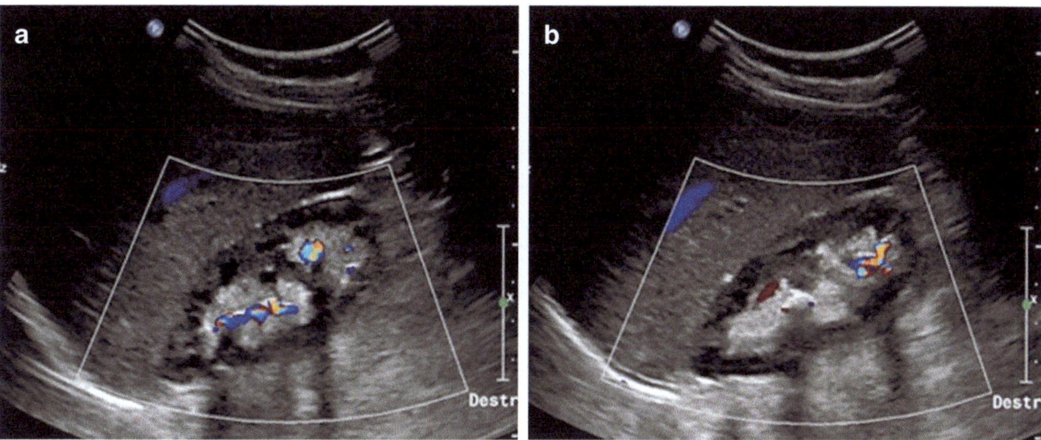

Fig. 3.3 (**a**, **b**) Color Doppler sonography: twinkling sign in stone renal disease

from the overall kidney volume. The potential of creating rendered views can serve as an excellent tool for comprehensive demonstration of complex pathology [8].

3.2 Doppler Sonography

Various *Doppler* techniques are routinely used in ultrasound studies of the urinary tract in children.

Color Doppler sonography (CDS) allows a quick and comprehensive overview of the vascular anatomy as well as an assessment of the velocity and direction of flow in the renal vessels. For this reason, CDS is also a fundamental examination for the follow-up of transplanted kidneys.

The twinkling sign, probably caused by crystal oscillations when hit by the US beam, has improved US potential in the depiction of stones in the urinary tract and renal or medullary calcifications and deposits (Fig. 3.3). A similar appearance is caused by high or turbulent flow inducing aliasing that improves CDS depiction of vascular pathologies such as renal arteriovenous fistula, renal artery stenosis, or renal venous vasculopathy [9].

CDS also improves detection and assessment of ureteral jet.

Duplex Doppler sonography (DDS) provides detailed information of flow profiles with a physiologically lower flow velocity, a higher resistive index (RI), and relatively lower diastolic flow velocity in infants and neonates. DDS is especially valuable in evaluating indirect signs of perfusion disturbance, e.g., in renal vein thrombosis with consecutively elevated arterial RI in the affected renal segment, or for depicting renal artery stenosis as well as flow changes in renal failure.

Power Doppler is based on the totally integrated Doppler spectrum. This technology demonstrates blood flow volume rather than blood flow velocity. The increased sensitivity for blood flow allows depiction of peripheral renal vasculature and diagnosis of focal perfusion defects (e.g., infarction, segmental acute pyelonephritis) or diffusely impaired cortical perfusion. High level equipment is essential and an experienced operator is needed to apply the correct power Doppler setting (Fig. 3.4) [1–5, 10, 11].

3.3 Voiding Urosonography (VUS)

VUS involves the administration of US contrast agent into the bladder for the diagnosis of vesicoureteral reflux. US contrast agents are not always available, and their use in children has been approved only in a limited number of countries, especially for their administration in the bladder. Despite these considerations, VUS is currently a viable alternative to other diagnostic tests such as voiding cystourethrography (VCUG) and radionuclide cystography. The study has become possible with the commercial introduction of

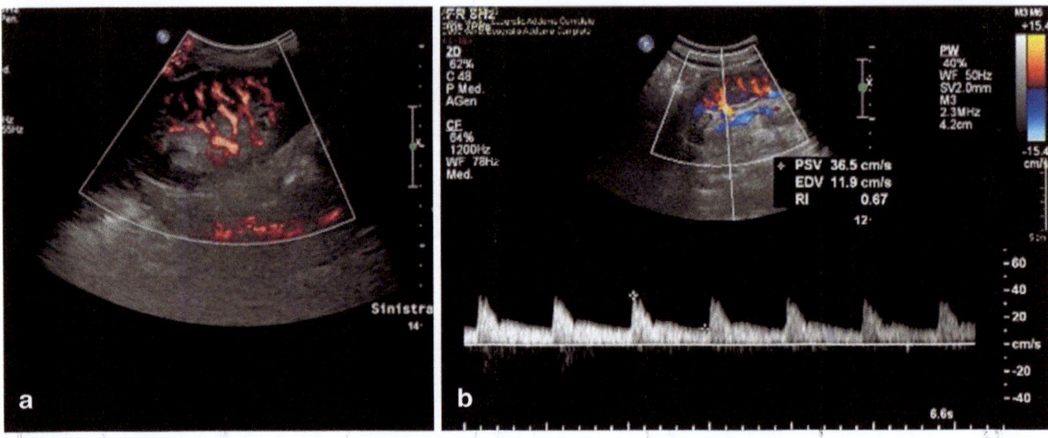

Fig. 3.4 Power Doppler sonography (**a**) and Duplex Doppler sonography (**b**) in a transplanted kidney

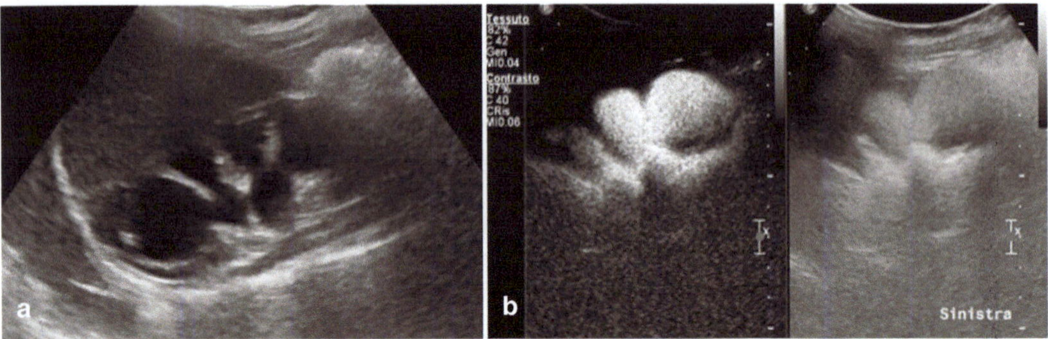

Fig. 3.5 Voiding urosonography: pre-contrastographic US study (**a**) and post-contrastographic US study (**b**) with optimal RVU visualization

second-generation contrast agents, consisting in stabilized sulfur hexafluoride phospholipid microbubbles (SonoVue, Bracco, Italy) [12–16]. These agents produce a high enhancement and a strong harmonic response, but above all they have greater resistance to the mechanical impact of the ultrasound beam, allowing longer investigation times, adequate for the detection of VUR. VUS consists of four main steps:

1. Pre-contrastographic standard US study of the urinary tract.
2. Administration of normal saline and US contrast agent after bladder catheterization.
3. Post-contrastographic US study of the urinary system.
4. Post-contrast examination of the renal pelvis and the terminal ureters during and after voiding. Transperineal US urethral examination can be considered in males.

Reflux is diagnosed when echogenic microbubbles are displayed in the ureters and into the pelvicalyceal system (Fig. 3.5). The severity of reflux is graded in a similar manner as the international reflux grading system for VCUG.

3.4 Voiding Cystourethrography (VCUG)

VCUG is the classic examination for the study of the bladder and urethra, particularly in males. It is able to highlight valves or urethral strictures, bladder diverticula, ureterocele, and vesicoureteral reflux [1–5].

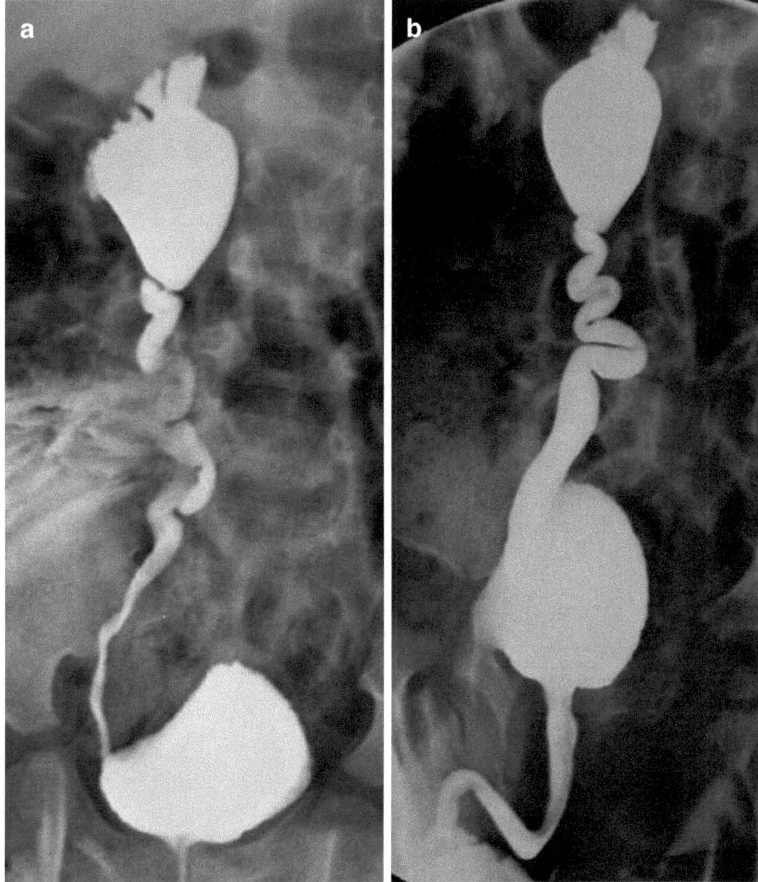

Fig. 3.6 VCUG shows a passive right RVU in the filling phase (**a**), increasing during voiding (**b**)

The examination is conducted prior to bladder catheterization performed under sterile conditions and preceded and followed by antibiotic prophylaxis. The catheters used are of the type Nelaton, devoid of balloon, and provided with side holes that are sufficiently large.

After placement of a bladder catheter, a soluble radiopaque contrast with high concentration is introduced into the bladder to reach a good bladder filling, which is essential, particularly in newborns and infants, because micturition occurs.

The radiogram of the VCUG must include all the urinary tract, from the kidney to the anterior urethra; lateral projections are essential for the study of the male urethra.

In the presence of reflux, the contrast medium rises along the ureter until the renal pelvis and calyces, which are more or less dilated; reflux may occur in the filling phase (passive reflux) or it may occur during voiding (active reflux); in most serious cases it can be intrarenal, an element that has always been considered important for the appearance of parenchymal scars. In the final phase of the survey, drainage dynamic contrast medium reflux must be assessed, from the cavity to the bladder (Fig. 3.6).

The severity of reflux is established on a scale defined by the International Reflux Study Committee. VCUG has became a standard procedure during which the bladder is filled in order to detect a greater amount of refluxes.

It is important to remember that the examination still involves a considerable radiation dose, especially for the inability to shield the gonads; this is especially true in cases with severe pathologies that require prolonged times of fluoroscopy and the acquisition of a greater number of images.

The recent introduction of pulsed fluoroscopy and the use of technology to capture the last image (last-image-hold technique) limit the number of spot films, resulting in a significant reduction in the dose of exposure.

Currently CVUG, performed according to the standard procedure, should be conducted only with technical fluoroscopy, pulsed fluoroscopy ideally with the lowest pulse setting, using solely or mainly the technique of capturing the last image [17].

However, it is important to consider that the indication for the cystography studies, whether it is performed in a standard way or more appropriately with fluoroscopy technique, has been drastically reduced over recent years; it is therefore necessary to carefully select the cases in which to perform the examination, in particular when there are equally suitable and reliable diagnostic alternatives, such as contrast-enhanced voiding urosonography (VUS).

3.5 Plain Film and Intravenous Urography

Plain film and *intravenous urography* are investigations that virtually disappeared from pediatric radiology. Urography in particular is no longer used in the neonatal period and very rarely during childhood, because similar and more detailed anatomical and functional information can be provided by ultrasonography, nuclear medicine examinations, and MR urography (MRU), studies less or not radiant.

Rare indications are represented by pre- or postsurgical studies and certain conditions when you can not perform in the territory MRU and scintigraphic studies. In such cases the IVU must be closely targeted to the clinical question so as to reduce the radiation dose to the lowest possible value.

The use of kidney-ureter-bladder plain radiographs may still have some role before lithotripsy interventions [1–5, 18].

3.6 Computed Tomography (CT)

Computed tomography has become the investigation of choice in the study of adult urology, both with the use of contrast medium (*Uro-CT*) and without injection of contrast medium for the detection of stones (stone-CT) [1, 3–5, 18–20].

However, the examination is highly radiant, and its diagnostic potential cannot be transferred blindly to children, who for more than adults have a higher *radiosensitivity*. In addition, children have lesser representation of adipose tissue, smaller structures, different diseases (e.g., fewer neoplasms, stones very rare and smaller), and different tissue composition (e.g., stones less calcified and more difficult to depict).

For this reason, pediatric CT does not achieve the same importance in pediatric uroradiology.

CT is currently considered particularly valuable for:

- Severe trauma of abdomen and pelvis
- Atypical or chronic inflammatory diseases, such as tuberculosis or xanthogranulomatous pyelonephritis
- Renal stone disease where US studies are not exhaustive
- Suspected or proven renal or pelvic malignancies (especially Wilms' tumor), particularly when MR is not available
- Congenital urogenital abnormalities, particularly for the study of anatomy bone in bladder exstrophy
- CT angiography studies, especially in certain conditions such as arterial complications after renal transplantation

Indisputable advantages of CT are:

- Perfect anatomical detail with spatial resolution of the order of 1 mm and the possibility of multiplanar reconstructions (MPR) and 3D
- High contrast resolution, useful in particular for the detection of stones unrecognized by ultrasound study
- Faster acquisition times with the overall reduction in the number of sedation or sedation time
- Wide availability
- Ability to use multiple windows tissue in the same study
- Simultaneous and easy evaluation of lung in malignant disease
- Good image quality in obese patients, although in most cases this is not a problem in children

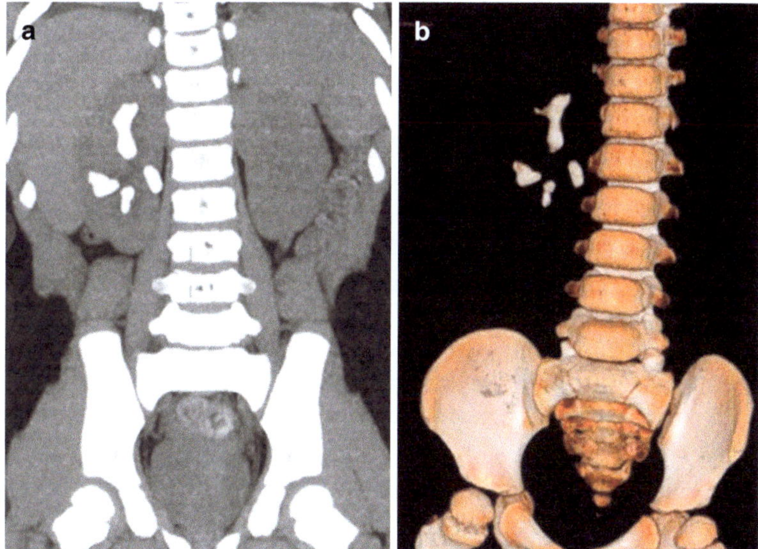

Fig. 3.7 Unenhanced CT: coronal MIP (**a**) and 3D VR (**b**) showing right kidney stone disease

The main disadvantage of CT is the radiation dose; a significant gonadal dose is unavoidable. Its iodinated contrast is also potentially nephrotoxic.

Compliance with the indications in the CT study is essential and of great importance. Never just "try a CT": when conducting a CT in a child, one should always ensure that the examination may provide therapeutically relevant information at the lowest radiation dose possible, in accordance with the ALARA principle. The CT scan should always be preceded by a thorough US ultrasound evaluation, which may obviate the CT study or, if it is necessary, allows you to perform the CT study with the most correct technique.

When CT is indicated, one must use pediatric protocols adapted to the weight and age of the patient, either as exposure parameters, generally available on the modern equipment, or as contrast medium. The scan area should be limited in relation to the clinical question, avoiding multiphasic scans.

Unenhanced CT is used almost exclusively when it is necessary or important to identify renal calcifications. In other cases its diagnostic contribution is minimal so that the unenhanced scan is omitted to reduce the radiation dose (Fig. 3.7).

Contrast-enhanced CT is realized after the fast injection of the contrast medium with the aim of obtaining optimal enhancement of the vessels (Fig. 3.8). The standard dose of contrast medium is 2 ml/kg of nonionic iodinated contrast.

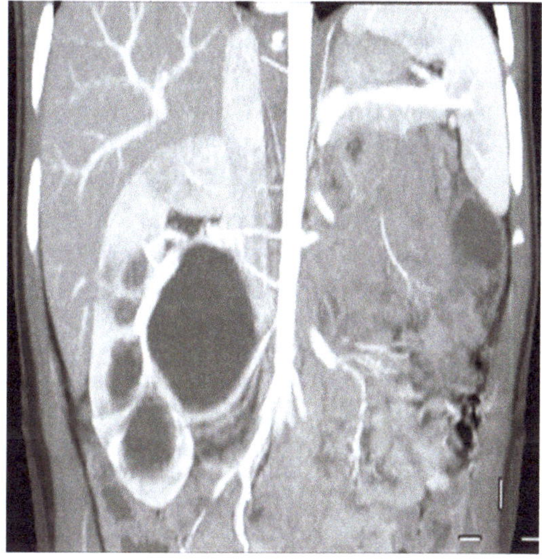

Fig. 3.8 Severe right hydronephrosis secondary to anomalousl vessels (inferior polar renal artery). Note the presence of three right renal arteries

With regard to the diagnostic question, CT scans are performed after a time between 20 and 60 s after injection of contrast medium. Urographic acquisition phase, after about 10 min after injection of contrast medium, may be necessary in cases of major traumatic events, in which a renal, ureteral, or bladder injury with contrast extravasation is suspected.

In some selected cases of nonsedated cooperative children, you can use an oral contrast, which is drunk gradually during the 45–60 min before to the examination.

3.6.1 MR Urography (MRU)

MRU has been introduced in the study of the urinary tract in children not more than 15 years ago, and although still a few centers routinely use it, its use is increasing [21–27].

It is currently the only test that provides superb anatomical information and functional imaging without the use of ionizing radiation. It allows an overall assessment of the excretory cavity, renal parenchyma, and surrounding tissue, as well as the main vessels. Although the dynamic contrast enhancement is similar to renal scintigraphy, MRU definitely ensures a higher contrast spatial and temporal resolution.

A meticulous attention to the preparation of the patient and an accurate scanning technique are fundamental in order to obtain really high-quality images.

It should be noted that MRU, especially in its functional part, is not yet standardized in various centers of pediatric radiology, resulting in various techniques and procedures related to each other.

3.6.1.1 Preparation of the Patient

To optimize the MRU, administration of fluid and furosemide is essential.

The basic information that must be necessarily known is the nonlinear relationship between the concentration of gadolinium and the signal intensity when T1-weighted gradient echo sequences that represent the basis for MRU are used. At low concentrations of gadolinium, T1 effects predominate, leaving the relationship relatively linear, whereas at high concentrations of the contrast agent, T2* effects predominate, resulting in a signal loss. For this reason, hydration and furosemide injection, diluting the contrast medium in excretory cavity, are the key elements to maintain a low and uniform concentration of gadolinium.

The standard dose of furosemide is 1 mg/kg up to a maximum of 20 mg/kg, administered 15 min before injection of the contrast medium, and this involves an additional benefit represented by the distension of the excretory cavities and by shortening the time of the study.

In some cases it may be appropriate to place a catheter to reduce discomfort resulting from overdistension of the bladder; further benefits include easier assessment of complex malformation and the elimination of potential RVU, which could confound interpretation of the image.

It is obvious that for specific questions the catheter can be clamped and images of the distended urinary bladder obtained. Children younger than 6–7 years of age need to be sedated; in older children able to cooperate, images are obtained either through quiet breathing or during breath-holding.

3.6.1.2 Pre-contrast Imaging (Static Fluid MRU or Water MRU)

Pre-contrast imaging is the most important phase for the anatomical evaluation of the urinary tract.

It is performed with coronal T2-weighted turbo spin-echo sequences (TSE T2 weighted) and 3D T2-weighted sequences; these last sequences are used to generate MIP (maximum intensity projection) and VR (volume-rendered) images, which allow the best visualization of the pelvicalyceal system and ureters.

The resulting images are very useful for the evaluation of obstructed collecting systems, duplex systems, and complex anatomical variants; its use is also fundamental in poorly functioning systems, up to the functionally excluded kidneys, which obviously have little or nothing displayed in contrastographic phase, similarly to what occurs with the *scintigraphic studies* (Fig. 3.9).

Axial T2-weighted turbo spin-echo sequences (TSE T2 weighted) are also acquired, from the kidneys to the pelvis, particularly useful for assessment of the renal parenchyma and for identification of bladder abnormalities, including ureteroceles and ectopic ureteral insertion.

3.6.1.3 Excretory MRU

It is the phase which allows the dynamic evaluation of the urinary tract.

In fact contrast-enhanced sequences are used to study the functions of concentration and excretion of the kidneys.

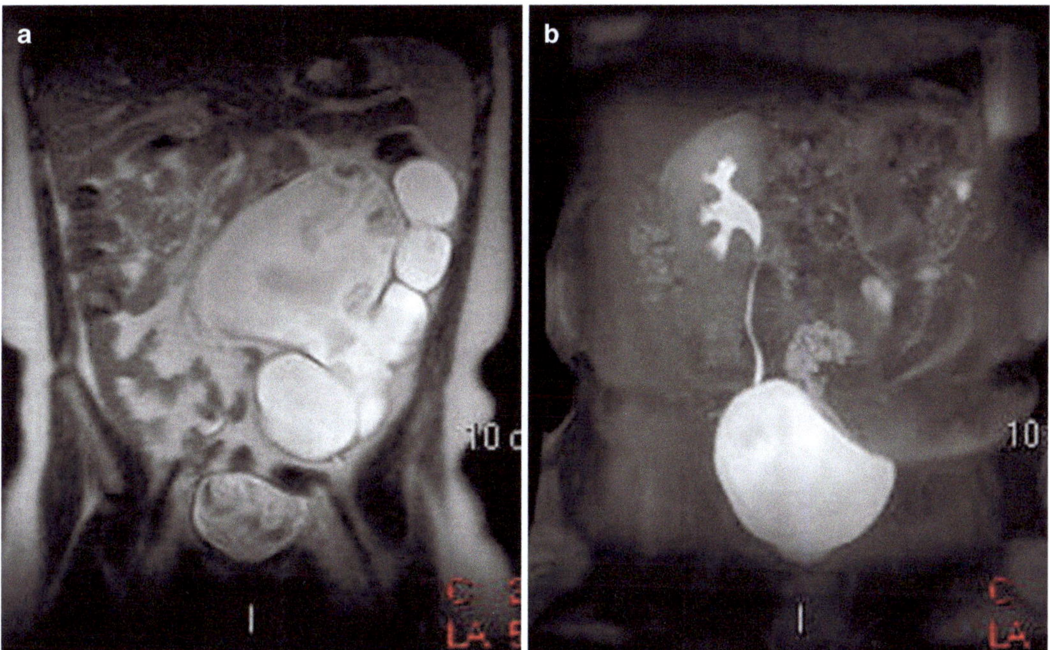

Fig. 3.9 Coronal T2-weighted MRU visualization of a left ureteropelvic junction obstruction (**a**). Post-contrast coronal 3D GE shows very poor urinary excretion by a potentially excluded kidney (**b**)

The knowledge of the relationship between the administration of paramagnetic contrast agent and nephrogenic systemic fibrosis requires great caution in its use in pediatric age and full compliance with all precautionary measures [28].

The contrast medium used was the gadolinium chelate, bound to the diethylenetriaminepentaacetic acid macromolecule (DTPA). The biodistribution of the contrast agent is determined solely by the macromolecule of DTPA, so that the gadolinium is filtered by the glomerulus, without significant tubular secretion or reabsorption. The standard dose used (0.1 mmol/kg) provides an excellent enhancement of the kidneys, allowing the evaluation of RM nephrogram by differentiating enhancing parenchyma from the background.

The signal intensity of the aorta is used as the arterial input function for calculating the curve of Patlak (index of the single kidney GFR). Therefore, to maintain the intensity of the aortic signal in a linear range, the contrast medium is injected very slowly, by means of power injector, at a standard speed of 0.1 ml/s without ever exceeding the speed of 0.25 ml/s.

The fundamental sequence for excretory phase is the 3D gradient echo, performed in a coronal oblique plane; fat suppression is recommended to enhance the visibility of the ureters. The acquisition time is approximately 8 s for each volume. Typically after the contrast administration, continuous dynamic images are acquired for about 10 min until the complete enhancement of the excretory system; such time may be extended up to 20 min in case of delayed visualization of the ureters. MIP (maximum intensity projection) images are automatically generated from each dynamic series. The high-resolution images obtained are excellent for 3D VR (volume rendering) reconstructions with the optimal visualization of the renal cortex, the medulla, the pelvicalyceal system, and the ureteral course into the bladder (Fig. 3.10).

3.6.1.4 Post Processing

It is the stage that allows measurements of various parameters of renal function and particularly the renal transit time, the calyceal transit time, the time-intensity curves, the differential renal

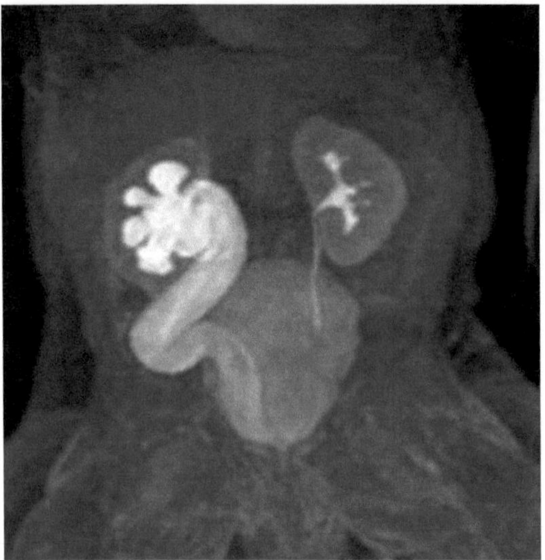

Fig. 3.10 Post-contrast MRU MIP reconstruction shows right obstructive hydroureteronephrosis

function, and the glomerular filtration rate (GFR) [27, 29–31].

For these functional analyses, we cite two software freely available online, the application of which requires an estimated time of about 10–15 min in dedicated independent console.

The first one is from the CHU Hôpitaux de Rouen, Rouen, France (www.univ-rouen.fr/med/MRurography/accueil.htm) and the second from the Children's Hospital of Philadelphia (CHOP), Philadelphia, PA, USA (www.chop-fmru.com).

Renal Transit Time (RTT)

The renal transit time is defined as the time taken by the contrast medium to pass from the renal cortical to the proximal ureters. The calculated time is used to distinguish systems that are not obstructed (RTT <245 s), systems obstructed (RTT > 490 s), or doubtful (RTT between 245 and 490 s). These values, though indicative, are significantly influenced by the urinary stasis, so that systems apparently obstructed drain easily when the patient is placed in the prone position with reduction of the calculated values.

Calyceal Transit Time (CTT)

It is similar to the previous and reflects the time taken by the contrast medium to pass from the renal cortex to the calyces. It is an expression of altered parenchymal phase in the dynamic contrast enhancement and has diagnostic value in unilateral diseases, simply categorized as rapid, symmetrical, or delayed compared to the healthy side.

Time-Intensity Curves

They represent the variations of the signal intensity of the various regions of the kidneys with respect to time, from the pre-contrast phase to the contrast phase up to washout of the parenchyma. Although the dynamic contrast enhancement can be directly displayed on imaging, it may be useful to reconstruct these changes graphically, in the form of time-intensity curves.

Differential Renal Function (DRF) and Glomerular Filtration Rate (GFR)

These are very important parameters, similar to those used in scintigraphic studies.

The differential renal function (DRF) can be calculated in two ways: the volumetric DRF (vDRF) and the Patlak DRF (pDRF).

- The *vDRF* is simply the volume of enhancing renal parenchyma above a threshold value defined by the user and is considered an expression of functional renal mass. The time point where it realizes the maximum parenchymal enhancement in each kidney is selected, which is the one immediately preceding the appearance of the contrast agent in the calyces. The point of maximum enhancement, used for the calculation of vDRF, can occur at different times in each kidney. Because you are using a threshold value, the calculated volume tends to be underestimated in poorly functioning kidneys.
- The *Patlak plot* represents an index of glomerular filtration rate (GFR). The Patlak number can be used to generate a pDRF. The Patlak number increases with the age and the size of the kidneys and can be followed sequentially as well as after surgical and medical intervention. The absolute Patlak number can be corrected according to body surface area using a simple weight-based correction factor. Although there has been validation of the Patlak technique in adults, the absolute

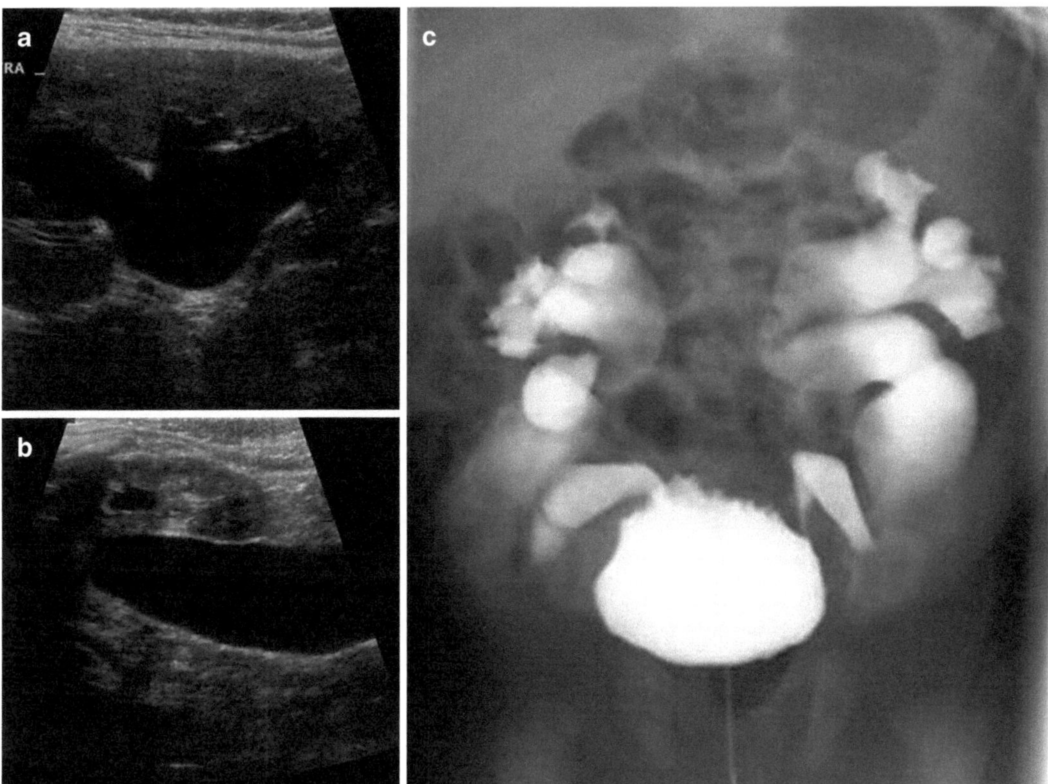

Fig. 3.11 Bilateral hydronephrosis in newborn, US study (**a**, **b**) and VCUG (**c**), that demonstrates severe bilateral reflux

Patlak number has not yet been validated in children. The pDRF is most useful, especially if the contralateral kidney is normal. The pDRF changes with acute alterations in GFR, whereas the vDRF appears to be relatively stable. Since the same renal segmentation is used in the Patlak analysis, similarly to the previous, pDRF underestimates the function of very poorly functioning kidneys.

In view of its vast potential, the *MRU* has virtually replaced the IVU in pediatric urology and has also become a first-line investigation in the evaluation of cystic kidney disease, when ultrasound is not exhaustive and does not settle questions clinically relevant. Additionally the MRU is increasingly used in the complications of urinary tract infections, in the diagnosis of equivocal renal lesions, in the assessment of post-traumatic complications, and in the evaluation of neoplastic diseases. Some recent works indicate a role in complicated stone disease.

3.7 Indications and Timing of Imaging

3.7.1 Hydronephrosis Diagnosed Antenatally

The postnatal imaging of hydronephrosis diagnosed antenatally is programmed according to the severity of prenatal findings [1, 2, 5, 11–17, 24–31].

In infants with prenatal diagnosis of severe bilateral hydronephrosis, sonography is required on the first day of life, especially in cases of hydroureteronephrosis and/or suspected abnormalities of the bladder or the urethra. In male children, standard US may be associated with a complementary assessment of the urethra with the perineal scan and voiding cystourethrography (VCUG) for suspected posterior urethral valves and to search for VUR (Fig. 3.11). In girls the spinal US study may be indicated in suspected neurogenic bladder, possibly followed by contrast-enhanced voiding urosonography (VUS) for VUR detection.

When an obstructive condition is diagnosed, further investigations are usually deferred until prior to surgery or after the sixth to eighth week of life, when the urinary tract is fully matured and MAG3 scintigraphy or MRU can provide reliable results.

In neonates with prenatal diagnosis of moderate hydronephrosis and/or unilateral with or without ureteral dilatation, US can be postponed to the fifth to seventh day of life due to the immaturity of the urinary tract and the risk of underestimating the pathological findings.

If the first US is normal, US study is repeated at the age of 1 or 2 months, but there is no required further diagnostic investigation.

If you found a significant hydronephrosis, as in UPJO, follow-up US is required at 3–6 weeks of age and a continuation of diagnostic work with MAG3 scintigraphy or MRU, to be performed at 6–8 weeks of age.

When there is a megaureter or other indirect signs of RVUs, for example, a thickened pelvic wall, it is indicated to perform a voiding *cystourethrography (VCUG)* in male or a contrast-enhanced voiding urosonography (VUS) in girls.

In complex urogenital anomalies, MRU is indicated.

3.7.2 Acute Neonatal Conditions

Pathological conditions in the newborn are considered including acute posterior urethral valves, pyonephrosis or urosepsis, acute renal failure, disorders of renal perfusion (e.g., renal vein thrombosis), and rare congenital renal tumors.

Acute renal failure can be prerenal (from systemic causes, e.g., asphyxia, cardiac arrest, hypotension), postrenal (e.g., severe obstructive conditions), or intrinsic. Among the causes of intrinsic acute renal failure should be considered: perfusion disorders such as hemolytic-uremic syndrome, or renal vein thrombosis; renal damage by toxic, metabolic, or systemic diseases (e.g., hyperoxaluria); neonatal glomerulonephritis; acute tubular necrosis and cortical and/or medullary necrosis; as well as preexisting conditions such as hypodysplasia or infantile polycystic kidney disease. All of these conditions can coexist and can be associated with various degrees of acute renal failure.

In all cases, an urgent US study should be performed, which often allows a precise diagnosis between different diseases. Usually sequential US is sufficient and does not need further investigation. It should be noted that in these studies US Doppler evaluation of renal perfusion is essential and that in neonates with oligoanuria conditions absence of hydronephrosis does not exclude an obstructive condition, so that a study of ultrasound after filling the bladder with perineal approach or a voiding cystourethrography is mandatory as well as follow-up US [2–5, 10, 11].

After the episodes of acute renal failure or in chronic renal failure, DMSA scintigraphic study is indicated, or increasingly MRU, to assess renal function and the presence of defects or scars and consequently determine the prognosis [21–31].

3.7.3 Urinary Tract Infections (UTI) and Vesicoureteral Reflux (VUR)

In children with acute urinary tract infection, fever, and signs of septicemia, urgent US should be performed to rule out obstructive conditions and find signs of a possible kidney involvement such as the increase in size of the kidney, abnormal echogenicity, "mucosal thickening," urolithiasis, or focal perfusion defects in power Doppler study.

If there is no evidence of dilatation or renal involvement and there is a good response to treatment, further investigation may be postponed [1–4].

All children with renal involvement are required to be submitted to VCUG or voiding cysto-sonography (VUS), once the infection is resolved [2, 5, 12–17].

Usually a DMSA scintigraphy is performed after 6–9 months for the evaluation of the parenchyma; in equivocal cases, renal scintigraphy or MRU is indicated since the discovery of renal involvement is the key aspect for planning subsequent monitoring and establishing a prophylactic antibiotic, although the latter concept is currently very controversial [22, 23].

In addition to the ultrasound study, imaging of complications of UTI requires ce-CT or, better, ce-MRU.

VUR has lost much of its importance, especially middle grade and not associated with urinary tract infection. The diagnostic algorithm reflects this new approach recognizing the high number of cases, mild-to-moderate, that spontaneously resolve without long-term sequelae or therapeutic consequences.

A meticulous search of VUR by voiding *cystourethrography* or *cistosonography* is still indicated [2–5, 12–17]:

- In children with significant hydronephrosis in the neonatal period, to differentiate obstructive from reflux disease and for the evaluation of the urethra
- In children with congenital dysplasia (potentially indicating congenital "reflux nephropathy"), with complex congenital malformations or syndromic disorders (e.g., duplex kidney with renal dysplasia or hydronephrosis, neurogenic bladder with myelomeningocele)
- In children with upper UTI, where VUR is a risk factor for renal scarring with all its implications

3.7.4 Obstructive Uropathy

Once diagnosed with *obstructive uropathy*, usually after a diagnosis of prenatal hydronephrosis and a neonatal ultrasound evaluation, the important task is to preserve bladder and kidney function [3, 5–11].

In posterior urethral valves, immediate bladder catheterization and an early surgical treatment are indicated.

In megaureter and dysplasia, the joint goal of imaging is to identify kidneys that are at risk, those intended for deterioration in growth and functionality.

Currently there is no imaging study that can reliably predict this negative trend, and therefore, periodic and regular controls are required that enable to capture early worsening of the obstructive condition and renal function, although it may be difficult to correctly distinguish the cases that may benefit surgical treatment from those that can be treated conservatively.

Usually we try to achieve this by performing repeated US studies and intermittent MAG3 scintigraphic studies, particularly if the ultrasound shows, as potential indicators of impairment, an increase in the thickness dilatation with parenchymal thinning and loss of corticomedullary differentiation, compensatory hypertrophy of the contralateral kidney, and an asymmetric impaired parenchymal perfusion.

In many centers MRU is increasingly replacing the *MAG3 scintigraphy* [1, 4, 5, 21, 23–26].

3.7.5 Other Malformations and Conditions Complex

The hypodysplasia is a congenital condition, different from acquired renal scarring resulting, for example, from hypoxia and infection [22]. US shows small kidneys with reduced or absent corticomedullary differentiation, with or without cysts, and often without hydronephrosis. Perfusion may be compromised with reduced vascularity at power Doppler and low flow velocity and altered RI (resistive index) on Doppler study [10, 11].

If hypodysplasia is unilateral, renal function remains in the global normal and even small kidneys can maintain a minimum residual function. Dysplasia is often found in the upper pole system of a duplex kidney that drains through a megaureter, eventually with ectopic insertion and sometimes with distal ureterocele. The lower pole system of duplex kidney tends to reflux; for this reason, children with these conditions undergo VCUG o VUS, especially when symptomatic (Fig. 3.12). Additionally, an MRU can be performed as it is becoming the complementary investigation of choice, as well as for the functional evaluation of kidneys, for the study of the ectopic kidneys, and/or for suspected ureteral ectopic insertions [4, 5].

It should be noted that renal abnormalities may be associated with abnormal genital

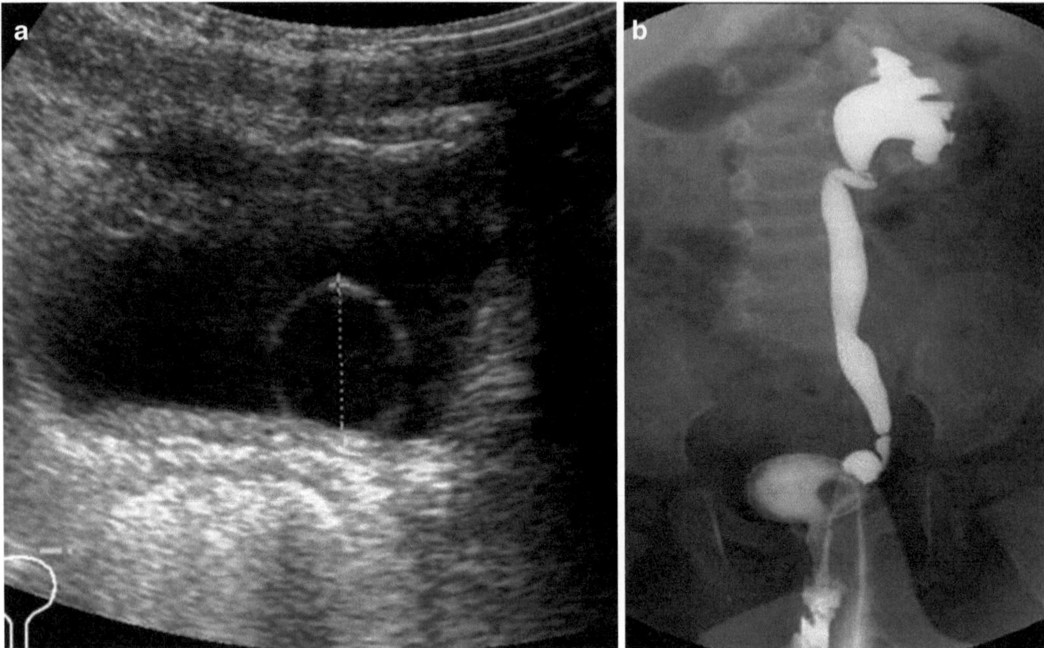

Fig. 3.12 US study (**a**) and VCUG (**b**) in left duplex kidney with distal ureterocele of upper pole system and reflux in the lower pole system

complex, and therefore, it is advisable to carry out meticulous investigations that enable early identification of such abnormalities, especially in girls; useful studies are US and magnetic resonance imaging.

3.7.6 Cystic Disease

There are various *cystic diseases* in children [2, 4, 5].

The most common condition is the nonfunctioning multicystic kidney (MCKD), characterized by the presence of numerous cysts of varying size, not communicating with the excretory cavity, possibly interspersed with small amounts of dysplastic parenchyma (Fig. 3.13). The differential diagnosis with extremely severe cases of UPJO can be difficult because MCKD may also represent the end point of obstructive conditions decompensated in the prenatal period. The multicystic kidney is unilateral; bilateral MCKD is incompatible with life.

If there are cysts of various sizes in both kidneys, in an otherwise normal renal parenchyma, in the absence of alteration of creatinine, the most likely diagnosis is that of autosomal dominant polycystic kidney disease (ADPKD), especially when cystic formations are also present in other organs. This congenital condition may manifest initially with one single cyst, so the finding of a

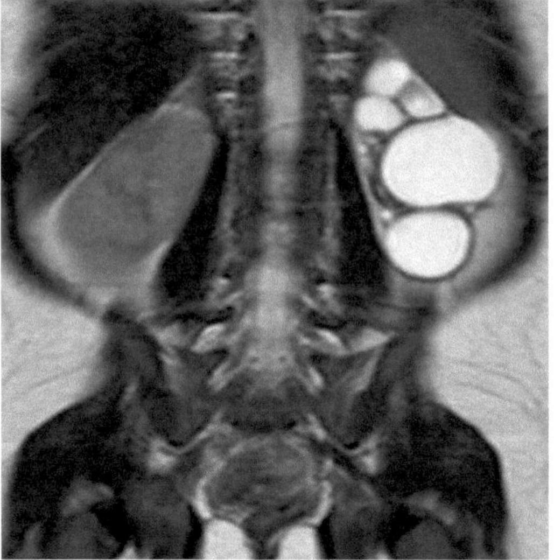

Fig. 3.13 Coronal T2 MRU: multicystic left kidney

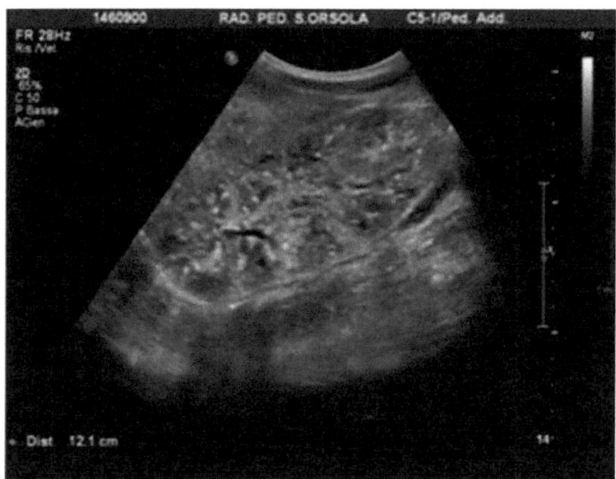

Fig. 3.14 US study: typical “salt and pepper” aspect and very large kidney in a 4-year-old male with ARPKD

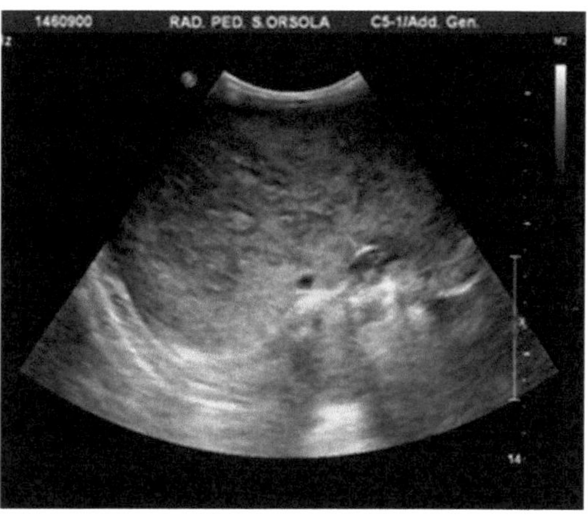

Fig. 3.15 US study: liver fibrosis in ARPKD

renal cyst in childhood should prompt a thorough clinical evaluation and family assessment.

The finding of large kidneys with diffuse and inhomogeneous increase of the echogenicity (“salt and pepper”) may indicate infantile autosomal recessive polycystic kidney disease (ARPKD) (Fig. 3.14). Initially, the microcysts are so small as not to be identifiable to the US study. When the ARPKD is suspected, it is essential to carry out a study of the entire abdomen and particularly additional ultrasound of the liver, to assess the presence of liver fibrosis (Fig. 3.15).

Other diseases include rare simple renal cysts and postinflammatory and post-traumatic cysts, which must be differentiated from calyceal diverticula, from urinoma, as well as from renal tumors such as cystic nephroma, cystic Wilms’ tumor, necrotic renal carcinoma, renal teratoma, or posthemorrhagic renal angiomyolipoma. All of these conditions require a study of the second level, CT, or preferably MR with contrast medium; delayed scan in MRU or delayed abdominal radiograph after CT is advisable to capture the late contrast medium accumulation in calyceal diverticulum.

3.7.7 Hematuria

Contrary to what occurs in the adult, rarely *pediatric hematuria* is an expression of malignant disease of the kidneys or bladder, conditions easily detectable at US study.

Microhematuria may be secondary to many pathological conditions, such as familial hematuria, glomerulonephritis, other kidney disease, UTI, urolithiasis, and hypercalciuria; even the VUR and obstructive uropathy may occur with hematuria. Therefore, the diagnostic algorithm varies in different conditions; sonography is generally sufficient, combined with a meticulous clinical/laboratory evaluation and a detailed family history. The result of all of these assessments will direct any further investigation [3–5].

3.7.8 Urolithiasis

It is a very rare condition in children than in adults, and because children have a higher radiosensitivity that prevents the free use of CT, the diagnostic protocols of the adult cannot be blindly transferred to the child.

In addition, children have smaller and less calcified kidney and ureter of small caliber, difficult to separate from the surrounding tissue due to the poor representation of fat; these aspects greatly reduce the diagnostic capability of the low-dose CT without contrast, routinely used in adults for the search of urinary stones. In children, US is the ideal technique able to detect stones localized in the pelvicalyceal system or

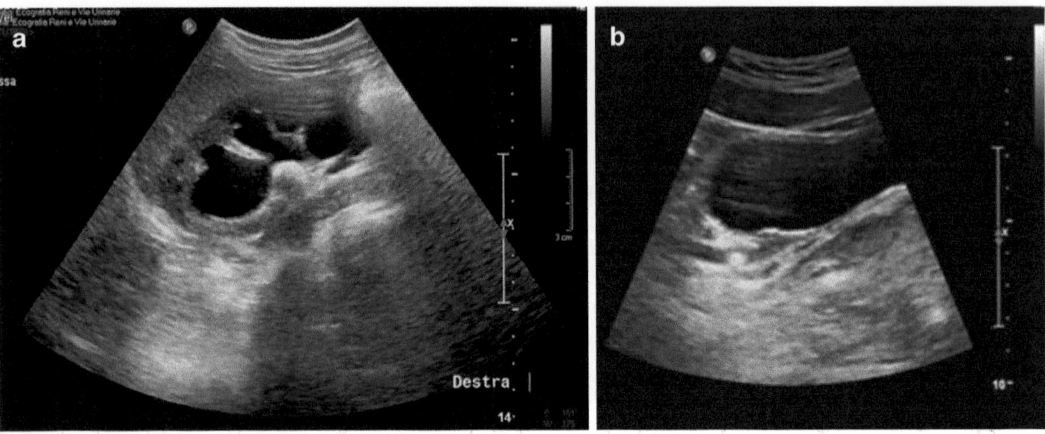

Fig. 3.16 Two different US studies showing a pelvic stone with hydronephrosis (**a**) and a distal ureteral stone (**b**)

proximal or distal ureter (Fig. 3.16). The study is preferably carried out in conditions of good hydration and adequate bladder filling. In some cases, an abdominal radiographs may be helpful (e.g., before a *lithotripsy*).

If for some reason IVU is still required, it will be conducted with the acquisition of as few images as possible; however, the examination is obsolete and almost disappeared from the centers of pediatric radiology.

The Uro-CT is used with much reluctance in children because it is highly radiant, and currently its use is restricted to cases in which the ultrasound study is nondiagnostic and unrelated to the clinic, in cases where there are indirect signs of the presence of the calculation that is not detected by US, in the complications of stone disease, as well as for presurgical imaging in the cases of percutaneous lithotripsy [1, 3, 5, 20].

3.7.9 Trauma

The *minor trauma* is rare in childhood. In these cases US is generally performed and always included with color Doppler study, possibly supplemented with CT or MRU for the evaluation of complex pictures. Ultrasound is also the investigation of choice in the follow-up.

Urethrography and cystography are used respectively for the evaluation of lesions of the urethra and bladder, which can lead to the suspicion of child abuse.

The major trauma is primarily evaluated with ce-CT study [20].

3.7.10 Urogenital Tumors

Although all benign and malignant neoplasms are primarily studied by ultrasound and echo-color Doppler, MR and CT are generally required in the subsequent investigation protocol, both for the evaluation of cancer themselves and for search of metastases, particularly lung metastases.

In any case for the definitive diagnosis, biopsy must be performed, even when imaging capabilities to orient a benign form; generally all bladder and kidney cancers are easily accessible for ultrasound-guided biopsy study [1, 4, 5, 20, 26, 28].

The cancers most often investigated in children are:

- Benign Tumors
- *Angiomyolipoma*, very rare in children but common in those with tuberous sclerosis (80 % of cases).
- Mesoblastic nephroma, the most common tumor in the neonatal period.
- Multilocular cystic nephroma, characteristically observed in male children aged <4 years.
- *Nephroblastomatosis*, defined by the presence of nephrogenic rests, associated with the risk

of Wilms' tumor. It can be in the form diffuse, focal, or multifocal in both kidneys, located in an intralobar or in a peripheral position. It is found in association with Wilms' tumor (present in 25 % of cases of Wilms' unilateral and in 100 % of cases of Wilms' bilateral), with the aniridia and the Beckwith-Wiedemann syndrome.

- Malignant Tumors*Wilms' tumor*, the most common abdominal malignancy in children aged <9 years with a peak between 2 and 3 years, typically large (diameter >12 cm), with at least a portion of the intrarenal component, usually sparing the collecting system; the neoplasia appears solid, often with a pseudo-capsule and well-defined areas of hemorrhage and necrosis. Less frequent are the calcifications (<15 %), while the renal vein thrombosis is reported in 5–10 % of cases (Fig. 3.17).
- Clear cell sarcoma occurs at 3–5 years of life, virtually indistinguishable from Wilms' tumor, metastatic to the bone (Fig. 3.18).

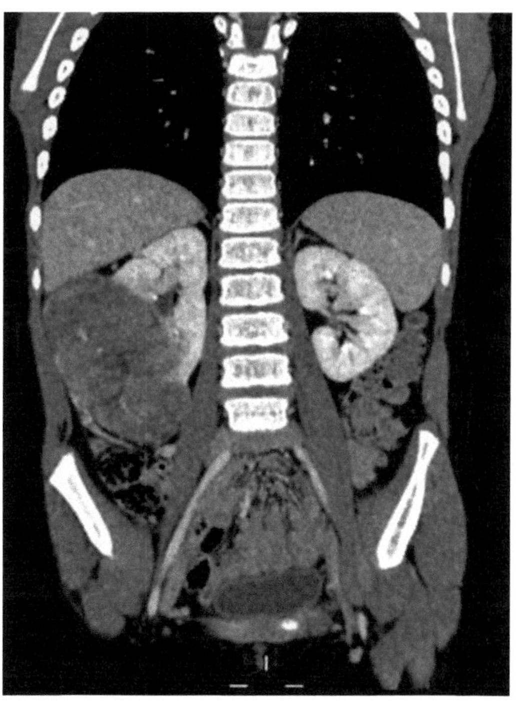

Fig. 3.17 Coronal CT scan: Wilms' tumor of the right kidney

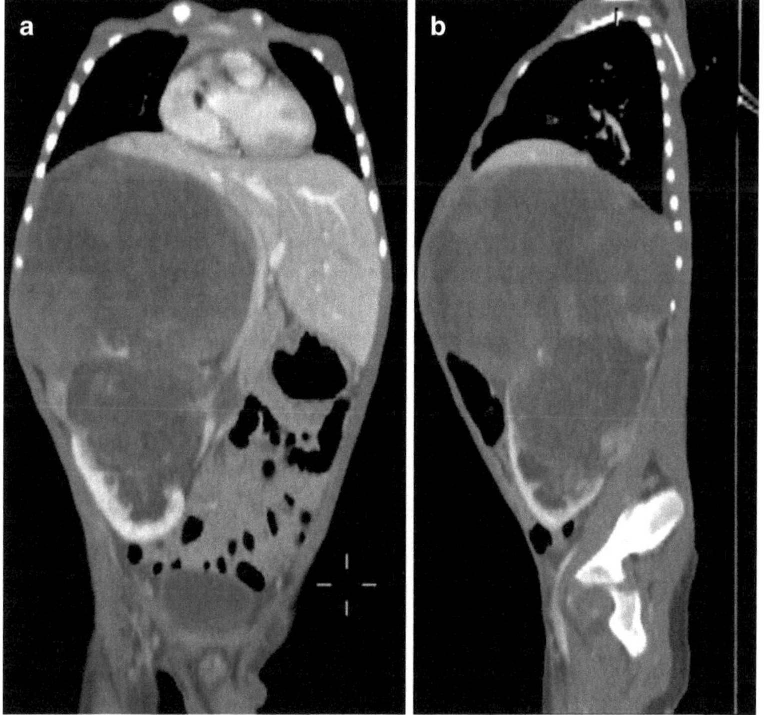

Fig. 3.18 Coronal (**a**) and sagittal (**b**) CT scans showing a massive clear cell sarcoma of the right kidney

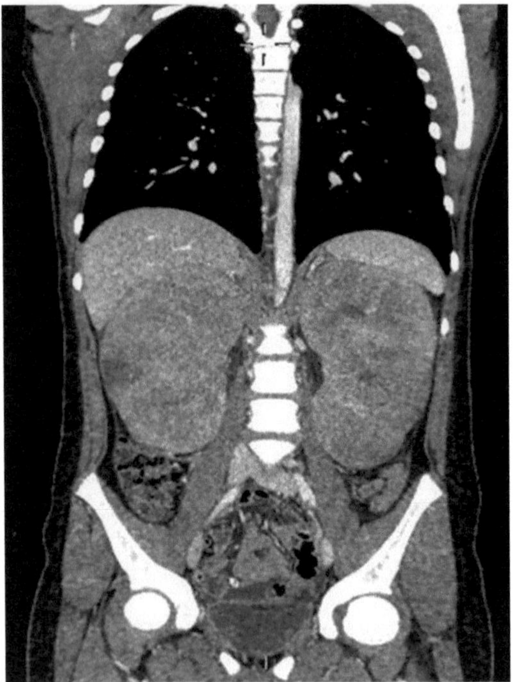

Fig. 3.19 US study (**a**) and coronal MPR CT (**b**) showing very large kidneys in renal leukemia

- Malignant rhabdoid tumor, heterogeneous intrarenal mass with thick capsule and a peripheral crescenting fluid collection in the subcapsular or perinephric space (median age 13 months). There is an association with tumors of the posterior cranial fossa.
- Renal cell carcinoma represents less than 1 % of renal tumors in children, indistinguishable from Wilms' tumor.
- Lymphoma/leukemia: different patterns of involvement, from diffuse forms characterized by symmetrical and massive enlargement of the kidneys with loss of corticomedullary differentiation (especially leukemia) to nodular forms most often seen in lymphomas, followed by direct invasion from adjacent adenopathy or lymphomatous retroperitoneal masses (Fig. 3.19).
- Rhabdomyosarcoma, the most common malignancy of the pelvis in children, frequently originates from the bladder wall at trigone, from the prostate or in paratesticular locations in male children. MRI is preferable to CT in the staging of pelvic lesions while US is essential for the assessment of the paratesticular masses. CT study is recommended for the evaluation of lung metastases, which are present in 10 % of cases at onset of disease.

References

1. Riccabona M (2002) Potential of modern sonographic techniques in paediatric uroradiology. Eur J Radiol 43:110–121
2. Riccabona M, Avni FE, Blickman JG et al (2008) Imaging recommendations in paediatric uroradiology. Minutes of the ESPR workgroup session on urinary tract infection, fetal hydronephrosis, urinary tract ultrasonography and voiding cystourethrography. Barcelona, Spain, June 2007. Pediatr Radiol 38: 138–145
3. Riccabona M, Avni FE, Blickman JG et al (2009) Imaging recommendations in paediatric uroradiology, part II. Minutes of the ESPR uroradiology task force session on childhood obstructive uropathy, high-grade fetal hydronephrosis, childhood haematuria, and urolithiasis in childhood. Pediatr Radiol 39:891–898
4. Riccabona M (2009) Urinary tract imaging in infancy. Pediatr Radiol 39:S436–S445
5. Darge K, Grattan-Smith, Riccabona M (2011) Pediatric uroradiology: state of the art. Pediatr Radiol 41:82–91
6. Riccabona M, Sorantin E, Ring E (1998) Application of M-mode sonography in pediatric patients. Eur Radiol 8:1457–1461
7. Bartram U, Darge K (2005) Harmonic versus conventional ultrasound imaging of the urinary tract in children. Pediatr Radiol 35:655–660
8. Riccabona M (2005) Pediatric three-dimensional ultrasound: basics and potential clinical value. Clin Imaging 29:1–5
9. Darge K, Heidemeier A (2006) US diagnosis of urinary tract calculi in children using the "twinkling sign". Ultrasound 14:167–173
10. Riccabona M, Ring E, Schwinger W et al (2001) Amplitude coded-colour Doppler sonography in pediatric renal disease. Eur Radiol 11:861–866
11. Mitterberger M, Pinggera GM, Neururer R et al (2008) Comparison of contrast-enhanced color Doppler imaging (CDI), computed tomography (CT), and magnetic resonance imaging (MRI) for the detection of crossing vessels in patients with ureteropelvic junction obstruction (UPJO). Eur Urol 53:1254–1260
12. Darge K (2008) Voiding urosonography with ultrasound contrast agents for the diagnosis of vesicoureteric reflux in children. I. Procedure. Pediatr Radiol 38:40–53
13. Darge K (2008) Voiding urosonography with US contrast agents for the diagnosis of vesicoureteric reflux in children. II. Comparison with radiological examinations. Pediatr Radiol 38:54–63

14. Darge K, Troeger J (2002) Vesicoureteral reflux grading in contrast-enhanced voiding urosonography. Eur J Radiol 43:122–128
15. Darge K, Moeller RT, Trusen A et al (2004) Diagnosis of vesicoureteric reflux with low-dose contrast-enhanced harmonic ultrasound imaging. Pediatr Radiol 35:73–78
16. Darge K, Ghods S, Zieger B et al (2001) Reduction in voiding cystourethrographies after the introduction of contrast enhanced sonographic reflux diagnosis. Pediatr Radiol 31:790–795
17. Ward VL, Strauss KJ, Barnewolt CE et al (2008) Pediatric radiation exposure and effective dose reduction during voiding cystourethrography. Radiology 249:1002–1009
18. Riccabona M, Avni FE, Dacher JN et al (2010) ESPR uroradiology task force and ESUR paediatric working group: imaging and procedural recommendations in paediatric uroradiology, part III. Minutes of the ESPR uroradiology task force mini-symposium on intravenous urography, uro-CT and MR-urography in childhood. Pediatr Radiol 40:1315–1320
19. Akay H, Akpinar E, Ergun O et al (2006) Unenhanced multidetector CT evaluation of urinary stones and secondary signs in pediatric patients. Diagn Interv Radiol 12:147–150
20. Maudgil DD, McHugh K (2002) The role of computed tomography in modern paediatric uroradiology. Eur J Radiol 43:129–138
21. Grattan-Smith JD, Little SB, Jones RA (2008) MR urography evaluation of obstructive uropathy. Pediatr Radiol 38:S49–S69
22. Grattan-Smith JD, Little SB, Jones RA (2008) Evaluation of reflux nephropathy, pyelonephritis and renal dysplasia. Pediatr Radiol 38:S83–S105
23. Perez-Brayfield MR, Kirsch AJ, Jones RA et al (2003) A prospective study comparing ultrasound, nuclear scintigraphy and dynamic contrast enhanced magnetic resonance imaging in the evaluation of hydronephrosis. J Urol 170:1330–1334
24. Grattan-Smith JD, Little SB, Jones RA (2008) MR urography in children: how we do it. Pediatr Radiol 38:S3–S17
25. Vivier PH, Blondiaux E, Dolores M et al (2009) Functional MR urography in children. J Radiol 90: 11–19
26. Riccabona M (2008) Potential of MR imaging in the paediatric abdomen. Eur J Radiol 68:235–244
27. Khrichenko D, Darge K (2010) Functional analysis in MR urography—made simple. Pediatr Radiol 40:182–199
28. Mendichovszky IA, Marks SD, Simcock CM et al (2008) Gadolinium and nephrogenic systemic fibrosis: time to tighten practice. Pediatr Radiol 38: 489–496
29. Grattan-Smith JD, Jones RA (2006) MR urography in children. Pediatr Radiol 36:1119–1132
30. Jones RA, Schmotzer B, Little SB et al (2008) MRU postprocessing. Pediatr Radiol 38:S18–S27
31. Hackstein N, Heckrodt J, Rau WS (2003) Measurement of single kidney glomerular filtration rate using a contrast-enhanced dynamic gradient-echo sequence and the Rutland-Patlak plot technique. J Magn Reson Imaging 18:714–725

Anesthesia in Pediatric Urology

4

Simonetta Baroncini, Monica Fae, Andrea Gentili, and Cristina Mondardini

4.1 Introduction

Urologic anesthesia is not a subspecialty but some aspects are typical to this type of surgery.

The majority of surgical urological pathologies, in pediatric age, are congenital.

Urologic surgery comprises different pathologies concerning the kidney and the upper intra-abdominal urinary tract but also malformations of the urethra and of the genitalia. Regarding the age in which the pathologies may be corrected, it is necessary to consider the potential neurotoxicity of anesthetic drugs.

Experimental studies showed apoptotic neurodegenerations and incomplete synaptogenesis with possible long-term cognitive deficiencies in young animals exposed to anesthetics. The mechanism of anesthetic drugs involves synaptic transmission of gamma-aminobutyric acid (GABA) or *N*-methyl-D-aspartate (NMDA) receptors. The toxicity is related to the dose and time of exposition to anesthetic drugs [1, 2]. There are many differences between the brain development in animals and humans, but it is important, while awaiting clinical evidences, to keep these studies in mind, in particular in the presence of minor urological pathologies that may be deferred.

4.2 Preoperative Evaluation

Clinical history and objective conditions are the only guide in choosing the investigation tests [3]. Children with urological conditions may suffer from renal insufficiency; furthermore, these pathologies can be associated with severe comorbidities such as congenital heart disease and craniofacial defects, and cardiologic visit with echocardiography test is considered appropriate.

Children with a neurogenic bladder, complex genitourinary anomalies, and multiple surgical procedures are at high risk for latex allergy, and allergic tests may be considered. In conditions of a high incidence of associated spinal abnormalities, for example, cloacal exstrophy, imaging should be evaluated before planning central neuraxial block for analgesia. When central blocks are indicated, coagulation tests are useful [4]. The preoperative evaluation must consider the anxiety and emotional problems that surgical treatments induce, in particular if associated with repeated procedures and due to the embarrassing nature of the genitourinary pathology.

Risk Evaluation and Informed Consent: The American Society of Anesthesiologists developed and modified later the ASA classification of physical status to define a correlation of clinical

S. Baroncini (✉) • M. Fae
A. Gentili • C. Mondardini
Department for Mother and Child Health,
S. Orsola-Malpighi University Hospital,
Via Massarenti 11, Bologna 40138, Italy
e-mail: simobar47@fastwebnet.it;
monica.fae@aosp.bo.it; andrea.gentili@aosp.bo.it;
cristina.mondi@libero.it

M. Lima, G. Manzoni (eds.), *Pediatric Urology: Contemporary Strategies from Fetal Life to Adolescence*,
DOI 10.1007/978-88-470-5693-0_4, © Springer-Verlag Italia 2015

condition and tolerance to surgery [5, 6]. The correct information about all possible anesthesia techniques (a pamphlet should be given before anesthesiological visit) and in particular of the benefit/risk of the purpose-tailored procedures must be provided before acquiring written consent for anesthesia. A specific risk such as difficult airway management or cardiac, respiratory, neurologic, and metabolic conditions should be annotated on the anesthesiological chart and on the operatory list.

4.3 Premedication and Preoperative Fasting

At the end of the global evaluation (history, objective clinical condition, laboratory tests if indicated, imaging, cardiologic tests), a pharmacological medication is considered. Parents are allowed to be present at induction of anesthesia. The sedative premedication is not always necessary, but when useful, midazolam 500 mcg/kg orally is currently the most frequently drug used. Midazolam can also be administered by nasal route (200 mcg/kg). Atropine in clinical practice is administered after vein placement only on demand. A local anesthetic emulsion (lidocaine 25 mg + prilocaine 25 mg) or medicated plaster (lidocaine 70 mg/tetracaine 70 mg, for children over 3 years) is applied on a detectable peripheral vein. Preoperative fasting is indicated for elective surgery and healthy patients, to avoid inhalation syndrome at anesthesia induction. Recent guidelines also consider the correct preoperative administration of drugs to decrease the risk for pulmonary aspiration in selected patients [7].

4.4 Specific Aspects

4.4.1 Latex Allergy

Latex allergy is an immunological reaction to natural rubber latex processed from the *Hevea brasiliensis* tree. Latex is used in the manufacture of many medical devices. Latex allergy has become a clinically important problem in recent years though is a not widespread phenomenon, but is more frequent in the risk groups. Allergy to latex is frequently implicated in pediatric intraoperative anaphylactic reactions [8]. High-risk groups for latex allergy in children include history of myelodysplasia with a neurogenic bladder, complex genitourinary anomalies, multiple surgical procedures, atopy, and allergies to balloons, bananas, avocados, chestnuts [9–11]. In children the signs and symptoms of the allergic reactions to latex vary from localized pruritus, rhinoconjunctivitis, and contact urticaria-angioedema to wheezing, severe bronchial asthma, cardiovascular collapse, and anaphylactic shock. Serious reactions are more likely to occur with parenteral or mucous membrane contact. The main problem of latex allergy is the development of anaphylaxis during surgical procedures or interventions. In pediatric urology an important issue concerns preventing patients from developing sensitization during repeated surgery, as well as the inhibition of symptomatic allergy development in already sensitized patients. Therefore, the preoperative identification of patients at risk is essential in the prevention of such allergy, reducing the possibility of sensitization and clinical reactions. Perioperative preventive measures have been suggested to reduce the risk. Many authors have outlined a preoperative, intraoperative, and postoperative checklist for latex-allergic patients, with the help of several specialists (anaesthesiologists, surgeons, allergologists, laboratory experts, and pharmacists) [12–14]. Perioperative management involves the recognition of the children at risk, appropriate allergological tests for these patients, chemoprophylaxis with H_1 and H_2 blockers and steroids graded according to the severity of symptoms. The perioperative minimizing of latex exposure especially in the operating room equipment, and educational training is necessary. The fundamental standard of latex-safe perioperative management is the continuity of treatment, always present in the consulting room, emergency room, wards, operating room, and pediatric intensive care: the patient must be accompanied by a medical card and is treated with latex-free equipment and items.

4.4.2 Fluid-Electrolyte Balance

Two aspects are important in designing a fluid therapy—fluid and volume replacement. Fluid replacement is necessary to maintain the hydroelectrolytic homeostasis and acid-base balance. Fluid distribution is regulated by osmotic pressure: hypothalamic nucleus is sensitive and responds to very low variations and this condition causes a hormonal response involving the secretion of ADH aldosterone. The dehydrated patient produces more ADH to preserve H_2O. It should be taken into account that during the preoperative period, ADH secretions may increase due to factors other than the osmotic ones (pain, stress, drugs). For a correct fluid intraoperative planning, consideration must be given to the metabolic requirement, preoperatory fasting, "third space" sequestration, blood loss related to surgery, and particular conditions such as the use of radiant lamps for neonates/preterms. Fluid requirements depend on the metabolic expenditure, which is higher in neonatal age. Under normal conditions 100 ml is required to metabolize 100 Kcal, but during GA the energy expenditure is 50 % [15] and lower than that calculated by Holliday and Segar [16]. The sequestration of fluid (extravascular, interstitial space) is different for each type of surgery: 1–3 ml/kg/h in minor surgery procedures till 10–20 ml/kg/h in major abdominal surgery procedures. Other mechanisms of fluid compartment regulation are needed to keep pH in the range 7.35–7.45 and electroneutrality. The amount of hydration solution required depends on preoperative conditions, fasting, and the restoration of "third space losses." To avoid the high risk of cerebral edema related to hyponatremia [17], the use of isotonic solution is suggested: the near ideal solution is a polyelectrolyte solution with glucose 0.8–1 %. The intraoperative use of glucose-free solution is not recommended in order to avoid hyperglycemia, which can determine osmotic diuresis and dehydration [18].

4.4.3 Renal Function

Many children submitted to urologic surgery, in particular for genitourinary procedures (orchidopexy, hypospadia, circumcision), are healthy, but it is possible that urologic pathologies have different comorbidities that require anesthetic implications [19]. When urologic major surgery is required, renal function must be evaluated. High creatinine and urea levels are often associated with acidosis or hyperkalemia; renal impairment can coexist with systemic diseases such as hypertension, cardiac failure, and decreased organ perfusion. Renal failure may require peritoneal or hemodialysis before surgery and the monitoring must be dedicated to volume and electrolyte status.

4.4.4 Hyperthermic Intraperitoneal Chemotherapy (HIPEC) for Rare Extensive Tumor Implants

Pediatric oncology therapy may be comprehensive of a program which provides care for patients with extensive abdominal tumor. These tumors in children are quite rare and therefore a specialized team is necessary for an optimal care. The types of tumors that can require this procedure include Wilms' tumor. The particularly high toxicity of this treatment suggests the need to maintain satisfactory urine output and avoid renal toxicity [20, 21]. The multidisciplinary care involves the collaboration between specialized pediatric oncologists, surgeons, radiation therapists, anesthesiologists, and intensivists.

4.5 Anesthesiological Management

The entire staff, involving different professional figures, should be trained and educated in order to improve safety, ensure treatment of possible side effects, and guarantee the management of emergencies.

4.5.1 Monitoring

Standard intraoperative monitoring is both invasive and noninvasive and is well described in the guidelines for safety in the operating room. Cardiovascular function is monitored by ECG (rhythm and frequency), NI systolic blood pressure (SBP), and diastolic blood pressure (DBP); if necessary a radial arterial catheter is cannulated not only for invasive monitoring but also for intraoperative and postoperative blood gas analysis and laboratory tests. When clinical conditions and the fluid requirements are difficult to evaluate, a central venous catheter (CVC) is placed by a superior cava approach for invasive monitoring of central venous pressure (CVP). The respiratory function is monitored by peripheral arterial oxygen saturation (SpO_2) and end-tidal CO_2 ($ETCO_2$). The mechanical ventilator permits the variation of all respiratory items including frequency, tidal volume (inspiratory and expiratory), minute volume, pressure, and mean airway pressure. Temperature measurement is a must in pediatric urological surgery and in particular in neonates. The temperature is tested with the esophageal probe during major surgery. The use of pre-warmed fluids and active warming systems (maîtresse, convective warm air blanket, radiant heater) is necessary. During uro-endoscopy many fluids are employed for irrigation, and this can determine hypothermia. GA and loco regional anesthesia (LRA) interfere with the thermoregulatory response in all ages.

4.5.2 Airway in Major/Minor Urologic Surgery

Comorbidity with urologic pathologies is observed in CHARGE, VACTERL, and DiGeorge syndromes, where craniofacial malformations suggest a difficult airway management. The evaluation of the difficult airway is recommended by the guidelines [22], and the Italian Health Ministry advocates particular attention to airway management and is a checklist point for safety in the operating room. The presence of all instruments and devices and expert anesthesiologists should guarantee the safety of difficult airway management.

Wilms' tumor may sometimes present inferior vena cava compression and diaphragmatic elevation due to the giant intra-abdominal mass: in this condition the induction to GA is at hight risk for inhalation, difficult ventilation, and circulatory collapse because of the very low venous return.

4.5.3 Vascular Access

Vascular access is necessary in all types of surgery. Adequate peripheral access is essential intraoperatively and also for fluid replacement in the postoperative period. One or two peripheral veins may be necessary.

If the intravenous induction to anesthesia is indicated, a topical anesthetic cream or plaster could be routinely applied on a visible vein to permit the cannulation without pain.

Clinical conditions and the type of surgery indicate the placement of a single- or double-lumen central venous catheter (CVC), appropriate for the size of the patient. This vascular access is required both for monitoring and for rapid and safe infusions of fluid and blood. The upper vena cava vein approach is mandatory for the oncologic retroperitoneal tumor, particularly when it has been extended to or into the inferior cava vein (rarely till the right atrium) and surgery may foresee vein clamping. The use of guidance ultrasonography during CVC placement has been demonstrated the better percutaneous procedure for decreasing the complication rate.

4.6 Anesthesia Techniques

General anesthesia is increasingly associated with regional anesthesia techniques, to optimize anesthesia and analgesia results throughout the perioperative period.

4.6.1 General Anesthesia (GA)

Anesthesia management can be performed by inhalation or intravenous hypnotics, associated with neuromuscular blocking agents, opioids, and adjuvant drugs if necessary. Anesthesiological management, today, foresees combined general-regional anesthesia.

Balanced anesthesia is the most common GA applied, in which a mixture of small amounts of several drugs, administered by different routes (inhalation + intravenous), permits a correct anesthetic plan for the surgery. Recently total intravenous anesthesia (TIVA) is chosen for pediatric patients, even in smaller children. In all pediatric ages and in particular in neonates, many drugs cannot be legally used. The bispectral index is designed to observe the anesthetic plan and drug consumption although results do not differ from those of conventional clinical practice [23].

4.6.1.1 Inhalation Agents

Sevoflurane is a halogenated general inhalation anesthetic drug and to date the most frequently drug employed in pediatric anesthesia. It is administered by vaporization vehicled by O_2/medical air at different FiO_2 (>0.5) [24]. The minimum alveolar concentration (MAC) in neonates (3.3 %) and children till 3 months (3.2 %) is similar, but older infants and children have a lower MAC of approximately 2.5 %. During mask induction the incidence of agitation is near 14 % but laryngospasm and bronchospasm are present in around 1 or 2 %. It is quite clear that the concomitant use of opioids requires a lower halogenated concentration. Inhalation anesthesia consents a rapid recovery but agitation is frequently present and is considered an adverse effect.

Particular attention must be given to the concentration of compound A (reaction with CO_2 adsorber in particular conditions) (A = alkene) which is suggested to be a potential cause of possible renal injuries (proteinuria, glycosuria).

4.6.1.2 Intravenous Agents

Thiopentone was considered in the past years the most commonly used intravenous agent for anesthesia induction; propofol is now the most frequently employed induction agent (1.5–3 mg/kg) in pediatric age. In Italy, the use of propofol in neonates is limited by a Health Ministry deliberation and written consent must be acquired. The current and recent literature contains many reports of good results in particular for anesthesia induction in procedural deep sedation [25–27]. In preterm neonates and in the first 10 days of life, there is a risk of propofol accumulation if given both for an intermittent bolus or infusion. It would seem sensible at present to limit its use to single bolus administration [28–31].

4.6.2 Regional Anesthesia (RA)

It is generally accepted that RA provides safe and effective pain relief, as it provides the block of sensory transmissions [32, 33]. Regional anesthetic techniques also in pediatric patients provide safe and effective pain relief during and after surgery with different techniques (Table 4.1) [34].

In 2010 the ADARPEF study revealed a low incidence of complications related to regional anesthetic techniques and concludes that RA has a good efficacy and safety [35]. The application of pediatric regional anesthesia blocks has increased in recent years, the neuraxial blocks are applied in all ages, and peripheral blocks are rapidly expanding especially in children aged 5 years or older. In pediatrics RA is performed under GA or deep sedation to reduce potential damages from a loss of behavioral control during the procedure and to keep hypnosis during surgery. However, RA reduces intraoperative anesthetic requirements, supporting recovery, early ambulation, and shortening the time to rehabilitation [36, 37]. A necessary condition to obtain the most benefits from RA is the knowledge and expertise of the specialist who chooses and applies the techniques and appropriate and adequate equipment and devices. Ultrasound guidance is the best clinical practice both for neuraxial and peripheral blocks. Ultrasonography could augment the success rate, since it allows anatomical structures and nerves to be visualized, permits the needle location to be identified, and reduces the amount of local anesthetic administered [38].

4.6.2.1 Neuraxial Blocks

Central neuraxial bock is suggested for patients undergoing major abdominal surgery. In the spinal approach, drugs are administered intrathecally into the cerebrospinal fluid and in epidural approach into the fatty tissues surrounding the dura [39]. Absolute contraindications are local

Table 4.1 Testicular torsion x only under II (Caudal Block) and VII (Systemic Analgesia) column

Pathologies	Epidural Catheter	Caudal Block	Penile N. Block	Ilio-ing. Ileo ipog	Rectus N. Block	Local W Infiltr.	Systemic Analgesia
Hypospadia		X	X[a]				X
Circumcision		X	X				X
Orchidopexy		X		X		X	X
Testicular torsion	X						X
Cystostomy		X					X
Laparoscopy for the upper urinary tract					1 LA retroperit. Intercostal B		X
Pyeloplasty	X						X
Nephrectomy	X						X
Bladder exstrophy	X[b]						X
Prune belly syndrome	X[b]						X

[a]Only in distal hypospadia
[b]Only after Rx

infection at injection site, hypovolemia, coagulopathy, high intracranial pressure, allergy to local anesthetics, and parent refusal. Relative contraindications include sepsis, neurological dysfunction, and anatomical abnormalities. Neurological injury, infection, ischemia, seizures, hypotension, and cardiac arrest are the risks of neuraxial anesthesia. It should be remembered that there are some anatomical differences between adults and children in the lumbosacral region.

4.6.2.2 Caudal Epidural Block

Epidural block by caudal route, the most popular technique in pediatrics, is suggested in hypospadias repair, ureteral reimplantation, orchidopexy, and surgical bladder procedures. The caudal space is easy to find in patients less than 7 years of age, when block is commonly performed. The sacral hiatus is found by searching for a triangle with the base formed by a line joining the right and left sacral cornea and the apex as lower IV sacral vertebrae. The sacral hiatus is situated higher in children than in adults. The dedicated needle passes, at a nearly 45° angle, through the sacrococcygeal ligament, and after loss of resistance, the local anesthetic is injected. This block is more frequently used as a "single shot." Adjuvants may be added to prolong the duration of analgesia. Over the past several years, caudal catheters were introduced upward even to thoracic level especially in neonates and infants, but this technique is no longer recommended, because of the risk of fecal soiling.

4.6.2.3 Lumbar Epidural Block

In contrast to the caudal block, lumbar epidural block is rarely used as a single injection; usually a catheter is inserted. Catheter placement is based on surgical incision location corresponding to segmental levels to target analgesia [40]. This technique should be performed by experienced anesthesiologists. In very small infants epidural needles are inserted below L4, so, to achieve the desired segmental level, the catheters should be threaded for a long segment, monitoring the efficacy of the pain relief. Currently the indication is to decrease the distance of insertion to as short as 3–4 cm inside the epidural space [41]. Central blocks have a history of more than 100 years in adults, but in pediatrics RA was rarely applied/described [42–44] and became an essential integrated, safe, and effective antalgic system producing excellent intraoperative analgesia, less than 20 years ago, when Anand published his work [45].

4.6.2.4 Peripheral Nerve Blocks

Peripheral nerve blocks are a valid alternative to the neuraxial technique with good sensory block and without the major complications of central block. Sympathetic block and hemodynamic changes are minimal as well as motor block and urinary retention. Use of neurostimulation and ultrasonography is recommended although, in the latter case, evidence is not strong. The length of block depends on the pharmacokinetics of the local anesthetic; long-acting anesthetics such as levobupivacaine or ropivacaine are preferred, while adjuvants as clonidine may extend the duration. For prolonged analgesia, catheters may be placed.

4.6.2.5 Penile Nerve Block

Dorsal penile nerve block is used in circumcision, phimosis, release of paraphimosis, and repair of penile lacerations. Intravenous analgesia is recommended before performing the nerve block. Various techniques have been proposed; nerves should be blocked as proximally to the base of penis as possible. It is necessary to note that the single injection at the base of the penis can cause injury of penis vessels as well as severe complications [46]. The approach most frequently used is described by Dalens as the "two-puncture procedure" [47]. The penile nerve block and caudal block provide similar pain scores and painless postoperative periods [48]. However, penile block may be preferable due to the possibility of temporary leg weakness after caudal block. Particularly interesting, a recent study reported that postoperative urethral fistula formation was more likely in children who received caudal epidural [49].

4.6.2.6 Ilioinguinal-Iliohypogastric Nerve Block

This block may be used for surgical procedures in the inguinal region, orchidopexy and varicocele, and herniorrhaphy. Using landmark technique, the puncture site is about 1 cm medial to the anterior superior iliac spine, but this traditional technique is burdened with high failure rates. The point of injection by ultrasound is more lateral and the trasversus abdominis/internal oblique fascial plane needs to be identified, where the nerves could be found [50].

4.6.2.7 Rectus Sheath Block

A rectus sheath block provides effective pain relief and muscle relaxation for laparoscopic surgery and other small midline incisions. It is performed bilaterally, between the rectus abdominis muscle and the posterior rectus sheath. The unpredictable depth of the posterior rectus sheath in children is a good argument for the use of ultrasound together with the advantage of allowing visualization of the bowel, which may decrease accidental puncture [51].

4.6.2.8 Transversus Abdominis Plane (TAP) Block

TAP block is effective in laparoscopic procedures and open surgery. Its use is limited by the need for bilateral blocks when the incision crosses the midline. This, like the other abdominal wall blocks described above, is effective for somatic pain but not for visceral pain. TAP block may be useful when epidural analgesia is contraindicated. Local anesthetic should be placed between the internal oblique and transversus abdominis muscles, the triangle of Petit is used as a landmark for injection, and a relatively large volume of anesthetic is required [52].

4.6.2.9 Local Wound Infiltration

Local wound infiltration is a component of multimodal postoperative analgesia. The single-shot infiltration of local anesthetics in laparoscopic working ports is more commonly performed than continuous wound infiltration for fear of complications. Also intraperitoneally instillation was rarely performed, although a systematic review and meta-analysis of its effectiveness in adults have given promising results [53].

4.7 Renal Transplantation

Children receiving a donated kidney undergo anesthesia and surgery while in chronic renal failure. Many have cardiac, hematological, respiratory, and metabolic problems secondary to their renal failure. The appropriate choice of anesthesia for patients undergoing renal transplantation requires minimal toxicity and accurate monitoring for patients at high risk for metabolic, cardiovascular, and respiratory perioperative complications. No specific data are available on the perioperative use of epidural analgesia in pediatric renal transplant patients and it appears to remain an uncommon practice. Epidural analgesia for pediatric renal transplantation remains controversial [54, 55] because of:

1. A theoretically increased risk of epidural hematoma and abscess formation
2. Perceived risks of vascular instability resulting in reductions in graft perfusion
3. Limited data on the profile of minor adverse effects

4.7.1 Induction

Standard anesthetic induction and monitoring is appropriate. If recently dialyzed, anticipate blood pressure (BP) drop on induction; depending on fluid status, patient should be treated with 20 ml/kg fluid bolus. Arterial monitoring in the upper limb is required if the transplant is to be anastomosed to the IVC/aorta (usually in children under 20 kg). Older children undergoing anastomoses to iliac vessels require arterial access according to comorbidity. Adequate peripheral access is essential intraoperatively and also for fluid replacement in the postoperative period. A large-bore peripheral venous catheter (in the upper limbs if IVC/aorta anastomosis is occurring) is required. Maintenance of the central venous pressure (CVP) is essential throughout surgery and during the postoperative period. Ideally this should not be performed via a Permcath. Insertion of a triple-lumen central venous catheter appropriate for the size of the patient is required (maintenance value for CVP is 7.5 mmHg/10 cmH_2O). Antibiotics should be given on induction, according to the protocol. Immunosuppression and premedication will have already been given in the ward. A urinary catheter should be inserted prior to surgery.

If anastomosis is to the IVC/aorta, dopamine will be required as an inotrope. Prepare dopamine 3 mg/kg in 50 ml 5 % dextrose (5 ml/h = 5 mcg/kg/min).

4.7.2 Intraoperative Management

Standard anesthetic maintenance is appropriate.

Prior to vascular unclamping, a 1–2 mg/kg furosemide bolus may be given if requested by the surgeon. Dopamine may be started at 5–10 mcg/kg/min and is indicated prior to vascular unclamping where anastomosis is onto the IVC/aorta. Rate is titrated to maintain BP parameters specified by the surgeon. Hyperkalemia may rarely be encountered intraoperatively. K^+ > 6 mmol is managed with salbutamol 4 mcg/kg, CaCl 0.2 ml/kg, bicarbonate 1 mmol/kg, and furosemide 1–2 mg/kg.

4.7.3 Intraoperative Fluid Management

Initial hypovolemia should be corrected with approximately 20 ml/kg of crystalloid (Ringer Lactate or NaCl). During vessel dissection/cross clamping and vascular anastomoses, the patient should be volume loaded with crystalloids and colloids (or blood if Hb <7 g/dl). With vascular unclamping, there is a large drop in systemic vascular resistance (particularly in smaller children) and a potential blood loss with anastomotic leak [56]. High blood flow through the graft immediately on clamp release is associated with improved early renal function. Maintain filling pressure and flow with fluid loading and inotropes as required [57]. Once renal perfusion is established, it is acceptable to allow the CVP to drift down to approximately 10 mmHg, but not lower for the duration of the surgery.

After ureteral anastomosis, urine production can be monitored and urine volume replaced with crystalloid.

4.7.4 Immediate Postoperative Management

Generally older patients should be extubated at the end of the procedure, with BP controlled in a range approximating to the donor's normal adult blood pressure. Postoperative ventilation is generally indicated in patients where the graft is anastomosed to the great vessels or where otherwise indicated clinically [58]. If dopamine has been started, it should be continued postoperatively and titrated to BP but may be stopped if hypertension occurs. Monitoring in pediatric intensive care unit should include BP, CVP, pulse, RR, half hourly peripheral and central temperature, and urine output.

Chest X-ray should be performed in recovery to check position of central venous line and renal graft ultrasound performed to assess blood flow.

Blood samples should be sent for full blood count, creatinine, urea and electrolytes, bicarbonate, calcium, phosphate, magnesium, albumin, glucose, and osmolality (repeat creatinine, urea, Na, K, and osmolality 2 h for 24 h).

4.7.5 Postoperative Analgesia

Morphine/fentanyl should be titrated until the child is comfortable and then a morphine/fentanyl continuous infusion is indicated.

4.7.6 Transfer from the Operating Room

Transfer of the patient is hazardous. Hypovolemia and graft thrombosis have been experienced and the following guidelines are suggested:

- Full monitoring should continue for transfer including CVP.
- Colloids or crystalloid should be running to maintain CVP at least at 7.5 mmHg.
- The patient should not leave the operating room with a low CVP.

4.7.7 Postoperative Fluid Management

Primary concern is the maintenance of CVP at 10 cm^2 of water (7.5 mmHg). Anticipate hypovolemia (low peripheral temperature, low CVP, tachycardia, BP may be low) and infuse colloids as rapidly as necessary to maintain a CVP at 10 cm^2 of water. Use blood, plasma, or normal saline according to the hemoglobin. A high urine flow is desirable (certainly over 2 ml/kg/h). Replace urine output and insensible losses (400 ml/m^2/24 h) initially with 0.45 % saline, volume for volume on an hourly basis. Check plasma and urine electrolytes 2 hourly for at least 24 h. If the plasma sodium is falling and the urine sodium is greater than 75 mmol/l, change to normal saline alternating with half normal saline, and continue to review results. Some children may become excessively polyuric post transplant, particularly after living donation. If so, consider replacing a proportion of the urine output rather than the full volume and/or weaning dopamine. Very rarely, a high blood pressure and vasoconstriction may represent raised intracranial pressure, particularly if associated with bradycardia. Always check the neurological observations in this situation.

If the potassium falls, knowledge of the urinary potassium excretion rate is helpful in calculating replacement. Appropriate anesthesia for pediatric renal transplantation requires stable intraoperative hemodynamics, optimal perfusion of the newly transplanted kidney, and good analgesia during recovery. Renal transplantation is the most effective renal replacement therapy for children with end-stage renal disease.

The contribution of anesthesia care to the success of the program may be measured in terms of intraoperative physiological stability and effective postoperative pain management.

Conflict of Interest None.

References

1. Kalkman CJ, Peelen L, Moons KG, Veenhuizen M, Bruens M, Sinnema G, de Jong TP (2009) Behavior and development in children and age at the time of first anesthetic exposure. Anesthesiology 110(4): 805–812
2. Wilder RT, Flick RP, Sprung J et al (2009) Early exposure to anesthesia and learning disabilities in a population-based birth cohort. Anesthesiology 110:796–804
3. Serafini G, Ingelmo PM, Astuto M, Baroncini S, Borrometi F, Bortone L, Ceschin C, Gentili A, Lampugnani E et al (2014) Preoperative evaluation in infants and children: recommendations of the Italian

Society of Pediatric and Neonatal Anesthesia and Intensive Care (SARNePI). Minerva Anestesiol 80(4):461–469
4. Gandhi M, Vashisht R (2010) Anaesthesia for paediatric urology. Contin Educ Anaesth Crit Care Pain 10(5):152–157
5. Han KR, Kim HL, Pantuck AJ (2004) Use of ASA classification to assess perioperative risk in patients undergoing radical nephrectomy for renal cell carcinoma. Urology 63:841–846
6. Freilich DA, Cilento BG Jr, Graham D, Zhou J, Retik AB, Nguyen HT (2010) Perioperative risk factors for surgical complications in pediatric urology: a pilot study in preoperative risk assessment in children. Urology 76(1):3–8
7. Committee ASA on Standards and Practice Parameters (2011) Practice guidelines for preoperative fasting and the use of pharmacologic agents to reduce the risk of pulmonary aspiration: application to healthy patients undergoing elective procedures: an updated report by ASA Committee on Standards and Practice Parameters. Anesthesiology 114:495–511
8. Murat I (2000) Latex allergy: were are we? Paediatr Anaesth 10:577–579
9. Bernardini R, Novembre E, Lombardi E et al (1999) Risk factors for latex allergy in patients with spina bifida and latex sensitization. Clin Exp Allergy 29:681–686
10. Ricci G, Gentili A, Di Lorenzo F et al (1999) Latex allergy in subjects who had undergone multiple surgical procedures for bladder exstrophy: relationship with clinical intervention and atopic diseases. BJU Int 83:1058–1062
11. Gentili A, Ricci G, Di Lorenzo FP, Pigna A, Masi M, Baroncini S (2003) Latex allergy in children with oesophageal atresia. Paediatr Anaesth 13:668–675
12. Holzman RS (1997) Clinical management of latex-allergic children. Anesth Analg 85:529–533
13. Gentili A, Lima M, Ricci GP, Pigna A, Fae M, Masi M, Baroncini S (2007) Perioperative treatment of latex-allergic children. J Patient Saf 3(3):166–172
14. Gentili A, Ricci GP, Di Lorenzo F, Pigna A, Tonini C, Baroncini S (2001) Latex allergy in pediatric age: an interdisciplinary perioperative management and case reports. Minerva Anestesiol 67(1–2):29–40
15. Lindahal SG (1988) Energy expenditure and fluid and electrolyte requirements in anesthetized infants and children. Anesthesiology 69(3):377–382
16. Holliday M, Segar W (1957) The maintenance need for water in parenteral fluid therapy. Pediatrics 19:823–832
17. Lönnqvist PA (2007) Inappropriate perioperative fluid management in children: time of solution. Paediatr Anaesth 17:203–205
18. Murat I, Dubois MC (2008) Perioperative fluid therapy in pediatrics. Paediatr Anaesth 18(5):363–370
19. Gregory GA (2012) Gregory's pediatric anesthesia. Wiley-Blackwell, Chichester
20. Hayes-Jordan A, Green H, Ludwig J, Anderson P (2012) Toxicity of hyperthermic intraperitoneal chemotherapy (HIPEC) in pediatric patients with sarcomatosis/carcinomatosis: early experience and phase 1 results. Pediatr Blood Cancer 59(2):395–397
21. Owesu-Aagymang P, Arunkumar R, Green H, Hurstd D, Landoski K, Hayes-Jordan A (2012) Anesthetic management and renal functional in pediatric patients undergoing cytoreductive surgery with continuous hyperthermic intraperitoneal chemotherapy (HIPEC) with cisplatin. Ann Surg Oncol 19(8):2652–2656
22. Gruppo di Studio SIAARTI "Vie Aeree Difficili", Frova G et al (2006) Recommendations for airway control and difficult airway management in paediatric patients. Minerva Anestesiol 72(9):723–748
23. Bresil P, Nielsson MS, Malver LP, Kraemer K, Schjørring O, Dethlefsen C, Lambert PH (2013) Impact of bispectral index for monitoring propofol remifentanil anaesthesia. A randomised clinical trial. Acta Anaesthesiol Scand 57(8):978–987
24. www.drugs.com/pro/sevoflurane.html
25. Ghanta S, Abdel-Latif ME, Lui K, Ravindranathan H, Awad J, Oei J (2007) Propofol compared with the morphine, atropine, and suxamethonium regimen as induction agents for neonatal endotracheal intubation: a randomized, controlled trial. Pediatrics 119(6): 1248–1255
26. Papoff P, Mancuso M, Caresta E, Moretti C (2008) Effectiveness and safety of propofol in newborn infants. Pediatrics 121(2):448–449
27. Shah PS, Shah VS (2011) Propofol for procedural sedation/anaesthesia in neonates. Cochrane Database Syst Rev (3):CD007248
28. Allegaert K, de Hoon J, Verbesselt R, Naulaers G, Murat I (2007) Maturational pharmacokinetics of single intravenous bolus of propofol. Paediatr Anaesth 17(11):1028–1034
29. Allegaert K, Peeters MY, Verbesselt R et al (2007) Inter-individual variability in propofol pharmacokinetics in preterm and term neonates. Br J Anaesth 99(6):864–870
30. Allegaert K, De Hoon J, Naulaers G, Van De Velde M (2008) Neonatal clinical pharmacology: recent observations of relevance for anaesthesiologists. Acta Anaesthesiol Belg 59:283–288
31. Skinner AV (2010) Neonatal pharmacology. Anaesth Intensive Care 12(3):79–84
32. Tobias JD, Flannagan J, Brock J, Brin E (1993) Neonatal regional anesthesia: alternative to general anesthesia for urologic surgery. Urology 41(4):362–365
33. Bernstein S (1993) Regional anesthesia for urological surgery. Int Anesthesiol Clin 31(1):57–66
34. Dalens B (2006) Some current controversies in paediatric regional anaesthesia. Curr Opin Anaesthesiol 19(3):301–308
35. Ecoffey C, Locroix F, Giaufre E (2010) Epidemiology and morbidity of regional anesthesia in children: a follow up one-year survey prospective of the French-Language Society of Paediatric Anaesthesiologists (ADARPEF). Pediatr Anaesth 20:1061–1069
36. Bordet AEF, Duflo F, Lanais S, Combet S, Taylor P, Pouyau A, Paturel B, James R, Allaouchiche B, Chassard D (2003) Patient-controlled epidural

analgesia versus continuous epidural infusion with ropivacaine for postoperative analgesia in children. Anesth Analg 97:1608–1611
37. Pavar D (2004) Regional anaesthesia in pediatric patients. Indian J Anaesth 48(5):394–399
38. Denny NM, Harrop-Griffiths W (2005) Location, location, location! Ultrasound imaging in regional anaesthesia. Br J Anaesth 94(1):1–3
39. Schug SA, Saunders D, Kurowski I, Paech MJ (2006) Neuraxial drug administration: a review of treatment options for anaesthesia and analgesia. CNS Drugs 20(11):917–933
40. Samol NB, Furstein JS, Moore DL (2012) Regional anesthesia and pain management for the pediatric patient. Int Anesthesiol Clin 50(4):83–95
41. Murrell D, Gibson PR, Cohen RC (1993) Continuous epidural analgesia in newborn infants undergoing major surgery. J Pediatr Surg 28:548–553
42. Ruston FG (1961) Epidural anaesthesia in paediatric surgery. Present status in the Hamilton General Hospital. Can Anaesth Soc J 11:12–34
43. Spiegel P (1962) Caudal anesthesia in paediatric surgery: a preliminary report. Anesth Analg 41:219–221
44. Fortuna A (1967) Caudal analgesia: a simple and safe technique in paediatric surgery. Br J Anaesth 39:165–170
45. Anand KJ, Sippell WG, Aynsley-Green A (1987) Randomized trial of fentanyl anaesthesia in preterm babies undergoing surgery: effects on the stress response. Lancet 1:62–66
46. Sara CA, Lowrt CJ (1984) A complication of circumcision and dorsal nerve block of the penis. Anesth Intensive Care 13:79–85
47. Dalens B, Vanneuville G, Dechellotte P (1989) Penile block via subpubic space in 100 children. Anesth Analg 69:41–45
48. Cyna AM, Middleton P (2008) Caudal epidural block versus other methods of postoperative pain relief for circumcision in boys. Cochrane Database Syst Rev 8(4):CD003005
49. Kundra P, Yuvaraj K, Agrawal K, Krishnappa S, Kumar LT (2012) Surgical outcome in children undergoing hypospadias repair under caudal epidural vs penile block. Paediatr Anaesth 22(7):707–712
50. Willschke H, Bösenberg A, Marhofer P, Johnston S, Kettner S, Eichenberger U et al (2006) Ultrasonographic-guided ilioinguinal/iliohypogastric nerve block in pediatric anesthesia: what is the optimal volume? Anesth Analg 102(6):1680–1684
51. Willschke H, Bösenberg A, Marhofer P, Johnston S, Kettner SC, Wanzel O, Kapral S (2006) Ultrasonography-guided rectus sheath block in paediatric anaesthesia-a new approach to an old technique. Br J Anaesth 97(2):244–249
52. Mai CL, Young MJ, Quraishi SA (2012) Clinical implications of the transversus abdominis plane block in pediatric anesthesia. Paediatr Anaesth 22(9): 831–840
53. Marks JL, Ata B, Tulandi T (2012) Systematic review and metaanalysis of intraperitoneal instillation of local anesthetics for reduction of pain after gynecologic laparoscopy. J Minim Invasive Gynecol 19(5): 545–553
54. Chalkiadis G (2003) The rise and fall of continuous epidural infusions in children. Paediatr Anaesth 13:91–93
55. Williams M, Milner QK (2003) Postoperative analgesia following renal transplantation – current practice in the UK. Anaesthesia 58:712–713
56. Dawidson I, Berglin E, Brynger H et al (1987) Intravascular volumes and colloid dynamics in relation to fluid management in living related kidney donors and recipients. Crit Care Med 15:631–636
57. Giessing M, Muller D, Winkelmann B, Roigas J, Loening SA (2007) Kidney transplantation in children and adolescents. Transplant Proc 39(7):2197–2201
58. Coupe N, O'Brien M, Gibson P, de Lima J (2005) Anesthesia for pediatric renal transplantation with and without epidural analgesia-a review of 7 years experience. Paediatr Anaesth 15(3):220–228

Endoscopy of the Urinary Tract

5

Michela Maffi and Mario Lima

5.1 Introduction

Direct visualization of urinary tract provided by cystourethroscopy is a useful tool for both diagnosis and treatment of several urinary pathologies. Technological advances enabled the miniaturization of many instruments making them accessible even in the pediatric age.

5.2 Instrumentation

The endoscopic instruments can be divided into rigid and flexible. Flexible tools offer the advantage of better inspection at any angle thanks to the deflection of the tip but provide a view of lower quality. Rigid endoscopes allow a better view, thanks to their lens system and to a larger lumen for water flow, and allow the use of additional tools, thanks to a wide operating channel and easier manipulation and directionality. Modern cystoscopes are one-piece units (Fig. 5.1). Rigid cystoscopes' calibers range from 5 Fr to adult sizes with a 2.5-3 Fr working channel that is wider in largest cystoscopes [1]. Every cystoscope has a connection for the camera and for the fiberoptic light source. Appropriate fluid flow is guaranteed by channels for the water input and output. This system creates a constant laminar flow that allows the correct execution of the procedure. Any urologic irrigant can be used for cystoscopy; most often, sterile water or saline solution is used. However, the latter should be avoided if electrocoagulation is planned [2]. Several instruments are available for both rigid and flexible endoscopes: graspers, Bugbee electrodes, hooks, biopsy forceps, stents, guidewires, catheters, needles, etc.

5.3 Operative Technique

5.3.1 Patient Preparation

Cystoscopy in children is performed under general anesthesia. The patient is at the end of the bed, to make possible the use of fluoroscopy, if necessary. The child lays in supine lithotomy position with legs supported by rolled up towels or appropriate stirrups (Fig. 5.2), while in infant, the froggled position is the most appropriate [1, 3]. The surgeon is at the end of the bed with a monitor in front of him while the nurse is on his right. Alternatively, small babies can be positioned transversally in the bed to let a safer management of the airways.

5.3.2 Preliminary Inspection

External genitalia should be inspected before the procedure is performed, to identify

M. Maffi • M. Lima (✉)
Department of Pediatric Surgery,
S. Orsola-Malpighi University Hospital,
Via Massarenti 11, Bologna 40138, Italy
e-mail: michela.maffi@libero.it; mario.lima@unibo.it

M. Lima, G. Manzoni (eds.), *Pediatric Urology: Contemporary Strategies from Fetal Life to Adolescence*,
DOI 10.1007/978-88-470-5693-0_5, © Springer-Verlag Italia 2015

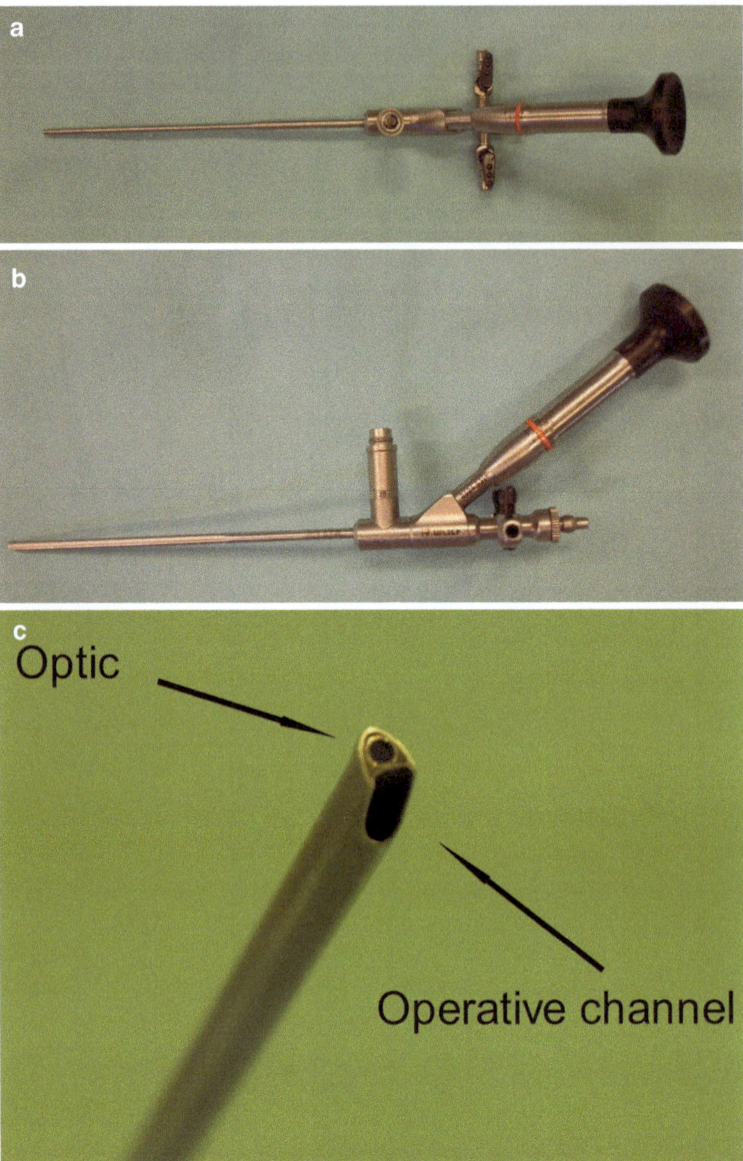

Fig. 5.1 (**a**, **b**) Rigid cystoscope; (**c**) detail of the tip

malformations, anomalies, masses, and the presence, the absence, and the position of the orifices presents. In the female, the urethral meatus may not be immediately visible. A better view can be obtained pulling on gently the labia majora. The inspection allows to evaluate the most appropriate caliber considering that the urethral meatus should accept a 7.5–8 Fr cystoscope in a term infant [1]. The instrument should be thoroughly lubricated, taking care not to grease the front lens. The surgeon must check the correct connection of the cystoscope to the camera and the light source and the proper functioning of the water flow.

5.3.3 Male Urethra

The penis should be straightened to form almost a right angle with the abdominal wall. The endoscope is inserted through the fossa navicularis, and both mucosal aspect and urethral caliber should be evaluated. An appropriate fluid flow has to be guaranteed to make the urethral lumen always visible avoiding urethral damages. If the lumen is not clearly visible, the cystoscope must be retracted till the view becomes better end the position of the instrument clearer. The bulbar urethra is recognizable by its larger diameter. When the tool passes at this level, the endoscope and the penis are

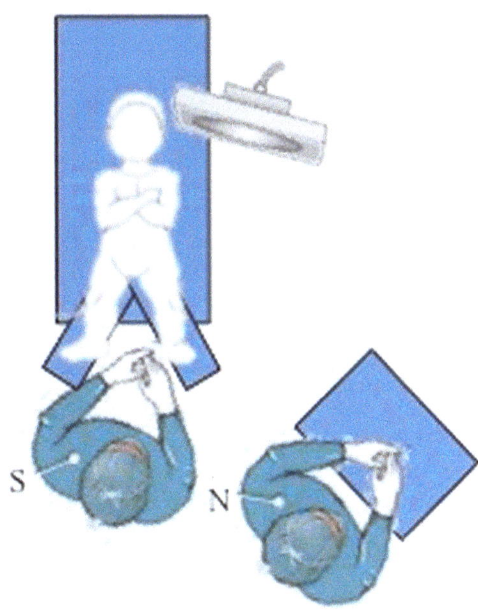

Fig. 5.2 Patient position

positioned parallel to the floor. This maneuver allows the passage of the instrument through the membranous urethra [2]. The external sphincter is identifiable by mucosal vascular striations radiating from a narrow lumen. A gentle pressure allows the passage in this area till the prostatic urethra. At this level, verumontanum appears as a hyperemic structure rising from the posterior wall of the urethra, and prostatic utriculus can be also evaluated. At the bladder neck, it may be necessary to depress the endoscope to enter into the bladder.

5.3.4 Female Urethra

The female urethra is significantly shorter than that of the male and can be inspected by inserting the endoscope under direct vision into the urethral meatus and by directing it straight towards the umbilicus till the bladder neck [2]. The mucosal aspect is similar to the posterior urethra of the male, sharing the same vascular striations.

5.3.5 Bladder

Once the endoscope is entered into the bladder, an exploration of the entire surface should be performed. Mucosal aspect and bladder structure can be evaluated. The interureteric ridge can be identified just inside the bladder neck along the trigone when the bladder is only slightly filled. Expert urologists can control the water flow to obtain a proper pressure allowing a correct view of the bladder's structures avoiding overdistension and mucosal bleeding.

The ureteric orifices are visible at each edge of the interureteric ridge, and a clear efflux of urine can be noted bilaterally. At the end of the inspection, the endoscope is gently removed and the bladder drained [1, 2].

5.3.6 Vagina

In female, the cystoscope can be inserted through the hymen in the vagina. A proper distension can be obtained thanks to a compression of the vaginal introitus. A homogeneous mucosa is normally seen, and in the distal part of the vagina, the cervical os appears.

Vaginoscopy should always be performed after cystoscopy to avoid bacterial contamination of the urinary tract with the vaginal flora.

5.4 Contraindications

Principal contraindications include a documented and active infection of the urinary tract and recent bladder surgery. Moreover, every anesthesiologic contraindication must be considered.

5.5 Indications and Findings

5.5.1 Hematuria

In most of the cases, hematuria in children has a medical cause, and it does not require cystoscopy. In fact, urinalysis and culture and ultrasounds or radiologic studies often lead to the diagnosis [3–5]. Some boys may present sporadic episodes of hematuria. In most of these cases, cystoscopy is negative and not indicated. Management is expectant with most children. Endoscopy is normally reserved for patients with significant and protracted bleeding. Vascular anomaly or polyps can be noted. A hemorrhagic cystitis can be present in children who undergo chemotherapy [6]. These children can benefit from cystoscopic removal of the clots and bladder irrigation.

5.5.2 Posterior Urethral Valves

Posterior urethral valves are two flaps starting from the verumontanum and extending distally and laterally [7]. After bladder filling via the cys-

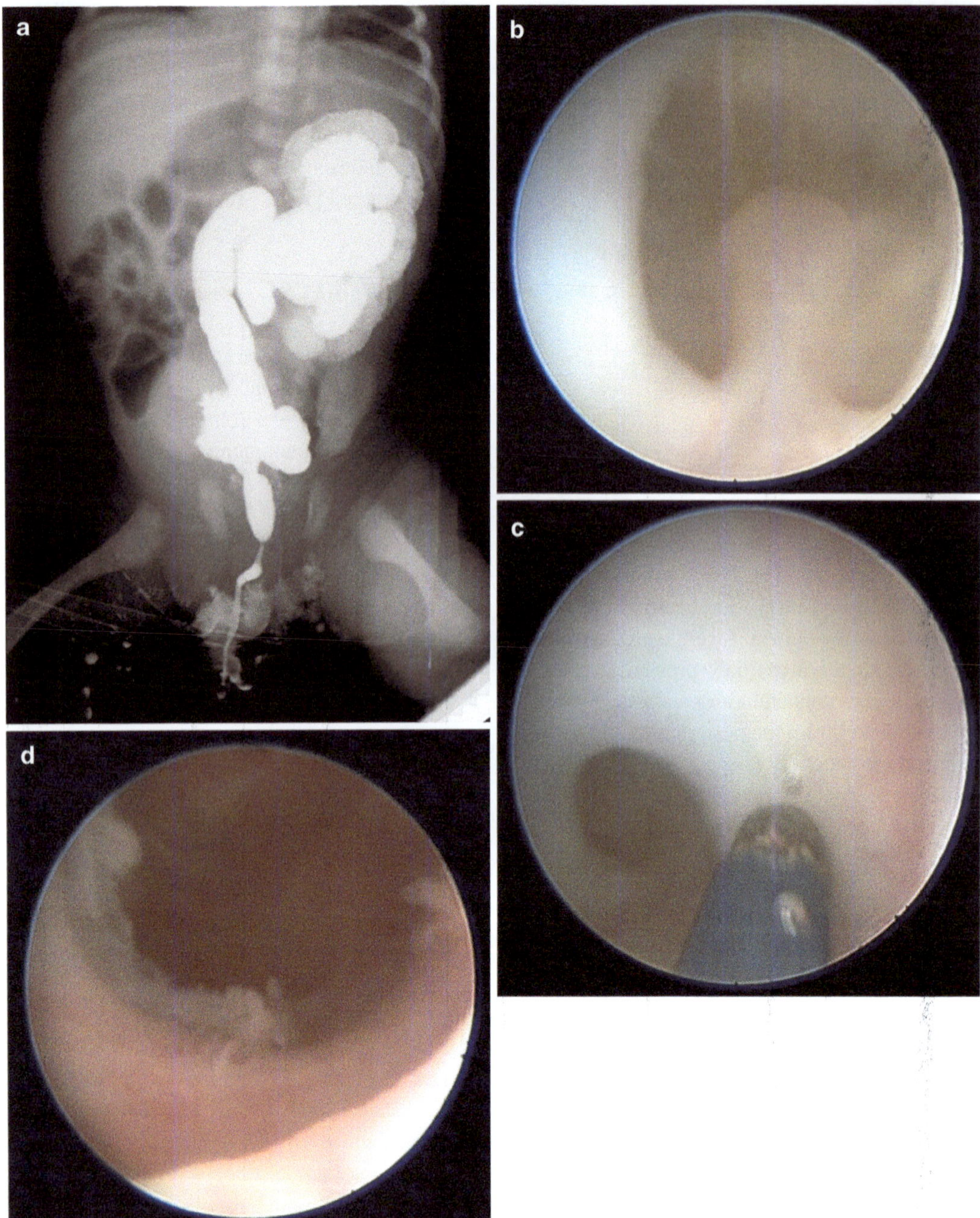

Fig. 5.3 Case of a boy with posterior urethral valves. (**a**) Cystogram (**b**) cystoscopic view of the valves (**c**) valves' ablation with Bugbee electrode (**d**) cystoscopic "second look"

toscope, Crede maneuver is performed to create an anterograde flow and opening the flaps. The valves can be treated with coagulating Bugbee electrode or resectoscope hooks or cold knife (Fig. 5.3) [1, 3, 8]. Incision is considered less aggressive than fulguration, but in expert hands both techniques are feasible.

In small preterm infants with severe obstructive pathology, the urethra may be too small to accept an endoscope. This problem can be solved performing an anterograde ablation via percutaneous cystotomy.

5.5.3 Anterior Urethral Valves

Anterior urethral valves are visible as a fenestrated diaphragm or a mucosal cusp arising from the ventral wall of the penile urethra (30 %), penoscrotal junction (30 %), and bulbar urethra (40 %) (Fig. 5.4) and associated to a urethral diverticulum [1, 3].

5.5.4 Trabeculation

Trabeculation appears as hypertrophic muscular bands under the vesical mucosa (Fig. 5.5). In these cases, obstructive pathologies, neurogenic causes, or voiding disorders must be searched.

5.5.5 Strictures

Urethral strictures in children may be congenital, but more often are acquired or iatrogenic. The most common causes are catheterization, trauma, hypospadias repair, and fulguration of posterior

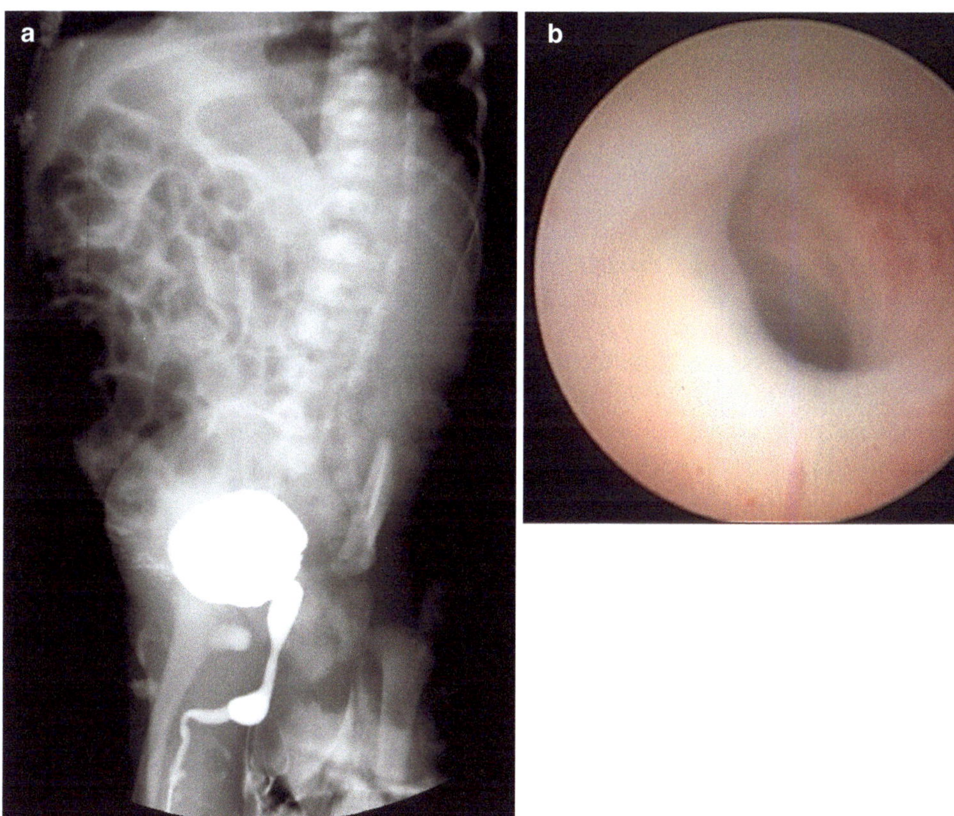

Fig. 5.4 Anterior urethral valves. (**a**) Cystogram showing urethral dilatation proximally to the valves (**b**) cystoscopic view of the valves

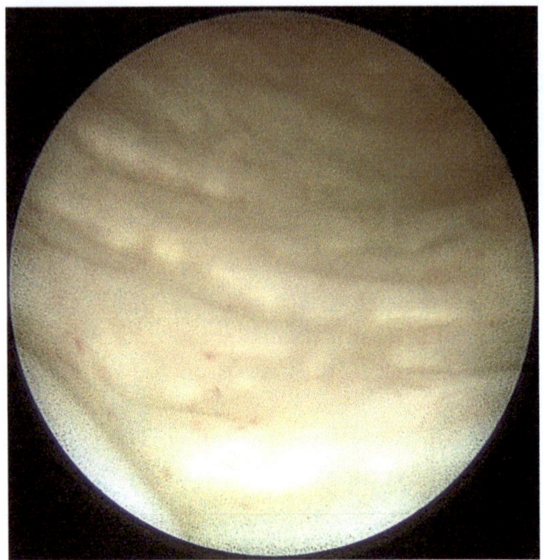

Fig. 5.5 Trabeculation. Hypertrophic muscular bands are visible under the mucosa

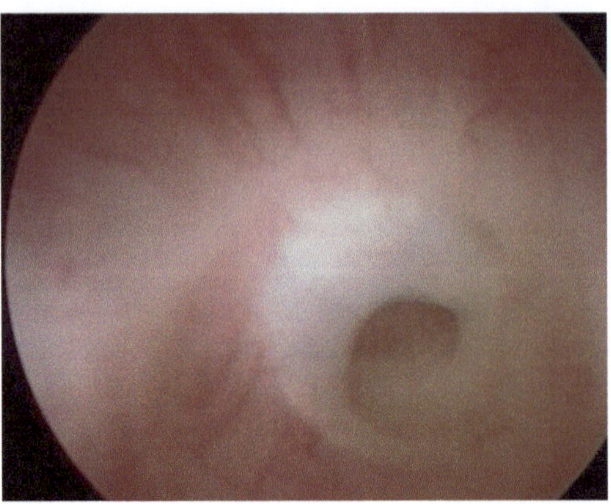

Fig. 5.6 Case of a boy with urethral stenosis after proximal hypospadia repair

urethral valves (Fig. 5.6). Endoscopic treatment consists of incision using a cold or hot knife, but recurrences are frequent especially in long strictures so open repair is often necessary.

5.5.6 Masses

Malignancies of the lower urinary tract are not frequent in children. The most frequent malignant tumor noted at this level is the rhabdomyosarcoma of the bladder. Cystoscopy can be used to evaluate the extension of the tumor and to obtain biopsies to confirm diagnosis.

Urethral polyps can also be noted in children. They often arise from the posterior wall of the urethra and are more frequent in males. Urethral polyps are universally benign, and endoscopic resection is curative [3].

5.5.7 Calculi

Bladder calculi are rare in children and often related to congenital malformation, neurologic bladder, or bladder reconstruction with pouches made of bowel. Once a stone is identified, it can be seized or broken and then removed with the aid of forceps. Catheters and/or baskets can be used to remove the ureteral stones (Fig. 5.7). Electrohydraulic lithotripsy or ultrasonic probes can also be performed to obtain stone fragmentation.

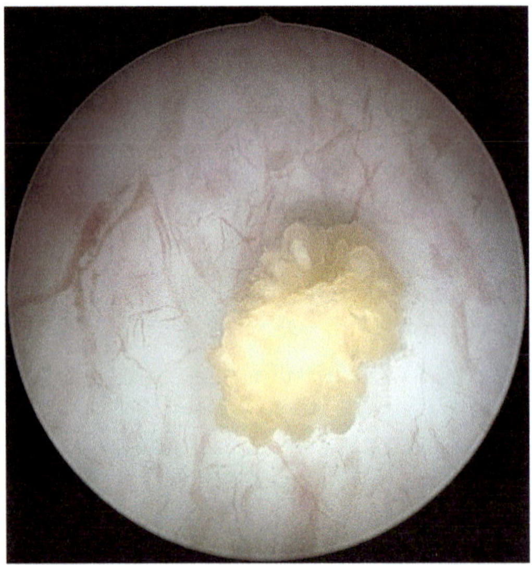

Fig. 5.7 Calculi

5.5.8 Ureterocele, Urinary Tract Duplication, and Ureteral Ectopia

Ureterocele is more frequently noted in a duplicated urinary system, but can also be present in a single urinary system. Cystoscopy can differentiate intravesical (orthotopic) ureterocele from the extravesical (ectopic) one. Ureterocele appears as a bulging structure, more visible with bladder slightly filled; in fact when the intravesical pressure grows, the ureterocele is compressed and became less visible. In the intravesical ureterocele, the meatus is often difficult to detect because it appears as a thin slit, while in the extravesical one, the meatus is larger and therefore more visible.

Incision is now considered the first approach in the treatment of the ureterocele. The incision or puncture should be performed as low as possible within the bladder neck (Fig. 5.8) [3, 9, 10]. In ectopic ureterocele, the urethral portion must be incised longitudinally to prevent urethral obstruction [11].

Puncture of the intravesical ureterocele is associated with high success rates, with minimal need for further procedures or surgery. In ectopic ureterocele, endoscopic treatment is less effective with a greater need for later curative surgery.

Ureteral ectopia must be searched carefully during urethral examination. Once identified ectopic meatus, its catheterization is considered useful for further reconstruction.

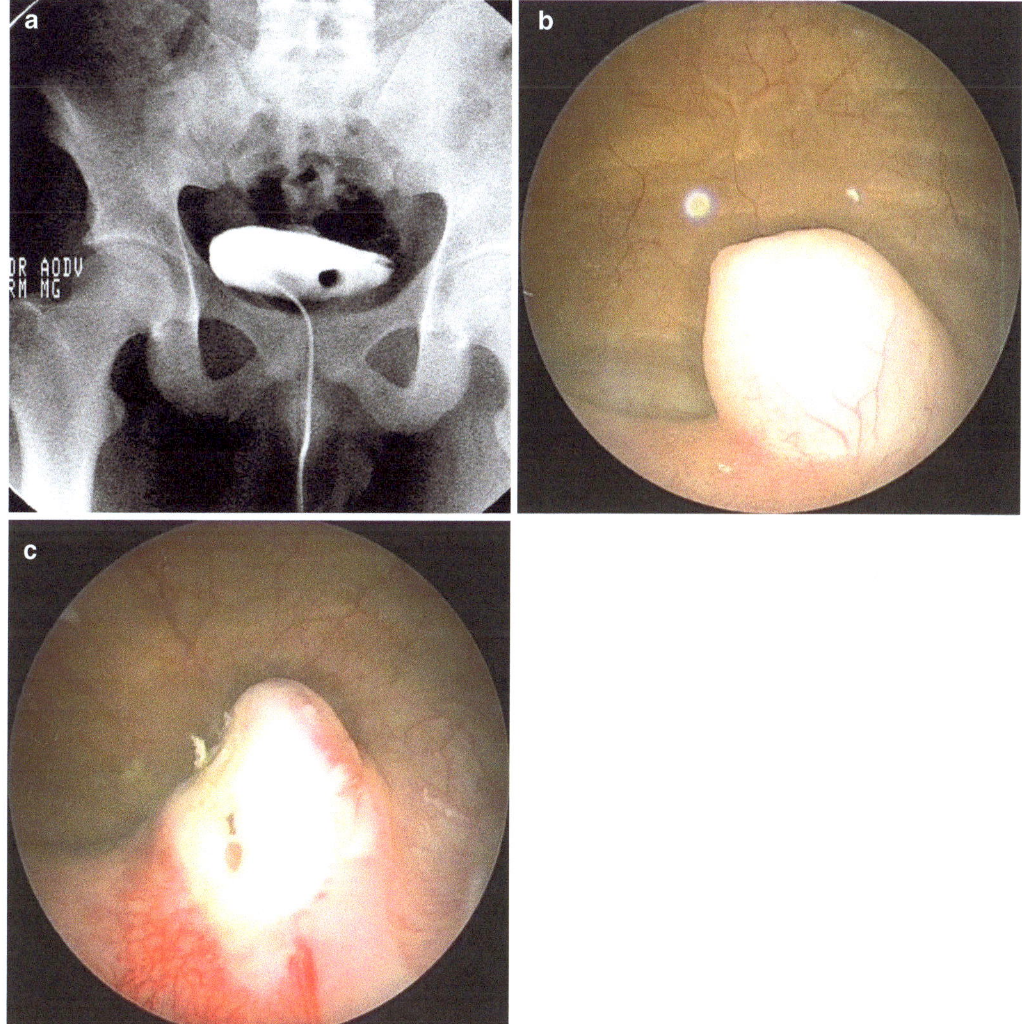

Fig. 5.8 Ureterocele can be seen with bladder slightly filled and can be opened with Bugbee electrode. (**a**) Cystogram showing the ureterocele as a filling defect; (**b**) cystoscopic view; (**c**) opened ureterocele

5.5.9 Vesicoureteral Reflux

Cystoscopy allows the direct view of ureterovesical junction (UVJ). Ureteral meatus can be identified at lateral edges of the trigone. Endoscopic data consist of the evaluation of meatal position and shape and of the length of the submucosal ureter. For several years, Lyon and colleagues' classification [12] regarding meatal shape (classified as normal or cone shaped, stadium shaped, horseshoe shaped, or golf hole shaped) has been considered a predicting factor for the reflux degree. Despite these assessments, a certain correlation between the anatomical aspect and the degree of malformation or prognosis does not exist [13]. On the contrary, meatal position (distinguished in normal, lateral, or ectopic) seems to be much more useful in the evaluation of reflux. In fact if a urethral meatus is located in ectopic position, probably the UVJ will be altered, the submucosal ureteral length will be shorter, and more easily the ureter will be refluxing. Submucosal ureteral length can be defined with the aid of a catheter. The limit of these classifications is the subjective evaluation even if comparison with the contralateral meatus can reduce subjectivity. Cystoscopy remains valid immediately before surgery to evaluate the UVJ and to rule out other diseases [3, 14].

Endoscopic approach can constitute a therapeutic option. The injection of biocompatible materials has been shown to be effective in the correction of reflux (Fig. 5.9). Teflon has been

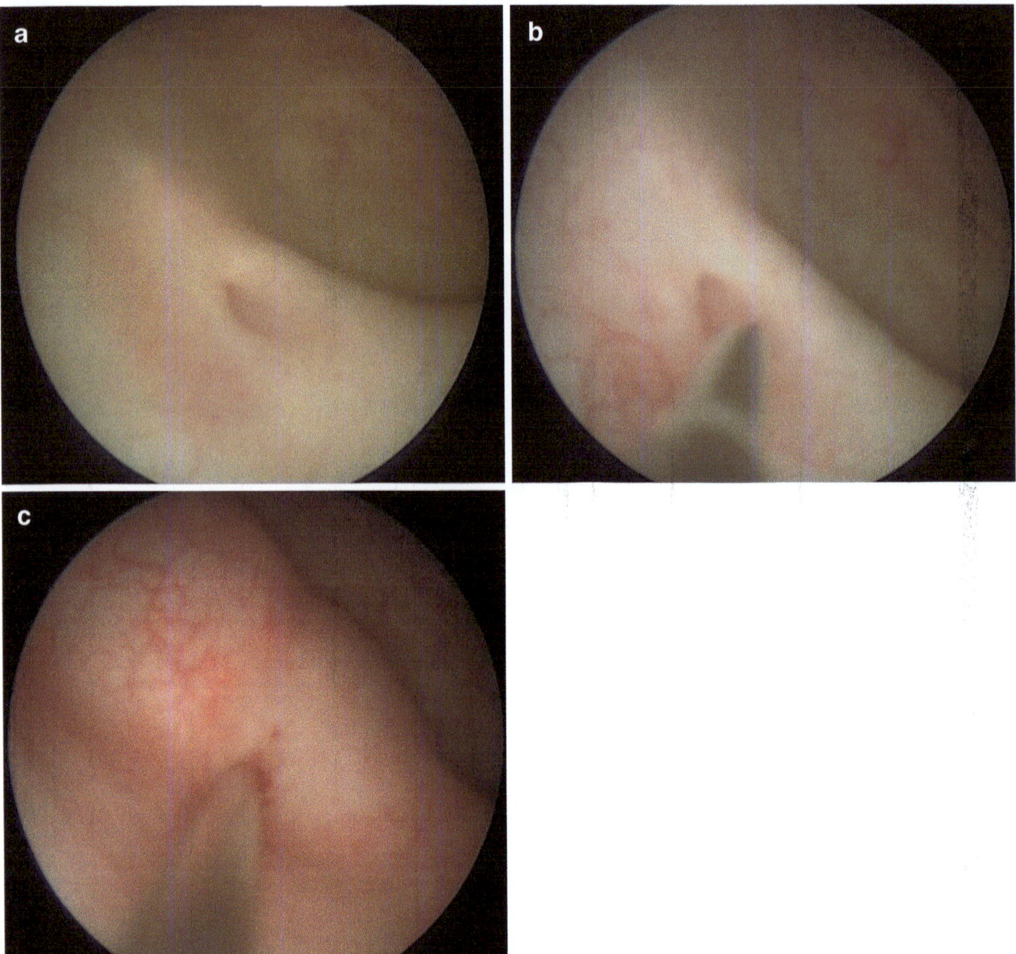

Fig. 5.9 (**a**) Refluxing meatus (**b**) submeatal injection of dextranomer (**c**) urethral meatus after injection

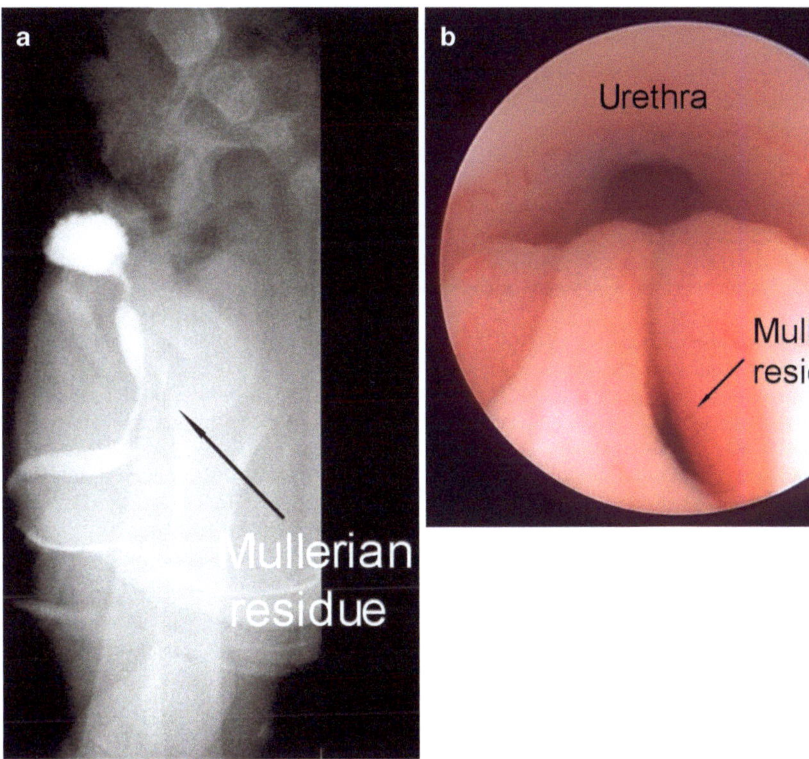

Fig. 5.10 (**a**) Cystogram reveals the presence of a müllerian remnant in a 1-year-old boy with ambiguous genitalia (**b**) cystoscopy shows the aditus of the residue

used for many years, but further studies revealed a long-term migration potential, so other materials have been proved. Bovine cross-linked collagen has been used, thanks to a greater compatibility, but its absorption often requires several procedures for a complete correction of the reflux. In the last years, dextranomer hyaluronidase has been approved for the management of VUR, and many institutes reported a high rate of success.

5.5.10 Ambiguous Genitalia

Endoscopic evaluation of ambiguous genitalia can guide the reconstruction planning. In females affected by congenital adrenal hyperplasia, cystoscopy is used to measure the length of the urogenital sinus. Vaginal orifice is not easily identifiable, but the water flow helps in vaginal distension making it visible. Vaginal catheterization is useful to guide the reconstructive procedures.

In proximal hypospadias, cystoscopy may visualize a Müllerian residue (Fig. 5.10).

5.6 Complications

Complications after cystoscopy are rare and include hemorrhage, dysuria, urethral trauma, and perforation. In particular the last complication is possible after complex reconstruction because of reduced compliance of the bladder.

References

1. Baker LA (2007) General principles of cystourethroscopy: Ch 11. In: Godbole PP (ed) Pediatric endourology techniques. Springer, London, pp 67–76
2. Carter HB, Chan DY (2007) Basic Instrumentation and Cystoscopy: Ch 6. In: Wein AJ (ed) Campbell-Walsh urology, 9th edn. Saunders Elsevier, Philadelphia
3. Mathews R (2010) Endoscopy of the lower urinary tract: Ch 6. In: Gearhart JP, Rink RC, Mouriquand

PDE (eds) Pediatric urology, 2nd edn. Saunders Elsevier, Philadelphia, pp 84–91
4. Gagnadoux MF (2012) Evaluation of microscopic hematuria in children. In: Niaudet P, Kim MS (eds) Wolters Kluwer Health. http://www.uptodate.com/contents/evaluation-of-microscopic-hematuria-in-children. Last updated 20 July 2012
5. Gagnadoux MF (2012) Evaluation of gross hematuria in children. In: Niaudet P, Kim MS (eds) Wolters Kluwer Health. http://www.uptodate.com/contents/evaluation-of-gross-hematuria-in-children. Last updated 20 July 2012
6. Efros MD, Ahmed T, Coombe N, Choudhury MS (1994) Urologic complications of high-dose chemotherapy and bone marrow transplantation. Urology 43:355–360
7. Holmes N (2013) Management of posterior urethral valves. In: Baskin LS, Kim MS (eds) Wolters Kluwer Health. http://www.uptodate.com/contents/management-of-posterior-urethral-valves. Last updated 25 Mar 2013
8. Diamond DA, Retik AB (2002) Endoscopic surgery of urethral valves and ureterocele: Ch 5. In: Frak JD, Gearhart JP, Snyder HM (eds) Operative pediatric urology, 2nd edn. Churchill, Livingstone
9. Monfort G, Morisson-Lacombe G, Coquet M (1985) Endoscopic treatment of ureteroceles revisited. J Urol 133:1031–1033
10. Rich MA, Keating MA, Snyder HM 3rd, Duckett JW (1990) Low transurethral incision of single system intravesical ureteroceles in children. J Urol 144:120–121
11. Coplen DE, Duckett JW (1995) The modern approach to ureteroceles. J Urol 153:166–171
12. Lyon RP, Marshall S, Tanagho EZ (1969) The ureteral orifice: its configuration and competency. J Urol 102(4):504–9
13. Duckett JW, Bellinger MF (1982) A plea for standardized grading of vesicoureteral reflux. Eur Urol 8:74–77
14. Messina P, De castro R, Appignani A (1986) Ruolo dell'endoscopia: Ch 13. In: De Castro R (ed) Chirurgia del reflusso vescico ureterale in età pediatrica. Monduzzi Editore, Bologna, pp 191–200

Laparoscopic and Retroperitoneoscopic Pediatric Urology

6

Francesca Destro and Mario Lima

6.1 Introduction

Minimally invasive surgery (MIS) in pediatric urology has gained a great interest in the past few years. Early uses of laparoscopy had diagnostic purposes and were related to the management of non-palpable testes (1970s). MIS is now used for more complex and challenging procedures, and it accounts for 10–15 % of all pediatric laparoscopic surgeries performed by urologists [1–6]. The evolution of pediatric MIS is the result of recent advances in camera technology and instrumentation and of the recognition of its safety. The benefits of laparoscopic surgery include reduced postoperative pain and hospital stay, quicker recovery, reduced complication rate, and excellent cosmetic results. MIS achieves good outcomes and high acceptance between parents despite the fact that there are still controversies [1–6].

Pediatric MIS is influenced by the unique features of pediatric patients. The relatively smaller size can be an advantage as it permits the access to both the upper and the lower urinary tract. However it makes the use of standard instrumentation and movements difficult. Technical problems of working in a relatively small space and high complication rate were common findings when laparoscopy was first introduced [7, 8]. It was immediately clear that techniques used in adults were not always applicable to small children. For instance, the use of a Veress needle to establish pneumoperitoneum (blind insertion of a Veress needle in the abdomen) may lead to extraperitoenal insufflation, surgical emphysema, and iatrogenic injuries. The open Hasson technique was introduced in children to limit organ damage, and it is the preferred method to access the abdomen and to obtain the pneumoperitoneum. To perform an open access, the skin is carved at the level of the umbilicus (supraumbilical, subumbilical, or tranumbilical incision), and the subcutaneous tissue is opened using electrocauterization. The underling linea alba is smashed with a blunt grasper that reaches the peritoneal cavity. The Hasson cannula is inserted after obtaining enough space. The cannula is then secured to the skin, or, in case of pneumathic anchorage trocars, the balloon is inflated to secure the trocar to the abdominal wall. The pneumoperitoneum is then created, and the trocars are inserted. All the instruments are placed under direct vision reducing the risk of damage. Gas inflation is performed with 0.5 L/min of flow in infants. It is completed in 30–60 s in small children (2–4 years) with 300 mL of gas. A 12–14-year-old boy requires 5 L to obtain full abdominal distension.

The other peculiar element of pediatric urology is that there is a wide spectrum of diseases and ages (from neonatal age to adolescence), and

F. Destro • M. Lima (✉)
Department of Pediatric Surgery,
S. Orsola-Malpighi University Hospital,
Via Massarenti 11, Bologna 40138, Italy
e-mail: francesca_destro@hotmail.com;
mario.lima@unibo.it

M. Lima, G. Manzoni (eds.), *Pediatric Urology: Contemporary Strategies from Fetal Life to Adolescence*,
DOI 10.1007/978-88-470-5693-0_6, © Springer-Verlag Italia 2015

Table 6.1 Indications for urological MIS

Upper urinary tract procedure	Nephrectomy
	Eminephrectomy
	Pyeloplasty
	Renal cyst excision/marsupialization
	Ureteroureterostomy–pyeloureterostomy
	Adrenalectomy
Lower urinary tract procedure	Uretral reimplantation
	Continent catheterizable channel
	Bladder augmentation
	Disorders of sex development
	Müllerian remnants
	Ovarian disorders

the urologist should be ready to adapt to different situations.

The main indications for MIS in children are shown in (Table 6.1).

Contraindications include the presence of coagulophaties, severe organ impairment (cardiological or respiratory disorders), and sepsis. The use of MIS for malignant diseases is still a matter of debate. Nephrectomy for Wilms' tumor requires open surgery (that allows the inspection of the entire abdomen and contralateral kidney, facilitates lymphnode sampling, and reduces the risk of spillage), while adrenal tumors may be approached laparoscopically. An exception is represented by patients with shrank Wilms' tumor after chemotherapy (<10 % of the patients' height). Investigations into the applicability of laparoscopy for malignancies have begun but require expansion in the future.

Once MIS has been identified as the technique of choice, the main problem is the choice of the most comfortable way to reach the affected urinary tract.

The *laparoscopic transperitoneal approach* is easier for surgeons who are at the beginning of their experience. It permits to approach the upper (the kidney is reached after the detachment of the colic angle and the opening of the Todd's fascia) and the lower urinary tract, as well as the testis and the spermatic vessels.

The alternative is the *retroperitoneoscopy* that permits the access to the retroperitoneal space without opening the peritoneum. One main problem is that the access to the bladder or the ureterovescical junction may be difficult in older children. The patient lies on the healthy flank (lateral decubitus position), and the incision (15 mm skin incision) is performed on the posterior axillary line at half distance between the last rib and the upper anterior iliac spine. Two important marker points are the superior part of the psoas and the lower renal pole that move with respiratory acts. The dissection should be performed near the psoas muscle in order to avoid peritoneal perforations and the passage of CO_2 in the abdomen. A 10 mm trocar for the 0° lens is inserted when the renal lower pole appears. Insufflation starts with 8–15 mmHg of pressure. The working chamber is obtained with the tip of the lens or with an endoscopic peanut. Two operative trocars are usually sufficient to complete the procedure. The trocars (5 or 3 mm) are inserted under direct vision when the posterior face of the kidney is freed. One is placed in the costo-spinal angle; the other one is placed just over the iliac crest. The third trocar is inserted if necessary only when there is adequate space. This is useful to retract the kidney up.

In recent years *robot-assisted laparoscopic surgery* (RALS) has been gaining acceptance. The technique permits a 3-dimensional vision and wide range of movements (6° of freedom) that are more precise than those of laparoscopy and lack tremors. For these reasons RALS can be used in case of complex reconstructive procedures. The problem with this new technology is that there is not an established set of criteria for adequate and standardized training, and instruments are still too big for children.

6.2 Anesthesiological Considerations

An optimal approach to the planning of anesthesia for laparoscopy depends on a knowledge of the technical requirements and an understanding of the physiological alterations associated with the procedure.

Physiologic changes during laparoscopic surgery are related to the changes associated with the increased abdominal pressure (IAP) associated with the inflation of the abdomen, the patient's postural modifications (head up or head down), the CO_2 absorption, and its general effects [9]. The magnitude of the physiologic perturbations associated with laparoscopy is influenced by the patient's age, the patient's underlying myocardial and respiratory function, and the administered anesthetic drugs.

The airways and cardiovascular system of a child have characteristics that differ from those of an adult: the former have less functional residual capacity (FRC), collapse volume is much closer to FRC, and both lung compliance and airway resistance are adversely related to lung size. Infants and young children have fewer alveoli than adults do. The number increases during childhood, from approximately 20 million after birth to 300 million by 8 years of age. Therefore, infants and young children have a relatively small area for gas exchange. The alveolus is small. Alveolar size increases from 150–180 to 250–300 μm during childhood. The infant's systemic vascular resistance is lower; heart rate plays a more important role in determining cardiac output, and there is a high metabolism and O_2 consumption [10–12].

Tension pneumoperitoneum causes an elevation in IAP which produces important effects on cardiovascular, pulmonary, renal, and metabolic function.

6.3 Upper Urinary Tract Procedures

They include nephrectomy, eminephrectomy, pyeloplasty, renal cyst excision/marsupialization, ureteroureterostomy–pyeloureterostomy, and adrenalectomy. Trocar position is usually the same for all surgeries performed at the level of the kidneys. In case of laparoscopic procedures, the placement of the first umbilical trocar should be performed carefully in order to avoid access complications that mostly occur at the umbilicus. The two operative trocars are separated by almost 8–10 cm. This is particularly important in robotic surgery to allow instruments movements.

6.3.1 Nephrectomy

It is the most common urological indication for MIS, and it was first performed in 1991. However laparoscopic nephrectomy is not as spread as in adults. The procedure is indicated in patients affected by benign diseases such as multicystic or dysplastic kidneys (associated with renal hypertension or failure to involute during follow-up), nonfunctioning kidneys (reflux or obstructive urophaty), xanthogranulomatosis, pyelonephritis, protein-losing nephropathy, nephrolitiasis, and nephropathy with severe hypertension. Contraindications include malignant tumors, previous intra-abdominal–retroperitoneal surgery, obesity (high kidneys), coagulopathies, and cardiopulmonary diseases. Hamilton et al. showed that laparoscopy compared to open surgery has a shorter hospital stay and less analgesic requirement, and it allows more extensive excision of the low ureteral stump, reducing the incidence of pyoureter and the need of another lower incision [13]. This is particularly true in case of ectopic ureters or vesicoureteral reflux that require complete ureteral stump removal. Laparoscopy also allows a better view of the anatomy thanks to the magnification of the technique, facilitating the dissection. In addition, the technique avoids ischemia related to excessive renal mobilization. Compared to the open nephrectomy, operative times are longer and related to surgeon's experience. According to Ku et colleagues, the nephrectomy can be performed through a retroperitoneal approach with operative times similar to the open approach and with shorter hospital stay [14]. The main advantage of retroperitoneoscopy is the easier access to the kidney and renal hylum (without the need for colonic mobilization), also in the presence of adhesions (related to previous pyelonephritis, hydronephrosis, etc.). Difficulties may be related to cephalad kidneys that make the triangulation between instruments and camera very difficult. The technique has also all the advantages of an extraperitoneal approach (lower risk for postoperative ileus, shoulder pain, omental evisceration, adhesions, urinary, or hematic abdominal collections), and it can be performed also in cases of previous abdominal surgery when the presence of adhesions is suspected. The fact that the peritoneum is left intact permits patients with end-stage renal disease to start dialysis immediately after surgery. The retroperitoneoscopy can be obtained with the posterior and the lateral approach. In the former approach, the patient lies prone with the affected side rotated down at 30–40°. The incision is in the midway between the iliac crest and the tip of the XII rib, lateral to the border of the sacrospinalis muscle. Ports are in the costovertebral angle on the XII rib tip. In the latter approach, the patient lies on the healthy flank. The incision is at the XII rib tip. The posterior approach allows a rapid access to the renal pedicle, while the lateral one necessitates constant traction over the pelvis to expose the vessels. The lateral approach guarantees a wider working chamber on the inferior and medial side (useful in cases of ectopic or horseshoe kidneys) and a better distal ureterectomy in children older than 5 years but a greater risk of tearing the peritoneum. Retroperitoneoscopic nephrectomy is applicable to all age groups with low conversion and complication rate.

The applicability of laparoscopic nephrectomy in infants is still an object of discussion. Infants seem to have higher complication rate, probably because of the narrowing working space or the renal susceptibility to pneumoperitoneum.

The use of robot-assisted nephrectomy is still debated, as it does not seem to have any advantages compared with traditional laparoscopy.

6.3.2 Heminephrectomy [15, 16]

Laparoscopic heminephrectomy has not gained the same popularity of nephrectomy in children, probably because of the difficulties in obtaining complete ureterectomy and high complication rates. Principal indications for heminephrectomy in children include pyeloureteral duplications with dysplastic superior unit for ureterocele, obstructive megaureter, or ectopic ureter; pyeloureteral duplications with dysplastic inferior unit for reflux nephropathy; or inferior pyeloureteral disease hydronephrosis (rare).

Recent upper urinary tract infections may be the cause of adhesions that make the dissection difficult and blood loss excessive.

Retroperitoneal heminephrectomy seems to be the preferable method (Fig. 6.1).

It does not require colon mobilization with reduced risk of organ injury and no risk of postoperative adhesions. It has however the disadvantages of a narrow working chamber and an unusual anatomical situation (the kidney is reached from behind). Laparoscopy guarantees a wider working chamber that makes it easier to perform sutures. The surgeon should choose between the two techniques on the basis of his experience. The first steps of the technique are the same as for nephrectomy. It is important to visualize the entire kidney and both ureters to completely understand the anatomy. It may be useful to place a ureteric catheter in the unaffected moiety to better identify it. Ureters and vessels should be carefully isolated. The vessels of the affected moiety are divided. The renal parenchyma that requires resection changes its color because of hypoperfusion. It can be transected with monopolar or bipolar coagulation. The proximal ureteral stump can be used to expose the anteromedial surface with additional vessels; the distal stump is removed as far as possible. The procedure seems to have 10–14 % of complication rate (especially urinary leakage).

Robotic-assisted laparoscopic heminephrectomy has the advantage of improved visualization reducing the risk of iatrogenic vascular injuries. Both the retroperitoneal and transperitoneal approaches can be performed. The retroperitoneal one reduces the risk of abdominal organ injury, but it is associated with small working spaces. Operative times are still long.

6.3.3 Pyeloplasty [17, 18]

Open Anderson–Hynes pyeloplasty is the technique of choice for the treatment of ureteropelvic junction obstructions (UPJO) in children. It has a success rate of 90–95 %. Alternatives to the classical open pyeloplasty are the laparoscopic pyeloplasty, retroperitoneal pyeloplasty, and robotic pyeloplasty. Some authors have recently proposed a video-assisted approach (OTAP) to overcome technical difficulties related to the narrow working chamber (see Chap. 9).

The use of laparoscopic pyeloplasty in children was described in 1995. Although the procedure requires expert laparoscopic surgeons, it gained acceptance and popularity being feasible and safe in older as well in smaller children and having success rates comparable with those achieved through the open approach. The indications for surgery are symptomatic pyeloureteral junction obstructions, worsening hydronephrosis on serial imaging, anteroposterior (AP) pelvis diameter >20 mm associated with calyceal dilatation, and renal function <40 % or AP pelvis

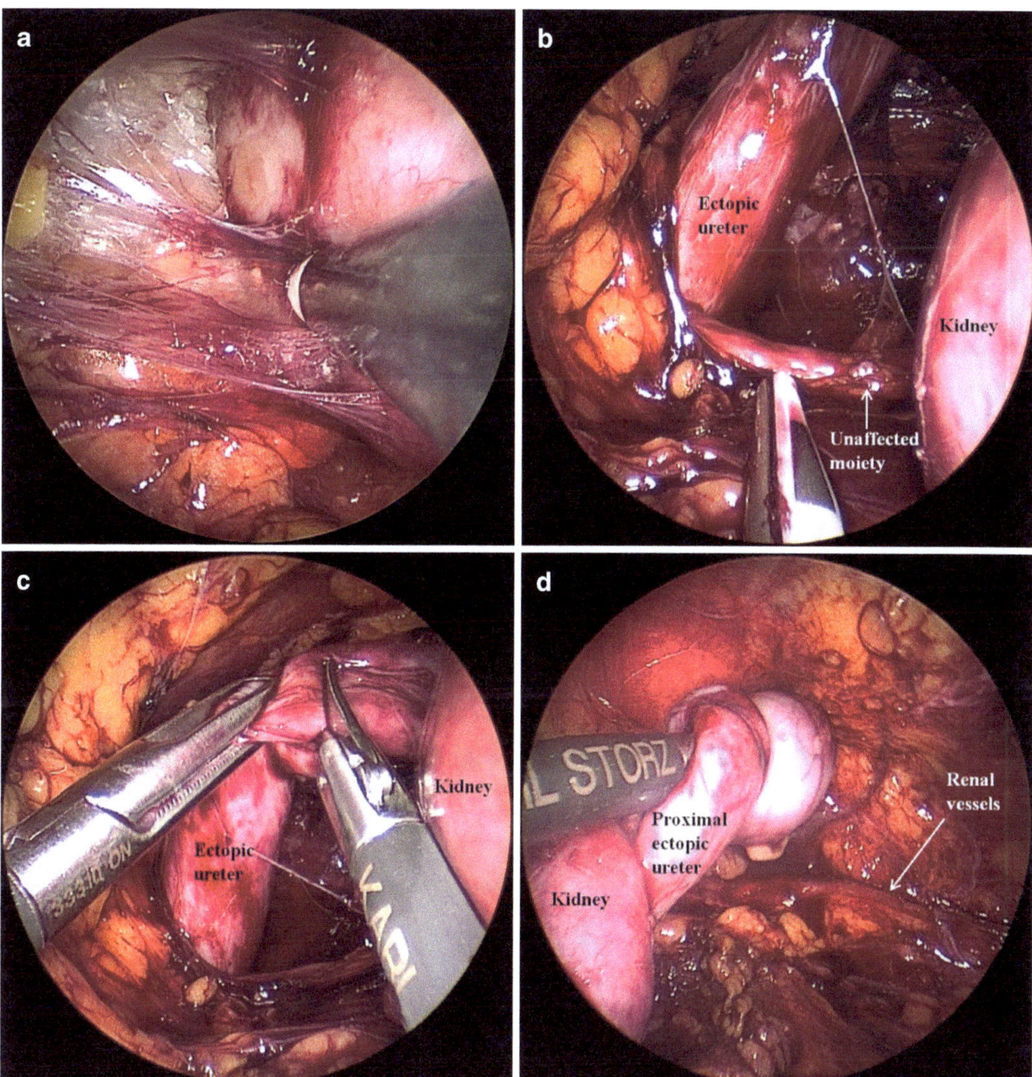

Fig. 6.1 Retroperitoneoscopic partial nephrectomy. An endoscopic peanut is used to expose and isolate the kidney, ureters, and vessels (**a**). The ureters appear at the end of the dissection. The ectopic ureter is huge and tortous. The presence of the endoureteral stent (inserted during previous cystoscopy) helps identifying the unaffected ureter (**b**). The ectopic ureter is dissected and legated as distally as possible (**c**). The cephalad part of the ectopic ureter is grasped and used to expose the renal pelvis and the upper renal pole (**d**). The small nonfunctioning upper renal pole is marked with electrocautery and removed with Ligasure™ (**e**)

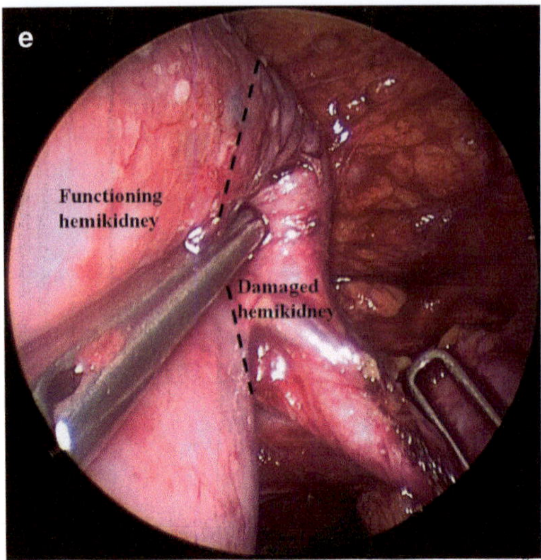

Fig. 6.1 (continued)

diameter >30 mm with calyceal dilatation. Contraindications are small extrarenal pelvis and anatomical variants. The procedure is performed with the patient in a lateral decubitus position. The lens in inserted through the umbilical port, and the two operative trocars are inserted under direct vision (under the costal margin and in the iliac fossa, both in the same side). The pyeloureteral junction is identified by reflecting the colon medially or through a transmesenteric window. Following the ureter may be useful. A suture through the abdominal wall is used as a "hitch stich" to stabilize and expose the renal pelvis. The renal pelvis is then dismembered and trimmed and the upper ureter spatulated. The anastomosis is performed and a transanastomotic ureteric double-J stent is left for a few weeks (4 weeks).

Laparoscopic pyeloplasty has a success rate of 82–100 % according to different series with rare intraoperative complications. Postoperative complications include ileus, urinary tract infections, omental hernia, and urinary extravasation. For these reasons laparoscopic pyeloplasty is becoming the gold standard in the management of PUJ obstruction in children. The main disadvantage is that the procedure is technically challenging, and it requires advanced suture skills (intracorporeal suture). The effect is that operative times are longer although they are trending towards shorter times with experience. As far as positive effects are concerned, it seems that older patients (>10 years) have the main advantages in terms of shorter hospital stay and decreased postoperative pain. The advent of small instruments has permitted the applicability of laparoscopic pyeloplasty also in infants. There is also the possibility to use a single-port system. This system does not reduce the risk of trocar insertion (bowel injury, bleeding, and hernias) that is due to the insertion of the first trocar.

The laparoscopic and retroperitoneal approaches have comparable results in terms of success rates, hospital stays, and narcotic requirements. Small workspace in retroperitoneoscopy may be the cause of failed pyeloplasty and makes the suture even harder leading to conversions.

The stead learning curve of intracorporeal suture has been overcome after the introduction of robotic-assisted laparscopic pyeloplasty (RALP). Unfortunately it is unclear whether RALP provides any advantage as it does not always decrease overall operative time, it lacks tactile feedback, and it is expensive. According to recent reports it reduces hospital stay and narcotic analgesic requirements.

When UPJO is due to crossing vessels (6–10 % of all cases with increasing incidence in older children), the vessels are usually transposed posterior to the anastomosis. Sometimes the vessels are the sole cause of obstruction and there is not intrinsic obstruction; it is thus sufficient to transpose the vessels without performing a pyeloplasty. This can be achieved through laparoscopic vascular hitch, as suggested by Cherian and Nemade [19].

6.3.4 Adrenalectomy [20]

Laparoscopic and retroperitoneoscopic adrenalectomy give various advantages over conventional open surgery. They have evolved into feasible and reproducible techniques since the first laparoscopic adrenalectomy in 1992. The techniques are associated with excellent hemodynamic stability and complete excision.

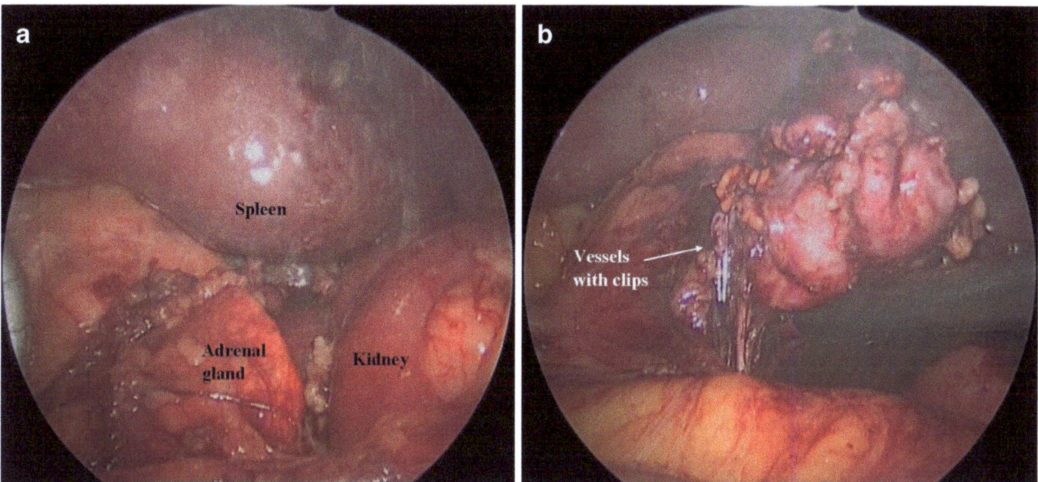

Fig. 6.2 Transperitoneal left adrenalectomy for adenoma. The adrenal gland is identified and isolated (**a**). The gland is then removed after vessel closure with endoclips (**b**)

Adrenalectomy indications include pheochromocytoma, adrenal adenoma, ACTH (adrenocorticotrophic hormone-dependent Cushing's syndrome), and neuroblastoma. The main contraindication is the tumor size. In case of adrenal masses larger than 6 cm, the open approach is preferable. Prior to surgery it is important to define the anatomy and the features of the mass (solid or cystic) with abdominal US or CT. Preoperative workup also includes the evaluations of adrenal vein and inferior vena cava looking for intravascular dissemination. Antihypertensive treatment is administrated in cases of pheochromocytoma.

The transperitoneal approach (Fig. 6.2) is more used than the retroperitoneal one, but the retroperitoneal approach provides direct access to the adrenal gland and easy visualization of the adrenal vein. However the access to the hylum may be difficult because of the kidney rotation and the small working space. During retroperitoneoscopic surgery the patient lies prone and the accesses are placed in the same way as for retroperitoneoscopic nephrectomy. The dissection starts over the kidney and does not involve lateral and inferior attachments that anchor the kidney and expose the upper pole. The adrenal gland appears at the superior medial border of the kidney. Adrenal vessels are identified and divided (first the artery and then the vein).

The vena cava on the right side acts as a landmark, but it may increase the risk of bleeding, in association with the short right adrenal vein that enters directly into the vena cava. Once it has been fully mobilized, the adrenal gland is removed through an Endobag.

6.4 Lower Urinary Tract Procedures

Lower tract procedures include ureteric reimplantation, creation of continent catheterizable channels, bladder augmentation, and others involved in disorders of sex development and of genitalia. All laparoscopic procedure use similar trocar placement: the lens in the umbilicus and two operative trocars at the midclavicular line bilaterally.

6.4.1 Antireflux Procedures [21, 22]

Traditionally open Cohen ureteral reimplantation is the treatment of choice for vesicoureteral reflux, with success rate around 98 %. Minimally invasive alternative approaches are the endoscopic subureteral injection of dextranomer/hyaluronic acid, the laparoscopic Lich–Gregoir extravesical reimplantation, and the laparoscopic intravesical route.

Endoscopic approaches have the disadvantages of requiring more injections.

The Lich–Gregoir technique does not require cystostomy because the antireflux mechanism is obtained tunneling the ureters extravesically. It is performed with three working ports in triangulation. A cystoscopy evaluates ureteral orifice location and determines whether there is enough tissue for extravesical detrusorraphy. The procedure starts with ureter identification and proximal isolation. In males it is important to incise the peritoneum caudal to the vas to avoid injuries. With the bladder distended, the tunnel was created with scissors and electrocautery, and it was closed over the ureter. The technique may be challenging in small children (<4 years), and it may cause voiding dysfunctions for pelvic plexus damage.

The alternative is the transvesical ureteral reimplantation that has been described with good results (Fig. 6.3).

The bladder is drained, inflated with carbon dioxide, and anchored to the abdominal wall. The camera port is inserted under cystoscopic vision as operative trocars. The procedure is then performed in the same way as the Cohen open technique. This approach is associated with improved cosmesis, less postoperative bladder spasm, and shorter hospital stay, but it is technically demanding as it involves suturing in a small cavity. Its overall success rate is 90 %.

Robotic assistance may be of benefits, but its application is still limited by working space.

6.4.2 Continent Catheterizable Channels (Mitrofanoff) [23]

Bladder dysfunctions may produce inefficient bladder emptying with subsequent damage of renal function. Patients with bladder dysfunctions may benefit clean intermittent catheterization (CIC) via the urethra. However some of them do not tolerate the maneuver. An alternative is the use of the appendix to create a connection between the abdominal wall and the bladder for catheter insertion. Continence is obtained with an intramural tunnel in the bladder wall. The effect is a successful method of continent catheterization.

The procedure has recently been proposed via MIS (laparoscopic procedures and robotics) resulting in reduced postoperative pain, shorter hospital stay, and improved cosmesis. In addition laparoscopy permits the access to the pelvis, peritoneum, and retroperitoneum through the same small incisions. One of the advantages is the possibility to combine multiple procedures (e.g., laparoscopic nephrectomy and ureterostomy as catheterizable channel).

6.4.3 Bladder Augmentation [2, 6]

Bladder augmentation is a procedure that aims at improving bladder capacity in patients with neurogenic bladder when conservative treatment fails. It is a challenging and rare procedure performed via traditional open surgery. It is often associated to other procedures to achieve social continence (e.g., bladder neck reconstruction or urethral sling). In this case laparoscopy has not been widely adopted, especially in pediatric age. The procedure requires very skilled surgeons with suturing ability.

On the other hand, robotic-assisted surgery has evolved, and it seems to be effective and feasible in small spaces.

6.4.4 Disorders of Sex Development [24]

Disorders of sex development (DSD) include a group of congenital conditions with atypical development of chromosomal, gonadal, or anatomic sex. The role of the pediatric surgeon in the management of these patients is part of a multidisciplinary team. Laparoscopy is a safe and reliable diagnostic method even if it requires a general anesthetic. It permits the direct and excellent visualization of the pelvic structures (uterus,

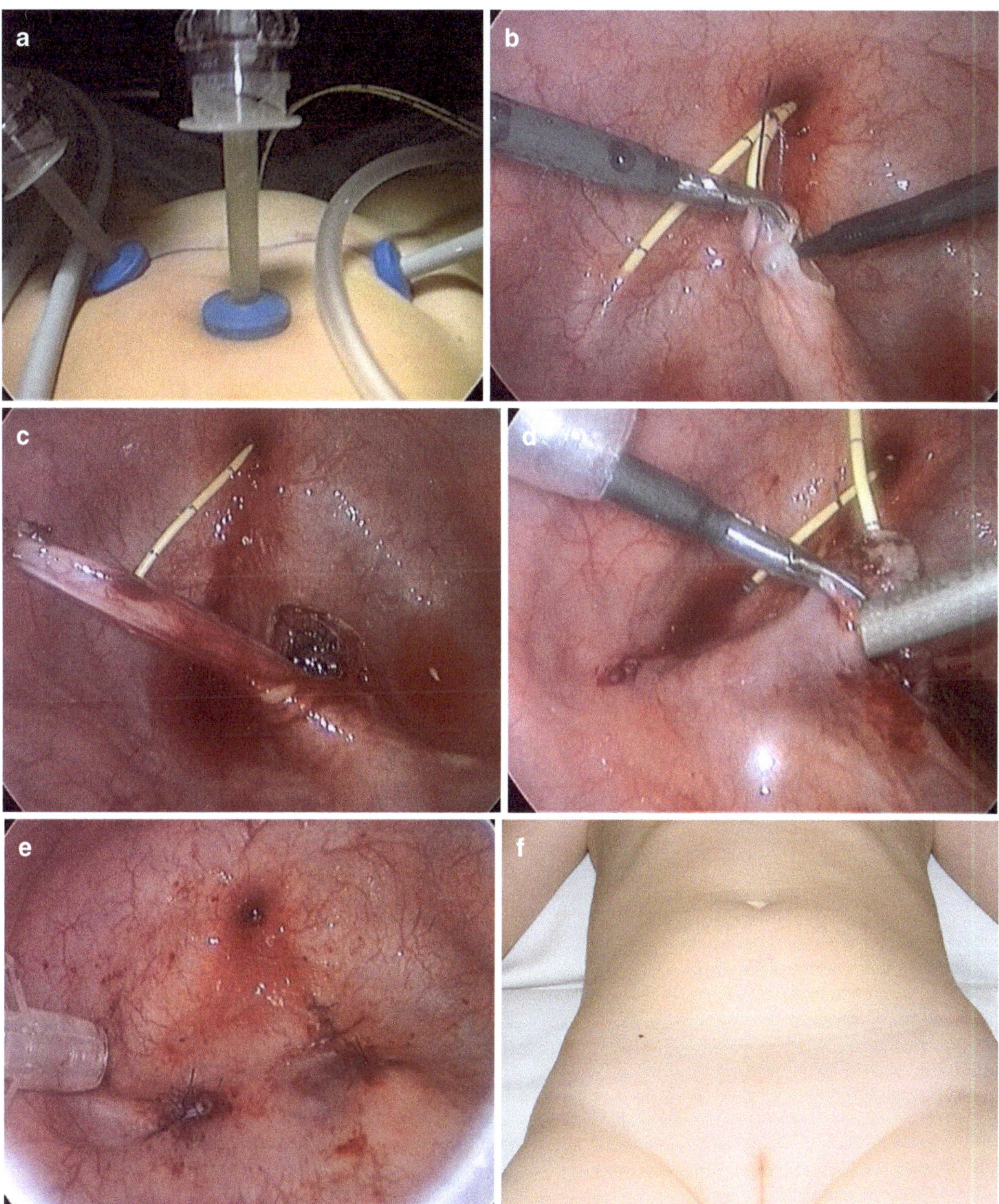

Fig. 6.3 Three trocars (**a**) are inserted in the bladder under direct vision (one for the lens and two for instruments). The affected ureter is isolated (**b**, **c**). After the creation of a submucosal tunnel, (**d**) the ureter is reimplanted in the bladder (**e**). Esthetical result is excellent (**f**)

müllerian duct remnants, gonads, and vasa deferentia) in infants and children contributing to the definition of the diagnosis. Diagnostic laparoscopy should be the investigation of choice in patients with complex DSD, it permits gonadal biopsies, and it is also a treatment procedure (removal of dysgenetic gonads, reconstruction of the external genitalia, timely gonadectomy, orchiopexy, etc.) (Figs. 6.4 and 6.5). Laparoscopy facilitates many procedures that are challenging with open surgery, such as the access to the male pelvis (too depth).

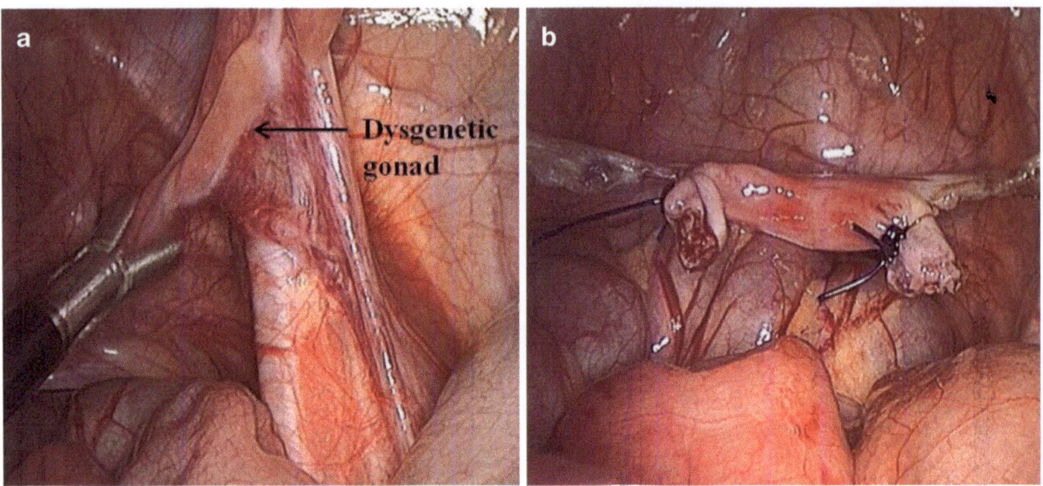

Fig. 6.4 Mixed gonadal dysgenesy with mosaicism 45 XO/46XY, SRY pos. The dysgenetic gonad is identified (**a**) and removed (**b**)

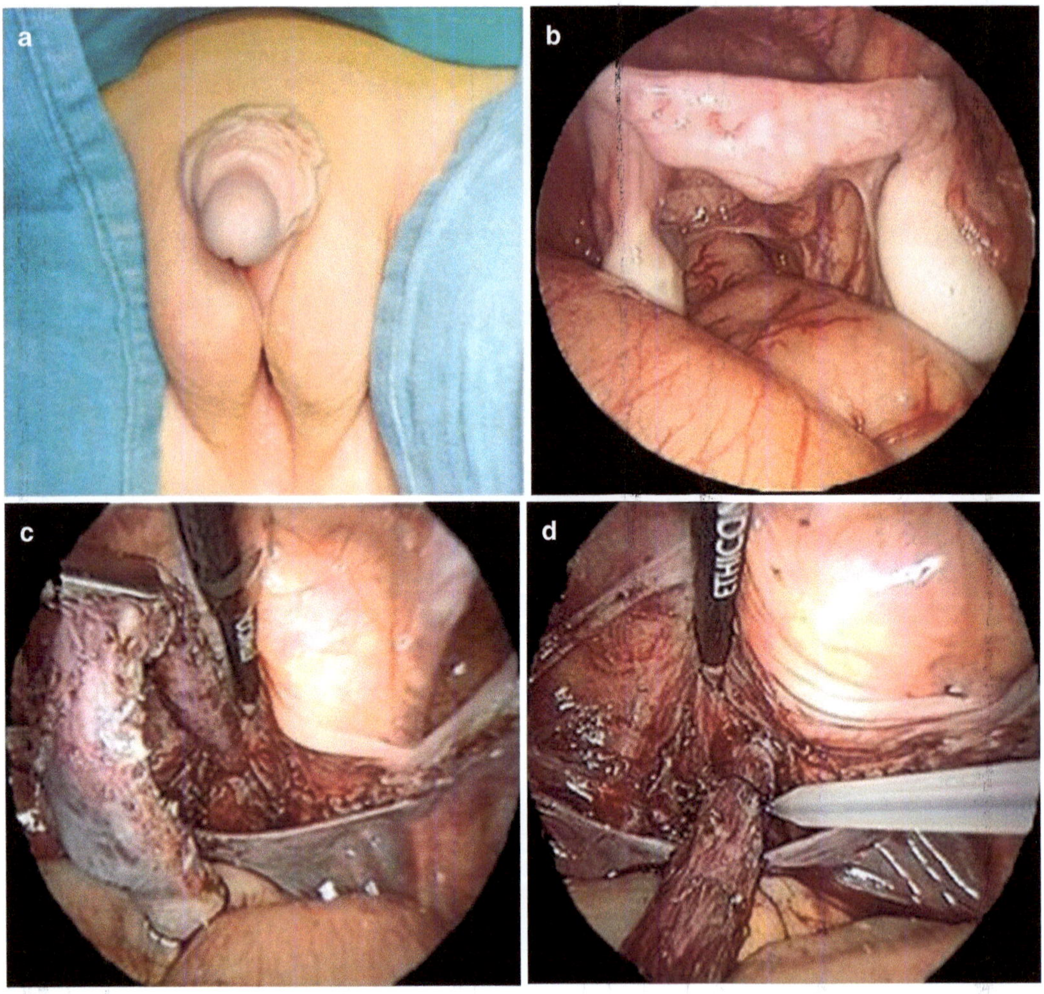

Fig. 6.5 Laparoscopic removal of a müllerian remnant in a patient with scrotal hypospadia. External genitalia (**a**). Laparoscopic identification of the müllerian remnant that looks like the uterus (**b**). Isolation of the remnant with an endo-peanut (**c**). Legation (**d**) and subsequent removal of the remnant

References

1. da Cruz JA, Passerotti CC (2010) Reconstructive laparoscopy in pediatric urology. Curr Opin Urol 20(4):330–335
2. Mushtaq I (2008) Laparoscopic paediatric urology. In: Thomas DFM, Duffy PG, Rickwood AMK (eds) Essentials of paediatric urology. Informa Healthcare, London, pp 317–329
3. Traxel EJ, Minevich EA, Noh PH (2010) A review: the application of minimally invasive surgery to pediatric urology: upper urinary tract procedures. Urology 76(1):122–133
4. Traxel EJ, Minevich EA, Noh PH (2010) A review: the application of minimally invasive surgery to pediatric urology: lower urinary tract reconstructive procedures. Urology 76(1):115–120
5. Esposito C, Valla JS, Yeung CK (2004) Current indications for laparoscopy and retroperitoneoscopy in pediatric urology. Surg Endosc 18(11):1559–1564
6. Orvieto MA, Large M, Gundeti MS (2012) Robotic paediatric urology. BJU Int 110(1):2–13
7. Thakre AA, Bailly Y, Sun LW et al (2008) Is smaller workspace a limitation for robot performance in laparoscopy? J Urol 179(3):1138–1142
8. Passerotti CC, Nguyen HT, Retik AB, Peters CA (2008) Patterns and predictors of laparoscopic complications in pediatric urology: the role of ongoing surgical volume and access techniques. J Urol 180(2):681–685
9. Rayman R, Girotti M, Armstrong K et al (1995) Assessing the safety of pediatric laparoscopic surgery. Surg Laparosc Endosc 5:437–443
10. Hamza J (1994) Physiologie périnatale. In: Saint-Maurice C (ed) Manuel d'anesthésie pédiatrique. Ed Pradel, Paris, pp 1–16
11. Motoyama EK, Finder JD (2011) Respiratory physiology in infants and children. In: Smith's: anesthesia for infants and children. Ed. Elsevier Mosby, Philadelphia (PA), pp 22–79
12. Strafford A (2011) Cardiovascular physiology in infants and children. In: Smith's: anesthesia for infants and children. Ed. Elsevier Mosby, Philadelphia (PA), pp 70–108
13. Hamilton BD, Gatti JM, Cartwright PC, Snow BW (2000) Comparison of laparoscopic versus open nephrectomy in the pediatric population. J Urol 163(3):937–939
14. Ku JH, Yeo WG, Choi H, Kim HH (2004) Comparison of retroperitoneal laparoscopic and open nephrectomy for benign renal diseases in children. Urology 63(3):566–570
15. Piaggio L, Franc-Guimond J, Figueroa TE et al (2006) Comparison of laparoscopic and open partial nephrectomy for duplication anomalies in children. J Urol 175(6):2269–2273
16. Chertin B, Ben-Chaim J, Landau EH et al (2007) Pediatric transperitoneal laparoscopic partial nephrectomy: comparison with an age-matched group undergoing open surgery. Pediatr Surg Int 23(12):1233–1236
17. Blanc T, Muller C, Abdoul H et al (2013) Retroperitoneal laparoscopic pyeloplasty in children: long-term outcome and critical analysis of 10-year experience in a teaching center. Eur Urol 63(3):565–572
18. Juliano RV, Mendonça RR, Meyer F et al (2011) Long-term outcome of laparoscopic pyeloplasty: multicentric comparative study of techniques and accesses. J Laparoendosc Adv Surg Tech A 21(5):399–403
19. Cherian A, Nemade H (2013) The 'double hitch' manoeuvre in laparoscopic pyeloplasty – early experience. J Pediatr Urol 9(4):524–526
20. Yankovic F, Undre S, Mushtaq I (2014) Surgical technique: Retroperitoneoscopic approach for adrenal masses in children. J Pediatr Urol. 10(2):400. e1–2.
21. Stanasel I, Atala A, Hemal A (2013) Robotic assisted ureteral reimplantation: current status. Curr Urol Rep 14(1):32–36
22. Lopez M, Varlet F (2010) Laparoscopic extravesical transperitoneal approach following the Lich-Gregoir technique in the treatment of vesicoureteral reflux in children. J Pediatr Surg 45(4):806–810
23. Farrugia MK, Malone PS (2010) Educational article: the Mitrofanoff procedure. J Pediatr Urol 6(4):330–337
24. Wünsch L, Holterhus PM, Wessel L, Hiort O (2012) Patients with disorders of sex development (DSD) at risk of gonadal tumour development: management based on laparoscopic biopsy and molecular diagnosis. BJU Int 110(11 Pt C):E958–E965

7 Robotic Surgery in Pediatric Urology: State of the Art and Future Horizons

Craig A. Peters

7.1 Background and History

Robotic surgery has been clinically available for surgeons since 2000 with the approval in the USA of the da Vinci (Intuitive Surgical Corp., Sunnyvale, CA) and Zeus Systems (Computer Motion-now defunct). Two robotic surgical systems emerged from research at the Stanford University and the Stanford Research Institute (now SRI). While the definition of robot can vary, with some feeling it must include some degree of programmable automation; others consider any electromechanical device including a computer that can perform some physical function to be a robot. The term has certainly moved into common usage, and classification systems are in process.

Early pediatric uses were in general surgery and urology, using the Zeus System and the da Vinci beginning in 2002 [1–5]. At this time, complex *laparoscopic surgery* in children was uncommon, although well described. This limited use, while adult applications were developing rapidly, was in part due to the complexity of the technique and the difficulty in developing sufficient skill to perform a reliable procedure that involved reconstructive elements. The potential to have the ability to use minimally invasive techniques to perform common operations with ease and general proficiency was appealing. The cost, however, limited access to the system to mainstream pediatric surgical subspecialists, except in a few institutions. A slow progression of reports demonstrated that the da Vinci System could be used in children safely and successfully. The Zeus System faded from use due to purchase of Computer Motion by Intuitive Surgical to halt several intellectual property lawsuits. The Zeus System had several features that made it more adaptable to children, however, including 5 mm instruments, a smaller footprint, and a lower price. Nonetheless, the da Vinci System became the only commercially available surgical robotic system by 2004.

As more children's hospitals acquired the da Vinci and more pediatric surgical specialists partnered with their adult colleagues in general hospitals, the use of the system in children steadily grew. This growth was nearly all in *pediatric urology*, however, as pediatric general surgery did not actively explore its utility except for isolated anecdotal cases [6, 7]. With increasing usage came increasing complexity and a wider range of ages being operated on, as well as the development of several instructional courses.

7.2 Current Technology

At present the da Vinci Surgical System, model Si, is the available technology. It consist of a *four-arm surgical unit* that includes one robotic

C.A. Peters, MD, FACS, FAAP
Surgical Innovation, Technology and Translation, The Sheikh Zayed Institute for Pediatric Surgical Innovation, Children's National Health System, Washington DC, USA
e-mail: crpeters@childrensnational.org

M. Lima, G. Manzoni (eds.), *Pediatric Urology: Contemporary Strategies from Fetal Life to Adolescence*, DOI 10.1007/978-88-470-5693-0_7, © Springer-Verlag Italia 2015

arm for the binocular endoscope, which is available in a 12 and 8.5 mm size and adapts to an Intuitive metal cannula or one of several plastic cannulae. Three arms are available for working instruments, but the fourth arm utilization can be difficult in smaller children, and it is not used regularly by many surgeons.

Working instruments are available in 8 and 5 mm sizes, each with a size-appropriate cannula that must be utilized. The 8 mm instruments are the original design and articulate smoothly by way of hinge joints very close to the tips of the instruments. In contrast, the 5 mm instruments were subsequently introduced and articulate by means of a series of partially articulated vertebra-like components. The articulation is less smooth and responsive and requires more room to turn. This can challenge their use in small spaces.

The 8 mm working instruments most commonly used include a *needle driver* that is rather blunt, a Maryland dissector that has bipolar cautery capacity, a curved scissor with monopolar cautery, and several different graspers for larger tissues or objects. A monopolar *hook cautery* instrument was the original cauterized instrument and continues to be a very useful tool for dissection, cutting, and hemostasis. There is also a very fine tip needle driver (diamond-tipped forceps) that can be used for very fine needles, although it is not very useful for tissue handling. A recent addition is the 8 mm *suction irrigator* with an articulated blunt tip that is very good for dissection. A needle driver with a scissor is available but can be difficult to use without inadvertently cutting the suture as it is being used to tie knots.

The 5 mm instruments include a needle driver that is blunt, a non-cautery curved scissor, a non-cautery Maryland dissector, and the hook cautery.

The 8 mm instrument *cannulae* include a reducing adapter to permit passage of smaller (5 mm) instruments without causing a gas leak as well as a plastic pointed but non-cutting obturator for introduction. The *obturator* is attached to the metal cannula with snaps to permit introduction and easy removal of the obturator. The 5 mm cannulae are not as well designed and have a rigid valve system that can snap off too easily, and the only obturator is metal, blunt tipped, and non-clipped. This makes introduction challenging and potentially dangerous as too much force may be applied in the absence of a pointed tip.

7.3 Basic Methods

7.3.1 Patient Positioning

Positioning is the first critical step in any robotic procedure. Renal procedures require the use of gravity to facilitate retraction and exposure. The method preferred by the author is to permit rotation of the patient with the endoscope in place to adjust the degree of lateral angulation. For *pyeloplasty*, this facilitates using the transmesenteric approach rather than having to mobilize the colon.

Patients are placed on an ipsilateral roll or wedge to raise the side and secured on the table with several straps, and the arms are placed along the sides and held in place by a strap or folded towel running behind the lumbar region and over each arm which is padded. A chest and thigh strap keeps the patient from moving. The operating table can be rotated to position the abdomen flat with the floor for access and then rotated to raise the ipsilateral side to the degree needed. This position is quick to set up, will hold infants to large adolescents securely, and is easily adjusted. It can permit rapid access to the abdomen in an emergency as well [8].

For bladder procedures, the patient is supine, and for larger children, a chest strap is used, as the *Trendelenburg position* is useful for exposure. Tall patients should be positioned with the legs split and carefully supported to allow the robotic surgical cart to fit between.

7.3.2 Port Placement

Many early users found challenges with the introduction of the working ports, although this can be simple with a systematic approach. *Open technique* is recommended for the initial port, although some use the *Veress technique*. The author's preferred method is to use an inferior intra-umbilical incision with stepwise cutting down to the peritoneum.

Once the peritoneum is entered and the field is visually clear, the size is stretched to accommodate the size of the cannula to be used. A fascial suture of 3-0 polyglycolic acid is placed in a *box stitch* manner using a CT-2 needle that has been curved to make it resemble a UR-6 needle or a 2-0 polyglycolic acid suture on a UR-6 is used in children over age 7 [9]. The box stitch then facilitates introducing the cannula into the peritoneum and will be used to close the fascia at the end of the procedure. The abdomen is insufflated, and the two or three working ports are placed under vision with a pre-placed fascial box stitch as with the initial port. The stitch facilitates placement and closure. It should be seen passing through the peritoneum to ensure a secure closure. Any assistant ports are placed at this time. Port placement should not take more than 10 or 15 min in most cases.

7.3.3 Dissection and Exposure

Dissection with the da Vinci System is similar to that used in conventional laparoscopy with a combination of sharp and blunt dissection, the sharp utilizing the hook cautery or the scissors. The surgeon should be aware that overly aggressive blunt dissection without *cautery* could cause bleeding that may obscure the field. The use of traction and countertraction greatly facilitates dissection. The advantage of the 3-D visualization and the articulation of the instruments is a subjective advantage over conventional laparoscopy, even in skilled hands. This is particularly the case with delicate exposure of renal vasculature and the ureter. At the same time, the absence of tactile feedback (*haptics*) can be troublesome if the surgeon is not carefully visualizing the tissues at all times. Excessive traction can be damaging, and overly aggressive dissection of delicate structures such as the ureter may risk devascularization. Similarly, great care needs to be paid to use of cautery, and all surrounding tissues should be away from the current, and awareness of the "hot" parts of the instrument should be constant. It is probably unwise to use a passive instrument such as a dissector to apply cautery by touching, as this risks contacting adjacent structures inadvertently.

Retraction is also a challenge, and the most effective tools are *hitch stitches*. These may be used by passing a suture through the body wall, through the object to be hitched, and then back out the body wall (Fig. 7.1). This permits adjustment of tension but is limited in its position. Intracorporeal hitches can be used for children with very thick abdominal walls, or a hook device can be rigged for adjustable and moveable hitching.

Passing *suture needles* into the field can slow down any procedure. The most efficient approach is to use small needles and make sure that the instrument being used to take the needle and suture inside is smaller than the cannula (i.e., 3.5 mm grasper for 5 mm cannula and a 5 mm grasper or needle driver for the 8 mm cannula). The suture should be grasped and not the needle to prevent the needle from pulling off.

7.3.4 Ureteral Stenting

Placing a double J stent for ureteral reconstruction may be accomplished either retrograde or antegrade. Retrograde placement is typically prior to the start of the robotic portion of the procedure in the usual fashion. This does require extra time but permits the use of an extraction string for stent removal without cystoscopy.

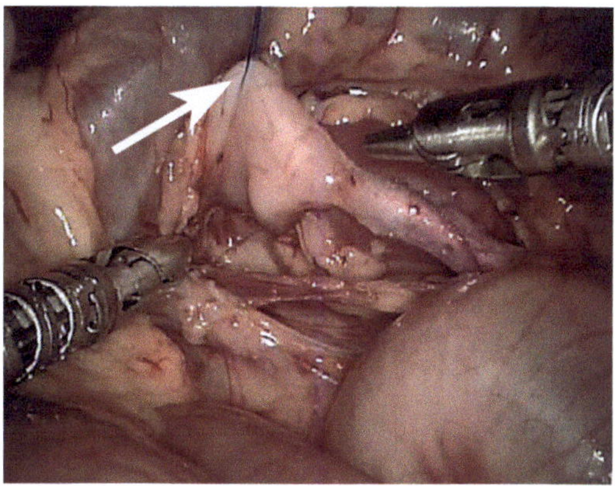

Fig. 7.1 Hitch stitch in place during robotic pyeloplasty. The renal pelvis is elevated and stabilized by the stitch (*arrow*), which is passed through the abdominal wall, through the medial aspect of the pelvis and out the abdominal wall

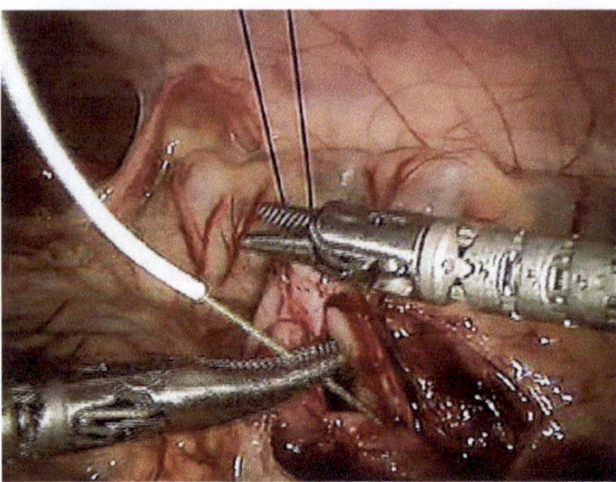

Fig. 7.2 Antegrade passage of a double J ureteral stent during pyeloplasty. The guidewire has been passed through a percutaneous angiocatheter and then down the ureter with the stent passed over the guidewire and directed into the ureter

Alternatively, *antegrade stent placement* can be very efficient. This is best performed by passing a 14 G angiocatheter through the abdominal wall at a location in line with the direction of the course of the stent and removing the needle. For smaller stents that can pass through a 14G angiocatheter (3.7 Fr and 4.8 Fr), the stent is pre-loaded on a guidewire with the flexible tip leading. This is passed through the angiocatheter then guided into the ureter (Fig. 7.2). The wire and stent are passed slowly down the ureter, watching for recoiling or excessive tension on the *ureter*. Usually this will pass very easily but can occasionally hang up. Using a smaller wire may help. The appropriate length can be estimated by the formula 10 cm plus age in years, and an extra 2 cm is useful. Some surgeons will fill the bladder with blue dye (indigo carmine or methylene blue) to signal when the bladder is entered, but this has not always been successful. Some have suggested an intraoperative US to identify the curl of the stent in the bladder, or a can be obtained in the operating room to confirm placement. Postoperative drainage is dependent upon the procedure and the surgeon's preferences.

7.3.5 Completion

Completion of the procedure should include a brief inspection of the operative field and the *peritoneum* to look for pooling of blood or irrigation or any inadvertent injury to an adjacent structure. This is usually done after the robot is disengaged and withdrawn. If significant dissection was undertaken, it can be useful to lower the intraperitoneal pressure for 2 or 3 min and reinspect for venous bleeding that was limited by the insufflation pressure. The working ports are removed under vision with the *pneumoperitoneum* in place to prevent catching any structures in the closure. The fascial sutures are tied, which closes the defect, and if there is no gas leak, this indicates a secure closure. The remainder of the insufflation gas is evacuated through the umbilical port, which is then removed, and the fascial suture is tied. Skin incisions are closed with a subcutaneous stitch followed by a subcuticular stitch if needed.

7.4 Principal Procedures

7.4.1 Pyeloplasty

The most common procedure in pediatric urology for which the da Vinci System has been used is *pyeloplasty*, and it is readily accomplished at all ages [10–12]. Three ports are used, with the endoscope and two *working ports*. Placement is typically umbilical for the endoscope and midline between the umbilicus and xiphoid for the first working port. The patient is then tilted to reveal the kidney and locate the UPJ to guide placement of the third port in the ipsilateral lower quadrant. It should not be too close to the site of the UPJ, or the instrument may not have enough room to maneuver. We have used a midline port placement in small children or those undergoing bilateral pyeloplasties, and this is very acceptable as long as the bladder is avoided. An alternative port placement strategy has been presented to limit any visible port site scars [13].

The left UPJ can be exposed *transmesenterically* in most cases, while on the right the hepatic flexure needs to be mobilized. Once the pelvis and ureter are identified, the ureter is lifted, the UPJ and pelvis further exposed, and the site of the hitch stitch identified. It should be

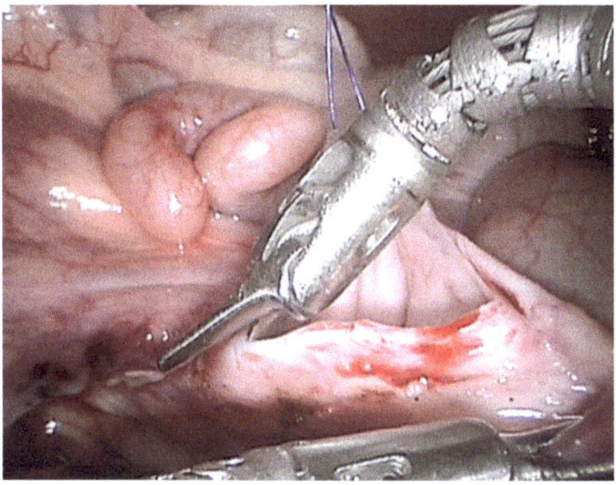

Fig. 7.3 Opening of the renal pelvis on a right-sided pyeloplasty. The hitch stitch is visible lateral to the pyelotomy. The UPJ is relatively low as seen by the presence of the appendix just lateral to the UPJ

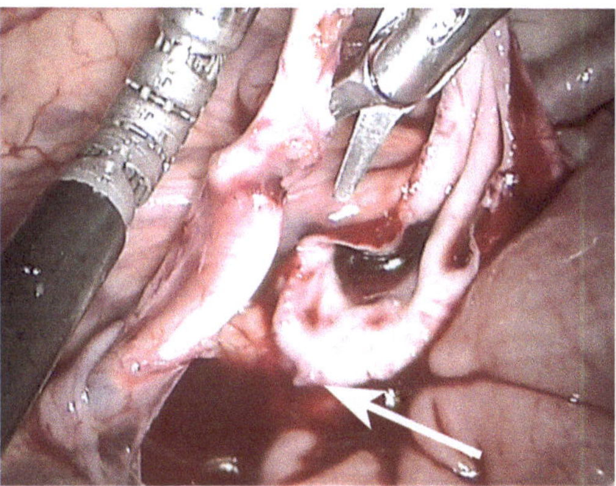

Fig. 7.4 Spatulation of the lateral aspect of the dismembered ureter using the 5 mm straight scissors. The open renal pelvis is visible with the most dependent portion indicated by the *arrow*

at the most medial aspect of the pelvis at the top of the planned pyelotomy. This provides orientation to the pelvis and what will be the most dependent portion of the pelvis. The *ureter* is not mobilized excessively. The pelvis is incised from either top down or bottom up and left on the ureter to serve as a handle (Fig. 7.3). The ureter is then spatulated on its lateral aspect, either by cutting through the UPJ or into the upper ureter. The length of the *spatulation* is best indicated by the visual opening of the ureter, which should admit the tips of the scissors (Fig. 7.4). If a stent has been pre-placed, it should be avoided.

The *anastomosis* is begun, usually on the dependent or posterior wall, starting with the inferior-most apex stitch (Fig. 7.5). Suture used depends on age and preference. Because it moves smoothly through tissues, an absorbable *monofilament* is favored in most cases, with 6-0 for infants and 5-0 for older children. This may be placed in a continuous manner, which is preferred due to uniform tension and watertightness (Fig. 7.6a, b). The anastomosis may be performed with interrupted suture as well, but this requires more time. If a stent is to be placed antegrade, this is done after the first side of the anastomosis. Otherwise, the anterior side of the pelvi-ureteric anastomosis is closed (Fig. 7.7). No other drains are usually used, and a bladder catheter is left in place overnight. Most children can be discharged home the next morning.

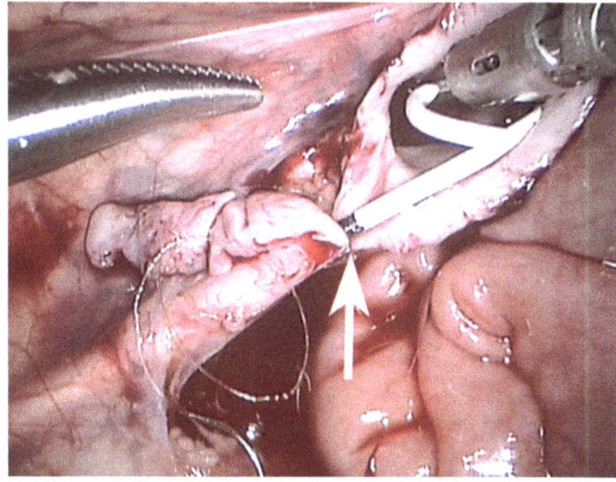

Fig. 7.5 Beginning the ureteropelvic anastomosis on a right-sided pyeloplasty. The inferior most apex suture has been placed (*arrow*). The pre-placed double J stent can be used to facilitate suture placement

7.4.2 Ureteral Reimplantation for Vesicoureteral Reflux

Robotically assisted *ureteral reimplantion* has been shown to have reliable success and be efficient [14–17]. The degree of advantage for younger children is uncertain, but for older children, this is an attractive option to limit the need for catheterization and inpatient stay. Bilateral reimplantations can be performed, and there is good evidence that the risk of *urinary retention*, as recognized in open extravesical reimplantation, is very low, but not absent [16, 17]. The principal means to avoid this is to avoid excessive

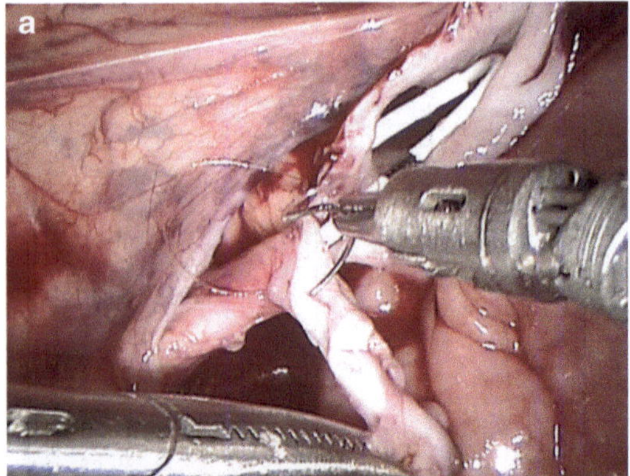

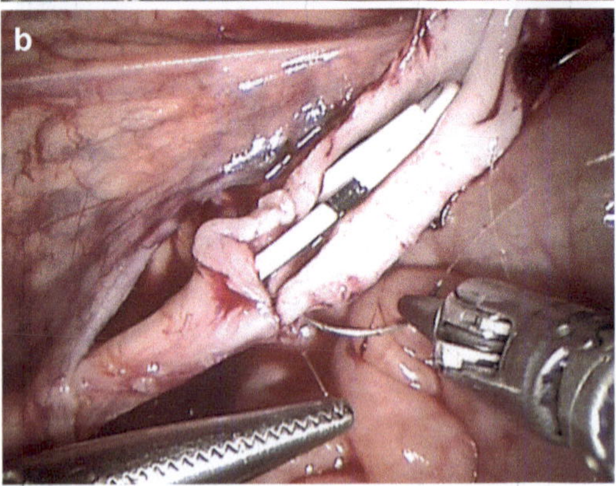

Fig. 7.6 (**a**) Anterior wall running anastomosis of a right-sided pyeloplasty using 5-0 absorbable monofilament suture. The part of the renal pelvis still attached to the ureter is used as a handle for manipulation to avoid injury to the anastomotic tissues. It will later be removed. (**b**) The posterior wall in this case is closed after the anterior due to positioning. Retracting on the tail of the suture stabilizes the tissues for suture placement

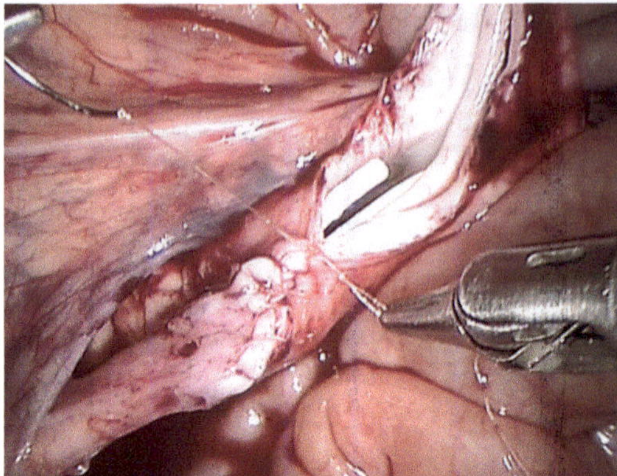

Fig. 7.7 The anastomosis is nearly complete with closure of the pelvis remaining

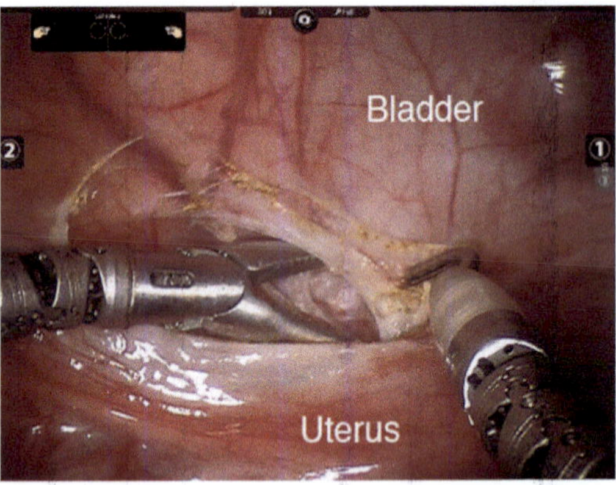

Fig. 7.8 Exposure of the left ureter in an extravesical reimplantation in a girl. The peritoneum between the bladder and uterus is incised transversely, and blunt dissection exposes the ureter

dissection away from the ureter and limit damage to the *perivesical nerves* [18].

Port positions include an umbilical port for the camera and in the midclavicular lines bilaterally at the umbilical level. In infants, the working ports should be just above the umbilicus to provide adequate room for the instruments.

Exposure of the ureter is initiated by incising the peritoneum transversely as it reflects onto the bladder anterior to the uterus in girls and just distal to the vas in boys (Fig. 7.8). Blunt dissection is used to develop the periureteral space, approaching the ureter just as it inserts into the bladder. There is always a small but distinct vessel that crosses over the ureter as either an inferior uterine or vesical artery. This is usually taken but occasionally can be preserved and mobilized superiorly as the ureter is mobilized. The hook cautery is most effective for ureteral mobilization with an initial elevation followed by progressive freeing of periureteral attachments, but not violating the ureteral adventitia (Fig. 7.9). The extent of *mobilization* is a judgment and usually amounts to about 5–6 cm and is just below the takeoff of the superior vesical branch of the *internal hypogastric artery*. The posterior attachments of the ureter cannot be directly seen behind the ureter but can be released by sliding the hook along the medial side of the ureter then directing it laterally under the ureter to catch these attachments, which are then cut with cautery.

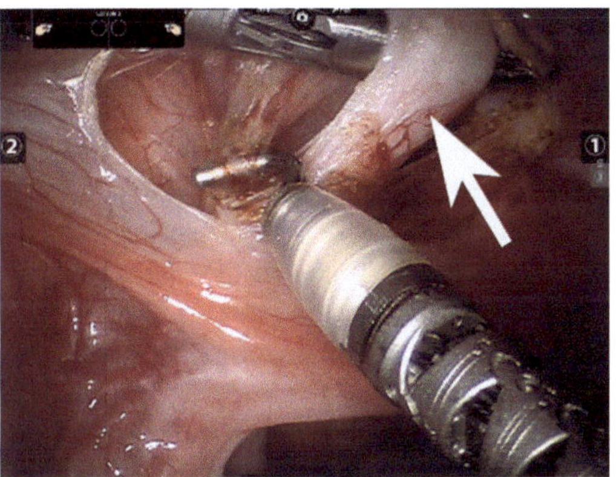

Fig. 7.9 Mobilization of the left ureter (*arrow*) using traction and hook cautery to release periadventitial tissues. Care is taken to stay close to the ureter without injury to the adventitial blood supply

Once the ureter is mobilized, the bladder is partially filled, and the line of the detrusor incision is marked based on where the bladder rolls over the ureter. The length is about 4 cm, but measurement is difficult as it varies with bladder filling or wall stretch. A *bladder hitch stitch* is then placed to lift and flatten the posterior wall of the bladder. The stitch (3-0 Vicryl) is passed on an SH needle through the abdominal wall just above the pubis and under internal vision. It should pass through near the obliterated umbilical artery. It is then passed through the bladder just superior and lateral to the top of the anticipated detrusor incision. The suture is looped around itself, and then a second bite of the bladder is made on the contralateral side and again looped. The location of the second bite is the same for unilateral and bilateral procedures. The needle is then passed outside and both ends lifted simultaneously (Fig. 7.10). The bladder is then filled to make the wall slightly tense, and the camera angle is shifted from 30° down to 30° up to facilitate the *detrusorotomy*.

The detrusor is incised from the top of the tunnel down to the hiatus. It is useful to first identify the depth needed to reach mucosa and then extend this by carefully holding the muscle and pushing the mucosa away inferiorly and laterally (Fig. 7.11). The freed muscle is then cut until the hiatus is reached, and a "V" incision made around the ureter. The hiatus is not incised circumferentially.

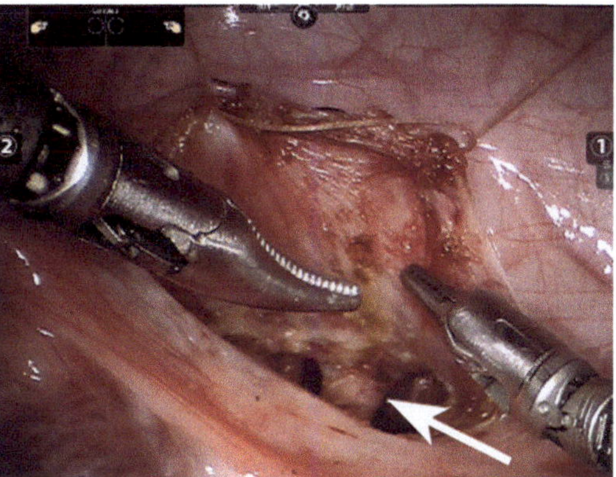

Fig. 7.10 Exposure of the back wall of the bladder and the mobilized ureter is facilitated by placement of a hitch stitch that is placed into two points of the bladder wall. This also stretches the bladder wall to facilitate creation of the detrusor tunnel. The mobilized ureter is indicated by the *arrow*

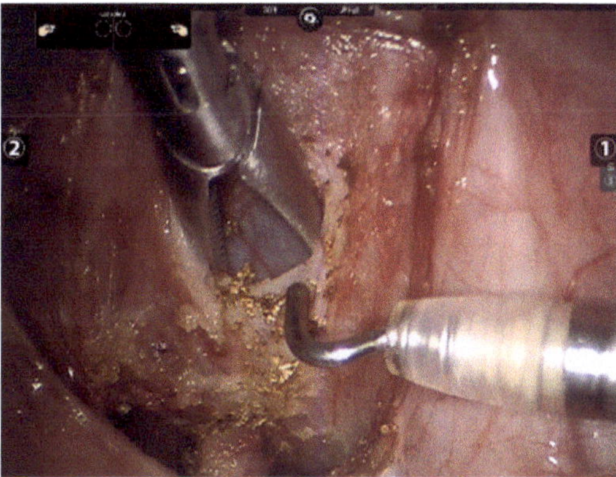

Fig. 7.11 Creation of the detrusor tunnel involves incision of the detrusor muscle without injuring the mucosa. The Maryland dissector can be used to gently spread the muscle fibers and lift them from the mucosa to permit incision with the hook cautery

Either the hook or 8 mm "hot shears" are used for this mobilization.

The detrusor edges are mobilized away from the mucosa slightly as flaps to cover the ureter. If the ureter is large, these should be made more generous. The *detrusor tunnel* is then closed with interrupted Vicryl suture (4-0 for young children, 3-0 for ages 8 and up) (Fig. 7.12). A total of five to seven stitches are usually sufficient. Once the tunnel is closed, the opposite side can be performed for bilateral, or the hitch stitch is cut, and the bladder filled partially to test for leaks. The

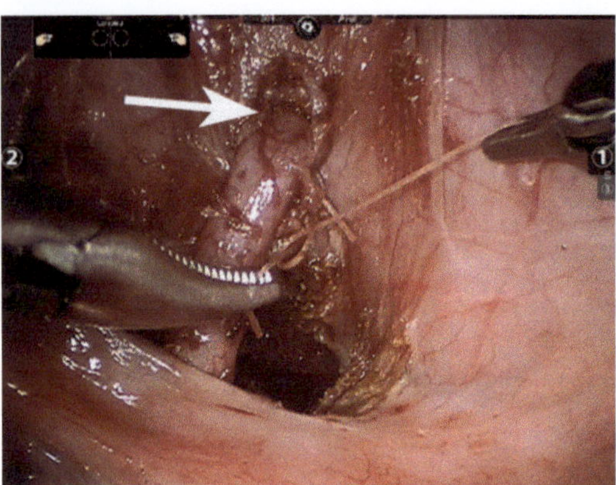

Fig. 7.12 Closure of the detrusor tunnel with interrupted absorbable sutures. The upper aspect of the tunnel and the ureter is indicated by the *arrow*

peritoneal incision is closed with a running 4-0 Vicryl.

A bladder catheter is not left in place for unilateral repairs if the mucosa has not been violated significantly, but for bilateral procedures, a catheter is left in place overnight. Parents are cautioned that some children will need to be re-catheterized if they fail a voiding trial, but this is seen in less than 10 %. A child with known and incompletely managed BBD may need the catheter in place longer.

7.4.3 Partial Nephrectomy

Robotic *partial nephrectomy* for *duplication anomalies* permits a precise control of the vasculature of the affected and remnant pole and definitive closure of the defect. Positioning and port placement are as with a pyeloplasty, although a right-sided upper pole partial nephrectomy will usually require a fourth port to lift the liver away. The colon is mobilized for both right and left procedures, and the affected ureter is identified near the lower pole. For most upper pole partial nephrectomies, it is dilated and is dissected free, ligated, and divided. It then serves as a handle to facilitate mobilization of the rest of the upper pole. Blunt dissection around the *ureter* in a cephalad direction under the hilum permits passing the ureteral stump superiorly and behind the vessels. It is then lifted to reveal the upper pole vessels, which are ligated. Either clips or suture may be used. If clips are used, care must be taken not to dislodge them. The plane between the upper pole pelvis and the lower pole parenchyma is developed bluntly, and then the thin renal parenchyma of the upper pole is incised with cautery or *harmonic scalpel*. If the upper pole collecting system is entered, one should ensure that any of the collecting system is not left in situ.

The defect from the upper pole is preferably closed using three *mattress sutures* over a tongue of retroperitoneal fat. While it is difficult to prove that this reduces the potential for a post-op *urinoma*, it seems reasonable and adds very little time. While this is more difficult with conventional laparoscopy and has not been done in many series, the incidence of urinoma seems higher in the laparoscopic reports compared to what has been reported with open [19]. While post-op urinomas have not been reported to cause clinical problems, they can become a concern to families.

No drain is routinely left in place, but if there is concern about violation of the lower pole, then a simple wound drain would be reasonable. No bladder catheter is left in place unless there is a similar concern.

7.4.4 Retrovesical Procedures

Robotic access to the retrovesical space is one of the areas of very clear value for this system. The articulated instruments are well suited to the tight working area and the need for care when dissecting in the deep pelvis. There are several early reports of robotic resection of *utricular cysts*, *seminal vesical cysts*, and persistent *Müllerian structures* using the robotic system [20].

The approach is with ports in position as with a ureteral reimplantation, and the peritoneum is incised between the bladder and rectum. The bladder remains attached anteriorly to keep it out of the field. For midline structures, it is important to stay directly on the structure to avoid injury to the lateral vasa or seminal vesicles. In some instances, the vasa will enter these abnormal structures and will need to be cut.

Table 7.1 Robotic pyeloplasty outcomes

Author	Study type	Patients	Age range	Success	Comment
Olsen [21]	Case series[a]	13	3.5–16.2	100 %	Retroperitoneal
Atug [22]	Case series	7	6–15	100 %	
Lee [11]	Case-control[b]	33 rob 33 open	0.2–19.6	97 %	Shorter hospital stay and narcotic use for robotic
Kutikov [23]	Case series	9	0.25–0.75	100 %	
Yee [24]	Case-control	8 rob 8 open	6.4–16.5	100 %	No significant differences but longer operative times
Franco [25]	Case-control	15 rob 12 lap	4–18	100 %	No significant differences between robotic and lap
Olsen [26]	Case series[a]	65	1.7–17.1	94 %	Retroperitoneal
Freilich [27]	Case series	5	3.4–14	100 %	Bilateral
Chan [28]	Case series	5	0.9–12	100 %	
Minnillo [29]	Case series[b]	155	10.5 mean	96 %	3 % required re-op
Rodriguez [30]	Case series	12	3.5–16	100 %	Stentless repair
Singh [31]	Case series	34	5–15	97 %	
Subotic [32]	Case series	19 rob 20 lap	>4 years robotic	100 %	Comparable outcomes between robotic and lap
Bansal [33]	Case-control[c]	9 rob 61 open	<12 months	100 % rob 98 % open	Infants only
Riachy [34]	Case-control[c]	46 rob 18 lap	rob 0.5–22; lap 0.25–18	100 % rob 87.5 % open	Operative time shorter for robotic, similar length of stay and narcotic use
Pelizzo [12]	Case series	3	<12 months	100 %	All infants under 10 kg

[a,b,c]Some of the same patients included in later report

They would not likely have been functional in any event. The structure is maintained intact for as long as possible but may need to be opened to permit determination of its distal extent. We usually try to remove the entire structure to where it enters the posterior *prostate* and suture ligate this neck with a figure-of-eight absorbable suture.

We have performed robotically assisted removals of large *ectopic ureters* that enter into the prostate or join the vas deferens, as well as seminal vesical cysts, typically associated with *dysplastic kidneys*. Some of these have been extremely large and very fibrotic, requiring careful tedious dissection, but the anatomic definition permitted by the endoscope and the controlled dissection makes this more efficient and certainly less morbid than an open procedure.

In the teenage male, they will have persisting postoperative pain and some bladder spasm for several days to weeks and may have a transient residual fluid collection.

7.5 Outcomes

Clinical outcomes for robotic procedures have been reported in various formats, predominantly as case series with a few comparative studies (Tables 7.1 and 7.2 for pyeloplasty and ureteral reimplantation). A formal prospective randomized trial has not been reported in the pediatric literature, and it may be nearly impossible to do so. In general, outcomes have been comparable to open or conventional laparoscopic approaches with some reduction in postoperative morbidity as measured by narcotic use and length of hospital stay. It must be recognized that these are very crude measures and do not capture the true impact of a surgical procedure. It is very clear from review of these studies that more sensitive and robust measures of the health impact of surgery on a child and their family are needed. It must also be recognized that the cost of robotic technology is an important factor in assessing its value, but this is a rapidly moving target that has many local

Table 7.2 Ureteral reimplantation – extravesical

Author	Study type	Patients	Age range	Success	Comment
Casale [15]	Case series[a]	41	1.3–7	97.6 %	Bilateral; no retention
Marchini [35]	Case-control	20 EV/19 IV 17 open EV 20 open IV	EV mean: 8.6 rob 6.1 open; IV mean: 9.9 rob 8.8 open	P2.2 % rob 93.2 % open IV; 100 % rob 94.2 % open	Multiple subgroups, including intravesical reimplants
Smith [17]	Case-control	25 EV 25 open EV	0.25–12	97 % rob 100 % open	3 transient retention in robotic group
Chalmers [36]	Case series	17 (6 bilat)	6.25 mean	90.9 %	No retention
Kasturi [16]	Case series[a]	150	2.25–9.3	99.3 %	Bilateral; no voiding dysfunction
Akhavan [14]	Case series	50 (28 bilat)	1.9–18	92.3 %	1 transient retention

[a]Some of the same patients included in later report

Table 7.3 Developmental robotic surgery in pediatric urology

Procedure	Descriptions	Comment
Intravesical ureteral reimplantation	[5, 35, 37, 38]	Remains challenging for access and maintenance of exposure
Continent catheterizable stoma	[39–43]	Effective and straightforward with appendix or ureter
Bladder neck reconstruction/sling	[44, 45]	Exposure of bladder neck is excellent and facilitates posterior dissection
Augmentation cystoplasty	[40, 46, 47]	Remains long operation. Advantages uncertain at present
Pyelolithotomy	[48, 49]	Limited application but useful for complex stone burden or when concomitant obstruction requires repair

variations in significance. Comparisons to conventional laparoscopy have limited value as this technology is used to such a limited degree in reconstructive pediatric urology and it may not evolve further if robotic systems remain available. It is unclear what impact and when competitive systems to the da Vinci System will have.

At present it is clear that robotic technology can provide for effective and safe minimally invasive reconstructive surgery for pediatric urology. Its applications have been growing with greater experience, and progressively more complex procedures are being reported with success, even if without efficiency.

7.6 Conclusions and Challenges

A number of other surgical procedures have been described using the robotic system in children but remain early in their development (Table 7.3). Continued exploration should be encouraged with careful and honest reporting of outcomes. There seems little doubt that the da Vinci robotic system offers enhanced ability to perform complex reconstructive and ablative urologic procedures in children, with reduced morbidity and equal efficacy. The value of the system, given its high cost, is not yet proven for all children. The adolescent shows a definite advantage in most renal and pelvis procedures, but the infant has a lesser degree of benefit. The dividing line is not at all clear.

It will also be very important to develop more robust measures of the impact of a surgical intervention on children and their families, as well as more accurate and relevant assessments of cost, to permit a better valuation of this technology as well as those that will surely follow.

The current da Vinci System is not at all designed for children but can be made to work effectively in the small child. There is a clear need for more pediatric-specific tools that reflect the types of procedures and tissues that are being manipulated. The smaller instruments (5 mm) are much less precise than the larger 8 mm ones. Integration with digital imaging technologies is an important emerging trend that will facilitate all pediatric urologic procedures.

The da Vinci platform is a clear *proof of principle* that *computer-assisted robotic devices* can enhance our surgical capabilities and offer reduced morbidity with equal and potentially even greater efficacy. The users of these evolving technologies need to be closely involved in the patterns of evolution and be rigorously honest with their appraisals, both to guide their development in appropriate and valuable direction and to maintain the credibility of their community.

References

1. Gutt CN et al (2002) Early experiences of robotic surgery in children. Surg Endosc 16(7):1083–1086
2. Lorincz A et al (2005) Totally minimally invasive robot-assisted unstented pyeloplasty using the Zeus Microwrist Surgical System: an animal study. J Pediatr Surg 40(2):418–422
3. Meininger DD et al (2001) Totally endoscopic Nissen fundoplication with a robotic system in a child. Surg Endosc 15(11):1360
4. Peters CA (2004) Laparoscopic and robotic approach to genitourinary anomalies in children. Urol Clin North Am 31(3):595–605, xi
5. Peters CA, Woo R (2005) Intravesical robotically assisted bilateral ureteral reimplantation. J Endourol 19(6):618–621; discussion 621–622
6. Meehan JJ, Meehan TD, Sandler A (2007) Robotic fundoplication in children: resident teaching and a single institutional review of our first 50 patients. J Pediatr Surg 42(12):2022–2025
7. Meehan JJ, Sandler A (2008) Pediatric robotic surgery: a single-institutional review of the first 100 consecutive cases. Surg Endosc 22(1):177–182
8. Chandrasoma S et al (2010) Straight-arm positioning and port placement for pediatric robotic-assisted laparoscopic renal surgery. J Robot Surg 4:29–32
9. Poppas DP, Bleustein CB, Peters CA (1999) Box stitch modification of Hasson technique for pediatric laparoscopy. J Endourol/Endourological Soc 13(6): 447–450
10. Autorino R et al (2014) Robot-assisted and laparoscopic repair of ureteropelvic junction obstruction: a systematic review and meta-analysis. Eur Urol 65(2):430–452
11. Lee RS et al (2006) Pediatric robot assisted laparoscopic dismembered pyeloplasty: comparison with a cohort of open surgery. J Urol 175(2):683–687; discussion 687
12. Pelizzo G et al (2014) Pediatric robotic pyeloplasty in patients weighing less than 10 kg initial experience. Surg Laparosc Endosc Percutan Tech 24(1):e29–e31
13. Gargollo PC (2011) Hidden incision endoscopic surgery: description of technique, parental satisfaction and applications. J Urol 185(4):1425–1431
14. Akhavan A, Avery D, Lendvay TS (2014) Robot-assisted extravesical ureteral reimplantation: outcomes and conclusions from 78 ureters. J Pediatr Urol pii:S1477–S5131
15. Casale P, Patel RP, Kolon TF (2008) Nerve sparing robotic extravesical ureteral reimplantation. J Urol 179(5):1987–1989; discussion 1990
16. Kasturi S et al (2012) Prospective long-term analysis of nerve-sparing extravesical robotic-assisted laparoscopic ureteral reimplantation. Urology 79(3):680–683
17. Smith RP, Oliver JL, Peters CA (2011) Pediatric robotic extravesical ureteral reimplantation: comparison with open surgery. J Urol 185(5):1876–1881
18. Dangle PP et al (2013) Is pelvic plexus nerve documentation feasible during robotic assisted laparoscopic ureteral reimplantation with extravesical approach? J Pediatr Urol 9(4):442–447
19. Mason MD et al (2013) Robotic-assisted partial nephrectomy in duplicated collecting systems in the pediatric population: techniques and outcomes. J Pediatr Urol. doi:10.1016/j.jpurol.2013.10.014
20. Passerotti C et al (2007) Minimally invasive surgical approaches to retrovesical structures. Int J Med Robot 3(4):307–311
21. Olsen LH, Jorgensen TM (2004) Computer assisted pyeloplasty in children: the retroperitoneal approach. J Urol 171(6 Pt 2):2629–2631
22. Atug F et al (2005) Robotic assisted laparoscopic pyeloplasty in children. J Urol 174(4 Pt 1):1440–1442
23. Kutikov A et al (2006) Robot assisted pyeloplasty in the infant-lessons learned. J Urol 176(5):2237–2239; discussion 2239–2240
24. Yee DS et al (2006) Initial comparison of robotic-assisted laparoscopic versus open pyeloplasty in children. Urology 67(3):599–602
25. Franco I, Dyer LL, Zelkovic P (2007) Laparoscopic pyeloplasty in the pediatric patient: hand sewn anastomosis versus robotic assisted anastomosis–is there a difference? J Urol 178(4 Pt 1):1483–1486
26. Olsen LH, Rawashdeh YF, Jorgensen TM (2007) Pediatric robot assisted retroperitoneoscopic pyeloplasty: a 5-year experience. J Urol 178(5):2137–2141; discussion 2141
27. Freilich DA et al (2008) Concurrent management of bilateral ureteropelvic junction obstruction in children using robotic-assisted laparoscopic surgery. Int Braz J Urol 34(2):198–204; discussion 204–205
28. Chan KW et al (2010) Early experience of robotic-assisted reconstructive operations in pediatric urology. J Laparoendosc Adv Surg Tech A 20(4):379–382
29. Minnillo BJ et al (2011) Long-term experience and outcomes of robotic assisted laparoscopic pyeloplasty in children and young adults. J Urol 185(4):1455–1460

30. Rodriguez AR, Rich MA, Swana HS (2012) Stentless pediatric robotic pyeloplasty. Ther Adv Urol 4(2): 57–60
31. Singh P et al (2012) Outcomes of robot-assisted laparoscopic pyeloplasty in children: a single center experience. J Endourol/Endourological Soc 26(3):249–253
32. Subotic U et al (2012) A minimal invasive surgical approach for children of all ages with ureteropelvic junction obstruction. J Pediatr Urol 8(4):354–358
33. Bansal D et al (2013) Infant robotic pyeloplasty: comparison with an open cohort. J Pediatr Urol 10: 380–385
34. Riachy E et al (2013) Pediatric standard and robot-assisted laparoscopic pyeloplasty: a comparative single institution study. J Urol 189(1):283–287
35. Marchini GS et al (2011) Robotic assisted laparoscopic ureteral reimplantation in children: case matched comparative study with open surgical approach. J Urol 185(5):1870–1875
36. Chalmers D, Herbst K, Kim C (2012) Robotic-assisted laparoscopic extravesical ureteral reimplantation: an initial experience. J Pediatr Urol 8(3):268–271
37. Olsen LH et al (2003) Computer assisted laparoscopic pneumovesical ureter reimplantation a.m. Cohen: initial experience in a pig model. APMIS Suppl 109: 23–25
38. Kutikov A et al (2006) Initial experience with laparoscopic transvesical ureteral reimplantation at the Children's Hospital of Philadelphia. J Urol 176(5): 2222–2225; discussion 2225–2226
39. Pedraza R, Weiser A, Franco I (2004) Laparoscopic appendicovesicostomy (Mitrofanoff procedure) in a child using the da Vinci robotic system. J Urol 171(4): 1652–1653
40. Gundeti MS et al (2008) Pediatric robotic-assisted laparoscopic augmentation ileocystoplasty and Mitrofanoff appendicovesicostomy: complete intracorporeal – initial case report. Urology 72(5):1144–1147; discussion 1147
41. Lendvay TS, Shnorhavorian M, Grady RW (2008) Robotic-assisted laparoscopic mitrofanoff appendicovesicostomy and antegrade continent enema colon tube creation in a pediatric spina bifida patient. J Laparoendosc Adv Surg Tech A 18(2):310–312
42. Thakre AA, Yeung CK, Peters C (2008) Robot-assisted Mitrofanoff and Malone antegrade continence enema reconstruction using divided appendix. J Endourol 22(10):2393–2396; discussion 2396
43. Nguyen HT et al (2009) Robotic assisted laparoscopic Mitrofanoff appendicovesicostomy: preliminary experience in a pediatric population. J Urol 182(4): 1528–1534
44. Storm DW, Fulmer BR, Sumfest JM (2008) Robotic-assisted laparoscopic approach for posterior bladder neck dissection and placement of pediatric bladder neck sling: initial experience. Urology 72(5):1149–1152
45. Bagrodia A, Gargollo P (2011) Robot-assisted bladder neck reconstruction, bladder neck sling, and appendicovesicostomy in children: description of technique and initial results. J Endourol/Endourological Soc 25(8):1299–1305
46. Passerotti CC et al (2008) Robot-assisted laparoscopic ileal bladder augmentation: defining techniques and potential pitfalls. J Endourol 22(2): 355–360
47. Rey D et al (2013) Feasibility of robotic double Yang-Monti ileal conduit with bladder augmentation: surgical technique. Urology 82:480–484
48. Lee RS et al (2007) Early results of robot assisted laparoscopic lithotomy in adolescents. J Urol 177(6):2306–2309; discussion 2309–2310
49. Ghani KR et al (2014) Robotic nephrolithotomy and pyelolithotomy with utilization of the robotic ultrasound probe. Int Braz J Urol 40(1):125–126

Part II

Kidney and Upper Urinary Tract

Congenital Ureteropelvic Junction Obstruction: A Pragmatic Approach

8

Craig A. Peters

Congenital UPJO is a well-known clinical entity that is readily diagnosed, with a well-described and highly successful surgical treatment yet continues to generate significant controversy as to the best means of diagnosis and timing of surgery. The clinical presentation has completely changed in the last 30 years with the advent of prenatal ultrasound, and in many ways, this diagnostic tool has radically changed our approach to this condition. This chapter will review the basics of clinical diagnosis and management and try to frame the controversy in such a way to permit a *pragmatic clinical approach* for children, based on reported outcomes, and a recognition that we do not have all the information regarding the natural history of UPJO, nor the best means to measure its impact.

8.1 Elements of the Clinical Decision

When managing a child with asymptomatic presumed UPJO, typically having presented with prenatal hydronephrosis, several key questions must be answered to permit a rational decision:

1. Why consider any intervention?
2. Can UPJO resolve spontaneously?
3. Can we predict if it will resolve?
4. If function declines, will it recover after successful surgery?
5. If function is low at diagnosis, can successful surgery improve it?
6. If we operate, what is the success rate?

C.A. Peters
Surgical Innovation, Technology and Translation, The Sheikh Zayed Institute for Pediatric Surgical Innovation, Children's National Health System, Washington DC, USA
e-mail: crpeters@childrensnational.org

1. *Why consider any intervention?*
   The rationale for *intervention* in UPJO is based on the known clinical fact that these children can develop symptoms of flank pain or, less commonly, UTI. Severe *bilateral UPJO* can cause renal failure, although this is very uncommon. Nonetheless, the basis for intervention is to prevent renal functional impairment. The degree of impairment and its clinical impact is highly variable. Numerous cases have been reported of unilateral kidneys showing deterioration in function as measured by *radionuclide imaging* or solitary kidneys with globally reduced function. When we see an older child with UPJ obstruction and poor function, we do not know when the functional impairment developed, however. Early studies [1, 2] suggested that early repair was more effective at protecting function than later repair, but this was not universal, and subsequent observations indicated that function might not be lost while awaiting *spontaneous resolution* [3–5]. At that time, early repair meant 2–4 weeks of age, but since then, a more observational approach has evolved, based on the evidence that a dilated kidney did not always show functional loss and might

M. Lima, G. Manzoni (eds.), *Pediatric Urology: Contemporary Strategies from Fetal Life to Adolescence*, DOI 10.1007/978-88-470-5693-0_8, © Springer-Verlag Italia 2015

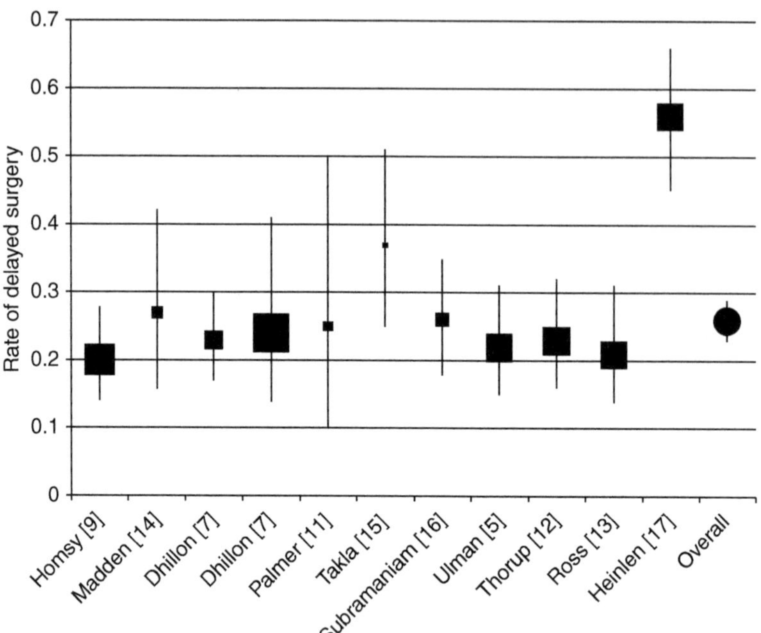

Fig. 8.1 Chart showing reported incidence of surgery in children being followed with prenatal hydronephrosis and apparent UPJ obstruction. Each study is represented by its reported incidence with the 95 % CI. The size of the marker is proportional to the number of patients. The overall incidence represents over 900 patients

revert to normal while retaining normal function.

2. *Can UPJO resolve spontaneously?*

   The critical observations that apparent UPJO can spontaneously improve changed the approach to this new population of children with *hydronephrosis* from prenatal detection. Numerous studies have assessed the likelihood of resolution and most will show, using roughly similar criteria, a rate of improvement between 70 and 80 % of more severe hydronephrosis. It has become well recognized that lesser degrees of dilation will almost always resolve in 12–24 months [5–17]. The time frame for improvement is roughly related to the severity of the dilation and can range from 12 to 48 months or more (Fig. 8.1).

   The mechanism of resolution remains unclear. Logical explanations include maturation of the smooth muscle peristaltic mechanism of the proximal ureter and pelvis. Milder degrees of hydronephrosis may be more the product of high bladder pressures in the immature boy, but this is unproven as well.

3. *Can we predict if it will resolve?*

   The likelihood of resolution is inversely proportional to the severity of hydronephrosis. Children with greater degrees of hydronephrosis are less likely to resolve in any particular time frame, although resolution can be seen with nearly any degree of dilation. For grades 1–2 dilation (on the SFU scale), resolution is likely to occur within 1–3 years, but some have persisted for longer periods. Persisting mild dilation is of unknown significance, and the strict need for monitoring is unknown. The clinically challenging cases of *grade 3 and 4 hydronephrosis* cannot be predicted individually as to time to resolution or risk of progression and therefore justify ongoing monitoring. Grade 3 dilation is uncommonly associated with decreased relative uptake at diagnosis [18]. When dealing with the individual, then resolution may be anticipated but cannot be certain, and ongoing monitoring is needed, based upon the severity of hydronephrosis and any functional abnormality on diuretic renography.

4. *If function declines, will it recover after successful surgery?*

   Relatively few studies have examined this situation, but these few have indicated that in most cases, a loss of relative uptake on diuretic renography will recover postoperatively [5].

This is not absolute, and it should be recognized in any observational management program that there is a risk for permanent loss of function [2, 19]. If the repair is delayed, then permanent loss of function is more likely. Ongoing *functional monitoring* in children at risk for loss is therefore advisable. The frequency of this monitoring, however, is not well defined.

5. *If function is low at diagnosis, can successful surgery improve it?*
   There are conflicting data as to this issue, yet most would suggest that when initial uptake or function is low, it is unlikely to improve [20–22]. The goal then of *surgical intervention* is to preserve the current state of function. Not all authors advocate intervention if the initial function is low and will recommend waiting for demonstration of further reduction in function. In some children with initially low functional levels, improvement without surgery has been reported [5]. This has not been the general reported experience in most series however, and the technical aspects of how function is assessed should be considered as possible reasons for this inconsistency.
6. *If we operate, what is the success rate?*
   Surgical success should be very high in terms of improving the degree of hydronephrosis and functional drainage parameters on diuretic renography. Estimates of 97–98 % success have been reported based upon either improved hydronephrosis or improved washout times on renography [23]. This is more apparent in younger patients, although even some older children will show marked improvement in the degree of dilation after pyeloplasty [24]. The lack of improvement or certainly worsening should prompt diuretic renography to assess more objectively the level of *drainage*, although interpretation may be controversial. The need for further intervention is subjective, and we have on occasion used temporary (6 weeks) ureteral stenting with subsequent improvement or further evaluation. The need for repeat pyeloplasty should be in the 1 % range for most cases [25].

Based upon these observations, the approach to the child with an apparent UPJO is dependent upon the clinical assessment, which is heavily weighted on the imaging evaluation. The full clinical assessment factors into surgical decision-making and ultimately into the choice of surgical intervention. These aspects will be discussed in more detail below.

8.1.1 Imaging Assessment

Current assessment of the child with apparent *UPJO* rests upon a determination of structure and functional studies. The most efficient approach that is usually adequate includes an *ultrasound* to define the severity of the *hydronephrosis*; the level of dilation defines the level of the obstruction and any associated structural anomalies of the urinary tract. A dilated ureter indicates that a more distal obstruction is likely present, although on occasion this can be present with a UPJO and concomitant VUR. The appearance of most kidneys with a severe UPJO is characteristic and has diffuse but uniform *caliectasis* that flattens and everts the papillae. More severe dilation effaces the parenchyma between the calyces and thins the parenchymal mantle due to distention. The renal pelvis can be massively dilated but may also be relatively small and nearly intrarenal. These cases nearly always have more severe intrarenal dilation and may pose more of a functional risk to the kidney. A massively dilated renal pelvis without significant caliectasis suggests a lesser degree of obstruction, and one should not base clinical decisions on the degree of pelvic dilation alone.

Ultrasound alone cannot define the severity of obstruction, but the appearance of the kidney is clearly related to the severity. Using quantitative imaging algorithms, we have been able to show that US can predict thresholds of obstructive severity based upon diuretic washout times [26]. Ultrasound can be used to follow patients under expectant monitoring with the presumption that increases or decreases in the severity of the dilation correlate with worsening or improvement in obstruction [13]. Ultrasound cannot reliably assess renal function as measured on renography. The need for functional assessment becomes important.

8.1.2 Diuretic Renography

The most reliable current method of assessing relative renal function is the *diuretic renogram* (DR) [27, 28]. When performed carefully and consistently, the DR remains the gold standard for assessing obstruction, but it is imperfect. The underlying principle of the DR is that the amount of early tracer uptake, measured at 2 min after injection, correlates with GFR. The relative uptake is then expressed as a fraction of 1 in percent. Numerous studies have demonstrated the reproducibility of the DR and its correlation with *DMSA* scanning. The correlation with more formal measures of renal function in experimental systems in the setting of hydronephrosis, however, may not be as reliable [29, 30]. Various factors may underlie this lack of correlation including the physical effect of the dilated pelvis to alterations in renal physiology in the face of obstruction [31]. It is also important to recognize that the "function" that is measured by DR is one of several renal functions, albeit a very important one. Renal tubular functions, including concentrating ability, acid base balance, and various hormonal functions, are not measured by DR. These rarely have a clinical impact in unilateral obstruction, however. The fact that the DR reports function as two percentages that always add up to 100 should not hide the fact that if both kidneys are abnormal, the sum is still 100 %. Using the DR to monitor *bilateral obstruction* can be difficult.

There is also the concern that the function measured by the DR may not fully reflect the status of the renal *parenchyma*. In biopsies of UPJO undergoing pyeloplasty, kidneys with normal uptake on DR did not always have normal histology, including both *interstitial fibrosis* and tubular loss [32–34]. Even in kidneys with no overt histological abnormalities, relative proximal tubular volume was decreased. These observations raise the real possibility that kidneys are able to compensate in the face of obstruction and maintain normal measured function yet be undergoing some degree of progressive injury that may not be evident for an extended period of time. Appropriate urinary *biomarkers* will likely be needed to assess the clinical significance of these findings [35].

The degree of *abnormal function* apparent on DR that is clinically significant remains undefined but in practice is typically less than 40 %. It should be borne in mind that it is unlikely that these kidneys, at first assessment, have lost function, but that this is impaired functional development [36]. They were never normal during development. One perspective is that if a kidney has not reached normal in the setting of obstruction, then it should be considered significantly obstructed if there is associated reduced drainage. Others take the view that evidence of loss of function in follow-up must be present to demonstrate obstruction [4]. While this may be an academic argument, one must define what is clinically considered to be significant and warrants surgical intervention. If the initial function is within 5 % of 50 %, then many are willing to observe these children for spontaneous improvement, even with reduced drainage. The ability of the washout time following diuretic to predict subsequent deterioration is inconsistent. The frequently stated 20-min threshold is not an accurate predictor, but washout times less than 20 min are more frequently associated with spontaneous improvement.

The *washout curve* must be interpreted carefully as there are differing patterns that may have significantly different outcomes [37]. The conventional method of measuring the washout is to administer the diuretic when the renal pelvis is full and the time to reach one-half of the renal pelvic counts is the t 1/2. If the tracer washout does not reach a half point, then a curve is extrapolated after 30 min. The methods to extrapolate this curve are varied and yield differing results [38]. This variation may reflect the occurrence of a *biphasic curve* where there may be an initially rapid washout that halts and then no further washout is seen (Fig. 8.2). A simple extrapolation of the initial phase of the curve would provide a very low $t_{1/2}$, which may not be at all reflective of

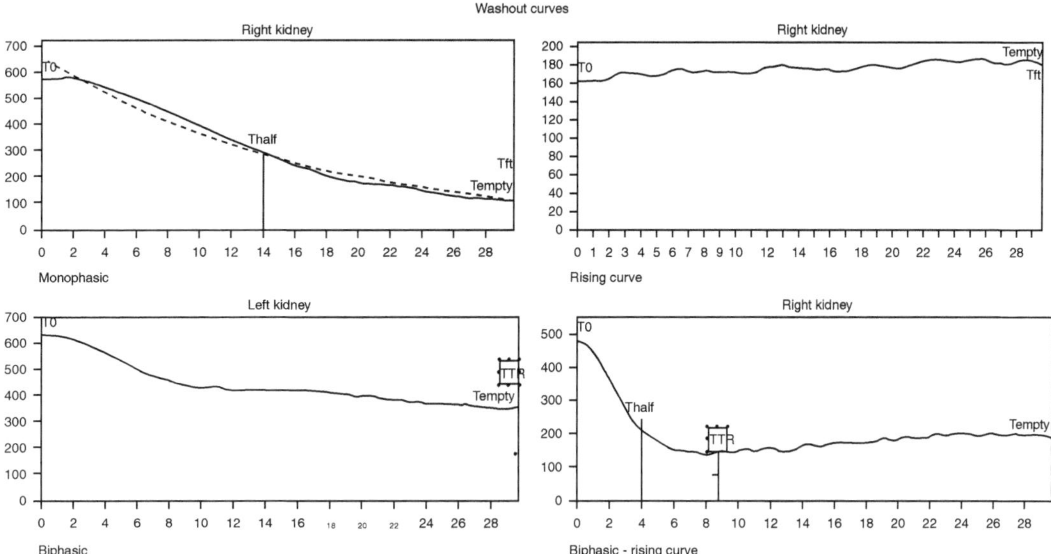

Fig. 8.2 Examples of diuretic renogram washout curves illustrating the concept of a biphasic curve with differing characteristics. A rising curve is almost always associated with significant obstruction

the system. The residual counts at 30 min may be a useful indicator as well. A rising curve is strongly indicative of high-grade obstruction, but even this has not been clearly correlated with functional deterioration. There is variability in the washout curve for an individual kidney over time, and this may reflect a dynamic obstructive process. A further parameter of the washout pattern that may offer useful clinical information is the amount of drainage after having the patient assume an upright position, suggesting that gravity can assist renal drainage [39]. This has been reported but not validated as a predictive factor in obstruction. Rapid drainage is probably an indicator of lesser degrees of obstruction.

The greatest value of the DR and *washout curve* is to monitor the status of the kidney over time, particularly when an observational approach is taken. The frequency of the testing can be defined by the initial severity, and some authors have used very frequent testing [5]. This is a burden on families and includes increased radiation. We would rarely repeat a MAG-3 before 6 months and often try to use an interval of 12 months.

There are no clear data-defined parameters for *clinically significant obstruction*, but pragmatic guides have emerged from practice. If function deteriorates more than 5 %, then intervention is likely warranted. Some will want to see a reduction of 10 % points. If the function is less than 35–40 % at initial testing and there is a significantly elevated washout time (probably greater than 30 min), then intervention should be considered. A simple increase in the washout time or the severity of hydronephrosis on ultrasound has been often used as an indication for surgery [13], but this is not necessarily associated with reduced function and can be seen to reverse itself. In the absence of clinical symptoms, the clinician will need to define for themselves and their patients thresholds for intervention with the recognition that there is little data to support these except that those parameters have usually been used as endpoints themselves.

It is well established that the *hydronephrosis* with a *UPJO* pattern can resolve spontaneously. The mechanism of this resolution is not defined, and it is often stated that this is *nonobstructive hydronephrosis*. This term begs the question of what caused the hydronephrosis, and there are no reliable answers. The fact of resolution suggests a maturational process either in the ureter itself or the bladder. This is supported by the higher frequency of hydronephrosis in boys correlated with the known pattern of high-pressure voiding seen in infant males. This was demonstrated in the sheep model with urachal ligation, which caused hydronephrosis in males only [40].

The clinical safety of an observational approach has been well documented as well, and our approach is that if initial function is above 40 % then the child can be observed, as long as the family recognizes that later surgery may be needed and that there is a risk of functional loss or the development of symptoms. It also carries the burden of follow-up testing, yet can avoid surgery in a large percentage of children. The child with more severe dilation and more delayed washout is more likely to not improve spontaneously or to deteriorate, and these parameters can be integrated into the discussion. There can be no single predictor of outcome with current technology, and as long as the family is aware of this and is reliable to return for follow-up, observation is the advisable approach. Loss of follow-up is a potential risk that must be included in the assessment of the child, however [12, 41].

While many have written of defining a kidney as obstructed or not obstructed, this suggests a black and white dichotomy that is not likely to reflect reality. These kidneys should more appropriately be seen as partially obstructed to varying degrees with the possibility of spontaneous improvement [36].

The search for adjunctive predictors of the outcome of congenital obstruction using *urinary biomarkers* has been ongoing, and yet no practical marker has come into use, despite numerous published reports of utility [35, 42–44]. It would seem highly probable that the various proteins in the urine of an obstructed kidney would reflect the condition of the kidney and its response to that obstruction. The complexity derives from the fact that congenital obstruction is dynamic and the kidney being affected is constantly changing. Various urinary proteins have been shown to vary greatly with age in the normal kidney, often with high levels in early infancy that decline rapidly with renal maturation [45]. The relative contribution of the urine (and its proteins) from the *obstructed kidney* compared to the other kidney is obviously affected by the severity of the obstruction, restricting urine drainage. Markers of pathological processes that are not present in normal kidneys would be logical targets but have not yet been confirmed to be sufficiently predictive. A further complexity has been in the definition of the clinical outcome that is to be predicted. Many reports state that surgery was the endpoint based upon criteria that, as discussed above, may be limited in their validity [46, 47]. It is also of less importance to distinguish obstructed kidneys from normals, but to define those hydronephrotic kidneys, which are likely to progress to functional deterioration. In this way, less invasive assessments can be used to monitor kidneys over time.

8.2 Surgical Decision-Making

A suggested algorithm for managing prenatally detected UPJO is shown in Fig. 8.3. Indications for *surgical intervention* may be strict or conditional. Strict indications include recurrent pain associated with increased hydronephrosis or characteristic MAG-3 findings, presence of a stone, pyelonephritis, and diminishing relative function on radionuclide scan. Increasing hydronephrosis or a worsening drainage pattern on MAG-3 to some is a strict indication, but in the absence of demonstrated functional deterioration, this is more of a conditional indication when isolated. Certainly in moderate dilation, transient increases in dilation do occur and may not predict functional deterioration. Increasing hydronephrosis and worsening drainage are associated with functional deterioration in clinical studies [13].

Conditional *indications* for surgical repair include reduced function at diagnosis, although to some this is not an indication at all [48]. When associated with severe hydronephrosis (grade 4), relative function below 40 % is an indication for surgery for the author. Persisting but stable dilation and function after several years of monitoring is a conditional indication for surgery and must be carefully discussed with the family. The burden of ongoing invasive imaging, including MAG-3 scans, will often be the motivating factor for families to move to surgery [41]. While

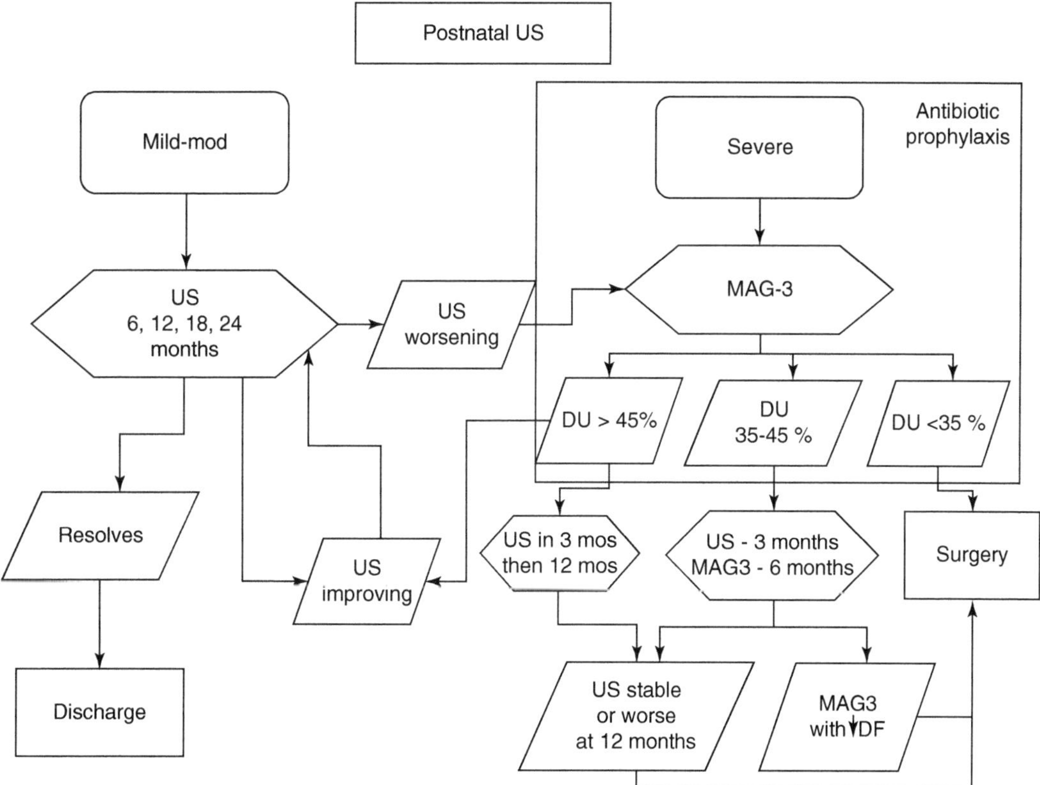

Fig. 8.3 Algorithm of a possible clinical approach to postnatal asymptomatic hydronephrosis. Antibiotic prophylaxis is frequently used during the first year of life for severe dilation

improvement in hydronephrosis has been reported at older ages, so has deterioration of function. If the family is comfortable with an observational approach and function remains stable, this is certainly reasonable. However, parental preferences should be honored, and to many, the uncertainty and burden of monitoring justify intervention. Since an *observational* approach for significant hydronephrosis with concern for *functional deterioration* requires ongoing functional assessment, the possibility of poor follow-up can be considered a conditional indication for surgery.

8.3 Surgical Correction of UPJO

The traditional method of correcting the obstructed UPJ remains the dismembered pyeloplasty (Anderson-Hynes), although numerous alternatives have been described. Minimally invasive techniques have become not only viable options but in some centers the preferred option. To date, there are limited data to validate the long-term efficacy of these approaches, yet it seems they are equally effective based on shorter-term reports.

8.3.1 Open Surgical Repair

The *Anderson-Hynes dismembered pyeloplasty*, described in 1949 for retrocaval ureter [49] and widely utilized and reported on, addresses the obstructive pathology by removal and subsequent reanastomosis. Once it was evident that ureteral peristalsis would return after dismemberment, this technique gained worldwide popularity. Several other open methods continue to be used in limited volumes. With reported success rates of 95–98 % for primary cases, it is difficult to understand why alternatives with less supporting clinical data would be used. Dismembered pyeloplasty can be approached in several ways. A lateral, muscle-splitting incision is widely used and offers excellent exposure with access to the mid-ureter if needed [50]. The incision is less painful than muscle cutting approaches. A more anterior incision can also be used with less disturbance of the lateral muscles and remains extraperitoneal, but the exposure is less direct. The dorsal *lumbotomy* approach is favored by the author for most open cases as it is a less noticeable incision, does not cut any muscle, and provides direct access to the posterior aspect of the renal pelvis. In infants this is a particularly efficient exposure as the bulging pelvis is readily accessed and brought into the field [51, 52]. The anatomy is not typically as familiar to many surgeons but can be readily learned.

Important determinants of successful *pyeloplasty* are the same for all types of procedures. These include adequate but not radical mobilization of the tissues. Excessive *mobilization* may compromise blood supply and produce fibrosis and obstructive scarring. Fully freeing the UPJ from surrounding adhesion, however, is important as the configuration of the UPJ is a clear contributor to obstruction in some cases. Adhesive bands that create sharp kinks in the proximal ureter may be contributors to intermittent obstruction. It is also important to ensure that a crossing lower pole vessel is not present and contributing to the obstruction. These are usually anterior to the ureter and have been missed with posterior retroperitoneal exposures. If there is any tension on the *anastomosis*, scarring may be produced so some mobilization of the proximal ureter and pelvis is needed. The pelvis is well vascularized and should be mobilized in favor of the ureter, but at times both must be freed.

Minimal tissue handling protects the anastomosis from excessive swelling. Stent placement is often used as an adjunct but should not be an excuse for rough handling of the tissues. Whenever possible, the tissues directly associated with the anastomosis should not be directly touched except by suture needles. Using the portion of the renal pelvis that will be discarded as a temporary handle for the proximal ureter is a practical way to limit tissue injury. Stay sutures are equally useful for open surgery but may become tangled in laparoscopic procedures.

Precise and uniform suture placement can facilitate successful pyeloplasty by limiting tissue constriction or necrosis and distribute tension equally. Both interrupted and *running suture anastomoses* are equally effective, but the author's preference has become running suture as it provides even distribution of tissue tension and a more watertight closure. Caution needs to be exercised to avoid bunching up of tissue or "purse-stringing" of the anastomosis by excessive tension on the running suture. Any absorbable suture is acceptable for pyeloplasty, but monofilament seems to produce less tissue injury and bunching, although monofilament is more difficult to use due to its stiffness and memory. The author uses poliglecaprone 25 (Monocryl; Ethicon) rather than polydioxanone (PDS; Ethicon) due to a more rapid absorption.

Drainage is a critical element of pyeloplasty, although there are several satisfactory options [53]. Non-stented repair is equally effective as stented and has been used for many years. It can be associated with acute leakage or transient obstruction, which can mandate some sort of intervention and does require use of a wound drain in the acute postoperative period. Internal stenting is very effective in the acute period but requires removal. A *double J stent* placed in an antegrade manner must be removed cystoscopically, which in children requires a general anesthetic. Stents placed retrograde with an extraction string are easily removed in the office or at home but require more time to perform the cystoscopy and stent placement just before the pyeloplasty. Antegrade placement of a *nephroureteral stent* permits temporary drainage and easy removal, but this requires placement through the renal pelvis or the renal parenchyma [54]. The author's preference is a retrograde stent with an extraction string as it permits preoperative imaging of the ureter if there is any question about ureteral anatomy. Postoperative bladder drainage is useful to limit leaking and discomfort, but not all surgeons use this. A bladder catheter is usually left in place overnight to improve upper tract drainage and has been shown to reduce postoperative wound drainage [55].

8.3.2 Minimally Invasive Pyeloplasty Techniques

Laparoscopic pyeloplasty was first described in children in 1995 [56] and the first series in 1996 by Tan and Roberts [57]. The first cases were technically challenging due to a general lack of expertise in delicate reconstructive laparoscopy as well as lack of defined operative algorithms for the procedure. While they generally followed the steps of open pyeloplasty, in retrospect, it is clear that specific setup and procedural steps have made it much more efficient. Initial results were generally comparable to open procedures, and patients subjectively recovered more rapidly. Use of the technique was limited, however, largely due to the difficult learning curve, and relatively few surgeons used the techniques. Several alternative laparoscopic methods were explored to limit the need for intraoperative suturing, which was the challenging and critical part of the procedure. These included reintroduction of the Fenger plasty, a Heineke-Mikulicz plasty of the UPJ [58], the Hellstrom procedure to transpose the UPJ below lower pole vessels [59], and a hybrid laparoscopic open procedure of mobilizing the UPJ to permit open repair [60]. While these repairs will continue to have their adherents, it is this author's concern that these techniques have never become widely accepted in open practice due to their being less effective than the traditional *Anderson-Hynes repair*. While they clearly can work in some cases, it is difficult to accurately predict in which children this is the case, and they limit the armamentarium of the surgeon intraoperatively. If the surgeon is not comfortable performing a sutured pyeloplasty laparoscopically, it makes little sense to start a procedure, "hoping" it will be a crossing vessel where the Hellstrom procedure could be used. What happens if it is not a crossing vessel? It seems more reasonable to provide the most certain repair for the child in one setting. Therefore, a dismembered pyeloplasty is the standard procedure performed in my practice with a few important exceptions.

8.3.2.1 Laparoscopic Pyeloplasty

A conventional *laparoscopic pyeloplasty* has been well described and is certainly an effective minimally invasive technique for repair of UPJO [61–63]. It does require significant practice to become efficient, yet does not require the technological resources of the robot. The operation is fundamentally the same as an open repair. *Port placement* is usually with an umbilical endoscope port (3.5–5 mm) with a midline upper working port of the same size and an ipsilateral lower quadrant port. An assistant port can be used but offers little extra value. The inferior port must be placed with consideration of the position of the actual UPJ, which, if very low, will be quite close to the port, hindering its efficacy. In those cases, the lower port may be placed in the midline.

The UPJ is exposed either *transmesenterically* by reflecting the small bowel away and identifying the UPJ through the thin mesentery. The colon is left in place, and a small peritoneotomy permits access to the pelvis. If the pelvis is not well seen or in right-sided cases, the colon is mobilized medially and the pelvis exposed. A hitch stitch is placed through the abdominal wall lateral and superior to the UPJ and passed through the pelvis at its medial edge and above the planned *pyelotomy*. This lifts and stabilizes the pelvis for repair. The pelvis is then incised in an oblique manner medial to lateral, superior to inferior to the point of most dependence just lateral to the UPJ. The pelvis is left in place on the ureter, and the lateral aspect of the ureter is spatulated to open the obstructed segment. The anastomosis is then begun at the inferior vertex of the spatulation, again with a running absorbable (preferably monofilament) suture (6-0 for infants and 5-0 for older children). Typically the anterior wall is anastomosed first to facilitate exposure of the second side. If a stent has been placed, it is useful to move the ureter as the initial sutures are placed. Prior to completion of the first side, the redundant renal pelvis is excised. The renal pelvis is irrigated of any clots prior to final completion. Drainage is similar to that for open surgery, but in general the author uses a double J stent and an overnight bladder catheter.

8.3.2.2 Robotic Pyeloplasty

The advent of the da Vinci Surgical System or *robot* (Intuitive Surgical, Inc., Sunnyvale, CA) has facilitated laparoscopic pyeloplasty in children and adults markedly, and it is now probably the most commonly used method to perform minimally invasive pediatric pyeloplasty in the USA [64–67]. The method is essentially identical to laparoscopic pyeloplasty with similar port placement and procedural steps as illustrated. Key elements to an efficient procedure include correct port placement, mobilization, and hitching of the renal pelvis and smooth running suturing of the anastomosis. With practice and an engaged team, these procedures can be completed in 1 h of robotic console time or less. Drainage and follow-up are the same as with open or laparoscopic repairs.

8.4 Outcomes

Open pediatric pyeloplasty should be associated with a high degree of clinical success and minimal need for further interventions. Although various reports use differing outcomes criteria, the anticipated success rate should be in the 97–98 % success rate for open surgery. Most reports of laparoscopic and robotic procedures are in this range as well, although the duration of follow-up and criteria for success varies. A recent meta-analysis supported this general contention [68, 69].

Complications are relatively uncommon but must be recognized [70, 71]. Minimally invasive methods, due to operating in the peritoneum, have been associated with rare GI injuries, some of which can have significant consequences. It is unclear how often this might occur in open surgery in real life, as these are not often reported. It should always be borne in mind that when working in the *retroperitoneal* space, either open or laparoscopic, the intra-abdominal structures, although not directly seen, are only millimeters away and are therefore susceptible to injury. With care, the wide view of an intraperitoneal approach lets the operator see all of the important structures.

Several reports have demonstrated that minimally invasive techniques can be successfully used in small infants [65, 66], although many surgeons limit their use to those over 6 months. We have not seen the need to use this limit but recognize that this is after a substantial experience with older children. The individual surgeon must be aware of her/his own experience and select the method best suited for their patients.

8.5 Outlook

The recent advent of advanced *minimally invasive techniques* to perform pyeloplasty in children has also offered the opportunity to perform progressively more complex operations and re-operative procedures with anticipated good success. This is one of the major arguments to continue exploration of these technologies, despite some of the concerns. Most of the objections raised reflect cost issues in the absence of demonstrable benefits. At this point in time, it may be premature to attempt to assess benefits or *cost-effectiveness* due to a significant lack of robust tools to assess benefits [72, 73]. Most reports use very crude measures of hospital length of stay, pain medication, and crude cost estimates. None of these accurately reflect the true impact of the type of procedure on the child and their family in the whole context of the encounter. Subjectively, these children seem to recover more quickly, but this is a very subjective assessment, and until we have more objective assessment techniques that reflect the physiological, psychological, and real financial impact of these technologies, we have to recognize the limitations on these claimed advantages.

8.6 Summary

Management of the presumed UPJ obstruction in a child has evolved substantially in the last three decades, although we remain limited in our ability to precisely predict who might need surgery. The evolution of a rational *observational management* strategy based on objective information has been a significant advance. We must remember, however, that this should not be seen as a reason to delay surgery in all children. It is very clear that UPJO can cause real harm to normal renal functional development, and our clinical tools are imprecise. If an observational approach is to be taken, it must be with the full understanding and partnership with the family to undertake the needed follow-up imaging and potential need to shift to a surgical approach. When surgery is needed, *minimally invasive technologies* have advanced markedly, and today highly predictable success can be expected using robotic technology or laparoscopic techniques in the hands of the highly experienced surgeon. UPJO will continue to challenge us in the sense of the need to identify the patient at risk for complications and those who can be safely observed as the underlying process resolves itself.

References

1. King LR et al (1984) The case for immediate pyeloplasty in the neonate with ureteropelvic junction obstruction. J Urol 132:636–640
2. King LR, Hatcher PA (1990) Natural history of fetal and neonatal hydronephrosis. Urology 35(5):433–438
3. Ransley PG et al (1990) The postnatal management of hydronephrosis diagnosed by prenatal ultrasound. J Urol 144(2 Pt 2):584–587; discussion 593–594
4. Koff SA (1998) Neonatal management of unilateral hydronephrosis. Role for delayed intervention. Urol Clin North Am 25(2):181–186
5. Ulman I, Jayanthi VR, Koff SA (2000) The long-term followup of newborns with severe unilateral hydronephrosis initially treated nonoperatively. J Urol 164(3 Pt 2):1101–1105
6. Josephson S, Dhillon HK, Ransley PG (1993) Postnatal management of antenatally detected, bilateral hydronephrosis. Urol Int 51(2):79–84
7. Dhillon HK (1998) Prenatally diagnosed hydronephrosis: the Great Ormond Street experience. Br J Urol 81(Suppl 2):39–44
8. Onen A, Jayanthi VR, Koff SA (2002) Long-term followup of prenatally detected severe bilateral newborn hydronephrosis initially managed nonoperatively. J Urol 168(3):1118–1120
9. Homsy YL et al (1990) Transitional hydronephrosis of the newborn and infant. J Urol 144:579–583
10. Arnold AJ, Rickwood AM (1990) Natural history of pelviureteric obstruction detected by prenatal sonography. Br J Urol 65(1):91–96
11. Palmer LS et al (1998) Surgery versus observation for managing obstructive grade 3 to 4 unilateral hydronephrosis: a report from the Society for Fetal Urology. J Urol 159(1):222–228
12. Thorup J et al (2003) The results of 15 years of consistent strategy in treating antenatally suspected pelviureteric junction obstruction. BJU Int 91(9):850–852
13. Ross SS et al (2011) Observation of infants with SFU grades 3–4 hydronephrosis: worsening drainage with serial diuresis renography indicates surgical intervention and helps prevent loss of renal function. J Pediatr Urol 7(3):266–271
14. Madden NP et al (1991) Antenatally detected pelviureteric junction obstruction. Is non-operation safe? Br J Urol 68(3):305–310
15. Takla NV et al (1998) Apparent unilateral ureteropelvic junction obstruction in the newborn: expectations for resolution. J Urol 160:2175–2178
16. Subramaniam R, Kouriefs C, Dickson AP (1999) Antenatally detected pelvi-ureteric junction obstruction: concerns about conservative management. BJU Int 84(3):335–338
17. Heinlen JE et al (2009) Operative versus nonoperative management of ureteropelvic junction obstruction in children. Urology 73(3):521–525; discussion 525
18. Erickson BA et al (2007) Newborn society of fetal urology grade 3 hydronephrosis is equivalent to preserved percentage differential function. J Pediatr Urol 3(5):382–386
19. Eskild-Jensen A et al (2003) Renal function may not be restored when using decreasing differential function as the criterion for surgery in unilateral hydronephrosis. BJU Int 92(7):779–782
20. Capolicchio G et al (1999) Prenatal diagnosis of hydronephrosis: impact on renal function and its recovery after pyeloplasty. J Urol 162(3 Pt 2):1029–1032
21. Salem YH et al (1995) Outcome analysis of pediatric pyeloplasty as a function of patient age, presentation and differential renal function. J Urol 154(5): 1889–1893
22. McAleer IM, Kaplan GW (1999) Renal function before and after pyeloplasty: does it improve? J Urol 162(3 Pt 2):1041–1044
23. Pohl HG et al (2001) Early diuresis renogram findings predict success following pyeloplasty. J Urol 165(6 Pt 2):2311–2315
24. Romao RL et al (2012) Early postoperative ultrasound after open pyeloplasty in children with prenatal hydronephrosis helps identify low risk of recurrent obstruction. J Urol 188(6):2347–2353
25. Rushton HG et al (1994) Pediatric pyeloplasty: is routine retrograde pyelography necessary? J Urol 152(2 Pt 2):604–606
26. Kang X et al (2013) Automatic analysis of pediatric renal ultrasound using shape, anatomical and image acquisition priors. Med Image Comput Comput Assist Interv 16(Pt 3):259–266

27. Conway JJ, Maizels M (1992) The "well tempered" diuretic renogram: a standard method to examine the asymptomatic neonate with hydronephrosis or hydroureteronephrosis. A report from combined meetings of The Society for Fetal Urology and members of The Pediatric Nuclear Medicine Council – The Society of Nuclear Medicine. J Nucl Med 33:2047–2051
28. Chung S et al (1993) Diuretic renography in the evaluation of neonatal hydronephrosis: is it reliable? J Urol 150(2 Pt 2):765–768
29. Homayoon K et al (1998) Relative accuracy of renal scan in estimation of renal function during partial ureteral obstruction. Can J Urol 5(4):611–619
30. Eskild-Jensen A et al (2004) Interpretation of the renogram: problems and pitfalls in hydronephrosis in children. BJU Int 94(6):887–892
31. Pippi Salle JL et al (2008) The importance of obtaining conjugate views on renographic evaluation of large hydronephrotic kidneys: an in vitro and ex vivo analysis. J Urol 180(4):1559–1565
32. Huang WY et al (2006) Renal biopsy in congenital ureteropelvic junction obstruction: evidence for parenchymal maldevelopment. Kidney Int 69(1):137–143
33. Zhang PL, Peters CA, Rosen S (2000) Ureteropelvic junction obstruction: morphological and clinical studies. Pediatr Nephrol 14(8–9):820–826
34. Kiratli PO et al (2008) Relation between radionuclide imaging and pathologic findings of ureteropelvic junction obstruction in neonatal hydronephrosis. Scand J Urol Nephrol 42(3):249–256
35. Chevalier RL (2004) Biomarkers of congenital obstructive nephropathy: past, present and future. J Urol 172(3):852–857
36. Peters CA (1995) Urinary tract obstruction in children. J Urol 154(5):1874–1883; discussion 1883–1884
37. Koff SA et al (2005) Renal pelvis volume during diuresis in children with hydronephrosis: implications for diagnosing obstruction with diuretic renography. J Urol 174(1):303–307
38. Connolly LP et al (2000) Variability of diuresis renography interpretation due to method of post-diuretic renal pelvic clearance half-time determination. J Urol 164(2):467–471
39. Piepsz A (2011) Antenatal detection of pelviureteric junction stenosis: main controversies. Semin Nucl Med 41(1):11–19
40. Gobet R, Bleakley J, Peters CA (1998) Premature urachal closure induces hydroureteronephrosis in male fetuses. J Urol 160(4):1463–1467
41. Eskild-Jensen A et al (2005) Congenital unilateral hydronephrosis: a review of the impact of diuretic renography on clinical treatment. J Urol 173(5):1471–1476
42. Decramer S et al (2006) Predicting the clinical outcome of congenital unilateral ureteropelvic junction obstruction in newborn by urinary proteome analysis. Nat Med 12(4):398–400
43. Decramer S, Bascands JL, Schanstra JP (2007) Non-invasive markers of ureteropelvic junction obstruction. World J Urol 25(5):457–465
44. Madsen MG et al (2011) Urinary biomarkers in prenatally diagnosed unilateral hydronephrosis. J Pediatr Urol 7(2):105–112
45. Lee RS et al (2008) Temporal variations of the postnatal rat urinary proteome as a reflection of systemic maturation. Proteomics 8(5):1097–1112
46. Bartoli F et al (2011) Urinary epidermal growth factor, monocyte chemotactic protein-1, and beta2-microglobulin in children with ureteropelvic junction obstruction. J Pediatr Surg 46(3):530–536
47. Taranta-Janusz K et al (2013) Urinary angiotensinogen as a novel marker of obstructive nephropathy in children. Acta Paediatr 102(9):e429–e433
48. Koff SA (2000) Postnatal management of antenatal hydronephrosis using an observational approach. Urology 55(5):609–611
49. Anderson JC, Hynes W (1949) Retrocaval ureter; a case diagnosed pre-operatively and treated successfully by a plastic operation. Br J Urol 21(3):209–214
50. Hensle TW, Shabsigh A (2004) Pyeloplasty (Anderson-Hynes). BJU Int 93(7):1123–1134
51. Onol FF et al (2009) Short stay pyeloplasty with transverse dorsal lumbotomy incision: our 10-year experience. Urology 74(6):1309–1312
52. Sheldon CA, Duckett JW, Snyder HM (1992) Evolution in the management of infant pyeloplasty. J Pediatr Surg 27(4):501–505
53. Bayne AP et al (2011) The impact of surgical approach and urinary diversion on patient outcomes in pediatric pyeloplasty. J Urol 186(4 Suppl): 1693–1698
54. Taveres A et al (2008) Insertion of an internal-external nephroureteral stent during pediatric laparoscopic pyeloplasty: description of the technique. Urology 71(6):1199–1202
55. Wollin M et al (1989) Priorities in urinary diversion following pyeloplasty. J Urol 142(2 Pt 2):576–578; discussion 603–605
56. Peters CA, Schlussel RN, Retik AB (1995) Pediatric laparoscopic dismembered pyeloplasty. J Urol 153(6):1962–1965
57. Tan HL, Roberts JP (1996) Laparoscopic dismembered pyeloplasty in children: preliminary results. Br J Urol 77(6):909–913
58. Polok M et al (2011) Nondismembered pyeloplasty in a pediatric population: results of 34 open and laparoscopic procedures. Urology 78(4):891–894
59. Schneider A et al (2013) Lower pole vessels in children with pelviureteric junction obstruction: laparoscopic vascular hitch or dismembered pyeloplasty? J Pediatr Urol 9(4):419–423
60. Farhat W et al (2004) Retroperitoneal-assisted laparoscopic pyeloplasty in children: initial experience. J Endourol 18(9):879–882
61. Braga LH et al (2010) Comparison of flank, dorsal lumbotomy and laparoscopic approaches for dismembered pyeloplasty in children older than 3 years with ureteropelvic junction obstruction. J Urol 183(1): 306–311

62. El-Ghoneimi A et al (2003) Laparoscopic dismembered pyeloplasty by a retroperitoneal approach in children. BJU Int 92(1):104–108; discussion 108
63. Tong Q et al (2009) Comparison of laparoscopic-assisted versus open dismembered pyeloplasty for ureteropelvic junction obstruction in infants: intermediate results. Urology 74(4):889–893
64. Franco I, Dyer LL, Zelkovic P (2007) Laparoscopic pyeloplasty in the pediatric patient: hand sewn anastomosis versus robotic assisted anastomosis–is there a difference? J Urol 178(4 Pt 1):1483–1486
65. Kutikov A et al (2006) Robot assisted pyeloplasty in the infant-lessons learned. J Urol 176(5):2237–2239; discussion 2239–40
66. Lee RS et al (2006) Pediatric robot assisted laparoscopic dismembered pyeloplasty: comparison with a cohort of open surgery. J Urol 175(2):683–687; discussion 687
67. Olsen LH, Rawashdeh YF, Jorgensen TM (2007) Pediatric robot assisted retroperitoneoscopic pyeloplasty: a 5-year experience. J Urol 178(5):2137–2141; discussion 2141
68. Braga LH et al (2009) Systematic review and meta-analysis of robotic-assisted versus conventional laparoscopic pyeloplasty for patients with ureteropelvic junction obstruction: effect on operative time, length of hospital stay, postoperative complications, and success rate. Eur Urol 56(5):848–857
69. Autorino R et al (2014) Robot-assisted and laparoscopic repair of ureteropelvic junction obstruction: a systematic review and meta-analysis. Eur Urol 65(2):430–452
70. Passerotti CC et al (2008) Patterns and predictors of laparoscopic complications in pediatric urology: the role of ongoing surgical volume and access techniques. J Urol 180(2):681–685
71. Nerli RB et al (2009) Complications of laparoscopic pyeloplasty in children. Pediatr Surg Int 25(4): 343–347
72. Peters CA (2004) Robotically assisted paediatric pyeloplasty: cutting edge or expensive toy? BJU Int 94(9):1214–1215
73. Peters CA (2009) Pediatric robotic-assisted surgery: too early an assessment? Pediatrics 124(6):1680–1681

One-Trocar-Assisted Pyeloplasty (OTAP)

9

Noemi Cantone, Francesca Destro, Giovanni Ruggeri, and Mario Lima

For several years open dismembered pyeloplasty through a retroperitoneal approach has been considered the gold standard for the treatment of pelvic ureteral junction obstruction (UPJO) in children and adults. In order to minimize the surgical morbidity of the open approach, many minimally invasive procedures have been introduced in the last decade in the field of pediatric urology [1, 2]. Both transperitoneal and retroperitoneal approach have been proposed [3–5]. All these procedures have been shown to be comparable to open pyeloplasty in success rates and operative time. However, the small operative space and the technical difficulties have strongly limited minimally invasive surgery. The first laparoscopic-assisted pyeloplasty was performed by El Gohary in 2004 [6]. Three ports were used to expose the ureteral junction obstruction (UPJ), and the pyeloplasty was performed in an open way.

Since 2005 in our center, we performed the one-trocar-assisted pyeloplasty (OTAP) [7]. This procedure was born to simplify the technique, combining the advantages of traditional surgery with those of a minimally invasive approach. Different from other techniques, we use only one port and an operative optic that allows the access in the renal lodge; after the exteriorization of the pyeloureteral junction through the small incision, we perform a classic pyeloplasty [8, 9].

9.1 Surgical Technique

The OTAP technique can be performed in every patient without absolute contraindications; relative contraindications are represented by huge pyelic dilatation, previous retroperitoneal surgery, and previous renal trauma.

General anesthesia by orotracheal intubation is used for all patients. The child is placed in lateral decubitus on the healthy flank over a roll with the omolateral arm elevated. An endourethral catheter is inserted. A 12 mm long incision is made on the prolongation of eleventh to twelfth rib (Fig. 9.1). The Gerota fascia and the perirenal fat are reached after blunt dissection through the muscles. We used a 10 mm trocar with a balloon-anchorage system and a 10 mm zero-degree lens operative telescope with a 5 mm operative channel. A retroperitoneal working chamber is created with peanuts and insufflations of CO_2 (8–10 mmHg of pressure and 0.5–1 l/min of flow depending on the patient's size). After identification of the kidney and the pelvis, the UPJ is anteriorly approached. It is isolated using an "L" dissector (Fig. 9.2) and exteriorized by a vessel loop through the lumbar incision (Figs. 9.3 and 9.4). Small vessels are coagulated by unipolar cautery. If necessary, the

N. Cantone (✉) • F. Destro • G. Ruggeri • M. Lima
Department of Pediatric Surgery,
S. Orsola-Malpighi University Hospital,
Bologna 40138, Italy
e-mail: noemicantone@hotmail.it;
francesca_destro@hotmail.com;
Mirella.mogiatti@studio.unibo.it;
giovanni_ruggeri@aosp.bo.it; mario.lima@unibo.it

M. Lima, G. Manzoni (eds.), *Pediatric Urology: Contemporary Strategies from Fetal Life to Adolescence*,
DOI 10.1007/978-88-470-5693-0_9, © Springer-Verlag Italia 2015

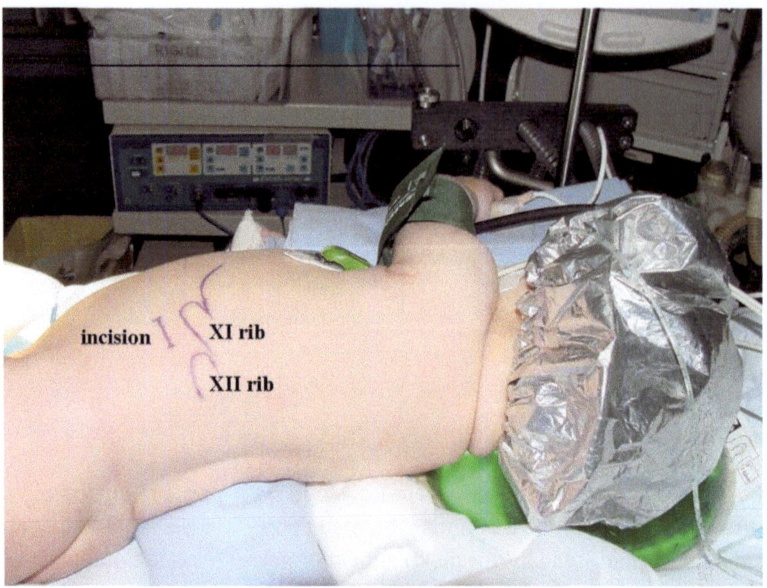

Fig. 9.1 Patient's position

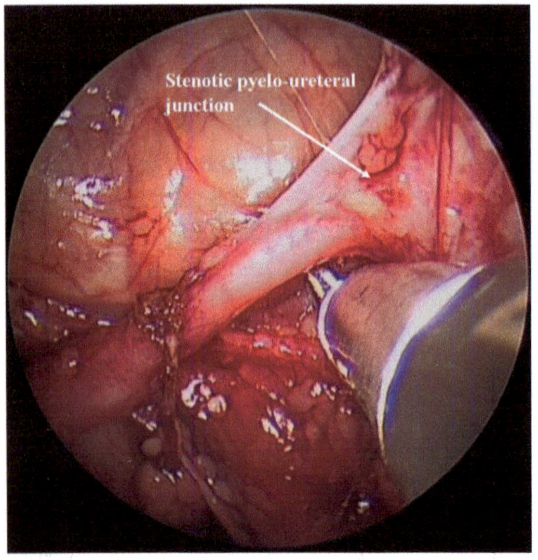

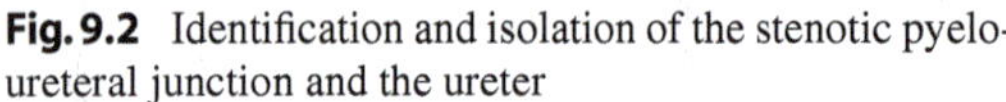
Fig. 9.2 Identification and isolation of the stenotic pyelo-ureteral junction and the ureter

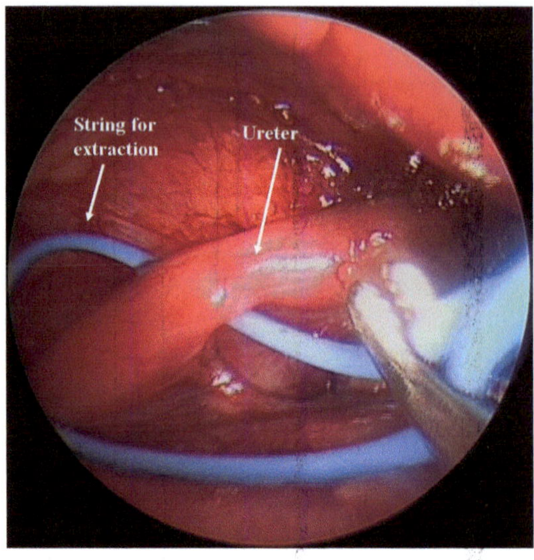

Fig. 9.3 The ureter is surrounded by a soft tape

giant hydronephrosis is aspirated by a needle. An Anderson–Hynes pyeloplasty is then performed in the traditional way using 6-0 or 7-0 polydioxanone suture. Any redundant renal pelvis is reduced before suturing (Figs. 9.5 and 9.6). In case of massive hydronephrosis, difficult pyeloplasty, or bad renal function, it is recommended to use a nephrostomic Mazeman catheter or a double pig-tail endourethral stent (Fig. 9.7); the correct position of the stent is checked by injection of methylene blue through the Foley catheter placed at the beginning. When the pyeloplasty is completed, the pelvis is repositioned in the renal lodge. The correct position of the pyeloureteral anastomosis and the absence of bleeding are checked at the end by a retroperitoneoscopic look (Fig. 9.8). A soft Penrose drain is left in place near the anastomosis and the wound is closed by absorbable suture.

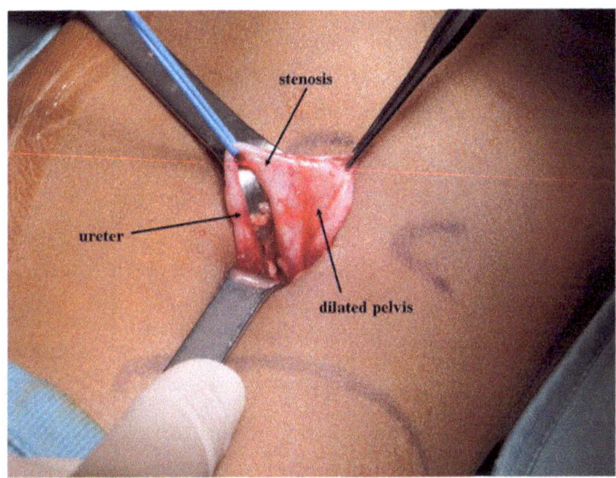

Fig. 9.4 The dilated pelvis and the proximal ureter are exteriorized through the lumbar incision

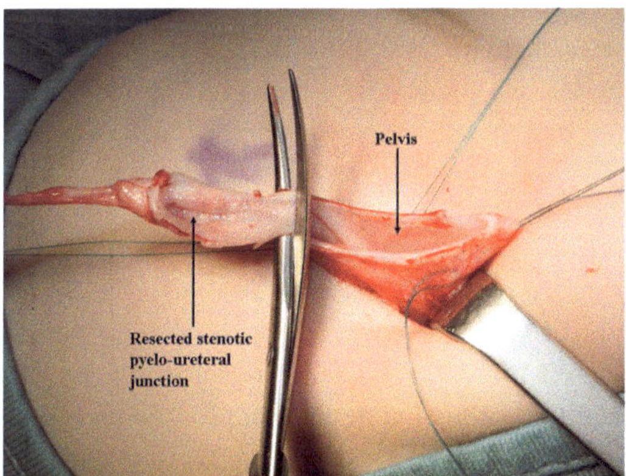

Fig. 9.5 Resection of the stenotic tract

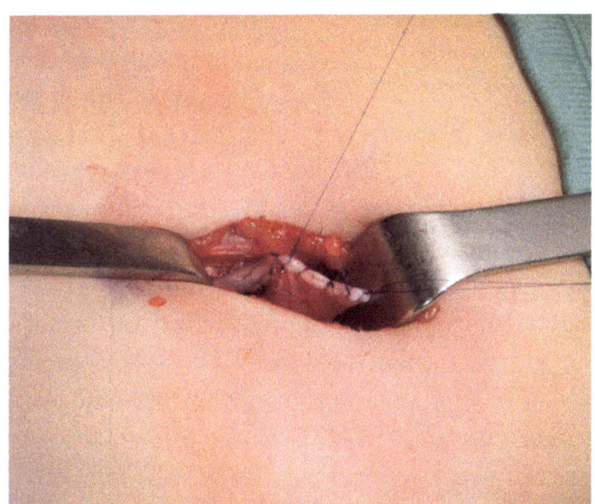

Fig. 9.6 The external image of Anderson–Hynes pyeloplasty

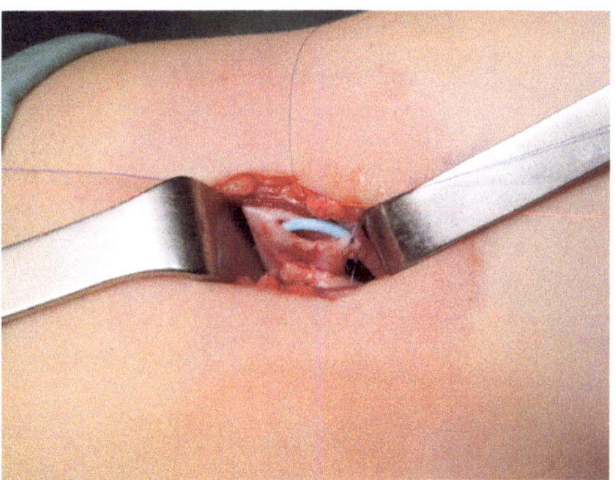

Fig. 9.7 A double-j stent is placed before completing the anastomosis

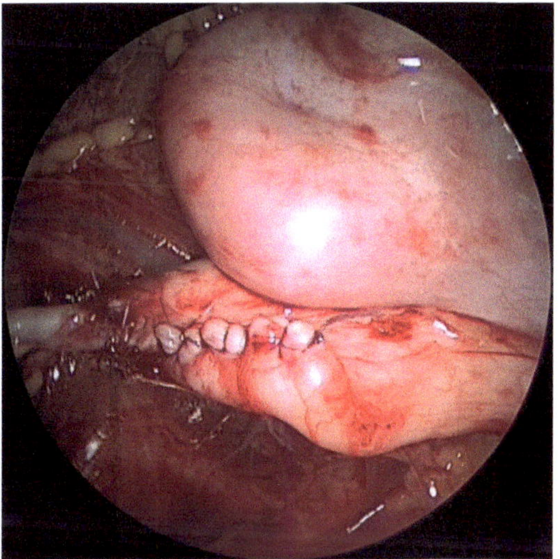

Fig. 9.8 The retroperitoneoscopic control at the end of the procedure

This technique is applicable both in case of intrinsic and extrinsic obstructions, e.g., the presence of a crossing vessel. In the last case, the vessel is de-crossed from UPJ before the exteriorization of the same; then the anastomosis is performed in the same abovementioned way (Figs. 9.9 and 9.10).

In case of difficult dissection one or two 3 mm instruments can be added.

In the postoperative time an appropriate dose of a prophylactic antibiotic (full dose for 5 days and 50 % dose after) must be given until Mazeman catheter or Double-J-stent is removed (on the 5th

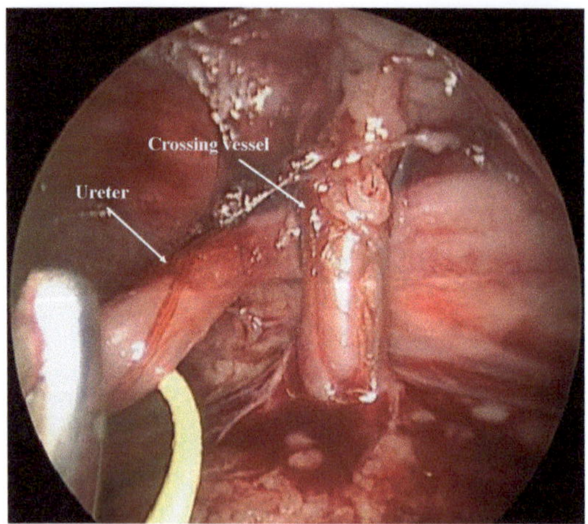

Fig. 9.9 Identification of an inferior polar renal vessel that compresses the proximal ureter

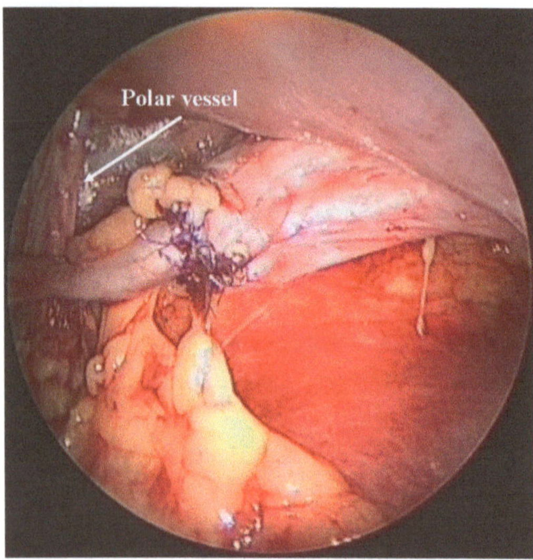

Fig. 9.10 Retroperitoneoscopic control: the polar vessel is behind the anastomosis

and 20th postoperative day respectively). The transurethral catheter is removed on the first postoperative day, whereas the drain is removed on the second postoperative day. The patient is discharged on the third postoperative day.

The *complication rate* is similar to the other techniques. The most common is the opening of the peritoneum (5.6 %), frequently when the operator is least experienced; in this case the pyeloplasty is performed in an open way. The event of a retroperitoneal urinoma is rare (3.4 %). Recurrence (1 %) should be due to fibrosis or ureter angles near the anastomosis; it is related to a difficult dissection that can cause ischemia and tension.

Follow-up consisted of a US evaluation after 1, 3, 6, and 12 months. A renal scan with MAG 3 is performed in selected cases, depending on radiological and clinical evaluation. The efficacy of the treatment is defined as absence of symptoms, decreased of pelvicaliceal dilatation on US, and improved renal drainage on renography.

OTAP is an efficacious alternative for the correction of UPJO in children. Despite the limited working chamber of the retroperitoneal approach, this procedure allows a rapid and direct access to renal pelvis with a good vessel exposition; otherwise, it maintains the advantage to realize the pelvic anastomosis in a comfortable space as in the traditional open technique. OTAP has all the advantages of a minimally invasive approach: feasibility, safety, less postoperative pain, short hospital stay, and good cosmesis. The high success rate is comparable to that of open pyeloplasty. Operative time is similar or even shorter than that of laparoscopic or retroperitoneoscopic approaches, including the time for the preoperative cystoscopy. Consideration of all, in our center, OTAP has replaced the standard technique.

9.2 Personal Experience

At our pediatric surgery department, we performed 88 OTAP in the last 8 years. The mean operative time was 139 min (range 60–225 min), and it was not influenced by aberrant vessels. Conversion to open repair was required in seven cases (mean age 19 months): five peritoneal opening and two technical difficulties. The postoperative course was characterized by urinary collection around the kidney ($n=3$) and recurrence ($n=1$). One patient among the three with urinary collection had a scarce urinary leakage and he was treated conservatively. In two cases the urinary collection required a reintervention with the placement of a transanastomotic stent to replace the former one that was accidentally removed. Follow-up was available in all patients (range 6–96 months). The comparison between preoperative and 3 months postoperative ultrasound showed a decrease of the severity of the hydronephrosis in 77 patients (87.5 %) and a stable disease in 11 patients (12.5 %). The success rate in symptomatic patients was 100 % (resolution of symptoms). All parents were satisfied with the aesthetical result.

References

1. El-Ghoneimi A (2004) Laparoscopic management of hydronephrosis in children. World J Urol 22:415–417
2. Gundeti MS, Kojima Y, Haga N et al (2013) Robotic-assisted laparoscopic reconstructive surgery in the lower urinary tract. Curr Urol Rep 14:333–341
3. Janetschek G, Peschel R, Altarac S et al (1996) Laparoscopic and retroperitoneoscopic repair of ureteropelvic junction obstruction. Urology 47:311–316
4. Reddy M, Nerli RB, Bashetty R et al (2005) Laparoscopic dismembered pyeloplasty in children. J Urol 174:700–704
5. El-Ghoneimi A, Farhat W, Bolduc S et al (2003) Laparoscopic dismembered pyeloplasty by a retroperitoneal approach in children. BJU Int 92:104–108
6. El Gohary MA (2004) Laparoscopic assisted pyeloplasty in children. Ped Endosurg Innov Tech 8:260–263
7. Lima M, Tursini S, Ruggeri G et al (2007) One trocar assisted pyeloplasty (OTAP): initial experience and codification of a technique. Pediatr Med Chir 29:108–111
8. Caione P, Lais A, Nappo SG (2010) One-port retroperitoneoscopic assisted pyeloplasty versus open dismembered pyeloplasty in young children: preliminary experience. J Urol 184:2109–2115
9. Scuderi MG, Arena S, Di Benedetto V (2011) One-trocar-assisted pyeloplasty. J Laparoendosc Adv Surg Tech A 21:651–654

Ureterovesical Junction Obstruction

10

Serdar Tekgul

10.1 Background

Leonardo da Vinci and Galen were the first who looked at the ureterovesical junction (UVJ) to identify causes of dilated ureter. Semblinow in 1883 made the first animal experiments to understand the pathophysiology of ureterovesical junction, which led to modern era of research to clarify the anatomy, function, and pathophysiology of UVJ anomalies.

In 1923, Caulk first described distal ureteral dilatation without evidence of hydronephrosis [1]. Thirty years later, Swenson postulated a neurologic etiology for both megacolon and megaureter [2]. Hendren later advanced the field of surgical management of megaureter through aggressive ureteral remodeling [3].

The clinical presentation of ureterovesical junction obstruction is the existence of a megaureter. The ureter that is dilated out of proportion is named as megaureter. Any ureter dilated more than 7 mm is considered to be a megaureter [4, 5]. The dilatation may be due to obstruction or reflux or neither (nonrefluxing, nonobstructed). The cause may be either primary (congenital) or secondary.

When a megaureter is diagnosed, the challenge is to be able to make the distinction whether this megaureter is really due to a significant obstruction or due to some other cause.

S. Tekgul, MD, FEAPU
Division of Pediatric Urology,
Department of Urology, Hacettepe University,
Sihhiye, Ankara 06100, Turkey
e-mail: serdartekgul@gmail.com

10.2 Pathophysiology and Classification

Congenital ureteral dilatation may be caused by vesicoureteric reflux, obstructive disease, high urine flow from non-concentrating kidneys, and maldevelopment of ureteral musculature. Bacterial toxins from infection within the system can increase the degree of megaureter and can even dilate a normal ureter by toxic paralysis of the muscle cells. A significant number of megaureters are diagnosed following an episode of urinary infection, and usually more than one of the above factors is present in any individual case. Thus, the exact contribution of reflux, infection, or ureteral malformation can be hard to quantitate in some cases of megaureter.

There are several classifications, varying from simple to complex. The international classification is based on evaluation of the urinary tract by ultrasonography and voiding cystourethrography [7]. In this classification, there are four categories of megaureters:

- Refluxing
- Obstructing
- Refluxing/obstructing
- Nonrefluxing/nonobstructing

Each category is further divided into primary or secondary, based on either intrinsic or extrinsic causes for their appearance.

M. Lima, G. Manzoni (eds.), *Pediatric Urology: Contemporary Strategies from Fetal Life to Adolescence*,
DOI 10.1007/978-88-470-5693-0_10, © Springer-Verlag Italia 2015

Primary obstructed megaureter is commonly caused by an aperistaltic segment of the distal ureter that fails to maintain urine flow effectively. This partial obstruction in the abnormal distal segment of the ureter leads to an impairment in ureteral drainage, functional obstruction. Progression to hydronephrosis occurs when the ureter no longer accommodates resistance to urinary drainage; pressure is then transferred more proximally. Complete obstructions are rare and are regularly associated with a nonfunctioning renal unit at diagnosis.

Different histopathologic variants including dense collagen deposition, distal circular smooth muscle hypertrophy, muscular dysplasia, and muscular derangement have been reported in different studies, which looked at the distal end of the dilated ureters [7–9].

Secondary obstructed megaureter occurs usually when ureteral dilatation is the result of a functional ureteral obstruction associated with elevated bladder pressures in posterior urethral valves (PUV) or neurogenic bladder.

Primary refluxing megaureter is related with severe vesicoureteric reflux (VUR) that changes ureteral efficiency by ureteral distention and by progressive increase of the volume of urine that needs to be pushed back into the bladder. The drainage of the ureter is usually normal. The megaureter-megacystis syndrome is an extreme form of the primary refluxing megaureters in which massive reflux prevents effective bladder emptying because urine is passed back and forth between the ureters and bladder (Fig. 10.1).

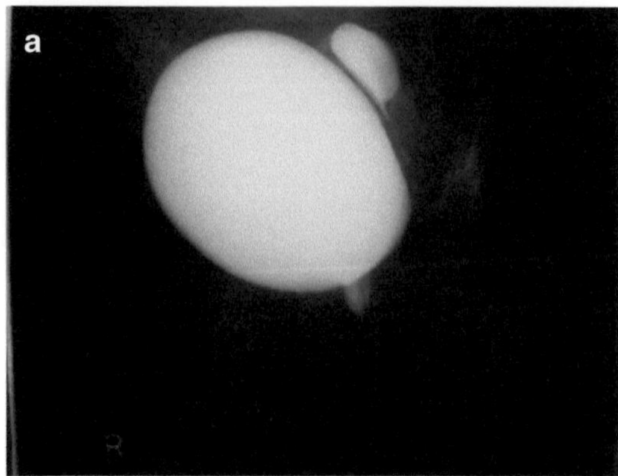

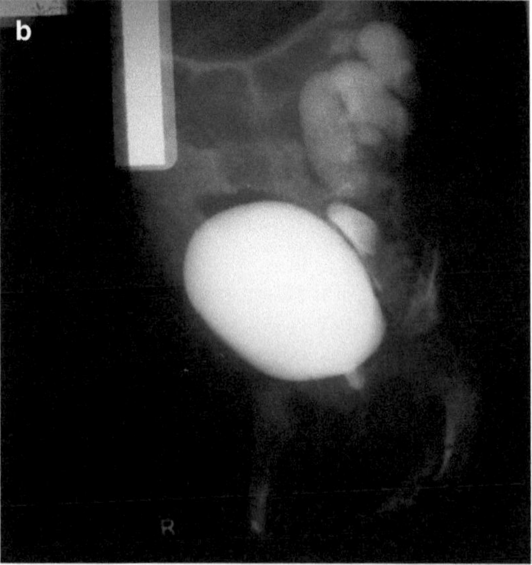

Fig. 10.1 (**a**, **b**) Refluxing obstructing megaureter; opaque can hardly reflux into the dilated upper tract because of obstructing segment at the distal end

Varying degrees of increased collagen deposition (predominantly collagen type III) have been shown in the refluxing megaureters; this was much more marked when compared to obstructed megaureters [10, 11]. All histologic abnormalities are more pronounced at the very distal portion of the ureter, which is an important concept to remember when doing reimplantation.

Secondary refluxing megaureter occurs secondary to elevated bladder pressures (like in PUV or neurogenic bladder). This results in decompensation of the ureterovesical junction (UVJ).

Primary nonrefluxing/nonobstructed megaureter is the dilated ureter when there is no evidence of obstruction or reflux. The etiology is unclear. The sudden increase in urine output in fetal life may overcome the dynamic ability of the ureter to transit urine and may cause a transient dilatation of the ureter. Many studies reported that spontaneous resolution of this condition over time. Time to resolution and degree of resolution were mainly based in the initial grade of hydronephrosis or degree of dilatation of the distal part of the ureter [12, 13].

Secondary nonrefluxing/nonobstructed megaureter occurs secondary to diabetes insipidus, in which high urinary flow rates may overcome the maximum transport capacity of the ureter by peristalsis. It may also be as a result of ureteral atony accompanying a urinary tract infection (UTI).

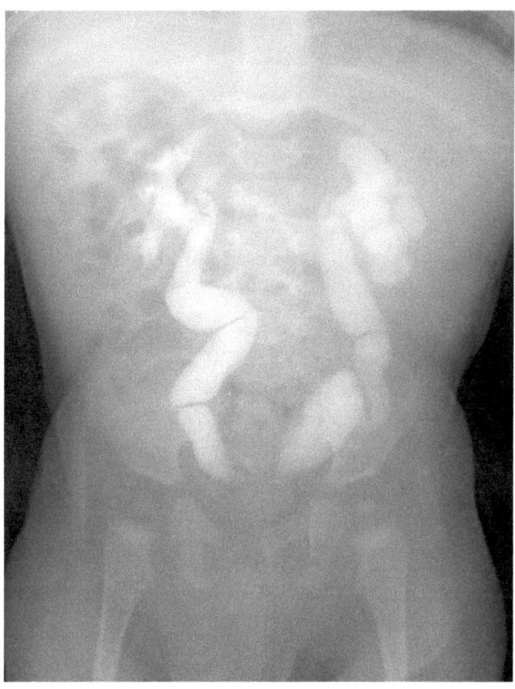

Fig. 10.2 Refluxing obstructing megaureter; following bladder emptying the opaque material in the upper collecting system does not freely flow back into the bladder because of obstruction at UVJ

In some cases ureterovesical junction (UVJ) is anatomically and functionally not normal in a way leading to reflux of urine associated with poor drainage of the urine back into the bladder. These are *refluxing and obstructed megaureter*, and this condition may have serious detrimental effect on the kidney (Figs. 10.1 and 10.2).These ureters should be considered for definitive repair, and the endoscopic injection is contraindicated in this condition as it may enhance obstruction.

10.3 Presentation

In patients with megaureters, there are usually no specific clinical signs. The use of prenatal US have dramatically increased the diagnosis of megaureters. Therefore, they usually present with an abnormal finding on routine prenatal ultrasound before being associated symptoms or infection. Before the era of prenatal US, all patients would have been seen with significant clinical symptoms [6]. Still some patients may present with symptoms like urinary tract infection (UTI), recurring abdominal pain, abdominal mass, and hematuria. In the remaining, the diagnosis may be incidental after imaging studies for unrelated symptoms. In advanced bilateral disease with renal insufficiency, megaureters may be discovered during the evaluation for hypertension or proteinuria.

10.4 Diagnosis (Diagnosis of Megaureters)

The main goal is to define the extent of the problem and make a distinction as regards which patients will require a surgical intervention and which will be observed.

It is important to exclude the presence of reflux and define the group of patients with obstruction, which may eventually lead to renal impairment. This will require imaging studies like ultrasonography US and voiding cystourethrography (VCUG) that will show the presence of reflux and anatomic details of the urinary system. Functional studies will be required to see the renal function status and urinary drainage.

Ultrasonography is the primary imaging modality and usually serves as the screening study in the prenatal period and the initial study in the symptomatic group.

The study should include assessment of the degree of hydronephrosis based on the Society for Fetal Urology grading of hydronephrosis (Table 10.1) and the distal ureteric morphology/ size.

One should evaluate the size, shape, tortuosity, and bulbar appearance of the ureter as well the peristaltic activity of the ureter. The course of the ureter should be evaluated from the kidney to its insertion to bladder. An obstructed distal segment can be recognized when the peristaltic activity stops at a point near the bladder. In obstructed, high-pressure systems, the peristaltic activity may be lost totally, and the whole ureter may be seen as dilated in its entire length.

Table 10.1 The Society for Fetal Urology hydronephrosis grading on ultrasonography

Grade I – Splitting of the renal sinus more than 10 mm
Grade II – Splitting of the renal sinus more than 10 mm in an extrarenal or intrarenal pelvis not extending to the calyces
Grade III – Dilatation extending into the calyces without cortical thinning
Grade IV – Dilatation extending into the calyces with cortical thinning

Ultrasonographic investigation may further provide information about the presence of calculi, echogenic debris suggesting infection, and condition of remaining renal units.

Voiding cystourethrography (VCUG) is performed to assess for the presence of vesicoureteric reflux and to further delineate the anatomy of the bladder and outlet. In cases with bilateral megaureter, any possible outlet obstruction or major bladder dysfunction must be excluded. In cases with high-grade reflux, a meticulous investigation of drainage of ureter after voiding should be done to exclude the presence of an also obstructing segment. This obstructing distal segment can be envisioned when the reflux of opaque material up into the collecting system or drainage of it back into the bladder is slow or compromised.

Functional studies will often be needed to get quantitative information about the function of each renal unit and to understand its dynamics. Diuretic renography is the most commonly used diagnostic tool to detect the severity and functional significance of problems with urine transport. 99mTc-MAG3 is the radionuclide of choice. It is important to perform the study under standardized circumstances (hydration, transurethral catheter) between the 4th and 6th weeks of life. Oral fluid intake is encouraged prior to the examination. At 15 min before the injection of the radionuclide, it is mandatory to administer normal saline intravenous infusion at a rate of 15 mL/kg over 30 min, with a subsequent maintenance rate of 4 mL/kg/h throughout the whole time of the investigation. The recommended dose of furosemide is 1 mg/kg for infants during the first year of life, while 0.5 mg/kg should be given to children aged 1–16 years, up to a maximum dose of 40 mg [13].

In cases in which anatomic definition is anticipated, intravenous urography (IVU) can be used if renal function is good and the degree of obstruction to the affected renal unit is mild. As IVU has technical limitations for providing a good imaging in infants, currently magnetic resonance imaging (MRI) is the method of choice to define the anatomic details. MRI can provide a three-dimensional depiction of the urinary collecting system. The requirement for special software to assess renal function accurately and the need for restraint, sedation, or general anesthesia limit its application in neonates and infants.

Despite the wide range of diagnostic tests, there is no single test that can accurately distinguish obstructive from nonobstructive cases. Therefore, serial studies will often be needed to understand the natural course of the disease and to understand if the condition is causing progressive renal damage.

10.5 Management

The management is mainly based on classification. If the dilatation of the ureter is secondary to outlet obstruction, neurogenic bladder, ureterocele, or diabetes insipidus, the treatment for the primary cause should be employed.

For the remaining primary megaureters, it is essential to exclude the presence of reflux. After reflux is excluded, any form of impaired drainage of the megaureter that is causing progressive hydronephrosis, loss of renal function, or symptoms needs to be identified and treated accordingly. All the rest should be followed up conservatively.

For the refluxing group, the initial management will also be conservative. If there are breakthrough infections despite prophylaxis, intervention for reflux should be considered. This may include less invasive procedures like endoscopic treatment, but eventually most symptomatic patients with refluxing megaureters will require reimplantation of the ureter.

If the patients with nonrefluxing megaureters are symptomatic (recurring UTI, pain, hematuria), then surgical correction should be considered at the first place. The different surgical options will be discussed below.

In all other cases, presenting with prenatal US or with incidental imaging conservative management is employed with periodic surveillance using US and functional studies. If a functional study reveals and confirms adequate ureteral drainage, conservative management is the best option for megaureters. Initially, low-dose prophylactic antibiotics within the first year of life are recommended for the prevention of urinary tract infections, although the evidence for the use of this course of therapy is poor.

There have been a good number of studies, which looked at the results of conservative management. In a group of 67 patients with megaureters who were followed up for a mean of 3.1 years, 23 dilated ureters (34 %) spontaneously resolved, while 33 (49 %) persisted. Repair was performed on 11 megaureters (17 %) because of breakthrough urinary infections in 3 and deteriorating renal function in 8 [14].

In a retrospective evaluation of a total of 75 patients (88 primary megaureters) followed for more than 6 months, 27 % required surgery up to 7 years. Indications for surgery were obstructive hydroureteronephrosis, functional impairment, and persistent symptoms. Surgery was not indicated in 82 % of primary megaureters with grades I or II hydronephrosis vs. 62.9 % of those with grade III or higher hydronephrosis. On multivariate analysis, age at presentation and washout pattern were significant predictors of spontaneous resolution [15].

In a prospective review of conservative management of primary megaureters, 50 ureteric units in 44 patients (six bilateral) were studied. Children were classified according to the lower ureteric diameter less than 10 mm vs. more than 10 mm. Antenatal diagnosis was achieved 84 % in the first and 58 % in the second group. In the first group, 76 % resolved completely over a median duration of 60 (18–204) months. Yet in the second group, only 17 % resolved completely over a median duration of 102 (42–210) months. Two patients developed ureteric calculi, and three other (with progressive worsening of hydronephrosis and debilitating infections) underwent ureteric tapering and reimplantation [16].

Most cases of primary megaureter resolve spontaneously or improve without loss of function or development of symptoms. Cautious observation will let surgery to be delayed beyond infancy in most patients. Resolution rate, degree of resolution, and time to resolution are related to the type and time of presentation, the initial grade of hydronephrosis, washout patterns on renal scans, and degree of dilatation of the distal part of the ureter [14, 16, 17]. If the megaureter remains stable without any progressive dilatation or loss in renal function, no intervention would be necessary. With spontaneous remission rates of up to 85 % in primary megaureter cases, surgical management is no longer recommended except for megaureters with recurrent urinary tract infections, deterioration in split renal function, and significant obstruction. Long-term follow-up is recommended because symptoms can develop years later. Urinary tract infections, pain, and/or stone formation within the collecting system may be the late presentations of this clinical problem.

When a surgical correction is required, there are a number of different approaches that one can take based on the clinical situation.

10.6 Temporary Diversion

In an obstructed megaureter presenting with UTI and fever, percutaneous nephrostomy is helpful because rapid drainage is required. Yet this is a temporary measure, and especially in infants maintaining nephrostomy tubes is difficult for more than a few weeks.

When a prolonged drainage is required, diversion of the ureter is the preferred choice in most young infants presenting with severely obstructed megaureters. This is an easy procedure with minimal morbidity. The ureter is approached using a 2 cm inguinal incision of the affected side. Although the identification of the ureter is usually quite easy because of its size, one should be cautious not to approach bowel by mistake as they look alike. A loop or an end ureterostomy is easy to perform, and decompression of the system is quite fast following the procedure [18].

The cutaneous ureterostomy could be undiverted later around 12–18 months of age.

Although external urinary diversion is a well-established temporizing measure in obstructed megaureters, there has been suggestion of some other innovative strategies for this condition. Lee et al. have suggested creation of a refluxing reimplant of the obstructed megaureter to the dome of the bladder as a temporary internal diversion in a freely high-grade refluxing fashion. This idea follows the principle that surgery can be safely deferred if vesicoureteral junction (VUJ) obstruction is exchanged for the less harmful VUR. They reported three cases, two of which benefited from the procedure. This advantage of this approach over a classical cutaneous ureterostomy is not clear, yet it could be a good option especially for bilateral cases as the cycling of the bladder could be maintained [19].

10.7 Insertion of JJ Stent and Other Endoscopic Procedures

Another innovative strategy has been the insertion of JJ stent across the UVJ. Compared to creating a refluxing reimplant, this is potentially a minimally invasive alternative to achieve temporary internal drainage of obstructed megaureter. The aim in this approach is to ensure unimpaired flow across the UVJ while waiting for spontaneous maturation of the junction, to stretch the stenotic ureteral segment, and/or to decompress the system and thus to make subsequent urinary excretion pattern reliable.

In a study by Castagnetti et al., they investigated the results of JJ stent insertion in two neonates and eight infants with a ureter greater than 10 mm and an obstructive excretion pattern. Open insertion was necessary in five cases (50 %). Seven patients (70 %) developed stent-related complications (five breakthrough urinary infections) requiring early stent removal in 2 (20 %). Five patients (50 %) underwent surgery at a median age of 14 months (range 13–27). None required ureteral tapering. None experienced any renal function loss with respect to the initial evaluation. They make the conclusion that although JJ stent insertion across the vesicoureteral junction allows for effective internal drainage of primary nonrefluxing megaureters, there was high morbidity rate (70 %) and various technical drawbacks [20].

In another study reviewing the results of JJ stenting for obstructed megaureters, Farrugia et al. looked at 16 infants with 19 obstructed megaureters who had been stented at a median age of 24 weeks for a median of 6 months. One-third of stents were inserted endoscopically. Drainage improved in ten ureters (56 %) following stent removal, and they did not require any further surgery. However, morbidity occurred in one-third of patients, and function deteriorated after removal of stent in two patients who later required a nephrectomy [21].

In another study looking at 31 patients (age range 2 months–15 years) and 38 renal units stented for obstructed megaureters, a resolution rate of 66 % and a complication rate of 22 % were reported [22].

For obstructed megaureters, JJ placement seems to be a good option with a resolution rate of more than 50 %. Yet the technique is not well defined. Some has to be done by open surgery (30–50 %), which makes the procedure not so attractive. It is quite evident that if endoscopic insertion were not possible, a forceful dilatation or incision of the ureteric orifice would be needed while stents are being placed during open surgery. There is no clear explanation of how stents are being inserted during open surgery in any report. Additionally there are no reports of reflux evaluation on those patients in whom open insertion has been done. Therefore, it is not clear whether the resolution is due to JJ stent or due to the procedure employed during the open insertion. For endoscopically placed ones, one may argue that actually the stenosis was not severe enough so JJ stent insertion was possible. Hence, the resolution may actually be due to the course of the disease rather than the effect of the stent.

The efficacy rate of JJ stent insertion is about 50 %, and how JJ stents are really effective is not well explained, and some of the resolution may actually be due to the natural course of the problem. Therefore, the evidence about its efficacy is weak. Also knowing the high associated morbidity of up to 20–70 %, one should be cautious in selecting the patients for this procedure. This procedure may have a role in symptomatic infants with significantly dilated megaureters with loss of function. However, one should be ready for high postoperative morbidity mainly breakthrough infections.

High-pressure balloon dilatation of the ureterovesical junction has also been studied in a total of 13 patients (median age 7 months, range 4–24) with primary obstructive megaureter. Of these patients, eight were diagnosed prenatally, and the others were diagnosed after a urinary tract infection. Significant postoperative improvement of hydroureteronephrosis was observed in 11 of 13 patients, and vesicoureteral reflux was found in two. Only three patients needed ureteral reimplantation after endoscopic treatment due to hydroureteronephrosis in two and high-grade vesicoureteral reflux in one [23].

In a study by Christman et al., a relatively older patient group of 17 who were all older than 1 year of age (mean age 7 years) underwent endoscopic management followed by double stenting. All patients underwent retrograde ureteropyelography to start the procedure. In segments less than 2 cm, balloon dilation was performed, and for those 2–3 cm, laser incision was added. Of the patients, 12 had marked improvement of hydroureteronephrosis on renal and bladder ultrasound. The remaining five patients had some improvement. All patients were followed for at least 2 years postoperatively and were noted to be symptom-free with stable imaging during the observation period [24].

In another study, five patients, aged between 6 and 12 months, were treated with endoscopic high-pressure balloon dilatation. In all patients, preoperative renal ultrasonography showed a distal ureteral dilation of more than 15 mm and an obstructive pattern on renal scan. All the patients showed an improvement on postoperative follow-up without any evidence of obstruction/reflux or any other complications [25].

Endoscopic procedures including balloon dilatation and laser endoureterotomy have been shown to be effective in different patients groups. However, based on the information available, it is difficult to define the group of patients who would benefit most from such procedures. One should bear in mind that endoscopic procedures might have some technical drawbacks especially in younger children and with significant stenosis of the UVJ where even a glide wire may sometimes be impossible to insert.

10.8 Definitive Repair

It is well known that the majority of congenital megaureters may be managed conservatively. Indications for surgical intervention include symptoms such as febrile UTIs or pain, and in the asymptomatic patient, a DRF below 40 % associated with massive or progressive hydronephrosis, or a drop in differential function on serial renograms. The definitive repair is reimplantation of the ureter with or without remodeling [26–29].

The definitive repair should not be considered before 1 year of age as this procedure may be challenging in infancy and may be detrimental for future bladder function if done bilaterally. If intervention is needed earlier in the first year of life, a form of temporary diversion (as discussed above) can be considered. The cutaneous diversion followed by definitive repair is the well-established method of choice. The innovative approaches like refluxing reimplant, JJ stent placement, and balloon dilatation should be considered as techniques that require further studies before being established options.

The basic aim of definitive treatment is to relieve obstruction, to gain normal drainage of the collecting system, to create a nonrefluxing vesicoureteral reimplantation, and to preserve renal development without long-term complications.

The initial approach to the ureter can be either intravesical, extravesical, or combined. The incision is chosen to access the upper ureter, the lower ureter, or the entire ureter. Straightening the ureter is necessary without devascularization. Preservation of the ureteral blood supply, which arises from the aorta, renal artery, gonadal artery, and internal iliac artery, is crucial particularly if undertaking extensive tailoring. If necessary, excision of the distal obstructive segment is employed. The ureter may need to be remodeled to a smaller diameter either by plication or tapering. Ureteral remodeling should enhance urinary flow into the bladder by restoring normal peristalsis with the reduction of ureteral luminal diameter. The ureter must be tapered to achieve a diameter for ensuring a nonrefluxing tunnel length. Neocystostomy tunnel lengths of 4:1–6:1 are recommended to prevent postoperative reflux. Postoperative drains or splints for the ureters are used at the preference of the surgeon.

There have been an extensive number of reports with different surgical techniques. When one tries to make an analysis, it is apparent that there is a lot of heterogeneity in the patient populations and the techniques employed in each paper. Thus, conclusive statements are not possible to make. Substantive differences are not statistically or clinically apparent. The type of remodeling excisional tapering or one of folding techniques can be used mainly based on surgeon's choice and experience. Majority would choose to place a JJ stent in the reimplanted ureter, which needs to be removed in the following weeks. In experienced hands, the success rates should be around 90 %. The success rates have been reported to be slightly higher with the folding group although none of the studies are controlled [30–34, 35–37].

The complications are not rare. The complications are not always due to a technical error but mostly to inherent characteristics of the ureter and the bladder function. The most common complications would be persistent obstruction or reflux. The obstruction can be due to edema early on and resolves in the follow-up. Persisting obstruction would be due to distal ureteral kinking at the entry to the bladder or ureteral ischemia, which can only be corrected by secondary surgery. Ipsilateral reflux occurs in 2–5 % of patients. If there is persisting reflux, initial approach would be conservative, and surgical correction should be considered if only there are clinical problems in the follow-up due to reflux [31, 36]. Contralateral reflux occurs more often but mostly resolves over time.

There is a growing trend toward minimally invasive surgery and the application of improved laparoscopic and robotic techniques to megaureter surgery as well [37–39]. Although they are not yet commonly established methods, there are centers, which report that robot-assisted reconstructive surgery of the distal ureter is feasible and can be used without compromising the generally accepted principles of open surgical procedures.

References

1. Caulk JR (1923) Megaloureter: the importance of the ureterovesical valve. J Urol 9:315
2. Swenson O (1955) Congenital defects in the pelvic parasympathetic system. Arch Dis Child 30(149):1–7
3. Hendren WH, Henderson BM (1969) Recent advances in pediatric surgery. Am J Surg 118(3):338–355
4. Cussen LJ (1971) The morphology of congenital dilatation of the ureter: intrinsic ureteral lesions. Aust N Z J Surg 41(2):185–194
5. Hellström M, Hjälmås K, Jacobsson B, Jodal U, Odén A (1985) Normal ureteral diameterin infancy and childhood. Acta Radiol Diagn (Stockh) 26(4):433–439
6. King LR (1980) Megaloureter: definition, diagnosis and management. J Urol 123(2):222–223
7. Hanna MK, Jeffs RD, Sturgess JM, Barkin M (1976) Ureteral structure and ultrastructure. Part II. Congenital ureteropelvic junction obstruction and primary obstructive megaureter. J Urol 116(6):725–730
8. Gosling JA, Dixon JS (1978) Functional obstruction of the ureter and renal pelvis. A histological and electron microscopic study. Br J Urol 50(3):145–152
9. Gee WF, Kiviat MD (1975) Ureteral response to partial obstruction. Smooth muscle hyperplasia and connective tissue proliferation. Invest Urol 12(4): 309–316
10. Gearhart JP, Lee BR, Partin AW, Epstein JI, Gosling JA (1995) A quantitative histological evaluation of the dilated ureter of childhood. II: ectopia, posterior urethral valves and the prune belly syndrome. J Urol 153(1):172–176
11. Lee BR, Silver RI, Partin AW, Epstein JI, Gearhart JP (1998) A quantitative histologic analysis of collagen subtypes: the primary obstructed and refluxing megaureter of childhood. Urology 51(5):820–823
12. McLellan DL, Retik AB, Bauer SB, Diamond DA, Atala A, Mandell J, Lebowitz RL, Borer JG, Peters CA (2002) Rate and predictors of spontaneous resolution of prenatally diagnosed primary nonrefluxing megaureter. J Urol 168(5):2177–2180
13. O'Reilly P, Aurell M, Britton K et al (1996) Consensus on diuresis renography for investigating the dilated upper urinary tract. Radionuclides in Nephrourology

Group. Consensus Committee on Diuresis Renography. J Nucl Med 37(11):1872–1876
14. Liu HY, Dhillon HK, Yeung CK, Diamond DA, Duffy PG, Ransley PG (1994) Clinical outcome and management of prenatally diagnosed primary megaureters. J Urol 152(2 Pt 2):614–617
15. Di Renzo D, Aguiar L, Cascini V, Di Nicola M, McCarten KM, Ellsworth PI, Chiesa PL, Caldamone AA (2013) Long-term followup of primary nonrefluxing megaureter. J Urol 190(3):1021–1026
16. Ranawaka R, Hennayake S (2013) Resolution of primary non-refluxing megaureter: an observational study. J Pediatr Surg 48(2):380–383
17. Baskin LS, Zderic SA, Snyder HM, Duckett JW (1994) Primary dilated megaureter: long-term followup. J Urol 152(2 Pt 2):618–621
18. Kitchens DM, DeFoor W, Minevich E, Reddy P, Polsky E, McGregor A, Sheldon C (2007) End cutaneous ureterostomy for the management of severe hydronephrosis. J Urol 177(4):1501–1504
19. Lee SD, Akbal C, Kaefer M (2005) Refluxing ureteral reimplant as temporary treatment of obstructive megaureter in neonate and infant. J Urol 173(4):1357–1360; discussion 1360
20. Castagnetti M, Cimador M, Sergio M, De Grazia E (2006) Double-J stent insertion across vesicoureteral junction – is it a valuable initial approach in neonates and infants with severe primary nonrefluxing megaureter? Urology 68(4):870–875; discussion 875–876
21. Farrugia MK, Steinbrecher HA, Malone PS (2011) The utilization of stents in the management of primary obstructive megaureters requiring intervention before 1 year of age. J Pediatr Urol 7(2):198–202
22. Carroll D, Chandran H, Joshi A, McCarthy LS, Parashar K (2010) Endoscopic placement of double-J ureteric stents in children as a treatment for primary obstructive megaureter. Urol Ann 2(3):114–118
23. García-Aparicio L, Rodo J, Krauel L, Palazon P, Martin O, Ribó JM (2012) High pressure balloon dilation of the ureterovesical junction – first line approach to treat primary obstructive megaureter? J Urol 187(5):1834–1838
24. Christman MS, Kasturi S, Lambert SM, Kovell RC, Casale P (2012) Endoscopic management and the role of double stenting for primary obstructive megaureters. J Urol 187(3):1018–1022. doi:10.1016/j.juro.2011.10.168. Epub 2012 Jan 20
25. Torino G, Collura G, Mele E, Garganese MC, Capozza N (2012) Severe primary obstructive megaureter in the first year of life: preliminary experience with endoscopic balloon dilation. J Endourol 26(4):325–329
26. Tekgül S, Riedmiller H, Hoebeke P, Kočvara R, Nijman RJ, Radmayr C, Stein R, Dogan HS (2013) European Association of Urology guidelines edition; guidelines on Paediatric Urology. www.uroweb.org/gls/pdf/21_Paediatric_Urology_LR_August2012.pdf
27. Keating MA, Escala J, Snyder HM III et al (1989) Changing concepts in management of primary obstructive megaureter. J Urol 142(2 Pt 2):636–640; discussion 667–668
28. Shokeir AA, Nijman RJ (2000) Primary megaureter: current trends in diagnosis and treatment. BJU Int 86(7):861–868
29. Farrugia MK, Hitchcock R, Radford A, Burki T, Robb A, Murphy F, On behalf of the British Association of Paediatric Urologists (BAPU) (2013) British Association of Paediatric Urologists consensus statement on the management of the primary obstructive megaureter. J Pediatr Urol 10(1):26–33
30. DeFoor W, Minevich E, Reddy P et al (2004) Results of tapered ureteral reimplantation for primary megaureter: extravesical versus intravesical approach. J Urol 172(4 Pt 2):1640–1643; discussion 1643
31. Hendren WH (1969) Operative repair of megaureter in children. J Urol 101:491
32. Hanna MK (1979) New surgical method for one stage total ureteral remodeling of massively dilated and tortuous ureter: tapering in situ technique. Urology 14:453
33. Wacksman J, Gilbert A, Sheldon CA (1992) Results of the renewed extravesical reimplant for surgical correction of vesicoureteral reflux. J Urol 148(2 Pt 1):359–361
34. Hanna MK (1982) Recent advances and further experience with surgical techniques for one stage total remodeling of massively dilated ureters. Urology 19:495
35. Kalicinski ZH, Kansy K, Kotarbinska B et al (1977) Surgery of megaureters-modification of Hendren's operation. J Pediatr Surg 12:183
36. Ehrlich RM (1985) The ureteral folding technique for megaureter surgery. J Urol 134:668
37. Musch M, Hohenhorst L, Pailliart A, Loewen H, Davoudi Y, Kroepfl D (2013) Robot-assisted reconstructive surgery of the distal ureter: single institution experience in 16 patients. BJU Int 111(5):773–783
38. Goh AC, Link RE (2011) Robot-assisted tapered ureteral reimplantation for congenital megaureter. Urology 77(3):742–745
39. Hemal AK, Nayyar R, Rao R (2009) Robotic repair of primary symptomatic obstructive megaureter with intracorporeal or extracorporeal ureteric tapering and ureteroneocystostomy. J Endourol 23(12):2041–2046

Ureteral Duplications and Ureteroceles

11

Marco Castagnetti and Waifro Rigamonti

11.1 Introduction

A duplex kidney refers to a kidney with two pelvicalyceal systems, generally referred to as upper and lower poles. The upper pole normally accounts for one third of the kidney, whereas the lower one for the remaining two thirds. Duplex systems occur in 0.8 % of cases in autoptic studies [1]. Anatomically, duplex systems can be incomplete (bifid pelvis or ureter) or complete. The former are four to five times more common than the latter.

From a clinical standpoint, ureteral duplications can be differentiated into uncomplicated and complicated. The former include duplex systems without any associated urinary tract dilatations. They never require treatment and often go undiagnosed for the whole life. In contrast, complicated ureteral duplications are duplex systems associated with other urological anomalies. Ureteral ectopia and ureterocele are the most common conditions associated with the upper pole of a duplex system, whereas primary vesicoureteral reflux (VUR) and ureteropelvic junction obstruction (UPJO) with the lower pole [2]. Upper pole UPJO and primary upper pole VUR are exceedingly rare for anatomical and embryological reasons. Complicated duplex system will be the focus of this chapter.

M. Castagnetti (✉)
Urology Unit, Section of Pediatric Urology,
University Hospital of Padua,
Via Giustiniani 2, 35128 Padua, Italy
e-mail: marcocastagnetti@hotmail.com

W. Rigamonti
Pediatric Surgery and Urology Unit,
Burlo Garofalo Hospital,
Via dell'Istria, 65/1, 34137 Trieste, Italy
e-mail: waifro.rigamonti@burlo.trieste.it

11.2 Presentation

Complicated duplex system anomalies can present either as an antenatally diagnosed asymptomatic hydronephrosis (HN) or with symptoms. In most of the cases diagnosed antenatally, the diagnosis is just of HN, as the presence of a dilated ureter (i.e., of hydroureteronephrosis, HUN) or of a ureterocele within the bladder are commonly overlooked on prenatal scans [3]. Postnatally, febrile urinary tract infections (UTIs) are instead the most common presenting symptoms. UTI occurs more commonly when a VUR is associated with the condition in any of the moieties but can occur also in patients with nonrefluxing HUN, as the infection is favored by the increased urinary stasis in a severely dilated urinary system and the extension of the dilated urinary reservoir to the bladder makes urinary contamination easier [4, 5]. Risk of infection might be higher in case of ureterocele, although it is still unclear whether this is due to the ureterocele itself or to the fact that VUR is often associated [5]. The risk of UTI is instead limited in patients with HN without any

M. Lima, G. Manzoni (eds.), *Pediatric Urology: Contemporary Strategies from Fetal Life to Adolescence*,
DOI 10.1007/978-88-470-5693-0_11, © Springer-Verlag Italia 2015

associated ureteral dilatation [5]. Finally, urinary incontinence is a rare but specific complaint in females with an ectopic ureter opening distally to the bladder neck. Such incontinence can be typically a nocturnal dribbling of urine with daytime continence [6].

11.3 Neonatal Management

The only reason prompting a surgical procedure in an infant with a complicated duplex system before accomplishment of a comprehensive workup is the presence of symptoms not amenable to medical treatment and posing a risk for the patient health, such as febrile UTI unresponsive to antibiotic treatment [7]. Otherwise, a complete workup should be accomplished before embarking on any surgical procedures [7]. We recommend starting the patient on antibiotic prophylaxis in case of ureteral dilatation in any moiety [4, 5]. In this way, the risk of febrile UTI seems comparable to that of patients undergoing early surgical treatment. Consistently, in patients with duplex system ureterocele (DSU), Husmann et al. observed the same infection rates at 6 months of age in 32 patients undergoing neonatal endoscopic decompression (infection rate 9 %) and 40 receiving antibiotic prophylaxis from birth (infection rate 8 %) [8]. In adjunct, a short cycle of antibiotic treatment should also be considered in case of diagnostic procedures requiring catheterization [5].

11.4 Workup

Basic diagnostic workup in patients with a complicated duplex system should generally include ultrasound scan (US) of the upper urinary tract and bladder and a renal nuclear scintigraphy. A voiding cystourethrography (VCUG) should be considered if a dilated ureter is visible on US. Additional imaging may be useful when anatomical information is still deemed necessary at the end of the basic workup.

The US of the urinary tract is generally the first investigation. In cases with a prenatally detected HN, it should be performed 5–7 days after birth to confirm the diagnosis. The US should define the laterality of the condition and identify the moieties that are dilated; the degree of the dilatation, whether or not ureteral dilatation is associated; and the aspect of the bladder including the presence of a ureterocele. In some cases of ureteral ectopia, the US can show the dilated ureter going distally to the trigone and below the bladder neck. Attention should be paid to the degree of bladder fullness during the exam, as ureteroceles can collapse and be overlooked in a full bladder. The size of the ureterocele and the thickness of the ureterocele wall are also important factors, as big or thick-walled ureteroceles might be more difficult to decompress and require more aggressive treatment, as detailed below.

VCUG should always follow but in case of isolated HN with no visible ureter, which essentially correspond to a suspicion of lower pole UPJO [9]. In order to rule out the presence of a ureterocele, a picture should be taken after injection of few cc of contrast into the bladder, at low-volume bladder filling, to prevent ureterocele collapse. In patients with ureterocele, VUR in the lower pole moiety is a common finding (Fig. 11.1a). Images taken during micturition can show the ureterocele sliding into the urethra potentially causing bladder outlet obstruction (BOO) (Fig. 11.1b). In patients with an ectopic ureter at the bladder neck, it is not unusual that the catheter inserted in the urethra for the VCUG instead of entering the bladder goes straight into the ectopic ureter. The injection of contrast actually results in a retrograde pyelography of the upper pole moiety (Fig. 11.2a). If the catheter goes into the bladder instead, the most common finding is an upper pole reflux when the bladder neck opens (Fig. 11.2b). Clinically, this situation is quite unfavorable, as the urine refluxing during micturition tends to remain trapped into the upper tract when the bladder neck is closed and this predisposes to the development of UTI.

Finally, an assessment of moiety function should be achieved by nuclear scintigraphy. The dynamic (99 m)Tc-mercaptoacetyltriglycine (MAG3) scintigraphy and the static (99 m) Tc-dimercaptosuccinic acid (DMSA) scintigraphy

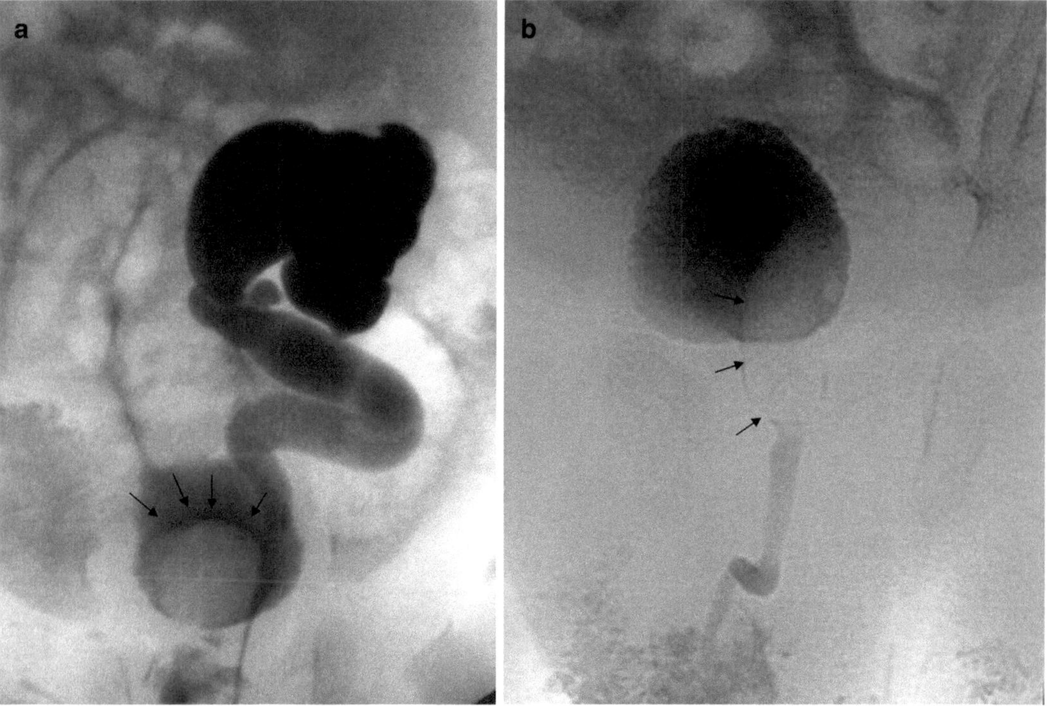

Fig. 11.1 (**a**) Ureterocele (*arrows*) with associated ipsilateral lower pole reflux; (**b**) ureterocele (*arrows*) sliding into the posterior urethra during micturition

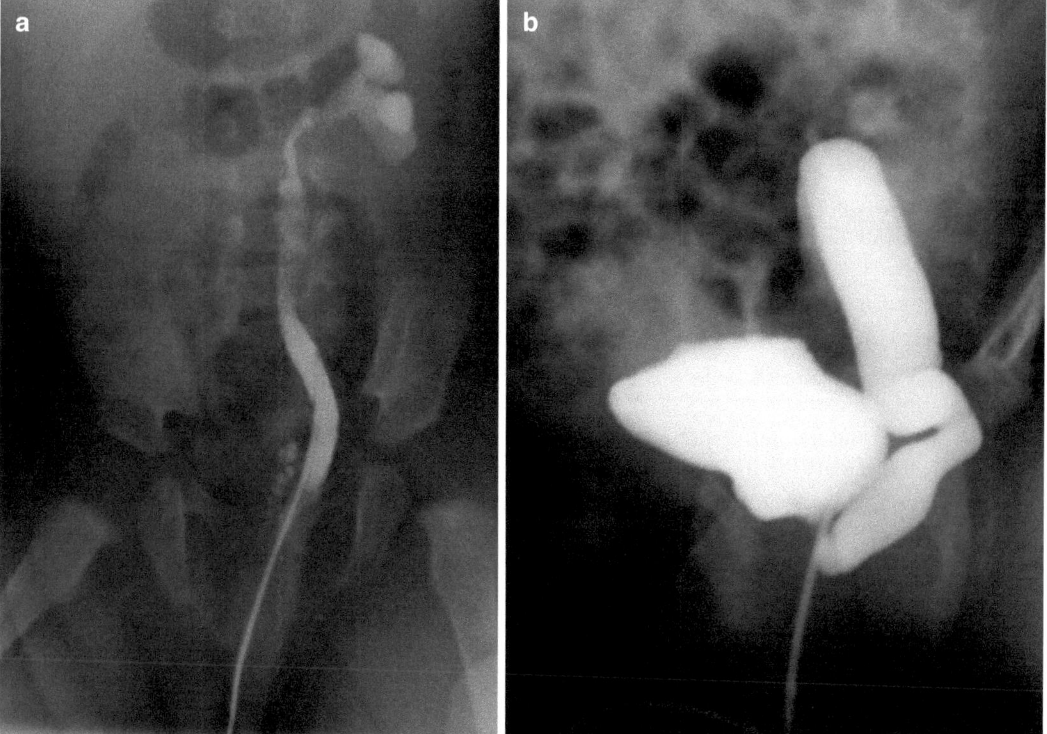

Fig. 11.2 Upper pole ectopic ureter: (**a**) retrograde pyelography of the ectopic moiety; (**b**) upper pole reflux during bladder neck opening

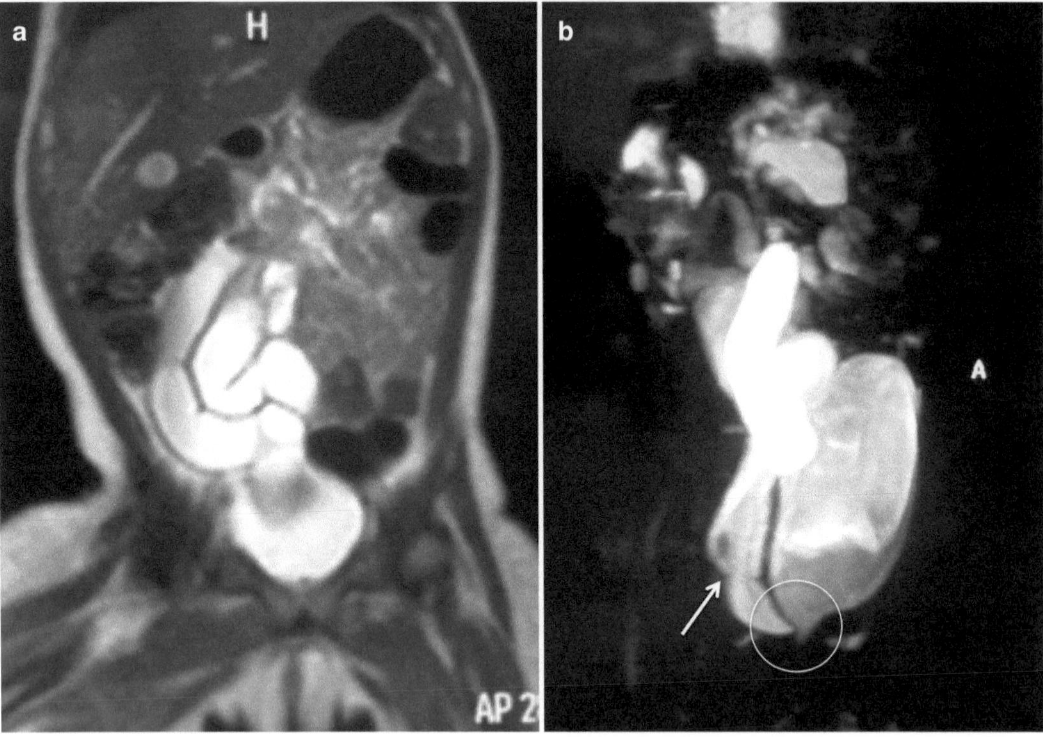

Fig. 11.3 Uro-MRI in a patient with ultrasound evidence of a duplex system with nonrefluxing dilatation of both ipsilateral moieties. (**a**) Coronal view showing the two dilated ureters; (**b**) transverse view showing the lower pole ureter opening into the upper pole one (*arrow*) and the latter ectopic at the bladder neck (within the *circle*)

are the alternative methods. The MAG3 has the putative advantage to allow for simultaneous assessment of cortical function and upper tract drainage; the DMSA possibly allows for a more accurate assessment of moiety function. In our practice, we favor the MAG3 scan in almost all the cases for two reasons. First, evidence suggests that the cortical images are not significantly different between the two tests [10]. Furthermore, the information necessary for the decision-making is not the assessment of cortical pyelonephritic scars, but the gross presence of any function in the moiety or its complete absence thereof. Second, the visualization of the urinary tract may help drawing the regions of interest pertaining to each moiety, thereby allowing for a somewhat more accurate assessment of the functional contribution of each moiety. Patients with primary lower pole VUR are the only exception, in our practice. Under these circumstances, we prefer using a DMSA scan for more careful search for parenchymal scars. We recommend, however, a MAG3 scan also in patients with VUR, if any trapping of contrast in the upper tract is seen on the VCUG, in order to rule out any concomitant obstruction that might contraindicate the injection of bulking agent as treatment of reflux, should recurrent febrile UTI occur.

Additional imaging can at time be useful to better define the anatomy of the condition. An example is the case of a massive nonrefluxing dilatation of both ipsilateral moieties, upper and lower one (Fig. 11.3), or if there is an apparent incongruence among the tests used for basic assessment, e.g., a dilated ureter is seen on US but no ureter is visible on the MAG3 scan. Under these circumstances, a uro-magnetic resonance imaging (MRI) is our investigation of choice. Since this investigation allows for simultaneous optimal anatomical definition and functional assessment, some centers have proposed its use as the first-line investigation [11]. In our opinion, however, it is a too expensive tool to be used for this purpose. Moreover, it requires deep sedation in some patients, and if a watchful waiting attitude is elected and the same investigation needs to be repeated several times during follow-up, these issues represent each time. In selected patients, when the indication for surgery is already clear after basic workup but a more accurate anatomical definition is deemed suitable for the choice of the surgical strategy, a retrograde pyelography to be performed at the beginning of the surgical repair can replace the uro-MRI.

11.5 Management

11.5.1 Lower Pole Conditions

In our practice, management of lower pole conditions does not differ essentially from the corresponding condition in a single system.

11.5.1.1 Lower Pole VUR

Although the chance for spontaneous resolution of primary lower pole VUR is lower than the same condition in a single system, in our opinion the first-line treatment remains watchful waiting with the adjunct of prolonged antibiotic prophylaxis in case of dilating reflux.

We offer surgical treatment to cases developing breakthrough febrile UTI or febrile UTI after discontinuation of prophylaxis. The latter is normally recommended in our practice 6 months after achievement of daytime continence. Endoscopic injection of a bulking agent in the lower pole ureter is our first treatment option irrespective of lower pole function. Effectiveness of endoscopic injection has much improved with the development of the technique of intraureteral injection after hydrodistention of the ureteral orifice, hydrodistention injection technique (HIT) [12]. In our practice, we consider successful any treatment that is not followed by recurrent febrile UTI. If symptoms do not recur, we do not even recommend a follow-up VCUG. If symptoms recur and the lower pole function is worth preserving, the endoscopic treatment can be repeated. Lower pole partial nephrectomy, instead, is offered to patients with a no/poorly functioning lower pole, if endoscopic treatment fails, i.e., in case of recurrent febrile UTI. Under these circumstances, we do not perform a complete ureterectomy, but rather resect the ureter at the level of the anterosuperior iliac spine and suture close. Massive endoscopic injection of the orifice draining the stump of the lower pole ureter can be considered at the time of surgery in order to minimize the risk of leaving a refluxing ureteral stump behind or can be offered later on in the rare event of symptoms (ureteral stump syndrome).

11.5.1.2 Lower Pole Ureteroelvic Junction Obstruction

In our practice, treatment is generally recommended in case of significant dilatation with parenchymal thinning, abnormal parenchymal uptake on the diuretic renography, or severely obstructive drainage pattern on the diuretic renography. In general, our attitude is slightly more aggressive in these patients than in those with UPJO in single systems, for two reasons. First, no specific cutoffs for differential renal function or for changes in differential renal function can be used, as the dilatation affects only a portion of the kidney and the borders of the lower pole cannot be neatly defined. Second, the underlying abnormality is less likely to improve spontaneously than in ordinary cases in single systems. If patients are anyway elected for watchful waiting, we do not recommend any antibiotic prophylaxis. An extrinsic obstruction due to abnormal vessels is common in patients with lower pole UPJO [13]. The most common cause of intrinsic obstruction is instead a ureteropelvic junction abnormality with a thin, dysplastic proximal ureteral segment joining in a Y fashion the upper pole ureter generally few mm below the ureteropelvic junction. Under these circumstances an end-to-lateral pyeloureteral anastomosis between the lower pole pelvis and the upper pole ureter can be the option [14].

11.5.2 Upper Pole Conditions

Upper pole conditions essentially include the upper pole ectopic ureter and the DSU.

11.5.2.1 Upper Pole Ectopic Ureter

Upper pole ectopic ureters generally open medially and distally to the lower pole one, which orifice is consistently located within the bladder. The most common form of ectopia is at the bladder neck, but ectopic ureters can also open in the vagina in females and in the genital tract in males. No investigation allows for an accurate identification of the site of opening of an ectopic ureter preoperatively, and the only reliable tool for an accurate identification is endoscopy. Nevertheless, also endoscopy can fail visualizing the ectopic orifice if it is stenotic, if it opens in the genital tract in males, or if it is located within the folds of the vaginal mucosa. Upper pole partial nephrectomy is the most common approach for upper pole ectopic ureters, based on the assumption that the upper pole is often dysplastic and poorly functioning [15, 16]. The degree of upper pole dysplasia is generally considered to directly correlate to the degree of ectopia; the more ectopic is the ureteral orifice, the more dysplastic the upper pole parenchyma [17]. Nevertheless, we performed pathology studies on specimens removed during upper pole partial nephrectomies and found that the histology of such specimens was more consistent with hypoplasia than dysplasia, i.e., we observed fewer nephrons than in normal cases, but otherwise normal [18]. Interestingly enough, these findings were not strictly correlated to the degree of ureteral ectopia [18]. This is consistent with the clinical observation that some upper poles are big on US and show reasonable function on renal scintigraphy (Fig. 11.4). Under these circumstances, reconstructive nephron-sparing surgery is appealing [18–20]. Options include diversion of the urinary stream from the upper moiety into the lower one or ureteral reimplantation [19–21]. If the latter is elected, an intravesical reimplantation is generally recommended and the two ipsilateral ureters are reimplanted en bloc based on the assumption that they cannot be separated as they share a common vascular supply. Nevertheless, over the recent past, in cases with a dilated upper pole ureter, we have started performing an extravesical, dismembered reimplantation of the ectopic ureter, as described below [22].

An endoscopy is performed to begin with in order to confirm the diagnosis, possibly determine the location of the ectopic ureter, and stenting the ureter in order to make subsequent dissection easier. In general, we prefer placing a 4 or 5 Fr ureteral stent in the lower pole ureter since this is the most difficult to identify during the dissection and the one that requires more careful handling. Afterwards, via a Pfannenstiel incision, the ureters on the affected side are identified above the bladder (Fig. 11.5a). At this level, the upper pole ureter is sectioned and the distal stump going behind the bladder is suture closed and abandoned. This avoids performing any dissection of the retrovesical space, which can harm peripheral bladder innervation, and allows leaving untouched the distal ureteral portion where the upper and the lower

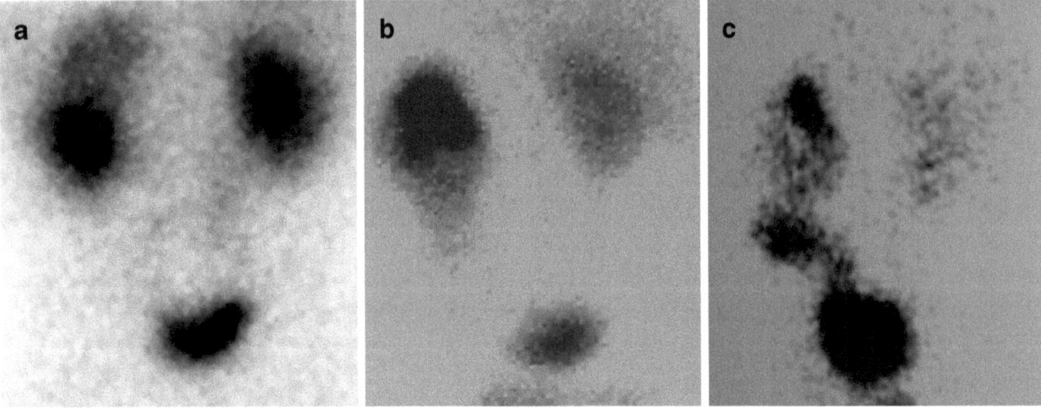

Fig. 11.4 Scintigraphic appearance of a large upper pole with preserved function (Reprinted from Castagnetti et al. [22] with permission from Elsevier)

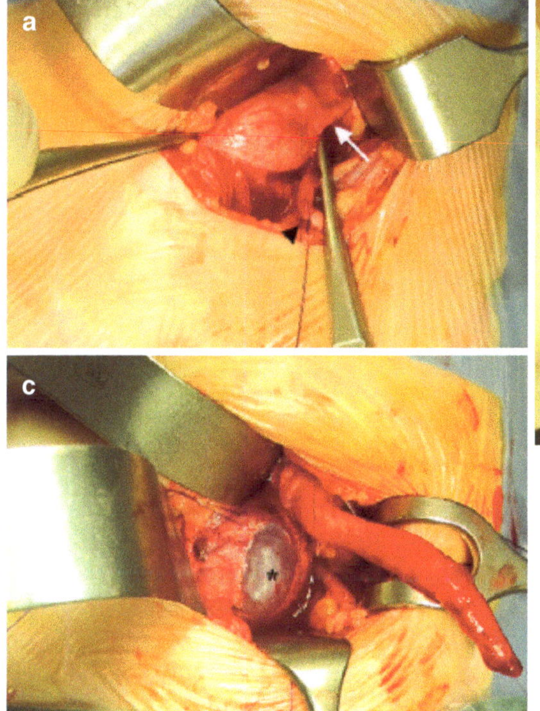

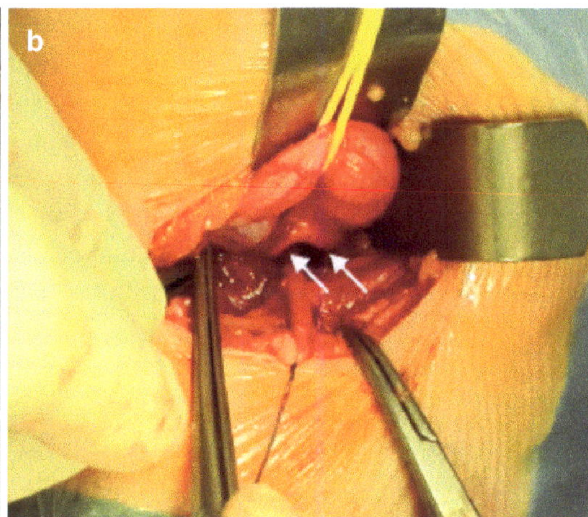

Fig. 11.5 Steps of dismembered extravesical reimplantation of a duplex system ectopic ureter. (**a**) dissection of upper pole and lower pole (*white arrow*) ipsilateral ureters together; (**b**) separation of the two ureters (the *white arrows* point to the lower pole ureter); (**c**) detrusortomy (*asterisk*) for extravesical reimplantation. For more details see text. (Reprinted from Castagnetti et al. [22] with permission from Elsevier)

pole ureters are most tightly adjacent. The required dissection is indeed not much different from that performed during ureteroureterostomy [15, 19] or refluxing ureteral reimplantation [23], two approaches that have recently been re-proposed as viable and easy procedures for similar cases. The ureteral length necessary for reimplantation is then obtained by proximal dissection of the upper pole ureter in the retroperitoneum with subsequent ureteral straightening (Fig. 11.5b). In general, these dilated ureters have quite a thick wall and the intramural vasculature makes them resistant to such a dissection. If necessary, the ureter can be tapered over a 12 Fr feeding tube. We recommend using an infolding technique (Starr plication) rather than an excisional tapering (Hendren tailoring) to prevent any ischemic injury to the dissected ureter. Finally, an extramucosal detrusorotomy is performed and the ureter reimplanted using an extravesical technique (Fig. 11.5c).

11.5.2.2 Duplex System Ureterocele (DSU)

DSU is the most complex condition associated with the upper pole of a duplex system and the main reason for such complexity is that it is no way just a ureteral pathology [7]. The ureterocele is located in the trigone and its presence can alter the function of the whole bladder particularly in duplex systems, where the trigone development is already partly abnormal due to the presence of two ipsilateral ureters [7, 24, 25]. The ureterocele can cause reflux or obstruction in the lower pole ipsilateral moiety and/or in the contralateral one(s). Moreover, the vast majority of ureteroceles in duplex systems extend into the bladder neck or posterior urethra, i.e., are ectopic. As such, they can cause BOO [7, 8]. After decompression, the portion of the bladder corresponding to the ureterocele results in an acontractile area, and this has two possible effects on bladder function.

It can alter detrusor contractility thereby leading to the development of large and poorly contractile bladders and, in ectopic ureteroceles, can act as a defect in the bladder neck potentially causing stress urinary incontinence [26, 27].

A complete anatomical repair of a DSU, particularly if ectopic, would involve ureterocele excision, reconstruction of the bladder base and neck, reimplantation of the lower pole ipsilateral ureter, and upper pole partial nephrectomy of the ureterocele moiety (if nonfunctioning). This is a feasible procedure in experienced hands, but remains formidable particularly in infancy [28]. Beganović et al. reported the largest long-term series of patients undergoing this procedure and showed persistent VUR in 13 % of cases and a secondary surgery rate of 36 % [29]. Moreover, it is of note that only two cases of stress urinary incontinence were reported in a large multicenter survey of continence problems in ureterocele patients who did not underwent lower urinary tract reconstruction as primary approach and neither resolved after bladder neck reconstruction. Therefore, stress urinary incontinence seems an exceptional phenomenon irrespective of primary approach and bladder neck reconstruction seems ineffective to fix it [27].

It is not surprising that historically surgeons have looked for easier alternative strategies to treat the condition. All these procedures rely on the decompression of the dilated ureterocele moiety rather than on the recreation of a normal anatomy. Decompression of the ureterocele moiety can be achieved in two ways. One is from the upper tract diverting the urinary stream from the upper into the lower pole via a high pyelo-pyelostomy or a lower ureteroureterostomy or most commonly (70 % of cases reported in the literature) removing the upper pole draining into the ureterocele [19, 20, 30, 31]. The second way to achieve ureterocele decompression is from the bladder opening somehow the ureterocele endoscopically [32]. Putative drawbacks of either approach include that they leave the muscular defect due to the ureterocele, have unpredictable consequences on the obstruction/reflux in the other moieties, and, in case of the endoscopic procedure, may possibly cause a de novo reflux in the punctured or incised ureterocele moiety [7]. In the following paragraphs, we will review the evidence about these points.

Endoscopic Decompression

The term endoscopic decompression includes a number of different procedures performed with different instruments [33]. The latter include Bugbee electrodes, stylet wires of ureteral catheters, Collin knives, and laser [33]. The ureterocele can either be punctured or incised. One major variation among the techniques for endoscopic decompression concerns the management of the ureterocele portion extending into the urethra in ectopic cases. Early reports suggested that this portion should be opened frankly in order to prevent any BOO [34]. Later on, it has become clear that once the ureterocele is decompressed, BOO is rare, and opening of the urethral portion of the ureterocele only increases the risk to end up with a de novo VUR into the ureterocele moiety [24, 35].

Many studies claimed that endoscopic treatment is seldom a definitive procedure, and ureterocele ectopic location and the number of moieties at jeopardy, i.e., with obstruction or VUR at presentation, were identified as the two major factors predicting a failure of the endoscopic treatment [36, 37]. Initial combined experience from Padua and Philadelphia corroborated these conclusions. Consistently, a first report quoted a secondary surgery rate of 27 % [34], which rose to 41 % after extended follow-up [37]. Additional surgery was required in 18 % of intravesical ureteroceles vs. 64 % of the ectopic ones [37]. Despite their merits, these reports were fraught with some limitations. To begin with, infants and older children were mixed up, as well as cases of single system and duplex system ureterocele. Second, a different incision technique was used in the two kinds of ureteroceles and ectopic ureteroceles were frankly opened, as described above. It is noteworthy that later on both groups independently reported comparable success rates in patients undergoing the same endoscopic technique for decompression irrespective of ureterocele location [24, 35, 38]. This conclusion is also supported by a recent meta-analysis, which showed that ureterocele ectopia does not represent a significant additional risk factor for failure of endoscopic decompression in patients with a duplex system [25]. Therefore, we now recommend an incision at the junction between the ureterocele and the bladder wall irrespective of ureterocele location. This creates a flap mechanism that prevents the development of reflux after decompression [39]. Creation of a small opening seems another crucial factor to prevent reflux, although this also increases the risk for the procedure to fail decompressing the ureterocele satisfactorily, as discussed below [24, 38].

Another major bias affecting early studies regarded the indications for secondary surgery. The latter was recommended in case of lack of function improvement in the upper pole or of persistent/de novo VUR in any moiety after endoscopic decompression. Over time, it has become evident that poorly or even nonfunctioning upper poles can be left in situ, if properly decompressed, and that VUR can resolve or be left alone [40]. Besides, in those cases with symptomatic VUR, the endoscopic treatment can fix the problem allowing for an "all endo" treatment [7, 41–43]. Taking that in mind, we reviewed the results in a series of patients treated in Padua between 2003 and 2010 [38]. In these patients the same endoscopic incision was performed, and the only indications for additional surgery included either the presence of symptoms or the persistence of severe dilatation. The secondary surgery rate dramatically dropped compared with previous series. Only 5 % of patients required additional bladder reconstruction because of symptoms once effective ureterocele decompression was achieved. The most common complication and reason for additional surgery was instead a failure to achieve effective decompression of the ureterocele moiety (22 % of cases), perhaps due to the fact that we always performed tiny holes into the ureterocele. Finally, we did not observe any case of urinary incontinence.

Upper Tract Approach

Despite our preference for the endoscopic decompression, we have not fully abandoned other treatment modalities such as the upper tract approach. Historically, controlled studies by Hussmann et al. suggested that this approach is significantly more effective than endoscopic decompression in patients with ectopic DSU and no associated VUR [44]. Under these conditions, it was reported to be definitive treatment in 80 % of cases [44]. More recently, the procedure has gained renewed interest due to the spread of minimally invasive surgery, but this approach can be formidable in infants where it carries the risk of lower pole injury and loss [45]. In our practice, we selectively offer an upper pole partial nephrectomy to ureterocele patients with severe upper tract dilatation and/or huge ureteroceles, if the function of the upper pole is negligible, or as secondary surgery if endoscopic decompression fails [38]. Admittedly, our definition of severe dilatation and huge ureterocele is indeed quite subjective and difficult to standardize.

Conservative Management of DSU

Finally, conservative management has recently emerged as an option in selected DSU patients. This approach was initially proposed in asymptomatic patients diagnosed antenatally [46]. Subsequently, its use was extended also to patients diagnosed after a UTI [47]. Studies have tried to identify the criteria to select the most suitable patients for conservative management. All the published series agree that this approach should be avoided in patients with evidence of BOO, severe HUN, or high-grade VUR, as these are risk factors for recurrent UTI if the system is not decompressed [47, 48]. Coplen and Austin also recommended the conservative management to be limited to patients with multicystic dysplasia in the upper pole [49], in keeping with the principle that a completely unimpaired drainage is preferable to preserve function. Other authors, instead, proposed that this approach could be pursued in cases where adequate upper tract drainage could be documented on diuretic renography, irrespective of ureterocele moiety function [47]. This is also our attitude and it is based on the assumption that the main aim of endoscopic decompression is to improve upper tract drainage; therefore, if good drainage is present, no additional procedure is necessary.

In infants elected for conservative treatment, antibiotic prophylaxis is generally recommended. Protocols are quite variable. Direnna and Leonard administered prophylaxis for a mean of 1.5 years [48]; Coplen and Austin until resolution of VUR or completion of toilet training [48]; and Shankar et al., finally, until age 5 years in cases with persisting VUR [46].

Conclusion

Surgery during the first months of life is seldom necessary in patients with a complicated duplex system. We recommend asymptomatic infants to be started on antibiotic prophylaxis and to undergo a basic workup including a combination of ultrasound scan of the urinary tract, voiding cystourethrography, and diuretic renography. Additional imaging can be used on a case basis. Management of lower pole conditions does not differ essentially from the corresponding condition in a single system. In case of ectopic ureters, we favor a dismembered extravesical reimplantation of the upper pole ureter. In case of ureterocele, conservative management is an option in selected cases. Otherwise, endoscopic decompression is generally our first choice, but in patients with big ureteroceles, severe upper tract hydroureteronephrosis, and poor upper pole function, upper pole partial nephrectomy seems more effective. In our experience, irrespective of the primary approach, once effective decompression is achieved, recurrent febrile urinary tract infections are rare, and so is the need for further surgical procedures. Incontinence is an exceedingly rare outcome.

References

1. Campbell MF (1970) Anomalies of the ureter. In: Campbell MF, Harrison GH (eds) Urology, 3rd edn. WB Saunders, Philadelphia
2. Whitten SM, Wilcox DT (2001) Duplex system. Prenat Diagn 21:952–957
3. Wiesel A, Queisser-Luft A, Clementi M et al (2005) EUROSCAN Study Group. Prenatal detection of congenital renal malformations by fetal ultrasonographic examination: an analysis of 709,030 births in 12 European countries. Eur J Med Genet 48:131–144
4. Nguyen HT, Herndon CD, Cooper C et al (2010) The Society for Fetal Urology consensus statement on the evaluation and management of antenatal hydronephrosis. J Pediatr Urol 6:212–231
5. Castagnetti M, Cimador M, Esposito C et al (2012) Antibiotic prophylaxis in antenatal nonrefluxing hydronephrosis, megaureter and ureterocele. Nat Rev Urol 9:321–329
6. Hizli F, Yilmaz E, Uygur MC (2011) Urinary incontinence in a young girl due to ectopic ureter: the importance of history in a diagnostic challenge. N Z Med J 124:88–92
7. Castagnetti M, El-Ghoneimi A (2009) Management of duplex system ureteroceles in neonates and infants. Nat Rev Urol 6:307–315
8. Husmann DA, Strand WR, Ewalt DH et al (2002) Is endoscopic decompression of the neonatal extravesical upper pole ureterocele necessary for prevention of urinary tract infections or bladder neck obstruction? J Urol 167:1440–1442
9. Kim YS, Do SH, Hong CH et al (2001) Does every patient with ureteropelvic junction obstruction need voiding cystourethrography? J Urol 165: 2305–2307
10. Othman S, Al-Hawas A, Al-Maqtari R (2012) Renal cortical imaging in children: 99mTc MAG3 versus 99mTc DMSA. Clin Nucl Med 37:351–355
11. Grattan-Smith JD, Jones RA (2006) MR urography in children. Pediatr Radiol 36:1119–1132
12. Molitierno JA Jr, Scherz HC, Kirsch AJ (2008) Endoscopic injection of dextranomer hyaluronic acid copolymer for the treatment of vesicoureteral reflux in duplex ureters. J Pediatr Urol 4:372–376
13. VanderBrink BA, Cain MP, Gilley D et al (2009) Reconstructive surgery for lower pole ureteropelvic junction obstruction associated with incomplete ureteral duplication. J Pediatr Urol 5:374–377
14. Avlan D, Gündoğdu G, Delibaş A et al (2010) Pyeloureterostomy in the management of the lower pole pelvi-ureteric junction obstruction in incomplete duplicated systems. Urology 76(76):1468–1471
15. Smith FL, Ritchie EL, Maizels M et al (1989) Surgery for duplex kidneys with ectopic ureters: ipsilateral ureteroureterostomy versus polar nephrectomy. J Urol 142:532–534
16. Plaire JC, Pope JC 4th, Kropp BP et al (1997) Management of ectopic ureters: experience with the upper tract approach. J Urol 158:1245–1247
17. Mackie GG, Stephens FD (1975) Duplex kidneys: a correlation of renal dysplasia with position of the ureteral orifice. J Urol 114:274–277
18. Meneghesso D, Castagnetti M, Della Vella M et al (2012) Clinico-pathological correlation in duplex system ectopic ureters and ureteroceles: can preoperative work-up predict renal histology? Pediatr Surg Int 28:309–314
19. Chacko JK, Koyle MA, Mingin GC et al (2007) Ipsilateral ureteroureterostomy in the surgical management of the severely dilated ureter in ureteral duplication. J Urol 178:1689–1692

20. Prieto J, Ziada A, Baker L et al (2009) Ureteroureterostomy via inguinal incision for ectopic ureters and ureteroceles without ipsilateral lower pole reflux. J Urol 181:1844–1848
21. el Ghoneimi A, Miranda J, Truong T et al (1996) Ectopic ureter with complete ureteric duplication: conservative surgical management. J Pediatr Surg 31:467–472
22. Castagnetti M, Canali R, Mastrocinque G et al (2013) Dismembered extravesical reimplantation of dilated upper pole ectopic ureters in duplex systems. J Pediatr Surg 48:459–463
23. Lee SD, Akbal C, Kaefer M (2005) Refluxing ureteral reimplant as temporary treatment of obstructive megaureter in neonate and infant. J Urol 173:1357–1360
24. Castagnetti M, Cimador M, Sergio M et al (2004) Transurethral incision of duplex system ureteroceles in neonates: does it increase the need for secondary surgery in intravesical and ectopic cases? BJU Int 93:1313–1317
25. Byun E, Merguerian PA (2006) A meta-analysis of surgical practice patterns in the endoscopic management of ureteroceles. J Urol 176:1871–1877
26. Abrahamsson K, Hansson E, Sillén U et al (1998) Bladder dysfunction: an integral part of the ectopic ureterocele complex. J Urol 160:1468–1470
27. Holmes NM, Coplen DE, Strand W et al (2002) Is bladder dysfunction and incontinence associated with ureteroceles congenital or acquired? J Urol 168:718–719
28. de Jong TP, Dik P, Klijn AJ et al (2000) Ectopic ureterocele: results of open surgical therapy in 40 patients. J Urol 164:2040–2043
29. Beganović A, Klijn AJ, Dik P et al (2007) Ectopic ureterocele: long-term results of open surgical therapy in 54 patients. J Urol 178:251–254
30. Cendron J, Melin Y, Valayer J (1981) Simplified treatment of ectopic ureterocele in 35 children. Eur Urol 7:321–323
31. Upadhyay J, Bolduc S, Braga L et al (2002) Impact of prenatal diagnosis on the morbidity associated with ureterocele management. J Urol 167:2560–2565
32. Monfort G, Morisson-Lacombe G, Coquet M (1985) Endoscopic treatment of ureteroceles revisited. J Urol 133:1031–1033
33. Ben Meir D, Silva CJ, Rao P et al (2004) Does the endoscopic technique of ureterocele incision matter? J Urol 172:684–686
34. Blyth B, Passerini-Glazel G, Camuffo C et al (1993) Endoscopic incision of ureteroceles: intravesical versus ectopic. J Urol 149:556–559
35. Hagg MJ, Mourachov PV, Snyder HM et al (2000) The modern endoscopic approach to ureterocele. J Urol 163:940–943
36. DeFoor W, Minevich E, Tackett L et al (2003) Ectopic ureterocele: clinical application of classification based on renal unit jeopardy. J Urol 169:1092–1094
37. Cooper CS, Passerini-Glazel G, Hutcheson JC et al (2000) Long-term followup of endoscopic incision of ureteroceles: intravesical versus extravesical. J Urol 164:1097–1099
38. Castagnetti M, Vidal E, Burei M et al (2013) Duplex system ureterocele in infants: should we reconsider the indications for secondary surgery after endoscopic puncture or partial nephrectomy? J Pediatr Urol 9:11–16
39. Rich MA, Keating MA, Snyder HM 3rd et al (1990) Low transurethral incision of single system intravesical ureteroceles in children. J Urol 144:120–121
40. Chertin B, Rabinowitz R, Pollack A et al (2005) Does prenatal diagnosis influence the morbidity associated with left in situ nonfunctioning or poorly functioning renal moiety after endoscopic puncture of ureterocele? J Urol 173:1349–1352
41. Chertin B, de Caluwé D, Puri P (2003) Is primary endoscopic puncture of ureterocele a long-term effective procedure? J Pediatr Surg 38:116–119
42. Adorisio O, Elia A, Landi L et al (2011) Effectiveness of primary endoscopic incision in treatment of ectopic ureterocele associated with duplex system. Urology 77:191–194
43. Jesus LE, Farhat WA, Amarante AC et al (2011) Clinical evolution of vesicoureteral reflux following endoscopic puncture in children with duplex system ureteroceles. J Urol 186:1455–1458
44. Husmann D, Strand B, Ewalt D et al (1999) Management of ectopic ureterocele associated with renal duplication: a comparison of partial nephrectomy and endoscopic decompression. J Urol 162:1406–1409
45. Wallis MC, Khoury AE, Lorenzo AJ et al (2006) Outcome analysis of retroperitoneal laparoscopic heminephrectomy in children. J Urol 175:2277–2280
46. Shankar KR, Vishwanath N, Rickwood AM (2001) Outcome of patients with prenatally detected duplex system ureterocele; natural history of those managed expectantly. J Urol 165:1226–1228
47. Han MY, Gibbons MD, Belman AB et al (2005) Indications for nonoperative management of ureteroceles. J Urol 174:1652–1655
48. Direnna T, Leonard MP (2006) Watchful waiting for prenatally detected ureteroceles. J Urol 175:1493–1495
49. Coplen DE, Austin PF (2004) Outcome analysis of prenatally detected ureteroceles associated with multicystic dysplasia. J Urol 172:1637–1639

Part III

Bladder

12 The Vesicoureteric Maze: The Reasons of Misunderstanding

Delphine Demède and Pierre Mouriquand

12.1 Introduction: What Are We Talking About?

Vesicoureteral reflux (*VUR*) remains one of the most controversial issues in pediatric urology. Several reasons can explain this confusion. The first one is the flooding of contradictory data found in literature with almost 9,000 hits on MEDLINE. As Sir Graham Hills (principal of the University of Strathclyde) said: "… too much knowledge generates hypotheses and theories not always rooted in reality" (the knowledge disease). The second reason is that modern medicine is locked in the evidence-based methodology which undermines individual experience and desperately tries to quantify and standardize situations which are beyond mathematical logic and protocols. Medicine is one of the fields where several answers can be given to one question, sometimes completely opposite although perfectly valid. The third reason is that the term VUR covers two entirely different entities: (1) "reflux disease" which is an abnormal construction of the urinary tract and more precisely of the ureterovesical junction and (2) the "reflux symptom" which is the visible part of the iceberg as it is the consequence of a lower urinary tract dysfunction (Table 12.1). "Reflux disease" is far more common in boys, often detected on prenatal ultrasound which shows dilated ureters. Cystography confirms a high-grade VUR (grades IV–V) and isotope studies commonly show an abnormal renal parenchyma. The resolution rate is low and surgery is often the recommended treatment. "Reflux disease" is rare and paradoxically more commonly taught at university than "reflux symptom" which is far more common and often misunderstood by doctors. This latter type of VUR is usually found during infancy in girls after recurrent *urinary tract infections* (*UTIs*). Ultrasound scans are usually normal as well as isotope studies. Cystography shows low-grade VUR (I–III). The resolution rate is high often accelerated by bladder training. Fig. 12.1 shows the various actors hidden behind these two types of VUR.

Table 12.1 VUR covers two different entities

	VUR "disease"	VUR "symptom"
Sex	Boy	Girl
Age	Newborn/Infant	Child
Presentation	Antenatal	UTI
U/S scan	Dilatation	Normal
Cystography	IV–V	I–II–III
DMSA	Abnormal	Normal
Resolution	<50 %	High
Etiology	Abnormal VUJ	Bladder dysfunction
Treatment	Surgery	Medical, reeducation
Frequency	+	+++++++++++++++
Teaching	++++++++++++	+

D. Demède (✉) • P. Mouriquand
Department of Pediatric Urology,
HFME Mother and Child Hospital, Lyon, France
e-mail: delphine.demede@chu-lyon.fr;
pierre.mouriquand@chu-lyon.fr

M. Lima, G. Manzoni (eds.), *Pediatric Urology: Contemporary Strategies from Fetal Life to Adolescence*,
DOI 10.1007/978-88-470-5693-0_12, © Springer-Verlag Italia 2015

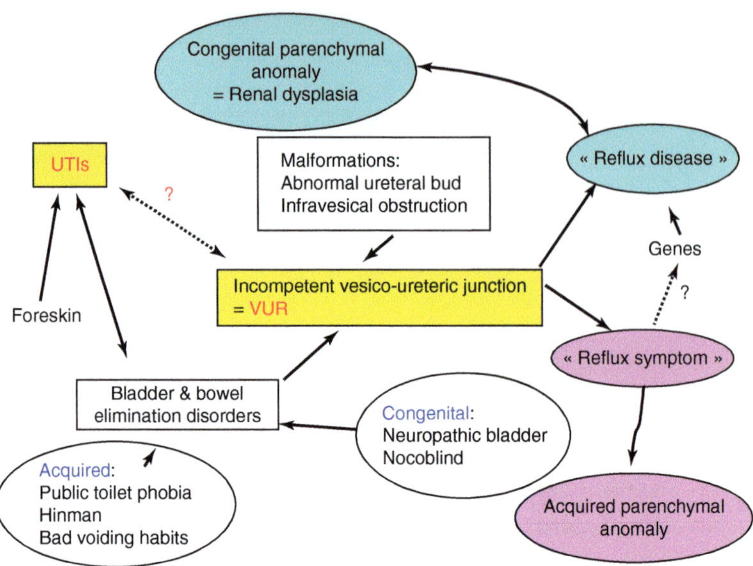

Fig. 12.1 The complex pathophysiology of VUR

12.2 Is VUR Dangerous?

12.2.1 VUR and UTI

Relationships between *VUR* and *UTI* are another source of confusion as VUR is often searched and found after several episodes of UTI. However, 90 % of VUR have sterile urine [1] and 60 % of febrile UTIs have no demonstrable VUR [2]. It is therefore unlikely that VUR causes UTIs, but it certainly aggravates the prognosis of an existing UTI by transporting infected urine from the bladder to the kidneys. Children with VUR are more likely to develop pyelonephritis and renal scarring as compared to those with no VUR, and children with VUR grade III or higher are more likely to develop scarring than children with lower grade of VUR [3]. There is a definite correlation between the degree of VUR and the development of the renal parenchyma. Correcting VUR does not really change the incidence of UTIs but certainly reduces the risk of febrile UTIs. The lesson to learn from this is that it is more important to find out the origins of a UTI than to treat an incidental VUR which is the only visible part of the iceberg. There is a consensus to say that UTI associated with VUR increases the risk of *renal parenchymal damage*, and although febrile UTI does not mean pyelonephritis, it is commonly considered prudent to treat any febrile UTI as a pyelonephritis. The only way to confirm the diagnosis of pyelonephritis would be to perform a DMSA scan during the acute phase of the infection which is practically difficult for many hospitals. Alternatively, an increase serum level of procalcitonin (≥1.0 ng/mL) would also be a sign in favor of a renal parenchymal involvement (sensitivity, 87.6 %; specificity, 89.3 %) and would be more accurate than the increase of CRP [4]. It is often postulated that pyelonephritis implies the ascent of bacteria along the ureter tract and implies therefore VUR although this is not evidenced. Fighting the causes of UTI implies to understand what the ingredients of a UTI are. Four actors need to meet: (1) nonflowing urine related either to acquired urine flow impairment mostly related to inadequate bladder emptying or related to congenital urine flow impairment; (2) the presence of a bacterial reservoir, a prepuce, or an overloaded bowel; (3) bacterial nastiness related to the microbiological profile of bacteria; and (4) the host receptivity dependent upon the biological profile of the individual.

12.2.2 VUR and Renal Parenchymal Damage

Abnormal renal parenchyma is commonly found on DMSA scan in children with VUR. Forty percent of prenatally detected VUR have an abnormal DMSA before any episode of UTI [5]. There is no available investigation which can identify *congenital parenchymal lesion* (dysplasia) from *acquired parenchymal lesion* ("reflux nephropathy"). Thirty to 50 % of VUR with renal damage will develop a high blood pressure on a long-term basis [6]. It is therefore recommended that damaged kidneys are regularly screened with ultrasound scan, measurement of urine microalbumin, and measurement of blood pressure. The impact of VUR on renal function and on end-stage renal failure is quite variably reported: 12–25 % of all children with *chronic renal failure* [7, 8] and 5–10 % of the Australian adult population [9]. According to the 2008 North American Pediatric Renal Trials and Collaborative Studies (NAPRTCS) report, reflux is the fourth commonest cause of chronic kidney disease, found in 8.4 % of the children and seen in 5.2 % of transplanted patients and 3.5 % of patients under dialysis [10]. There is a relationship between the severity of VUR and its bilaterality and the nephrological prognosis [4]. It does not seem that modern management of VUR has significantly changed the nephrological outcome [11].

12.3 Relationship with Bladder Dysfunction

12.3.1 Infants

Higher voiding pressures and a dyssynergic pattern of micturition were reported to be associated with primary VUR in infants when compared to the normal lower urinary tract [12]. This association, which predominated in male children, may have some relevance in the pathogenesis of VUR and may influence its resolution.

12.3.2 Older Children

A strong correlation exists between *dysfunctional voiding* and UTI found in 60 % of cases, as well as VUR found in 20 % of patients. It largely predominates in girls [13]. The IRS study showed that dysfunctional voiding correlates with persistence of VUR and UTI whatever treatment used [14].

12.4 If, When and How Should VUR Be Looked for?

If finding VUR impact management, i.e., if the kidneys are at risk, VUR screening should then be recommended. Four circumstances should be discussed: (1) *Prenatal upper urinary tract dilatation* is related to VUR in 15–20 % of cases [15]. These VUR are severe, associated with bilateral dilatation and congenital renal damage (60 %), and predominate in males (75 %) and have lower rates of spontaneous resolution (50 %) [5]. (2) The first *febrile UTIs* are associated with VUR in 40 % of cases [16]. Most would no longer recommend systematic VUR screening in this group, (3) in siblings of a child with VUR, and (4) in most associated uropathies.

1. Contrast cystography remains the investigation of reference and provides the clearest anatomy of the lower urinary tract. However, its morbidity is well established with significant irradiation, discomfort, and a risk of iatrogenic UTI following bladder catheterization [17]. Despite the current tendency to demonize cystography, many would prescribe it when the ureters are dilated, when the bladder and/or posterior urethra looks abnormal, or when in case of pyeloureteral duplication with or without ureterocele. There is no consensus on cystography in case of dilated renal pelvis without dilated ureter or in case of prenatal dilatation without postnatal dilatation (Table 12.2).

Table 12.2 The place of cystography in prenatally dilated urinary tract

Is cystography indicated in prenatally dilated urinary tract?	
Yes	No
15–30 % are VUR	Unpleasant (catheter)
This is the best investigation to exclude PUV (4 %) which requires an urgent treatment	Significant morbidity (1 % UTI)
VUR may be an indication for AB prophylaxy/circ.	Radiations ++
It is a reliable investigation when performed by a paediatric radiologist	RVU diagnosis is unnecessary in asymptomatic children
U/S scan is poor investigation to detect VUR	The role of antibioprophylaxis remains unclear

2. Isotopic cystography delivers much less irradiation and is a highly performant investigation to detect VUR [18]. However, it does not provide good anatomical pictures of the lower urinary tract.
3. *DMSA* is the gold standard to detect parenchymal renal lesions but is unable to distinguish acquired or congenital renal parenchymal anomalies [19].
4. *Ultrasound scan* has a very poor sensitivity to detect VUR (10 %) [16], and there is no correlation between ultrasound findings and VUR severity [20]. Seventy five percent of VUR (including high-grade VUR) have no ultrasound dilatation [21]. It is also a poor investigation to detect renal scars [22].
5. Etiologic diagnosis of VUR is crucial. In the majority of cases, assessment of bladder and intestinal behavior including history, uroflowmetry, post-voiding residue, and bladder wall sonographic assessment is sufficient to distinguish dysfunctional from malformative VUR.

All in all, is it important to detect VUR? No if the child is asymptomatic, if bladder emptying is complete (no postmicturition residue on BladderScan™), if relative renal function is stable or improves on repeated DMSA scans, and if the upper tract dilatation is stable or improves on repeated ultrasound scans. The answer is yes if one of these requirements fails or if antibioprophylaxis is advocated especially in case of severe VUR.

From these facts, it appears clear that kidney-bladder connection is essential to understand VUR. An abnormal functioning kidney associated with an abnormal functioning bladder is a time bomb. It is therefore quite logical to interrogate the kidney and the bladder to identify patients in potential danger. One way to do this is the *"top-down"* approach which starts with the first febrile UTI and the patient receiving the usual antibiotic treatment. An ultrasound scan is performed to detect any underlying anomaly of the urinary tract, followed by a DMSA scan 3–6 months later. If both ultrasound scan and DMSA are normal, there is no need to perform a *cystography.* If the ultrasound scan and/or DMSA is abnormal, a cystography is performed [23]. Some will argue that it is not necessary to start investigations after one single febrile UTI. Starting investigations at the first febrile UTI is supported by Ransley's "Big Bang" theory [24] which showed that there is no reason why a first UTI should be innocent for the renal parenchyma if bacteria are getting into it. While retrospective and prospective studies have demonstrated that the use of the top-down approach could reduce the number of cystographies performed, high-grade VUR might be missed in a minority of children [23, 25, 26]. A recent meta-analysis has shown that DMSA performs poorly at detecting high-grade reflux, with a sensitivity and a specificity of 79 and 53 %, respectively [27]. The rationale behind the "top-down approach" is based on the essential studies from Godley et al. [28] in London which demonstrated that VUR resolution is extremely high in infants with normal DMSA and normal *bladder functions*. These findings have been confirmed by other teams [5, 29]. This comes back to the introduction of this paper where VUR "disease" is more likely to require a radical treatment than VUR "symptoms" which should better respond to bladder training.

Several reports have shown promising results using serum *procalcitonin* levels to identify patients with significant VUR and renal damage in an effort to reduce the use of cystography [30].

12.5 VUR Treatments

The question is not how to treat VUR but why. The history of VUR treatment is interesting as attitudes have completely swung several times over the past three decades. In the 1960–1970s, restoring "anatomy" was the sine qua non condition to cure VUR which was thought to be the cause of UTIs. UTIs implied intravenous urography and cystography. If VUR was demonstrated, it was fixed by surgery. Surgical procedures were already well established and considered to be reliable enough to be performed in most cases. In the 1980s came the English wave showing that function was more important than anatomy. VUR was treated only if it impacts renal function. The kidney-bladder connection was put under the spotlights. Cystographies were less performed, whereas isotope studies became the central investigation killing the intravenous urography. It was also the period during which antibioprophylaxis appeared to be a safe measure to prevent UTIs and renal parenchymal damage [31]. After the 1980s came the endoscopic treatments of VUR whose easiness to perform supported by strong commercial pressure swept away most scientific rationale behind the treatment of VUR. The wave of endoscopic treatments increased again with the FDA agreement in the USA. At the same time, antibioprophylaxis became more contested. Several wise people tried to clarify the therapeutic indications of VUR but mostly showed that whatever you do, it does not make much difference in terms of outcome.

12.6 Antibiotic Prophylaxis

The subject of *antibiotic prophylaxis* in VUR is undergoing a raging debate because of serious doubts about its usefulness as well as concerns about the risk of antimicrobial resistance, patient compliance, and costs of medication. Many VUR will spontaneously resolve with age. At 10 years, *resolution* rates went up to 52 % of children with severe grade [32]. In the last 6 years, five prospective randomized trials evaluated the role of antibiotic prophylaxis in the prevention of recurrent UTI and renal scarring in children with or without reflux [33–37]. Three studies reported no benefit with prophylaxis in children with or without VUR [33–35]. Craig found a decrease of UTIs under prophylaxis in comparison to placebo [36]. None of these studies showed any difference in the rate of scarring with prophylaxis versus no prophylaxis.

The 2010 *Swedish study* [37] compared the outcome of 203 VUR grades III and IV submitted to either prophylaxis, endoscopic treatment, or simple surveillance. All patients were reassessed 2 years after inclusion with a new cystography and DMSA. This study clearly demonstrated that prophylaxis and endoscopic treatment were efficient to reduce febrile UTIs. Children who did not receive antibiotic prophylaxis were three times more likely to develop a febrile UTI than those maintained on prophylaxis. This was more pronounced in girls over 1 year of age. Prophylaxis was the best treatment to stop new renal damage.

The AUA published its guidelines on management of primary reflux in children in 2010. For children less than a year old, it is a recommendation to use prophylaxis for all grades of VUR diagnosed after a UTI and in grade III–IV VUR diagnosed through screening, whereas it is an option in grade I–II VUR. In children older than a year, prophylaxis is a recommendation if VUR is associated with recurrent febrile UTI, bladder-bowel dysfunction, or renal cortical abnormalities, in the absence of which it is an option [38].

For the National Institute for Health and Care Excellence, antibiotic prophylaxis should not be routinely recommended in infants and children following first time UTI and may be considered in those with recurrent UTI [39].

12.7 Treatment of Bowel Bladder Dysfunction (BBD)

Chasing *BBD* is important as it is often associated with an increased risk of recurrent UTI and reduced chances of spontaneous VUR resolution [40]. Possible treatments include bladder training, behavioral therapy, biofeedback, anticholinergic medications, alpha-blockers, and treatment of constipation [38].

12.8 Is There Still a Place for a Radical Treatment of VUR?

Commonly accepted *indications* are the persistence of febrile UTIs despite antibioprophylaxis and deterioration of relative renal function on serial isotope studies. Endoscopy supporters claim that subureteral injections of biocompatible substance are more efficient to reduce the risk of febrile UTI than *conventional surgery*. Evidence for this is quite slim. Meta-analyses demonstrated that, on average, 77 % of ureters injected with dextranomer/hyaluronic acid are VUR-free 3 months after injection [41, 42]. In the Swedish reflux trial [43], 20 % of previously successfully treated children presented with recurrent VUR after 2 years of follow-up, despite relatively high success rates (86 %). Surgery has not been shown to be superior to antibioprophylaxis as far as recurrence of UTI or renal scar is concerned. This was demonstrated by the Birmingham study, the International Reflux Study, and the Swedish reflux trial [43–45]. Surgical options include laparoscopic or open surgical ureteral reimplantation, the latter being the gold standard to stop reflux with about 98 % success rate.

The best illustration of the contradictory approaches of VUR is on one side doctors who tend to neglect VUR considering that it is a completely anecdotal event and on the other side surgeons who track and correct all VUR using the PIC cystography (positioning the instillation of contrast at the ureteral orifice) and even offering endoscopic treatment when VUR is not detectable. This is the VUR paradox for which John Woodward used to say that VUR treatments have been established a long time before knowing their indications. Many questions remain unanswered, mostly the place of antibioprophylaxis, the management of asymptomatic VUR, and the place of endoscopic treatments which seem to be efficient on low-grade VUR which probably do not need any treatment except bladder training.

References

1. Gross GW, Lebowitz RL (1981) Infection does not cause reflux. Am J Roentgenol 137(5):929–932
2. Sargent MA (2000) What is the normal prevalence of vesicoureteral reflux? Pediatr Radiol 30(9):587–593
3. Shaikh N, Ewing AL, Bhatnagar S, Hoberman A (2000) Risk of renal scarring in children with a first urinary tract infection: a systematic review. Pediatrics 126:1084–1091
4. Sun HL, Wu KH, Chen SM, Chao YH, Ku MS, Hung TW, Liao PF, Lue KH, Sheu JN (2013) Role of procalcitonin in predicting dilating vesicoureteral reflux in young children hospitalized with a first febrile urinary tract infection. Pediatr Infect Dis J 32(9):348–354
5. Yeung CK, Godley ML, Dhillon HK, Gordon I, Duffy PG, Ransley PG (1997) The characteristics of primary vesico-ureteric reflux in male and female infants with pre-natal hydronephrosis. Br J Urol 80(2):319–327
6. Goonasekera CDA, Dillon MJ (1999) Hypertension in reflux nephropathy. BJU Int 83:1–12
7. Chantler C, Carter JE, Bewick M, Counahan R, Cameron JS, Ogg CS, Williams DG, Winder E (1980) 10 years' experience with regular haemodialysis and renal transplantation. Arch Dis Child 55:435–445
8. Ardissino G, Dacco V, Testa S, Bonaudo R, Claris-Appiani A, Taioli E et al (2003) Epidemiology of chronic renal failure in children: data from the ItalKid project. Pediatrics 111:382–387
9. Mathew TH (1987) Reflux nephropathy as a cause of end stage renal failure. In: Twelfth report of the Australian and new Zealand combined dialysis and transplant registry. Disney APS, Ed Australian Kidney Foundation, Woodville, pp 115–121
10. NAPRTCS (2008) North American Pediatric Renal Transplant Cooperative Study (NAPRTCS); Annual report 2008
11. Craig JC, Irwig LM, Knight JF, Roy LP (2000) Does treatment of vesicoureteric reflux in childhood prevent end-stage renal disease attributable to reflux nephropathy? Pediatrics 105(6):1236–1241
12. Yeung CK, Godley ML, Dhillon HK, Duffy PG, Ransley PG (1998) Urodynamic patterns in infants with normal lower urinary tracts or primary vesicoureteric reflux. BJU 81:461–467
13. Schulman SL, Quinn CK, Plachter N, Kodman-Jones C (1999) Comprehensive management of dysfunctional voiding. Pediatrics 103:E31
14. Van Gool JD, Hjälmas K, Tamminen-Mobius T, Olbing H (1992) Historical clues to the complex of dysfunctional voiding, urinary tract infection and vesicoureteral reflux. The International Reflux Study in children. J Urol 148:1699–1702
15. Dhillon HK (1998) Prenatally diagnosed hydronephrosis: the Great Ormond Street experience. Br J Urol 81:39–44
16. Hoberman A, Charron M, Hickey RW, Baskin M, Kearney DH, Wald ER (2003) Imaging studies after a first febrile urinary tract infection in young children. N Engl J Med 348:195–202
17. Agrawalla S, Pearce R, Goodman TR (2004) How to perform the perfect voiding cystourethrogram. Pediatr Radiol 34:114–119
18. McLaren CJ, Simpson ET (2001) Direct comparison of radiology and nuclear medicine cystograms in young infants with vesico-ureteric reflux. BJU Int 87:93–97
19. Elison BS, Taylor D, Van der Wall H, Pereira JK, Cahill S, Rosenberg AR et al (1992) Comparison of DMSA scintigraphy with intravenous urography for the detection of renal scarring and its correlation with vesicoureteric reflux. Br J Urol 69:294–302
20. Foresman WH, Hulbert WC Jr, Rabinowitz R (2001) Does urinary tract ultrasonography at hospitalization for acute pyelonephritis predict vesicoureteral reflux? J Urol 165:2232–2234
21. Blane CE, DiPietro MA, Zerin JM, Sedman AB, Bloom DA (1993) Renal sonography is not a reliable screening examination for vesicoureteral reflux. J Urol 150:752–755

22. Roebuck DJ, Howard RG, Metreweli C (1999) How sensitive is ultrasound in the detection of renal scars? Br J Radiol 72:345–348
23. Preda U, Jodal R, Sixt E, Stokland, Hansson S (2007) Normal dimercaptosuccinic acid scintigraphy makes voiding cystourethrography unnecessary after urinary tract infection. J Pediatr 151:581–584
24. Ransley PG, Risdon RA (1975) Renal papillary morphology and intrarenal reflux in the young pig. Urol Res 3:105–109
25. Hansson S, Dhamey M, Sigstrom O et al (2004) Dimercapto-succinic acid scintigraphy instead of voiding cystourethrography for infants with urinary tract infection. J Urol 172:1071–1073
26. Herz D, Merguerian P, McQuiston L, Danielson C, Gheen M, Brenfleck L (2010) 5-year prospective results of dimercapto-succinic acid imaging in children with febrile urinary tract infection: proof that the top-down approach works. J Urol 184:1703–1709
27. Mantadakis E, Vouloumanou EK, Georgantzi GG, Tsalkidis A, Chatzimichael A, Falagas ME (2011) Acute Tc-99m DMSA scan for identifying dilating vesicoureteral reflux in children: a meta-analysis. Pediatrics 128:169–179
28. Godley ML, Desai D, Yeung CK, Dhillon HK, Duffy PG, Ransley PG (2001) The relationship between early renal status, and the resolution of vesico-ureteric reflux and bladder function at 16 months. BJU Int 87(6):457–462
29. Sillén U (2008) Bladder dysfunction and vesicoureteral reflux. Adv Urol 2008:815472
30. Leroy S, Romanello C, Galetto-Lacour A et al (2007) Procalcitonin to reduce the number of unnecessary cystographies in children with a urinary tract infection: a European validation study. J Pediatr 150:89–95
31. Smellie J, Edwards D, Hunter N, Normand IC, Prescod N (1975) Vesico-ureteric reflux and renal scarring. Kidney Int Suppl 4:65–72
32. Smellie JM, Jodal U, Lax H, Mobius TT, Hirche H, Olbing H (2001) Outcome at 10 years of severe vesicoureteric reflux managed medically: report of the International Reflux Study in children. J Pediatr 139:656–663
33. Garin EH, Olavarria F, Garcia Nieto V, Valenciano B, Campos A, Young L (2006) Clinical significance of primary vesicoureteral reflux and urinary antibiotic prophylaxis after acute pyelonephritis: a multicenter, randomized, controlled study. Pediatrics 117:626–632
34. Pennesi MTL, Peratoner L, Bordugo A, Cattaneo A, Ronfani L, Minisini S, Ventura A (2008) Is antibiotic prophylaxis in children with vesicoureteral reflux effective in preventing pyelonephritis and renal scars? A randomized, controlled trial. Pediatrics 121:1489–1494
35. Montini G, Rigon L, Zucchetta P et al (2008) Prophylaxis after first febrile urinary tract infection in children? A multicenter, randomized, controlled, noninferiority trial. Pediatrics 122:1064–1071
36. Craig JC, Simpson JM, Williams GJ et al (2009) Antibiotic prophylaxis and recurrent urinary tract infection in children. N Engl J Med 361:1748–1759
37. Brandstrom P, Esbjorner E, Herthelius M et al (2010) The Swedish reflux trial in children: I. Study design and study population characteristics. J Urol 184:274–279
38. Peters CA, Skoog SJ, Arant BS Jr et al (2010) Summary of the AUA guideline on management of primary vesicoureteral reflux in children. J Urol 184:1134–1144
39. National Institute for Health and Clinical Excellence (NICE). Urinary tract infection in children: diagnosis, treatment and long-term management. Accessed June 2011
40. Sillen U, Brandstrom P, Jodal U et al (2010) The Swedish reflux trial in children: V. Bladder dysfunction. J Urol 184:298–304
41. Elder JS, Diaz M, Caldamone AA et al (2006) Endoscopic therapy for vesicoureteral reflux: a meta-analysis. I. Reflux resolution and urinary tract infection. J Urol 175:716–722
42. Routh JC, Inman BA, Reinberg Y (2010) Dextranomer/hyaluronic acid for pediatric vesicoureteral reflux: systematic review. Pediatrics 125:1001–1009
43. Holmdahl G, Braandstrom P, Lackgren G et al (2010) The Swedish reflux trial in children: II. Vesicoureteral reflux outcome. J Urol 184:280–285
44. Birmingham Reflux Study Group (1987) Prospective trial of operative versus non-operative treatment of severe vesicoureteric reflux in children: five years' observation. Br Med J 295:237–241
45. Wheeler D, Vimalachandra D, Hodson EM, Roy LP, Smith G, Craig JC (2003) Antibiotics and surgery for vesicoureteric reflux: a meta-analysis of randomised controlled trials. Arch Dis Child 88:688–694

Strategy and Tactics in the Management of Bladder Exstrophy

13

Philip Ransley and Alfredo Berrettini

13.1 Introduction

Bladder exstrophy (BE) remains one of the greatest technical and philosophical challenges in pediatric urology technical because of the well-known reality of failure (we have all seen the exstrophy bladder closed once, twice, and even thrice before wiser counsel is brought to bear) and philosophical because the surgery undertaken depends on one's understanding of the underlying anomaly and the steps to be taken to correct or circumvent the tissue abnormalities. Indeed the technical challenges really begin once a successful quality closure has been achieved and is then guided by the philosophy of treatment.

The cause of the spectrum of the exstrophy group of abnormalities remains obscure, and although we regard them as variations of a common stem, their origins may indeed be different in different cases. The superior vesical fissure and the true exstrophy but with a normally positioned umbilicus do not fit easily into a single entity. Certainly the bladders are not all the same at birth. They range from the beautifully smooth glistening mucosa of an everted bladder of good size, which immediately shows a wave of muscle contraction when touched, to the tiny inelastic plate with polypoid mucosa and extensive dysplasia (Fig. 13.1).

In the former, there is a rapid change after birth with loss of contractility and mucosal thickening, and those who have seen an exstrophy bladder at the moment of birth will understand. In this modern world of prenatal diagnosis, every exstrophy surgeon should seek every opportunity of witnessing the nature of the adversary at the time of birth and not just wait for transfer to the unit hours later. Although there may be arguments for delayed closure, to be discussed later, there is no doubt that witnessing the perinatal changes is for one of us (PGR) a powerful argument for maintaining early postnatal closure as a principle tactic but only as part of an overall strategy of early, staged, selective reconstruction.

For the moment let us go back to the discussion of causation. It is really surprising how little we know and perhaps as a consequence how little we understand about the abnormality and indeed where does the *fundamental* problem lie that leads to the phenotype of an open bladder, wide pubic bones, and an epispadiac urethra. Early theories examined the idea of failure of mesodermal migration into the cloacal membrane, and this could be reproduced in a chick model by physically preventing migration in the embryo and did indeed give rise to exstrophy [1].

P. Ransley
Division of Pediatric Urology, Civil Hospital, Sindh Institute of Urology and Transplantation, Karachi, Pakistan
e-mail: pgr3@me.com

A. Berrettini (✉)
Pediatric Urology Unit, Fondazione IRCCS Ca' Granda – Ospedale Maggiore Policlinico, Via della Commenda 10, Milan 20122, Italy
e-mail: alfredo.berrettini@policlinico.mi.it

M. Lima, G. Manzoni (eds.), *Pediatric Urology: Contemporary Strategies from Fetal Life to Adolescence*,
DOI 10.1007/978-88-470-5693-0_13, © Springer-Verlag Italia 2015

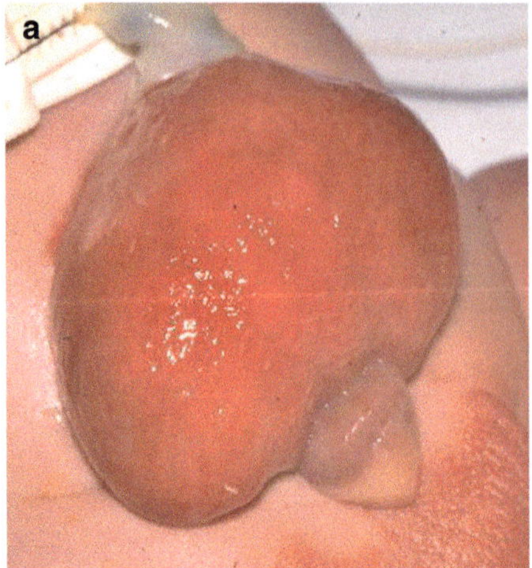

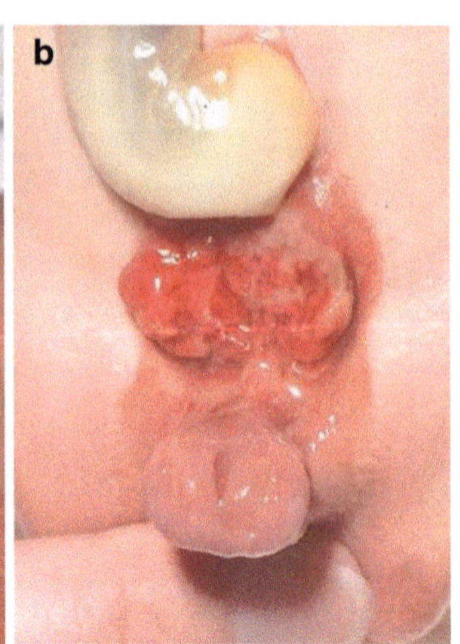

Fig. 13.1 An illustration of the variations in morphology (and therefore possibly future function) of the exstrophic bladder at birth. (**a**) Good size, everted, with smooth mucosa and visible contractions of detrusor in response to touch. (**b**) Small, contracted, and fibrotic bladder plate with polypoid dysplastic mucosa

However, this did little to help in understanding the reason for the failure or in formulating a clinical strategy. More recently it has been suggested that there may be a genetic defect, which affects cell signaling from the mucosa that should control muscle differentiation in the mesenchyme and that for some inexplicable reason this is more pronounced anteriorly than posteriorly, leading to the bladder defect [2]. As a speculative explanation of the entire abnormality, one has to then conclude that the other features and particularly the open pelvic ring are a physical consequence of the initial bladder abnormality.

Such a perception has important practical implications for the reconstructive surgeon for it means that other pelvic structures may be normal and therefore restored to normal position and function by the exhibition of surgical skill. This idea is supported by MRI studies showing well-differentiated pelvic and sphincter musculature [3] and the recent suggestion that the anterior bony pelvis is of normal length at birth and not deficient as previously thought [4]. But there is a philosophical catch. If the other structures are normal and are restored to normal anatomy, how will an abnormal bladder respond? Is it realistic to expect it to compensate for its abnormal origins and to function "normally"? By contrast, the idea of exstrophy as a field defect proposes that none of the elements involved are normal (for whatever reason) and that however skilled the anatomical reconstruction, the system simply doesn't work. Maybe both are true and differing origins explain differing responses to a single pattern of treatment. We know from decades of surgical endeavor that continence with natural voiding by detrusor contraction at normal intervals (implying normal capacity but not necessarily so) and dry at night (without getting up during the night) can be achieved. But it is rare and exceptionally rare for all these elements to be present consistently over a prolonged period of time; yes, think decades. Lesser degrees of success in a physiological sense are compatible with a very "normal" life, but for some (and maybe the majority) the outcome is less satisfactory and the unwarranted pursuit of an unachievable goal has led to many patients suffering kidney damage and some tragically pushed into chronic renal failure. Since continent diversion has such a good short- and medium-term outcome, this must enter the treatment algorithm as part of an overall strategy and not simply as a last resort when other methods have been pushed to the limit and failed. The senior author's first augment/Mitrofanoff was constructed 35 years ago and is still working well with the same channel and reservoir. Experiences like this weigh in significantly as the balance of probabilities is assessed in early childhood.

One final factor needs to be recognized. The vast majority of exstrophy cases have been and still are being born (approximately 10/day or one every 2–3 h) and treated in the less privileged parts of the world. Indeed the classical clinical descriptions, classification, and treatments emanate largely from a handful of centers located principally in the Western world treating a tiny fraction of the exstrophy population. Their population sampling may not be representative and their treatments not transferable to the wider group. An expert on malaria living in Sweden can be an expert but not if they depend only on the cases arising locally.

We would like to address the exstrophy problem as a sequence of argued decisions in an overall strategy that seeks to select the ultimate surgical solution as early as possible in order to provide a childhood which is not interrupted by repeated surgical interventions and allows full participation in the wide range of contemporary social activities which are a part of modern life.

13.2 The Newborn with Bladder Exstrophy

Although the prenatal ultrasound features of bladder exstrophy are well described [5] with the absence of a bladder and a low insertion of the umbilical cord as the principle signs, it is a rare anomaly and it is not surprising that cases are missed and become evident only at birth [6]. However, when the diagnosis is confirmed before birth, there is the opportunity and the need for a clear outline of treatment and prognosis to be provided honestly in order to allow the parents to make informed decisions. Undoubtedly this requirement for calm discussion, somewhat in the abstract, has honed the need for a postnatal strategy to be presented in a logical and sequential form, and this contrasts with the distressed discussion which takes place at birth when it is easier to focus on the immediate need for closure and to leave the future somewhat vague. The exstrophy surgeon must approach the problem with a clear plan which encompasses immediate and future surgery.

So, how should the newborn exstrophy be approached? The first question, of course, is whether or not immediate closure should be undertaken. It is perhaps ironic that the greatest numbers of bladder exstrophies worldwide are to be found in underdeveloped countries where attendance at a suitable hospital let alone neonatal surgery is not possible and surgeons there are familiar with the late presenting case often up to 5 or even 10 years later. It is worth remembering that such cases have normal kidneys and one of us (PGR) has even seen (*and* in Europe) a 75-year-old married male with untreated exstrophy and two normal kidneys!

There are arguments both ways. One of the benefits from closure in the first 24 to 48 h is the ease with which the symphysis can be approximated, whether or not relaxin plays a part and another is the rapid healing with minimal scar formation characteristic of the fetus. The response of the newborn bladder to continued exposure is very variable. Some display squamous metaplasia polyp formation and bladder plate contraction, while others evert, maintain their size or even enlarge, and show relatively little in the way of mucosal changes. However, there is no reason to think that prolonged exposure does anything except adversely affect potential bladder function.

There are several practical details which can make a difference to healing and therefore to success. The first of these is satisfactory immobilization. The authors gave up traction in all its various forms and the totally inadequate mermaid bandaging a long time ago. They were ineffective immobilizers and created difficulties with the wound especially if there was any leakage around the stents or pooling of urine from the urethra in the area of the midline closure. A frog plaster (*full internal rotation of the femurs with slight hip abduction and knee flexion; the plaster extends from the thigh to the ankle with a bar across at the knees*) (Fig. 13.2) was a significant improvement in providing much better stability and immobility with better access to the wound, and the sheer weight of the plaster itself prevented the repeated hip flexion, which was such a bugbear in the postoperative period. The disappearance of conventional plaster of Paris and its replacement with modern lightweight polymers are not seen as progress by the exstrophy surgeon!

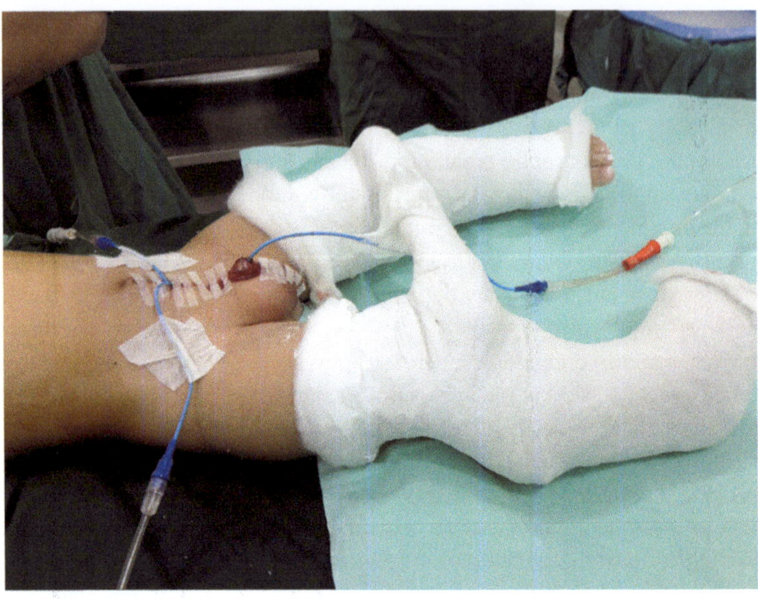

Fig. 13.2 The frog plaster. The femora legs are maintained in internal rotation which greatly relieves tension in the midline closure. The weight of the plaster prevents regular flexion at the hips

We have been fortunate to witness and benefit from the enormous advances in pediatric and neonatal anesthesia and intensive care over the last 20 years, and this has allowed for maintaining the closed exstrophy patient paralyzed and ventilated for a number of days. The precise number is not defined, but it should probably be of the order of 5–7 days. It is a significant advance in the immediate care of neonatal exstrophy closure and should be deployed wherever and whenever possible. Mushtaq et al. have explored this approach in a major center and in a retrospective review confirmed its effectiveness but could not demonstrate significant benefit over ward management postoperatively with an indwelling epidural catheter [7]. However, the partition to ward or ICU with ventilation was allocated selectively, based on difficulty of closure as well as surgeon preference and so it is hard to draw any generalized conclusion. It remains clear that immobilization by paralysis and ventilation is a major step forward and allows the quasi fetal healing to proceed rapidly and securely.

The authors' preference is for simple neonatal closure in the first 24 to 48 h with very limited dissection beyond the bladder neck in males, and this is conducted without osteotomies or penile reconstruction. Postnatal ventilation is maintained for 5–7 days and then a frog plaster for 2 weeks.

The arguments against neonatal osteotomy are several. Firstly with early intervention it is generally possible to close the pelvic ring satisfactorily by simple internal rotation of the femora and medial compression during the operation, and even with newborn osteotomies the diastasis recurs with growth. Attempts at using an external fixator in the newborn period are generally unsuccessful. The bones are too thin and fragile to support the pins, and they work completely loose in a matter of a few days. That is not to say that osteotomy has no place in longer-term management, but there is little value in adding to the burden of neonatal intervention.

13.3 Post Closure Follow-up

There is a great deal of satisfaction, tinged with relief, to see a securely healed neonatal exstrophy closure, and it enables the family to return home and begin to enjoy life with the new addition while facing far fewer problems than would be encountered caring for an exposed bladder. However, there should be no complacency and follow-up is crucial, seeking a good clinical history of wet nappies and an ultrasound of the kidneys showing no upper tract dilatation at 1 and 3 months following surgery. Although it is fortunately rare, there can be upper tract consequences from neonatal closure with bladder size, thickness, compliance, and the tension of closure all being possible factors which can change with time. Stenosis of the bladder outflow can be a disaster, and conversely a partial dehiscence of the bladder closure with bladder prolapse can be equally dangerous as the ureters can become obstructed as they prolapse through a narrow defect. A precautionary ultrasound is all that is required during this period in order for everyone involved to sleep soundly.

13.4 Subsequent Intervention

What happens next varies enormously from center to center and has changed with time over the decades. In the classical sequence the next step may well have been epispadias repair at around 2 years of age with the expectation that the increased resistance would generate some further development of bladder capacity and allow for a bladder neck reconstruction at a time "when the child is old enough to cooperate" [8]. Failure resulted in urinary diversion, originally incontinent and subsequently continent. Reported success rates in terms of voiding continence varied wildly from <20 % to over 75 %, but the variables in selection, treatment sequence, and assessment make any meaningful comparisons very difficult [9]. It is also noteworthy that the struggle for voiding continence was not without hazard for the upper tract, and many patients have suffered upper tract dilatation and renal damage as continence procedures are applied to bladders which fail to develop adequate capacity and/or fail to empty. Not only that but the consequence of such a program is that repeated surgery is performed in the older child and that if the final outcome is in fact continent diversion, then this solution is applied after the child has suffered many years of wetness with or without upper tract risks. It is the authors' contention that this sequence can be compressed in time and the ultimate solution defined before school starts and allows for an unfettered childhood. The secret lies in analyzing the needs and objectives of each component of the surgical reconstruction and then seeing how they best fit together before critically monitoring progress *and being not only prepared but positively willing to consider undertaking the surgery for continent diversion at an early age.*

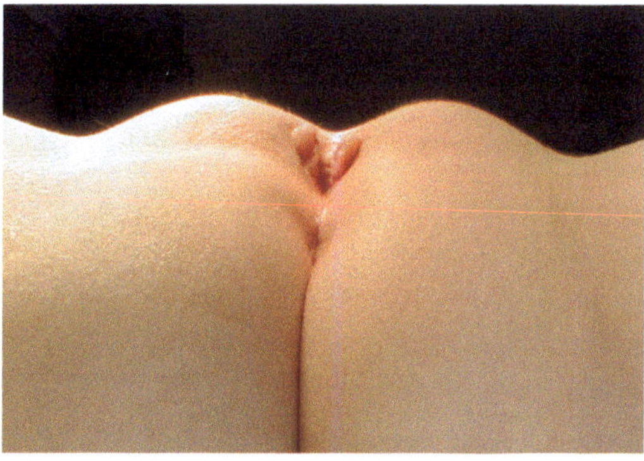

Fig. 13.3 Highline view of the female perineum. Forward projection of the pubic bones with a depressed midline scar. This is best corrected by osteotomy. Many examples can be worse than this illustration

13.4.1 Osteotomies

The practical difficulties with neonatal bone and the poor outcomes from neonatal osteotomy have led to its abandonment in most places, while others were wise enough never to engage. Nevertheless osteotomy may still have a significant role to play, particularly in females and in those cases where the bladder shows encouraging signs of being a dynamic organ and voiding continence is a serious objective.

In females, there are great benefits for cosmesis. The widely separated protruding pubic tubercles and a large triangular hairless midline scar in a young female are prevented by a satisfactory early osteotomy and extremely difficult, if not impossible, to correct later (Fig. 13.3). A good osteotomy should produce the appearance of a mons pubis with normal hair distribution. Theoretically the anterior pelvic floor travels

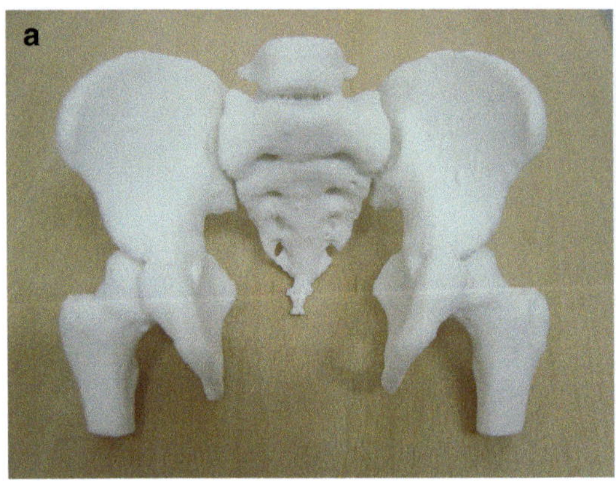

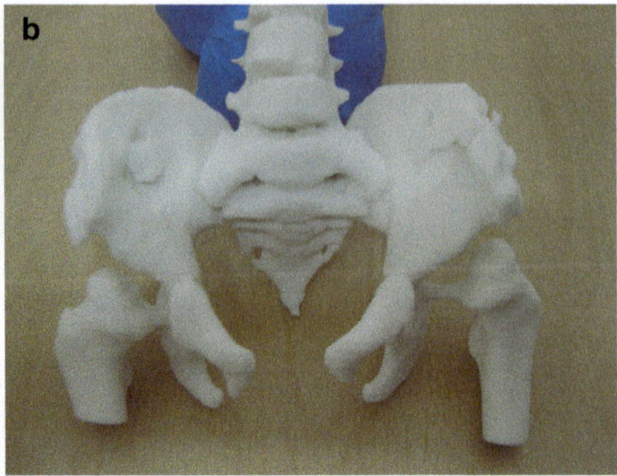

Fig. 13.4 Three-dimensional reconstructions from CT scans. (**a**) Pre-osteotomy. (**b**) Post-osteotomy in the first year of life. The anterior pelvis can close medially without caudal displacement (see text)

medially with the bones and might be helpful in preventing long-term vaginal and uterine prolapse which can otherwise be a terrible affliction for the adult exstrophy patient and often ends in hysterectomy [10].

For boys, an osteotomy has the potential to contribute a little benefit to the position of the penis by bringing the bony attachments of the corpora closer together. It does not add to length in the way which was so graphically illustrated in many classical texts on exstrophy reconstruction [11], and indeed it can make the penis appear shorter. This happens when the anterior pelvis rotates not only medially but inferiorly and carries the short penis with it so that it is even more hidden in the scrotum and the penile appearance after osteotomy can be worse than before. There is no draftsman's treatise on this subject, but it is a very subjective observation that the inferior rotation becomes much more marked when the osteotomy is performed after weight bearing. Before weight bearing the pelvis seems to move medially much more easily, without caudal migration, and the difference probably lies in the sacrotuberous ligaments which either become much stronger or shorter once an erect posture is adopted (Fig. 13.4).

Bearing all these considerations in mind, it seems logical to consider undertaking an osteotomy in both males and females when the gap has widened significantly following neonatal closure and that this should be performed once the bones are stronger but before weight bearing. This gives a window for action at 6–9 months of age.

13.4.2 Bladder Neck Surgery and Epispadias Repair

This section refers almost exclusively to boys. One of the recurring themes in the discussion of exstrophy reconstruction has always been the need to relocate the posterior urethra, prostate, bladder neck, and sphincter complex deeply into the pelvis/perineum beneath the arching corpora cavernosa. This was recognized by Mitchell in the evolution of the total disassembly operation, and his ideas and technique are soundly based [12]. However, by confining it to the newborn reconstruction, an additional element of complexity was added and the technique did not translate easily into the wider world. The classical modified Cantwell procedure [13] was limited in its success by approaching only from the front and does not result in the deep seating of the bladder neck region as much as other techniques even though the urethra is securely ventral. Any technique leaving the urethra dorsally placed is not adequately addressing the requirements for functional reconstruction, and such procedures are largely confined to history.

Today, there are essentially three approaches to obtaining adequate mobilization and deep placement of the BN/prostate/sphincter complex, and the final solution may come from utilizing elements of each together in a hybrid operation.

The first is osteotomy. The classical modified Salter osteotomy [14] is well established and is referred to as "anterior" to distinguish it from the old vertical "posterior" osteotomy. Some units have combined both for enhanced pelvic mobility [15]. Whichever way it is done, the resultant medial movement anteriorly contributes a component to the soft tissue mobility and its satisfactory placement and reconstruction. Less attention has been given to the idea of truly anterior osteotomies, i.e., combined superior and inferior ramotomies bilaterally. A superior ramotomy alone seems to have little to commend it as it does not contribute to the deep soft tissue mobility, but the combination could be effective in this regard. The inferior ramotomy is not easy but might be combined with the Kureel perineal approach (vide infra).

The second is the Kelly procedure which evolved over more than 30 years through the painstaking efforts of one man, Justin Kelly, initially in Boston and subsequently in Melbourne [16, 17].

This operation aims to benefit the penis externally while at the same time allowing the bladder neck to sink deeply. These aspects are usually in conflict, and although the Kelly procedure circumvents this problem, it does so at the price of requiring a perineal urethrostomy. However, it could be said that this becoming necessary is in itself a measure of its success in satisfying both of these two conflicting requirements.

The principle of the operation is that the two corpora cavernosa are completely relieved of any attachments to the inferior pubic rami and that the neurovascular bundles supplying them are also mobilized out of the pudendal canals. This results in a midline structure consisting of the corpora, urethra, prostate, and bladder neck from which all lateral tension has been relieved and which is mobile independent of the bones. With a perineal urethrostomy the corpora can move up and out while the bladder neck moves down and back and the sphincter/bladder neck region can be reconstructed without tension. The technique is under long-term evaluation in small numbers at Great Ormond Street Hospital in London and possibly elsewhere. It remains to be seen which aspects are most valuable in the long term and whether or not there are any long-term disadvantages to complete disconnection of the corpora.

Like the Mitchell complete disassembly before it, it is possible that the Kelly technique is a delicate wine that drinks well at home but does not travel and does not translate easily into a widespread treatment for the thousands of exstrophy patients around the globe. Kureel in Lucknow sees a large number of exstrophy patients from northern India and has also sought to provide good soft tissue relaxation and recession by radical mobilization [18]. His technique also involves radical corporal mobilization from virtually the whole of the inferior pubic ramus in the subperiosteal plane but without complete detachment. This is achieved via the perineum through a midline incision which extends down through the midline of the scrotum and with lateral extensions out to the pubic tubercle on each side in front of the anus. This provides a very clear view of the posterior urethral/prostatic/bladder neck anatomy, and it is impressive to see the sphincter identified by the use of a muscle stimulator both before and after reconstruction (Fig. 13.5). The soft tissue relaxation is of the same order as with the Kelly and can be enhanced by osteotomy. It is easy to see from the perineum that this approach could be combined with superior and inferior

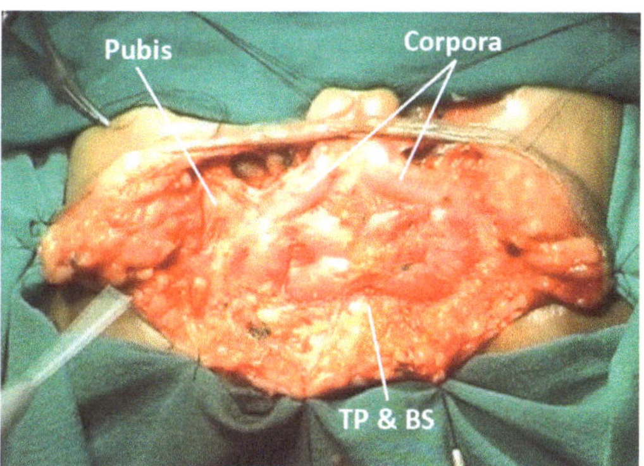

Fig. 13.5 Intra-operative view via the perineal approach showing the easy access for corporal mobilization and to the sphincter/bladder neck area (H.N. Kureel with permission). *TP & BS* = Transverse Perinei & Bulbospongiosus muscle

ramotomy which would result in the same independent midline block of tissue as created with the Kelly. Either way, the ease of soft tissue reconstruction with this technique is impressive and can be combined with a modified Cantwell epispadias repair with or without the need to disconnect the urethra and form a perineal urethrostomy. In that it can also be combined with osteotomy (either ischial or pubic), it makes for a very versatile approach.

13.4.2.1 Bladder Neck Reconstruction

It is necessary to include some discussion of what is loosely termed "bladder neck reconstruction." In so far as it is a procedure which in the reconstructive phase for bladder exstrophy may be conducted from the perineal/lower abdominal approach, it differs from the operation for bladder neck reconstruction in epispadias which is an entirely suprapubic, transvesical procedure. However, they remain in principle the same operation aimed at tubularizing the posterior urethra up to the normal bladder neck position and restoring the verumontanum to its correct location in the posterior urethra.

Both the concept and the technique of bladder neck reconstruction have changed a great deal in recent years. In classical texts it followed some time after bladder closure and epispadias repair and sought to provide a resistance sufficient to prevent urinary leakage by creating a narrow tube *out of bladder tissue* through which the bladder could be emptied by a combination of detrusor contraction and abdominal straining. This is, of course, not a functional bladder neck but a fixed resistance just sufficient to prevent incontinence. But a fixed resistance of this nature creates huge problems. Firstly the bladder must increase in capacity extremely rapidly and at least sufficiently to accommodate the overnight urine volume or there is the potential for a dangerously high pressure to exist within the bladder for many hours overnight. Secondly it must resist stress incontinence. For it to be sufficiently tight to achieve, this must result in obstructed voiding which in turn must lead to detrusor failure in the long term. Indeed, in that era, it was often observed that in those cases where the delicate balance was achieved providing voiding to completion with dryness, in time detrusor failure sets in and ultimately some other form of emptying was required. In its final incarnation the *Young-Dees-Leadbetter* bladder neck reconstruction included the reimplantation of the ureters at a higher level allowing the whole trigone to be tubularized (Fig. 13.6) [19]. This had the potential for denervating the bladder apart from providing a long resistance which often became fibrotic. This type of operation in principle and in practice is valuable for providing a leak proof channel while maintaining access via the urethra in cases undergoing bladder augmentation with a Mitrofanoff channel for emptying but *has absolutely no role in functional reconstruction aimed at voiding.*

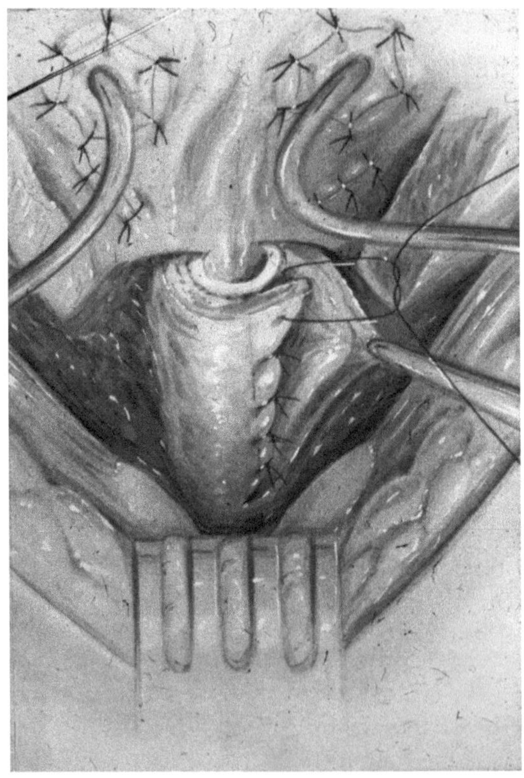

Fig. 13.6 The Young-Dees-Leadbetter bladder neck reconstruction illustrating the destructive nature of the lateral incisions into the bladder and trigonal tubularization (Reproduced from Hohenfellner [24])

Returning to the concept of functional reconstruction, as stated previously, the concept of bladder neck reconstruction is simply that, i.e., tubularization of the posterior urethra up to the normal bladder neck position which inevitably

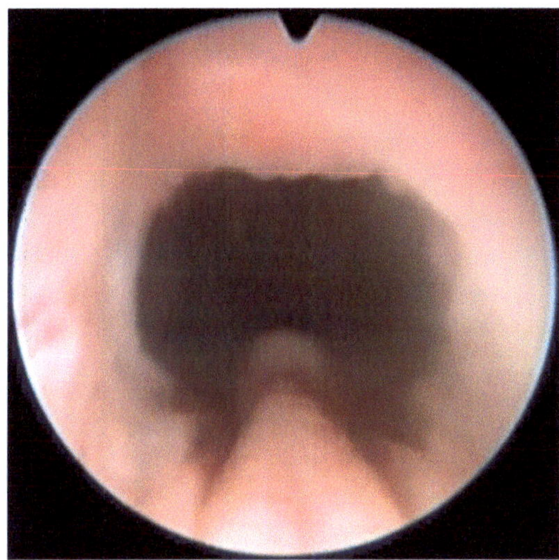

Fig. 13.7 Endoscopic view showing the verumontanum lying proximal to the "bladder neck" and therefore effectively inside the bladder lumen following primary exstrophy closure

includes reconstruction of the external sphincter and not trespassing on the intravesical trigone. As the bladder expands in those early months of life, it also includes the posterior urethra, and very often, in fact almost routinely, the veru comes to lie inside the bladder when the bladder is full (Fig. 13.7). The tubularization of the posterior urethra restores the veru to its normal position and attempts to reconstruct the normal sphincter and bladder neck. For guidance this can be taken as the point approximately half way between the veru and the ureteric openings. One of the major benefits of doing this must be to help protect against future episodes of epididymitis due to vasal reflux. The procedure is most easily conducted as part of the urethral reconstruction but can be undertaken independently, as in epispadias, via the transvesical route.

A Gil-Vernet ureteric advancement can complement the procedure to prevent reflux and avoid the need for formal reimplantation in these difficult bladders [20].

13.4.2.2 Assembling the Jigsaw

Every case will be different: the size of the bladder and the outcome of neonatal closure with regard to the bones and the bladder. Male and female, penile size, and upper tract dilatation are all variables which impact upon the decision with regard to the next major intervention.

Following neonatal closure it is imperative that the system is assessed by ultrasound to detect upper tract dilatation at 3 months and 6 months. At the 6-month point this should be accompanied by a cystoscopy and filling cystogram under anesthesia. Screening the bladder during slow filling and rapid emptying (with a syringe) will give a good estimate of the true bladder capacity which may often be different from the system capacity as there is commonly reflux into distensible upper tracts. One word of caution is necessary and needs to be repeated often and that is that capacity alone tells you nothing about contractility and the ability to empty. The cystoscopy will also assess the length of the posterior urethra resulting from primary closure in both males and females and the position of the veru in males. In truth the urethra is always very short as the original closure deliberately limited dissection in the region of the bladder neck. In males it is the authors' practice to give male patients a testosterone boost between 4 and 6 months (i.e., following the normal postnatal testosterone surge) up to a maximum of 25 mg × three doses.

The stage is now set for a second selective major intervention which is aimed at promoting voiding continence and, of course, repairing the epispadias in males. This is in many ways analogous to the complete disassembly technique deferred to a time when the structures involved are more robust and more easily identifiable but employs the Kureel technique of radical mobilization from the perineum.

The philosophy governing this second intervention is fairly simple and basically revolves around the subjective assessment of bladder size/quality and bony position. Where osteotomy is being considered, there is some urgency in the decision for males as there is the wish to accomplish this prior to weight bearing but less urgency in females where the benefit is for the pelvic floor and cosmesis and the timing seems to be less critical. A second principle is that in the quest for voiding continence, it is appropriate to introduce some better bladder cycling at an early stage, and a third is that in those cases with a clearly hopeless bladder, an elective continent

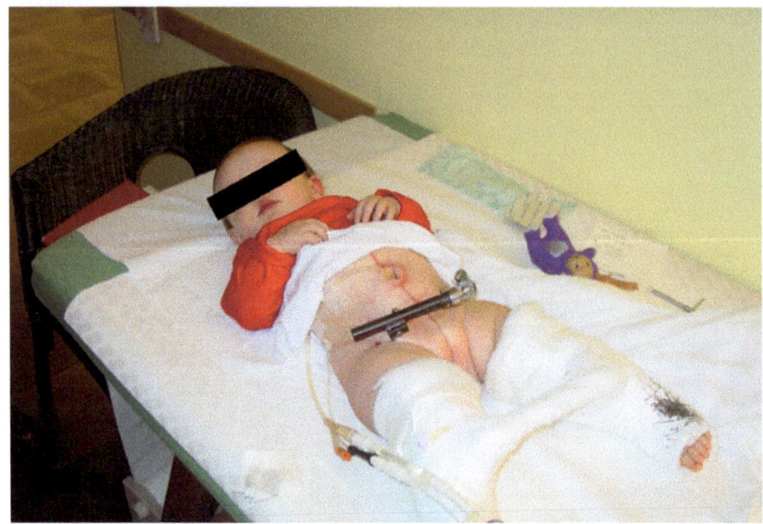

Fig. 13.8 Female infant with bladder exstrophy and a bladder similar to that in Fig. 13.3. She has undergone definitive surgery at the age of 13 months with bilateral osteotomies, bladder neck reconstruction, colocystoplasty, omphaloplasty, and a Mitrofanoff channel in the right iliac fossa and a VQZ stoma as a single-stage procedure. She is seen here at 6 weeks immediately prior to removal of the fixator

diversion will be undertaken early, in the 12–18-month window.

The permutations are enormous and there can be no single guideline for the next step, but with experience the fundamental decisions are fairly easy to make and one may consider four sample scenarios to illustrate the process.

1. *A female infant with a very poor bladder.* Here the decision is quite simple. She will be managed by an early continent diversion with a Mitrofanoff some time in the 12–18 m window. If the bony position is poor, then osteotomy will be included at the time of that reconstruction for cosmesis and pelvic floor security (Fig. 13.8). Nothing more is required in the first year of life, but it would be wise to maintain ultrasound surveillance.
2. *A male infant with a very poor bladder.* This child's destiny is also an augmentation/Mitrofanoff in the second year of life, but it is beneficial to have the genital surgery completed beforehand. It is very unlikely that osteotomy will be part of his reconstruction unless the bony position is extremely poor. In most such cases the requirement will be for a simple epispadias repair utilizing the Kureel approach with a modified Cantwell reconstruction. The surgery in the region of the bladder neck must be extremely conservative in this group and allow for free drainage of urine or the upper tracts will be placed at great risk. Osteotomies can be added where there is extreme separation of the bones and the extent of the corporal mobilization will be governed by penile anatomy. The threshold for converting to a perineal urethrostomy in order to maximize penile length is lower in this group who will not be voiding.
3. *A female infant with a good or at least encouraging bladder.* The philosophical requirement here is for some surgery to increase outflow resistance, i.e., urethral lengthening and ipso facto bladder neck reconstruction. The threshold for adding osteotomy is low and may be added to the intervention whenever the bony position is less than optimal in order to maximize cosmetic benefit and pelvic floor security.
4. *A Male infant with a good or at least encouraging bladder.* This is a target population where every effort is going to be made to secure voiding continence and perhaps fortunately is generally the largest group. A radical epispadias repair is required with osteotomies incorporating maximal mobilisation by the Kureel approach and careful reconstruction of the external sphincter (identifiable with a stimulator), posterior urethra and bladder neck. This is facilitated by osteotomy in all but those with an excellent bony position resulting from the neonatal closure. The threshold for formation of a perineal urethrostomy is

high and every effort is made to preserve the urethra in continuity.

The first year of life has therefore seen these infants kept under close observation and completing all the reconstructive surgery relating to the *anatomical* abnormality of the exstrophy itself. What follows is functional assessment and the management of urinary continence.

13.5 The Second Year of Life and Beyond

The parents of an exstrophy child are faced at birth with a whole new world of uncertainties and ambitions. There is no doubt that the relentless pursuit of unrealistic ambition is both extremely distressing and potentially very harmful. Many children have suffered renal damage, even to the point of chronic renal failure, through the failure to acknowledge that their particular exstrophy bladder cannot function as an adequate storage organ on its own, and with experience it becomes relatively straightforward to recognize those bladders which do not respond to the challenge of increasing outflow resistance and to seek an alternative solution other than the dogged pursuit of voiding continence. It is always a balance and there are no hard and fast rules, but the advice given in early life must have the child's long-term best interests at heart. One example of the burdens thrust upon a child is well illustrated by a patient seen by the authors at the age of 29 years. By all accounts he represents success and could be summarized as a patient with bladder exstrophy who underwent closure and continent reconstruction in infancy. He empties his bladder by voiding spontaneously, and since puberty he has been completely dry day and night. What more could you ask for from a difficult and challenging problem? Of course the devil lies in the detail. He is dry day and night but this is achieved only by a disciplined *hourly* voiding schedule during the day, and he has got up to void at least *four times per night every night of his life*. Clearly his bladder capacity is a limiting factor, and in his life he consciously avoids

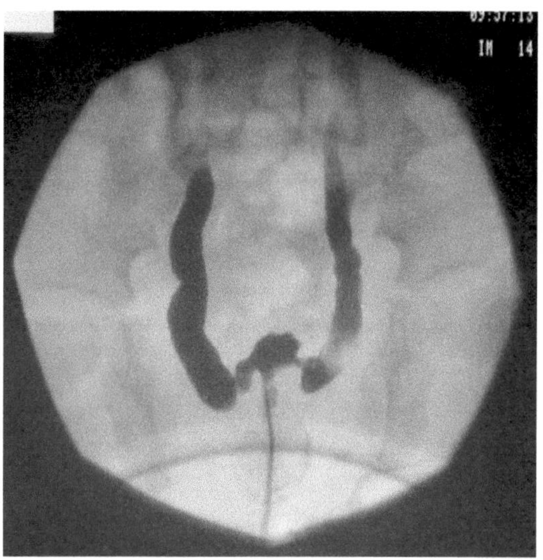

Fig. 13.9 Filling cystogram under anesthesia showing a tiny bladder following neonatal closure. This bladder is destined for augmentation/Mitrofanoff and this decision can be made comfortably in the first year of life (see text). It is essential that the bladder drains freely prior to augmentation to prevent upper tract consequences

planes, trains, and going to the cinema. It cannot be said that continent voiding has given him the best quality of life and a secure continent diversion may have been preferable. This story will strike a chord with many people involved in exstrophy reconstruction, and there is no doubt that the continent diversion has been instrumental in giving many patients a better quality of life than that which can be achieved with the native bladder alone.

Recognizing the uncertainties which exist at birth, we always tell the parents that we are going on a journey together and that we will always be there to advise and help them along the way. However, our destination at the outset is unknown and we must make choices as we progress as to where we are finally going. Continuing our analytical pathway we have now reached 1 year of age with several different groups of fellow travelers seeking direction.

There is one group who are fairly easy to counsel. They identified themselves early on with very poor bladders (Fig. 13.9) and are now diverting to the path of continent bladder augmentation with a Mitrofanoff channel for intermittent catheterization. There are so many advantages to early augmentation. It is an easier surgery and the child grows up regarding intermittent catheterization as normal. True, it ties the child to a competent third party for catheterization (usually the parents and grandparents but can also be an au pair or a nursery school assistant) in the early years, but it is remarkable how often they can take responsibility for the catheterization process themselves from about the age of 4–5 years, and all that is needed for support is someone to indicate the time that catheterization is required. They are going to be joined by new companions who set out on a different path with functional reconstruction but in whom it is very clear early on that they are not going to respond.

Following the major surgery for the functional group at 6–9 m, critical follow-up at 1 year is absolutely essential. This includes ultrasound of the urinary tract with the bladder full and empty and a dynamic isotope scan should also be performed. From these two investigations an understanding of how the system transports and stores urine is gleaned and can be interpreted alongside any measurements of voided volumes and bladder capacity on cystography. A cystoscopy is performed to assess the anatomical result from reconstruction and particularly with regard to any stricture formation, the position of the verumontanum, and the nature of the bladder neck. This last observation is of importance when considering the possible use of bulking agents to boost outflow resistance. It is imperative that there should be space to inject above the verumontanum. Increasing outflow resistance below the veru increases the risk of troublesome epididymitis in the long term. At the same time a filling and emptying cystogram is performed under anesthesia which provides one of the benchmarks for bladder progress. Bulking agents may be used to correct reflux with advantage.

From these observations our fellow travelers divide easily into three loose groups. There are those who have failed to develop and can immediately be directed to join those already headed for continent diversion from a very early stage. There will be a group whose progress is splendid. Good anatomy, a responding bladder, and safe upper tracts allow them to follow their own path and to be seen again to check their progress after an interval of up to 12 months.

In the middle will be a group who fall into neither category. It may be that they have not been sufficiently challenged and that some bulking agent at the bladder neck can be added to further challenge and fine-tune the system (Fig. 13.10). On the other hand, and this is more common, the outlet reconstruction and the resistance are satisfactory, but the bladder does not seem to be responding adequately. These are patients at some risk and require regular ultrasound review and reassessment under anesthesia after 6 months. They will declare themselves with time depending on bladder development, but regular observation over a few years will generally make things clear, and those requiring augmentation can be selected and completed before serious school begins.

13.6 Augmentation

Frequent reference has been made to continent diversion throughout this chapter which is really aimed at outlining a selective approach to the exstrophy problem. Here is not the place to get involved in a detailed discussion of the various techniques which may be employed in order to establish safe urine storage in the exstrophy population, but a few words outlining the authors' preferences are appropriate. The first point for discussion is the position for the Mitrofanoff channel [21]. It is our contention that, in contrast with the neuropathic population, this is best placed in the right iliac fossa (even taking account of handedness) and using the appendix whenever available (one advantage of early diversion is the relatively longer appendix in younger children) as the most robust channel for the long term and that this is concealed in a VQZ stoma [22]. The medial end is implanted into the bladder whenever possible

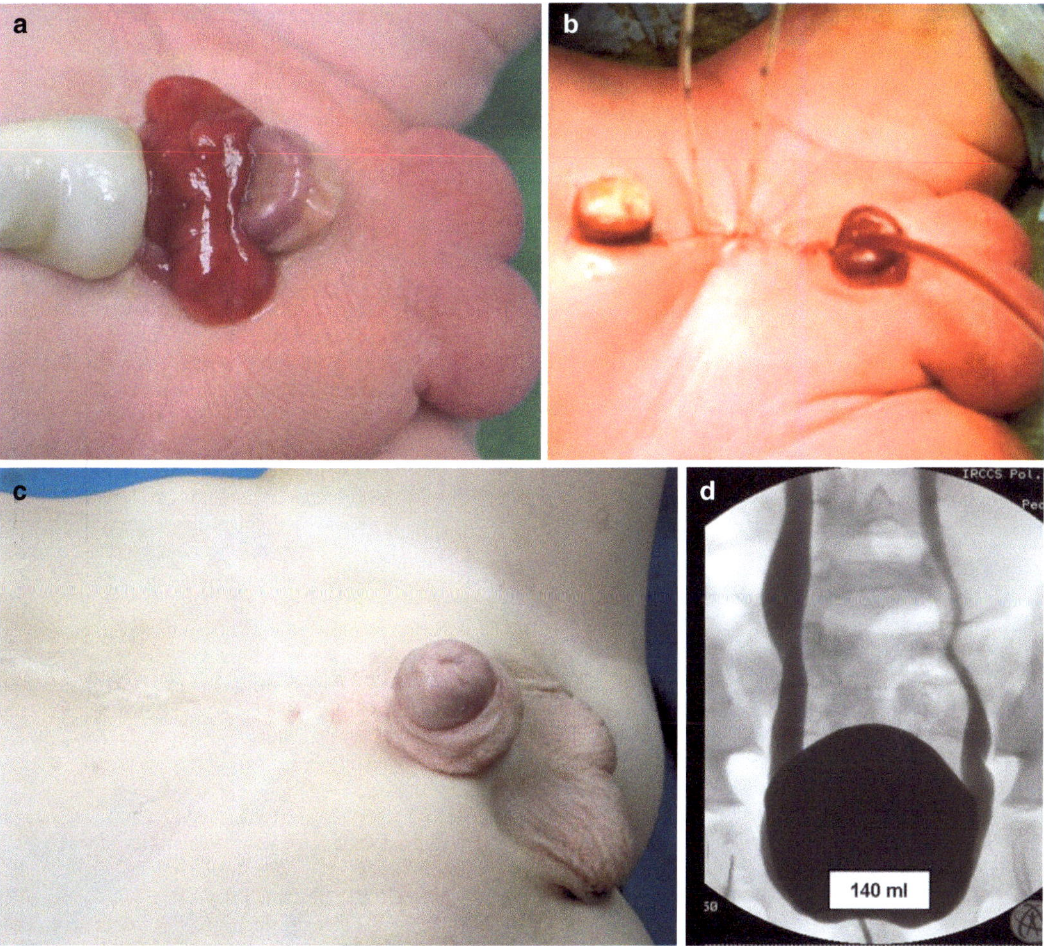

Fig. 13.10 Sequence of images in the first few years of life. (**a**) The newborn exstrophy (**b**) following neonatal closure and ventilation for 5 days. (**c**) Appearance following the second intervention at 9 months and (**d**) cystogram under anesthesia at 3 years. Voiding with increasing dry interval and a bladder capacity of 140 ml. He will require some fine-tuning at the bladder neck by endoscopic injection of bulking agent

together with the ureters if these need to be moved during bladder neck surgery. This has the advantage of a low bladder entry for the catheter and for a siphon effect to work easily which assists in complete bladder emptying and mucus clearance. The added bowel then simply functions as a reservoir and after detubularization may be configured to the surgeon's preference. Ours remains the use of the splenic flexure and descending colon based on the left colic vessels and reconfigured as a cup before anastomosis to the bladder margins. This is simple and has stood the test of time.

No reconstruction is complete without a neoumbilicus. However, although a temporary illusion may be created during closure of early midline scars, the definitive reconstruction should be deferred until the final intra-abdominal reconstruction has been performed [23].

This program seeks to allow the child with exstrophy to begin his or her school life with a safe and well-established system for urinary tract management (Fig. 13.11). They will take for granted the satisfactory function of whatever system they have adopted, and if they ever say "thank you," it will be for the umbilicus!

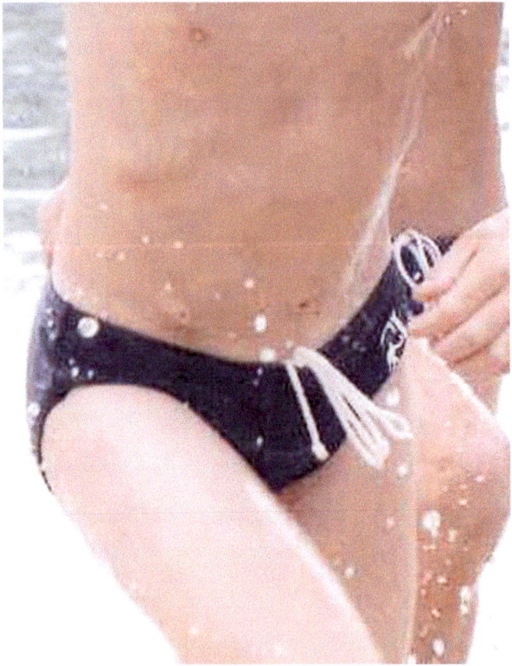

Fig. 13.11 A child born with bladder exstrophy competing in a triathlon at the age of 10 years. An augmentation/Mitrofanoff was performed after the bladder failed to respond to the challenge of bladder neck reconstruction. The omphaloplasty and Mitrofanoff stoma are clearly visible

References

1. Thomalla JV, Rudolph RA, Rink RC et al (1985) Induction of cloacal exstrophy in the chick embryo using the CO_2 laser. J Urol 134:991–995
2. Manner J, Kluth D (2005) The morphogenesis of the exstrophy-epispadias complex: a new concept based on observations made in early embryonic cases of cloacal exstrophy. Anat Embryol (Berl) 210:51–57
3. Kureel SN, Gupta A, Gupta RK (2011) Surgical anatomy of urogenital diaphragm and course of its vessels in exstrophy-epispadias. Urology 78:159–163
4. Williams AM, Solaiyappan M, Pannu HK, Bluemke D, Shechter G, Gearhart JP (2004) 3-dimensional magnetic resonance imaging modeling of the pelvic floor musculature in classic bladder exstrophy before pelvic osteotomy. J Urol 172(4 Pt 2):1702–1705
5. Evangelidis A, Murphy JP, Gatti JM (2004) Prenatal diagnosis of bladder exstrophy by 3-dimensional ultrasound. J Urol 172:1111
6. Goyal A et al (2012) Antenatal diagnosis of bladder/cloacal exstrophy: challenges and possible solutions. J Pediatr Urol 8(2):140–144
7. Mushtaq I, Garriboli M, Smeulders N, Cherian A, Desai D, Eaton S, Duffy P, Cuckow P (2014) Primary bladder exstrophy closure in neonates: challenging the traditions. J Urol 191(1):193–197
8. Gearhart JP, Jeffs RD (2007) The bladder exstrophy-epispadias complex: Chapter 119. In: Walsh PC et al (eds) Campbell's urology, 9th edn. WB Saunders, Philadelphia
9. Purves JT (2011) Modern approaches in primary exstrophy closure. Semin Pediatr Surg 20:79–84
10. Anusionwu I, Baradaran N, Trock BJ, Stec AA, Gearhart JP, Wright EJ (2012) Is pelvic osteotomy associated with lower risk of pelvic organ prolapse in postpubertal females with classic bladder exstrophy? J Urol 188:2343–2346
11. Silver RI, Yang A, Ben-Chaim J, Jeffs RD, Gearhart JP (1997) Penile length in adulthood after exstrophy reconstruction. J Urol 157(3):999–1003
12. Grady RW, Mitchell ME (1999) Complete primary repair of exstrophy. J Urol 162:1415–1420
13. Ransley PG, Duffy PG, Wollin M (1988) Bladder exstrophy closure and epispadias repair. In: Spitz L, Nixon HH (eds) Rob and Smith's operative surgery pediatric surgery. Buttersworth, Boston, pp 620–622
14. Sponseller PD, Jani MM, Jeffs RD et al (2001) Anterior innominate osteotomy in repair of bladder exstrophy. J Bone Joint Surg Am 83-A:184–193
15. Gearhart JP, Forschner DC, Jeffs RD, Ben-Chaim J, Sponseller PD (1996) A combined vertical and horizontal pelvic osteotomy approach for primary and secondary repair of bladder exstrophy. J Urol 155:689–693
16. Kelly J (1995) Vesical exstrophy: repair using radical mobilisation of soft tissues. Pediatr Surg Int 10:298
17. Jarzebowski AC, McMullin ND, Grover SR, Southwell BR, Hutson JM (2009) The Kelly technique of bladder exstrophy repair: continence, cosmesis and pelvic organ prolapse outcomes. J Urol 182:1802–1806
18. Kureel SN, Gupta A, Kumar S, Singh V, Dalela D (2011) A novel midline scroto-perineal approach facilitating innervation preserving sphincteroplasty and radical corporal detachment for reconstruction of exstrophy-epispadias. Urology 78:668–674
19. Leadbetter GW (1964) Surgical correction of total urinary incontinence. J Urol 91:261–266
20. Gil-Vernet JM (1984) A new technique for surgical correction of vesicoureteral reflux. J Urol 131:456–458
21. Mitrofanoff P (1980) Trans-appendicular continent cystostomy in the management of the neurogenic bladder. Chir Pediatr 21:297–305
22. Ransley PG (2002) The "VQZ" plasty for catheterizable stomas. In: Frank JD, Gearhart JP, Snyder HM III (eds) Operative pediatric urology, 2nd edn. Churchill Livingstone, London, pp 109–114
23. Vallasciani S, Berrettini A, Minoli DG, Manzoni GA, Ransley PG Neo-omphaloplasty in bladder exstrophy: further experience. In: ESPU 24th annual congress "video session", April 2013, Genoa, Italy
24. Hohenfellner R, Stein R (1996) Primary urinary diversion in patients with bladder exstrophy. Urology 48:28–830

Cloacal and Urogenital Sinus Anomalies

14

Francesca Destro, Noemi Cantone, Giovanni Ruggeri, and Mario Lima

The persistence of cloacal and urogenital sinus remains one of the most challenging problems for the reconstructive pediatric urologist [1, 2].

Cloaca is a Latin word for sewer and it is a normal condition in some birds, reptiles, and some fish.

In children it has a relatively rare incidence (1/40,000–50,000 patients). It comprises 10 % of anorectal malformations (ARMs) in females and 2–4 % of all ARMs [3, 4].

ARM constitutes a spectrum in females including: rectovestibular fistula, persistence of urogenital sinus, persistence of cloaca, and cloacal exstrophy.

Urogenital sinus (UGS) anomalies include complex genitourinary malformations with anomalous confluence of the urethra and the vagina. It is caused by the altered embryological evolution of organs that end in the vulva. In particular the separation of the UGS into the urethra and the female genital tract is more or less incomplete, with the urethra and vagina sharing a distal common channel to the perineum. The single orifice is usually in the perineum or rarely at the top of a hypertrophic clitoris. The anus and the rectum are normal and well placed. It is thus simple to differ this condition from the persistence of the cloaca where intestinal and genitourinary tracts end in a single perineal orifice (clover syndrome).

F. Destro • N. Cantone • G. Ruggeri • M. Lima (✉)
Department of Pediatric Surgery,
S. Orsola-Malpighi University Hospital,
Via Massarenti 11, Bologna 40138, Italy
e-mail: Francesca_destro@hotmail.com;
Noemi.cantone@hotmail.it;
Giovanni_ruggeri@aosp.bo.it; Mario.lima@unibo.it

14.1 Embryogenesis and Sexual Differentiation

From 4 to 6 weeks of gestation (g.w.), there is a critical time of the development of cloacal structures [5]. The 4-week embryo has a cavity (internal cloaca) where the allantois, the rectum, and the Wolff ducts end. The cloacal membrane closes the cavity at the caudal end and it is still intact.

Then there is a progression of the urorectal septum that gradually separates the cloaca (6 g.w.) in the urogenital sinus (anterior) and the rectum (posterior).

The developmental failure of the UGS in female patients gives rise to the.

The complete separation of the UGS is related to the absence of androgens. Androgens inhibit the development of the UG sinus. Therefore patients with congenital adrenal hyperplasia (CAH) can develop a persistence of UGS.

In case of early maldevelopment and rupture of the cloacal membrane just before everything is separated, there is the development of cloacal exstrophy.

During this altered process the uterus and the vagina often fail to fuse in the midway. Therefore duplications of the Müllerian structures are very

M. Lima, G. Manzoni (eds.), *Pediatric Urology: Contemporary Strategies from Fetal Life to Adolescence*,
DOI 10.1007/978-88-470-5693-0_14, © Springer-Verlag Italia 2015

common in patients with cloaca along with vaginal atresia.

Sexual differentiation starts after the 9th g.w. depending on the presence or absence of the Y chromosome (cr) or better of a part of the Y cr called SRY (sex-determining region Y) on the Y short arm. It is now clear why there are male patients with XX or female patients with XY.

SRY gene promotes the gonadal differentiation into the testes. The testis starts the production of androgens (Leydig cells produce testosterone) that stimulate the transformation of the Wolffian duct (vas deferens, epididymis, and seminal vesicles) and promotes the growth of external genitalia. At the same time, Sertoli cells of the testes produce the Müllerian-inhibiting factor (MIF) that stops the development of the uterus.

The absence of the Y cr and the presence of two X stimulate the development of female internal genitalia (ovary and Müllerian structures as the fallopian tubes, uterus, and part of the vagina) and the regression of Wolffian system.

14.2 UGS Persistence

Persistence of the UGS is related to two conditions:

- UGS persistence with ambiguous genitalia – disorders of sex development (46,XX DSD, previous female pseudohermaphroditism, ovotesticular DSD, previous true hermaphroditism, mixed gonadal dysgenesis)
- UGS persistence alone (female hypospadias, urovaginal confluence, UGS with high transverse septum)

14.2.1 UGS Persistence Associated with Ambiguous Genitalia (Chromosomopathies or Disendocrinopathies)

(a) 46,XX DSD = an endogenous or exogenous hyperandrogenism gives a picture of female pseudohermaphroditism that overlaps the congenital adrenogenital syndrome. It is related to an enzymatic deficit (21-hydroxylase deficit in 95 % of cases) in the cortisol synthesis. The effect is an increment of intermediate metabolites (usually androgens) that leads to virilization of external genitalia. Time and intensity of stimulation are responsible for the severity of the clinical picture: from clitoris hypertrophy to complete labioscrotal fusion with penile clitoris. Internal genitalia (uterus, fallopian tubes, and proximal vagina) are always normal, while the entry point of the vagina in the uterus (UGS) varies. The UGS can be low (near the perineum) or high (near the external urethral sphincter) or intermediate between the two (Fig. 14.1).

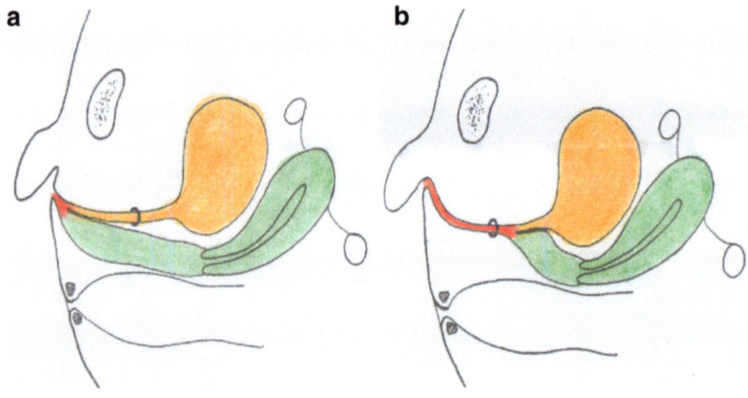

Fig. 14.1 Two extreme forms of UGS in CAH. (**a**) Low form: early division of the UGS. (**b**) High form: the UGD is long with cranial division

(b) Ovotesticular DSD = True hermaphroditism is defined by the presence of both ovarian and testicular tissues, either separately or, more commonly, together as ovotestis. Karyotype is 46,XX in almost 60 % of true hermaphroditism; it is 46,XY in 10 % and it is mixed (XX/XY) in 30 % of cases. The translocation of the Y cr short arm over the X explains the presence of the testis in XX patients. Internal genitalia are the same of the ipsilateral gonad. The testis has its own epididymis and vas deferens, while the fallopian tubes are well developed in the ovarian side. Both systems are represented in case of ovotestis. There is often a rudimentary uterus. True hermaphrodite has usually a wide vaginal opening in the urethra near the perineum or in the perineum with its own orifice.

(c) Mixed gonadal dysgenesis = patients with mixed gonadal dysgenesis have a testis on one side and a dysgenetic gonad or a streak on the opposite side, persistence of Müllerian-derived structures, genitalia asymmetry, and mosaicism (45, X/46, XY). External genitalia are ambiguous in 80 % of cases. The aspect of internal genitalia is related to the gonad. The vas deferens and epididymis are well developed at the side of the testis (which is usually undescended), while the fallopian tubes and uterus are at the side of the streak. In all these cases there is a wide vaginal opening in a short UGS.

14.2.2 UGS Persistence (Idiopathic)

It is a rare condition affecting females with normal set of chromosome (46,XX) and a unique external vulvar orifice for both the urethra and the vagina. They are related to an arrest of the vaginal differentiation process with a different anomaly degree (female hypospadia, urovaginal confluence, UGS persistence).

(a) Female hypospadia = the vaginal vestibule is normal and the urethral orifice ends on the anterior vaginal wall, one or two centimeters over the vaginal opening. There are no continence problems, but "vaginal urination" may lead to vaginal dilatation, stagnation of urine and false incontinence, vulvovaginitis, dysuria, and lower urinary tract infection.

(b) Urovaginal confluence = the bladder directly opens in the vagina with an incompetent bladder neck or through a short urethra. There is always urinary incontinence. There are urinary (unilateral renal agenesis)-associated and genital (proximal vagina and bifid uterus)-associated anomalies.

(c) UGS with high transverse septum = There is a single vulvar orifice that is wide and seems to be part of the external urethral orifice (indeed it leads to the bladder). This tract is actually the distal part of the vagina (there is a common channel or UGS) that does not communicate with the vagina because there is a transverse septum. The septum makes the vagina a close organ. The condition can be identified in the neonatal period as an abdominal mass (accumulation of vaginal and uterine secretions) under maternal hormonal stimulation (hydrometrocolpos) or it can be diagnosed in pubertal age.

14.2.3 UGS Management

The management of the patient with UGS persistence is certainly multidisciplinary with a team working with the parents and the child [6]. The diagnosis is often made in the neonatal period because most patients have ambiguous genitalia. Physical examination should include careful inspection of external genitalia (position of labioscrotal folds, location and size of the gonads, and consistency of the phallic tissue), perineum (presence or absence and location of the anus, number of orifices), abdomen, and the back searching for masses or abnormalities. Prior to surgery endoscopic (Fig. 14.2) and radiological (contrast x-ray studies) evaluations delineate the anatomy, in particular the length of the sinus, the location of the bladder neck and the vaginal introitus, the presence of a cervix and the contour of the bladder.

Ultrasonography is useful to evaluate the internal genital and higher urinary tract. MRI is used

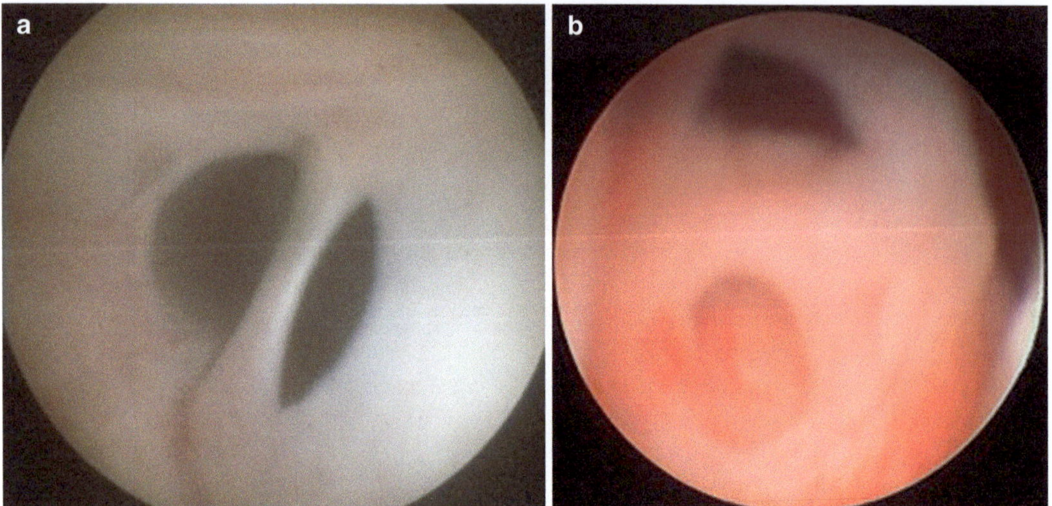

Fig. 14.2 Endoscopic evaluation with identification of two openings in a common channel

when the anatomy remains confusing. Gonadal biopsy is rarely necessary.

The initial management includes dilatation of UGS and intermittent catheterization (in the vagina or in the bladder) or vaginostomy/vesicostomy in case of failure of catheterization.

14.2.4 UGS Treatment

The anatomy of the UGS (caliber and length of the common channel) defines the surgical strategy.

14.2.4.1 UGS Associated with Disorders of Sex Development

The former belief that early surgery to "normalize" the masculinized genitalia helps promoting attachment between parents and infants is not so clear anymore. The feminizing genital surgery is very controversial. Timing and type of reconstruction are currently in question [7–9]. The aim of surgical techniques is to offer nice cosmesis preserving the sensation and function. We leave the deepening of this discussion to the chapter on intersexes.

Feminizing genitoplasty include: clitoridoplasty, vaginoplasty, and labiaplasty.

The radiological (cystourethrogram, retrograde genitogram) and endoscopic evaluation of the confluence level of the urethra and vagina is important. The higher is the level of masculinization, the higher the vagina ends into the UGS. Classical distinction divides low and high forms depending on the position of the vaginal opening compared to the external urethral sphincter. However, it is more correct to use the terms intermediate, high (40 %), and low (60 %).

Clitoridoplasty

It can be performed prior or after UGS correction in high forms or be contemporary to vaginoplasty in low forms. The objectives are to preserve the neurovascular integrity of the glans clitoris, prevent painful erections, and provide feminine cosmesis (Fig. 14.3). A traction suture is placed on the glans clitoris. The clitoris is then bared with a circumferential incision made 2 cm below the glans and two longitudinal medial incisions (dorsal and ventral). Corpora cavernosa are freed up to their bifurcation isolating the dorsal neurovascular bundles. Then they are resected preserving the spongiosum. The glans is sewn to the bifurcation of the corporal bodies. Skin flaps, obtained with the clitoris-covering skin (prepuce), are used to make the labia minora.

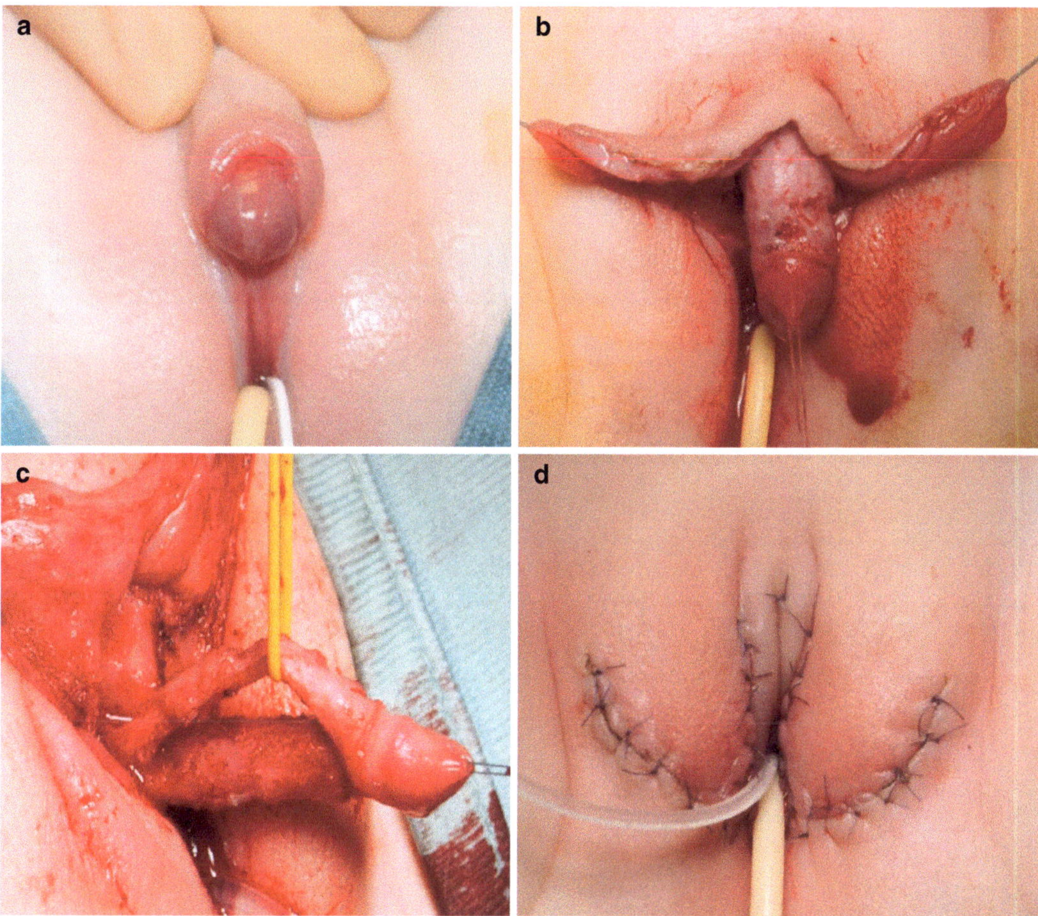

Fig. 14.3 Clitoridolabioplasty in a case of CAH. The aspect of genitalia is shown in (**a**). The clitoris is bared (**b**). Corpora cavernosa are freed up to their bifurcation isolating the dorsal neurovascular bundles (**c**). Skin flaps, obtained with the clitoris-covering skin (prepuce), are used to make the labia minora (**d**)

Vaginoplasty

The type of vaginoplasty (Fig. 14.4) depends on the anatomical location of the vaginal entrance into the UGS. The procedure is preceded by an enema or a total bowel preparation. In case of CAH steroid administration should be suited based on scheme therapy by the endocrinologist. Endoscopic evaluation is performed prior to surgery to assess the level of the vaginal entrance. A Fogarty catheter is placed into the vagina and a Foley one into the bladder. The entire lower body of the child is then prepared to obtain a surgical field that will allow both the perineal and abdominal steps (if necessary).

(a) Low forms

Cutback vaginoplasty = it is used for isolated labial fusion (it is not used anymore for common UGS). The UGS is opened through a vertical incision. The vagina is then marsupialized to the perineal skin.

Flap vaginoplasty = the urethral meatus is exposed through a median skin incision. The skin flap is obtained with an "inverted U" incision with the base anterior to the anus and just below the sinus. The flap is folded posteriorly. The dissection (in deep tissues) involves the posterior vaginal wall that is separated from the rectal wall. At the end of the dissection, the

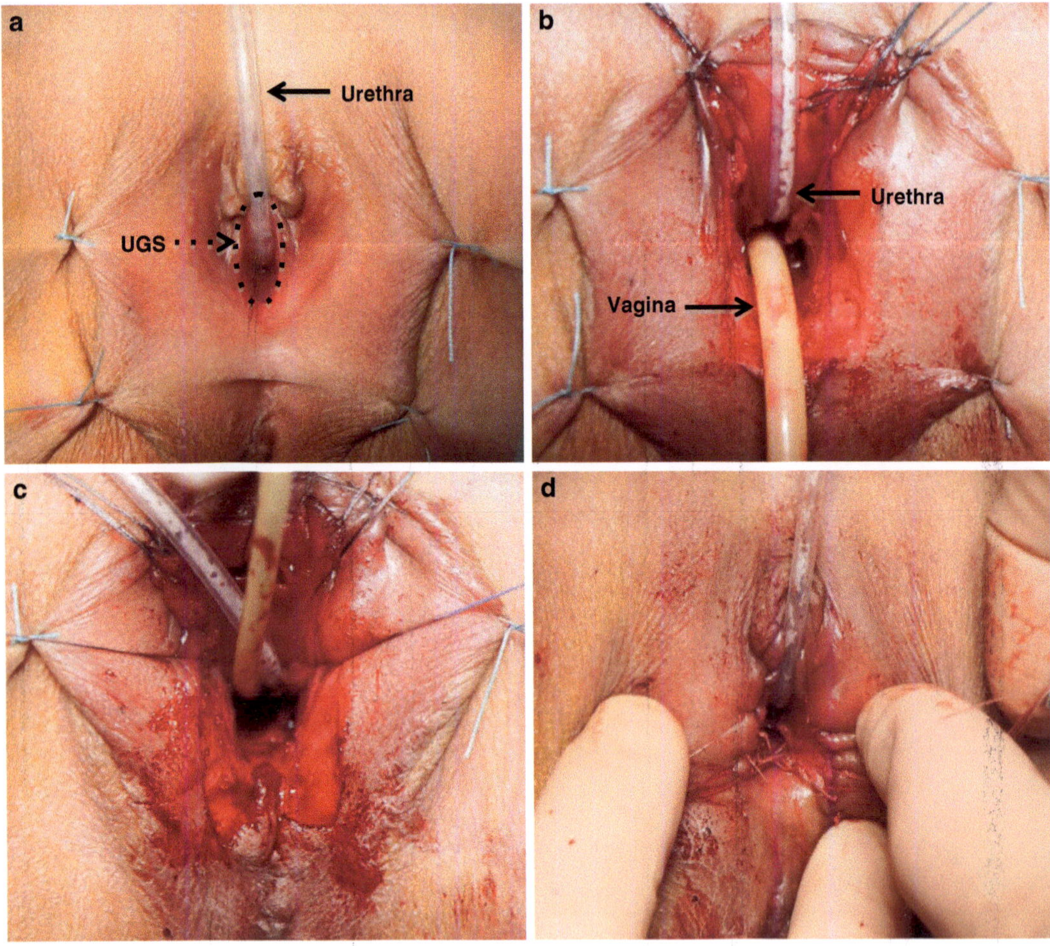

Fig. 14.4 Vaginoplasty. The urethra is catheterized endoscopically (**a**). The urethra and vagina are separated and brought down to the perineum (**b**, **c**). Final aspect (**d**)

posterior vaginal wall is opened in the midline and the skin flap interposed in order to obtain vaginal exteriorization. The vagina is then attached to the neo-vulva. The vulva has been previously reconstructed in all its parts (preputial skin has been advanced to create the labia minora and labia majora that have been shaped by Y-V plasty). Dilatations are performed after 2 weeks for 6 months and then once a month till sexual activity begins. A Foley catheter is left indwelling and a Penrose drain is left in the vagina for the first 2–3 days. Stenosis is one of the most frequent complications.

(b) High forms

This group includes very masculinized patients with hyper- and hypoplastic vaginas. The presence of a common urethrovaginal wall and the attempts for preserving the external urethral sphincter make this surgery very complex. The procedure of choice is the vaginal pull-through, simplified by urogenital mobilization (total or partial).

Hendren pull-through vaginoplasty [10] = the surgery is preceded by clitoridolabioplasty (previously performed in the first surgical step). The dissection is performed through the perineum, after the introduction of a Fogarty catheter in the vagina and of a rigid probe in the urethra. You create two skin "U" flaps in the perineum (one with a posterior and the other with an anterior base). Dissection proceeds below the posterior flap toward the junction of the urethra and vagina. Once the posterior vaginal wall is reached, the Fogarty catheter is removed. It is then possible to separate the vagina from the urethra under direct view. The urethra is closed transversally. The vagina is then completely mobilized and incised on four quadrants. A wide vaginal opening is obtained suturing the vagina with four skin flaps (two principle flaps – anterior and posterior – and two lateral accessory flaps). Dilatations are performed after surgery to avoid stenosis.

Jones vaginoplasty [11] = it provides a combined abdominoperineal approach. Two skin "U" flaps are obtained in the perineum (one with a posterior and the other with an anterior base). A probe is inserted through the abdomen (minimal laparotomy) in the uterus and in the vagina until it reaches the perineum. Then the surgical procedure is completed with the same modalities described for the Hendren approach.

Gonzalez vaginoplasty [12] = clitoridolabioplasty and vaginoplasty are performed together in order to use the foreskin for anterior vaginal wall reconstruction. The vagina is isolated through the perineum. An "inverted U" skin flap (with the apex at the UGS opening) is obtained in the perineum and it is used for posterior vaginal wall reconstruction. You perform two openings on the foreskin flap that has been transposed posteriorly and sutured to the vagina (anterior wall). The clitoris and the urethral opening are sewn in these openings. Posterior (skin) and anterior (foreskin) flaps are then sutured together to form the distal vaginal tract.

Passerini-Glazel vaginoplasty [13] = the foreskin and the penis are used with part of the urethra to replace the distal vagina. The clitoris skin is mobilized and the spongiosum is separated from the cavernosa. The urethra is opened vertically. Clitoridoplasty is then completed. The clitoris skin is divided in two parts that are rotated and sutured to the flap obtained from the opening of the urethra and the spongiosum. This way you obtain a wide rectangular flap that is tubularized and sutured to the vagina that has been previously prepared through the perineum or through the bladder (transtrigonally).

Peña vaginourethroplasty, total sagittal transanorectal approach [14] = this is a total mobilization firstly described for cloacal correction (see below). The technique permits the vagina to reach the perineum without tensions thus reducing the risk of vaginal stenosis. Peña proposed a transanorectal sagittal approach with easier visualization of the confluence and less demanding separation of urethra and vagina. The child is placed prone on pelvic rolls. The incision extends from the sacrum to the external UGS opening, through the anorectum. The levator ani, the muscle complex, and the external sphincter are opened in the midline and the anterior and posterior rectal wall are opened too. Posterior UGS wall is identified and opened exposing the urethral and vaginal openings. After the placement of a urethral catheter, vagina and urethra are separated. This phase is delicate because the two structures have a common wall. It may be useful to place traction stitches over the anterior vaginal wall. The dissection reached the bladder neck and the vagina is mobilized up to the uterine neck preserving the vascular pedicles that allow vaginal pull-through. The neourethra is then reconstructed with UGS walls and the mobilized vagina is sewn to the perineal skin, near the urethral neo-orifice. Then the perineal body is reconstructed and the rectum walls as well as all muscles are sutured. Vaginal dilatations are not necessary and vesical catheter is kept for 2 weeks. These infants usually have a protective colostomy, performed in a previous surgical time. The colostomy is closed after 2 months.

Domini ASTRA, anterior sagittal transanorectal approach (Fig. 14.5) [15] = the anorectum is opened just in its anterior wall. The anatomical vision is still excellent, the reconstruction is simplified, and

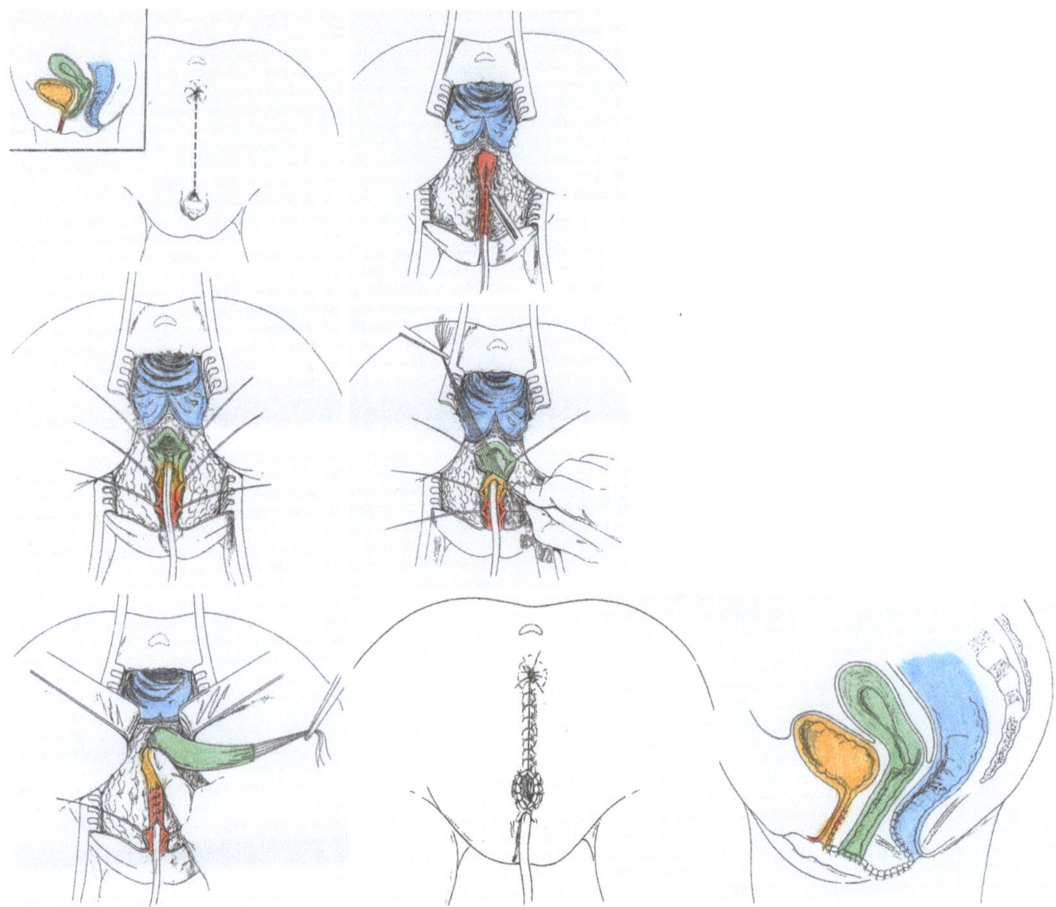

Fig. 14.5 ASTRA technique. Transanorectal incision (*upper, left*). The anterior wall of the rectum is incised in the midline (*upper, right*). The complete opening of the UGS allows the visualization of the vagina and urethra (*center*). The vagina is separated from the urethra (*down, left*). Final suture after anastomosis of the three structures to the perineum (*down, center*, and *right*)

neuromuscular structures are preserved. ASTRA is an easier way to separate high UGS without major disruption of the pelvic floor. It was proposed since the vaginal pull-through can have problems related to vaginal separation: it is technically difficult, it may result in vaginal ischemia, and it may create vesicourethral fistulas and urinary incontinence. The patient is placed in the prone position with a Fogarty catheter in the vagina and then approached transrectally. The technique is then the same as for Peña vaginoplasty with no need for protective colostomy. An important point is to give preoperative estrogen therapy to create a much more robust vagina that is easier mobilized. Another advantage of the ASTRA is that you can reconstruct the urinary sphincter. Clitoridolabioplasty is performed after 2 months.

Total urogenital and partial mobilization, TUM/PUM (Fig. 14.6) [16] = the UGS is circumscribed and suspended by traction sutures. The urethral plate may be divided below the glans clitoris, dissected and mobilized with the UGS. An incision is then performed posterior to the UGS, in the midline. All the attachments between the rectum and the UGS are divided

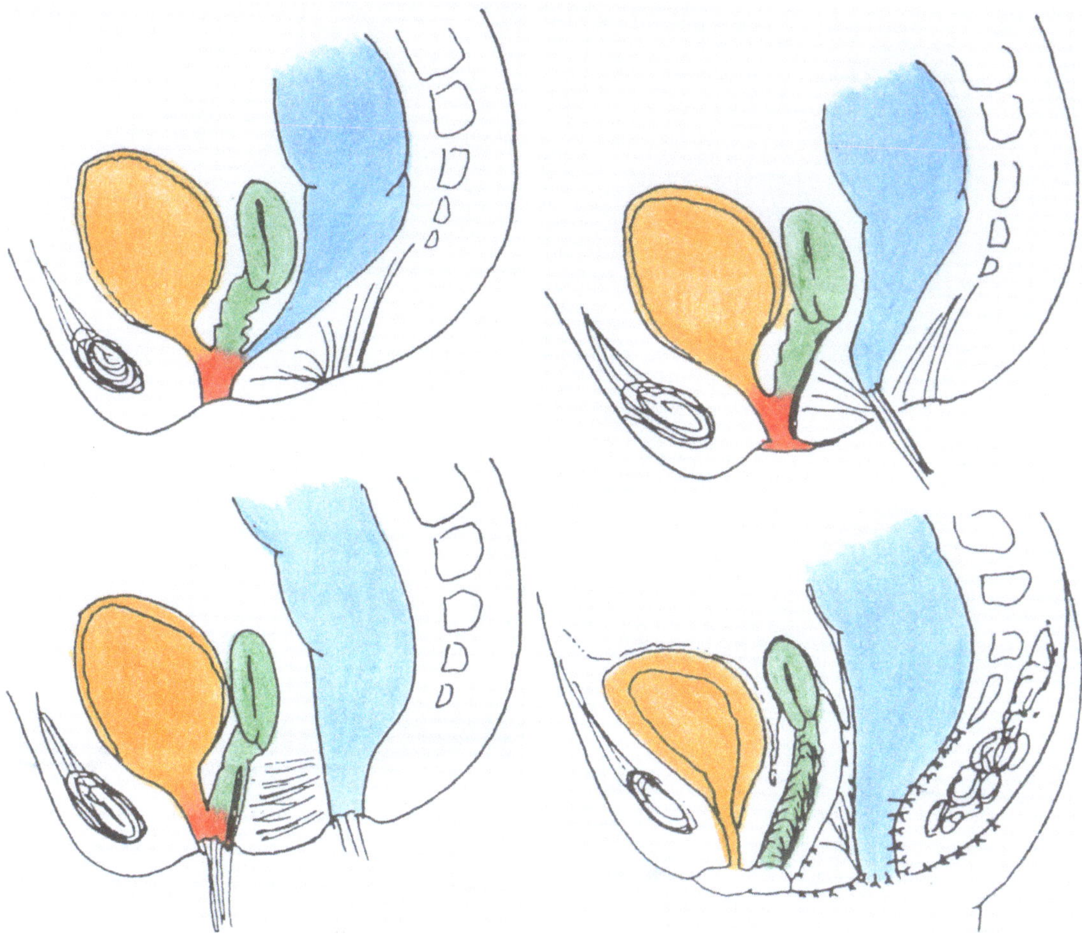

Fig. 14.6 TUM for correction of defects with short common channel. The rectum is separated from the UGS. The sinus is isolated with blunt dissection. At the end of the dissection, the urethra and vagina are sutured with the skin

without injuring the rectum or the sinus. The dissection proceeds near the posterior vaginal wall until the peritoneum is reached and swept superiorly. Meanwhile the sinus has been mobilized anteriorly and divided from the pubis. In PUM the dissection stops at the pubourethral ligament. The posterior wall of the vagina is opened near the confluence. If the vagina reaches the perineum, it is pulled through and the redundant tissue is used to create a vestibule. If the vagina does not reach the perineum, the anterior vaginal wall should be separated from the urethra after the baby has been turned prone. In this situation the redundant tissue is used to create a Passerini flap. At the end a Penrose drain is left in the vagina and the Foley catheter is left in the urethra.

14.2.4.2 Idiopathic UGS

(a) Female hypospadia = these forms do not usually require any treatment. Sometimes it is useful to obtain a complete separation between urethra and vagina using inverted perineal skin flaps sutured to the vagina.
(b) Urovaginal confluence = the aim is to reconstruct the urethra and restore the continence. These forms are characterized by an almost normal vagina in which a short urethra ends. The problem is essentially the urethra. The urethroplasty can be performed with vaginal

flaps. The ASTRA technique is not applicable because the vagina already reaches the vulva. The anterior wall of the vagina is used to restore the urethra when the bladder neck is competent. Bladder skin urethroplasty is used when the urethra and the bladder neck are absent. This is a suprapubic surgery that ends with a perineal step. The anterior bladder wall is exposed until the bladder enters the UGS. The bladder is separated from the sinus and the vagina is reconstructed using the UGS tissue. The pseudo-bladder neck is closed. A bladder flap (3.5×8 cm) is obtained from the anterior bladder wall and it is tubularized forming the neourethra. The neourethra is lowered behind the pubis and sutured to the vulva over the vaginal introitus (ex-UGS).

(c) UGS with high transverse septum = this condition is very rare. The most used surgery consists of vaginal lowering through a combined via (abdominovulvar). The anterior vaginal wall is opened through the abdomen. Then the UGS is used as urethra. Another possibility is to perform the ASTRA technique that can be used also for these cases.

14.2.4.3 Urethrovaginal Fistula

It is a post-traumatic acquired pathology. It can be corrected with the ASTRA technique.

14.3 Cloacal Persistence

It was once defined as "UGS persistence associated with anorectal malformation." It represents an independent clinical entity (just in females). Three systems (urinary, genital, and intestinal) lead into a common channel that opens in the perineum (Fig. 14.7) [17]. This means that there is a connection between the vagina, the rectum, and the bladder at different levels and stages of development. The level at which the three parts unite in the cloaca varies (there are high and low forms) and it affects the complexity of the anomaly.

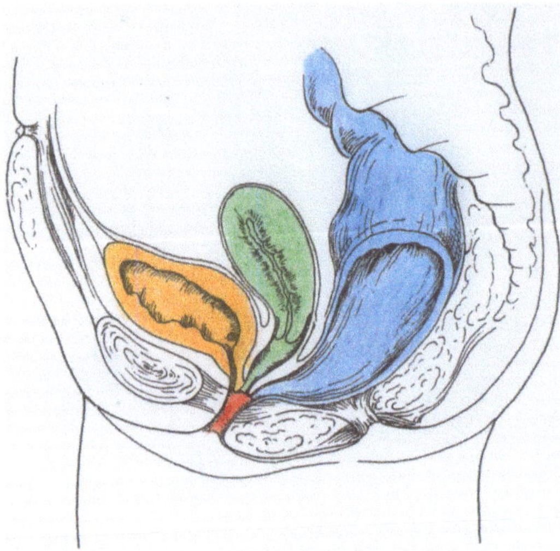

Fig. 14.7 Cloaca: the rectum (*blue*), the vagina (*green*), and the urethra (*yellow*) converge in the same channel (*red*)

The diagnosis of cloaca is clinical. The perineum of a neonate with simple cloaca has a single orifice below the clitoris (which is often hypertrophic), imperforate anus, and diminished labia. The complex cloaca (long cloacal channel), on the other side, can be characterized by a posterior displacement of the single opening and flat buttocks. The posterior cloaca itself can be rather bizarre with a single opening that is displaced posteriorly in a variety of anatomical findings that can be quite difficult to delineate initially. The evaluation of children with cloaca is similar to that described for UGS, but these children might have severe associations.

Cloacal malformation can present as ambiguous genitalia. It is important to remember that girls with a single perineal opening, even if they have weird genitalia, should be considered as girls with cloacal abnormalities until proven otherwise.

Hydrocolpos is associated with cloaca in 30–60 % of cases. It is related to the narrow UGS or cloacal channel and to the bad vaginal drainage (obstructive process that dilates the upper part). In severe cases the abdominal mass gives diaphragmatic compression with respiratory distress, decreased venous drainage for lower extremities, or urine loss in the peritoneum due to retrograde flow of urine through the genital tract (peritonitis with urinary pseudocysts, ascites). Prenatal very distended hydrocolpos may lead to prune-belly abdomens.

Müllerian anomalies are often associated with cloacae that contribute to determine the prognosis, like other associated anomalies. For instance, vaginal absence, which is present in 9 % of cases, worsens the picture. Cloacae can also present with vulvar abnormalities or with hemangiomas. In the latter case the hemangioma can extend proximally involving internal structures.

The overall incidence of associated anomalies is high. In particular urologic anomalies are present in 70 % of cases, spine and lumbosacral spinal cord anomalies in 30 %. Other cardiac anomalies and gastrointestinal alterations such as tracheoesophageal fistula, duodenal atresia, and rectal duplication have been seen in children with cloacae. All these anomalies and the cloaca itself worsen the functional outcome, especially in terms of continence.

Many cloacae are now diagnosed antenatally, especially those with hydrocolpos or with some kind of distended structures (e.g., cystic pelvic dilatations as well as bilateral hydronephrosis are common findings) that are identified on prenatal US. The presence of some elements (hydronephrosis, an intrapelvic collection of fluid, dilated distal bowel, spinal and/or sacral malformations, absent kidney) on prenatal US of female fetuses is highly suggestive for cloacae. A reason for pregnancy termination is the association with spinal dysraphism that is present in 50 % of cloacae. Renal agenesis, ectopia, and dysplasia can also be present, and dysplasia is the reason why 20 % of patients develop end-stage renal disease. There can be also ureteral reflux (50 %) and rarely urethral duplications (whose treatment is simple and consists of opening the midline creating a normal mucosal strip between the glans, clitoris, and urethra). Spinal abnormalities account for 50 % of associated malformations. The child should be turned prone for back evaluation, since sacral anomalies are so frequent. One third of patients will develop a postoperative neuropathic bladder requiring clean intermittent catheterization (CIC) or Mitrofanoff.

In the first 24 h of life, it is fundamental to identify the associated anomalies that threaten the life of the baby and to exclude the presence of hydronephrosis or hydrocolpos. Ultrasounds may show very distended bladder, rectum, and vagina. Very distended vaginas lead to hydronephrosis by compression. This is an important issue, as hydronephrosis caused by a distended hydrocolpos does not improve after vesicostomy. The vagina, which is what compresses the ureter, should be drained instead of the bladder. Adequate management of neonatal hydrocolpos and hydronephrosis is essential to avoid further renal damage. You should drain the dilated vagina before contemplating vesicostomy. Vesicostomy is only occasionally required when the baby is not capable of emptying the bladder. Hydronephrosis may also be related to vesicoureteral reflux that is assessed by injecting water-soluble contrast after catheterization (hopefully of the urethra). The urologic evaluation is considered completed if the kidneys are normal and there is no hydrocolpos. An echocardiogram and a plain radiograph of the sacrum rule out cardiac and spinal malformations.

Babies with cloaca should be investigated with abdominal x-ray that is important to see where the gas fills the abdomen, and it may reveal a pelvic mass and linear calcification in case of ascites or granular calcifications (meconium from urine washing into the rectum).

After US and plain x-ray investigations, a combined cysto-vagino-cologram should be performed prior to reconstruction, once a colostomy has been performed and the patient is stable. This test is crucial for future reconstruction because it shows the type of UGS (high or low).

Prior to surgery it is useful to perform a cystoscopy and to place a catheter in the bladder and vagina. Investigation with cysto-vagino-cologram and endoscopy is important for surgical planning and to avoid injuries to adjacent structures.

The length of the cloacal channel can be used as a prognostic factor [18]. The real important part is the length of the urethra and the size of the vagina that should be endoscopically evaluated in order to decide whether an intra-abdominal or posterior sagittal approach should be done. MRI and CT reconstruction are done occasionally especially in older patients and in patients with complications.

14.3.1 Cloacal Management

It is obvious that given the complexity of the anomaly, the treatment should be individualized.

In general you have to decompress the gastrointestinal and genitourinary tract. Later on you should perform definitive correction of both the genitourinary abnormalities and the cloacal malformation. These procedures are simultaneous in most instances, as delayed vaginoplasty often requires remobilization of the rectum in a scarred tissue. The optimal age for surgery has not been established. The repair in the neonatal age seems to be safe and effective in healthy infants, but the choice for many surgeons is a delayed repair between 6 and 12 months.

In newborns it is essential to treat the hydrocolpos. Intermittent catheterization is the best way to achieve vaginal decompression if the cloacal channel is large enough to allow it and the family is compliant. In other cases you can do a vaginostomy. The management can include:

- Divided high sigmoid colostomy that is performed promptly after delivery and stabilization of the child. Colostomy decompresses the gastrointestinal tract and prevents the flow of stool into the cloaca. A right transverse divided colostomy allows future rectal pull-through and potential vaginoplasty, but it leaves the large distal colon and a large area for exchange of urinary electrolytes. Peña suggests performing a divided colostomy in the proximal descending colon. To decide where to put the colostomy is important especially if the vagina is very small and it will require a piece of colon.
- Endoscopy should be performed with colostomy to define the anatomy and to decompress the bladder and vagina.
- Dilatation of cloacal channel
- Vesical (or vaginal) intermittent catheterization
- Vaginostomy is required if hydrocolpos has not responded to catheterization of the cloaca. Percutaneous tube vaginostomy is better than the open vaginostomy because the vagina is not tendered to the abdominal wall, and once you have to do the pull-through or the mobilization of the vagina, it is easier.
- Vesicostomy

In infants the management depends on the complexity of the anomaly and on anatomical findings and it aims to definitive repair (PSARVUP – posterior sagittal anorectovaginourethroplasty).

14.3.2 Cloaca Treatment

The aim of surgery is to achieve a normal anatomy and function (aspect of the perineum, urinary and fecal continence, and sexual activity) of the three organs involved in the malformation.

In cloacae (and in ARMs), the striated muscle of the pelvic floor is represented by a complex funnel-shaped structure extending from its pelvic insertions (pubis, pelvic rim, and sacrum) to the perineal skin. This structure is composed by:

(a) A superior part: the elevator ani
(b) An intermediate part: vertical muscle fibers that run parallel to the rectum (muscle complex)
(c) An inferior part: parasagittal fibers that cross around the anus forming the external sphincter

Fecal continence is the result of the synergy between these components. Striated urethral sphincter constitutes the anterior extension of this funnel-shaped structure. This sphincter is around the cloacal sinus and should be restored after urethral reconstruction. The section over the midline permits the identification of these muscular planes and of the cloacal sinus.

Definitive PSARVUP (Fig. 14.8) repair is preceded by a new cystoscopy because the endoscopy done in the newborn period is not ideal.

PSARPVUP procedure is performed with the infant in prone position with elevated pelvis. The exception is related to patients with common channels longer than 3 cm or with the need of the intestine to reconstruct the vagina. These conditions require also an abdominal approach to complete the repair and reach all the very high structures (rectum, vagina, or both) or the intestinal segment chosen for vaginoplasty. The procedure starts with a sagittal incision made in the midline, from the sacrum to the posterior edge of cloacal external orifice. The first thing to do is the identification of the muscle planes and their half division. The posterior wall of the rectum and the cloacal channel are then identified and opened showing the three orifices (rectum, vagina, and urethra). The vagina

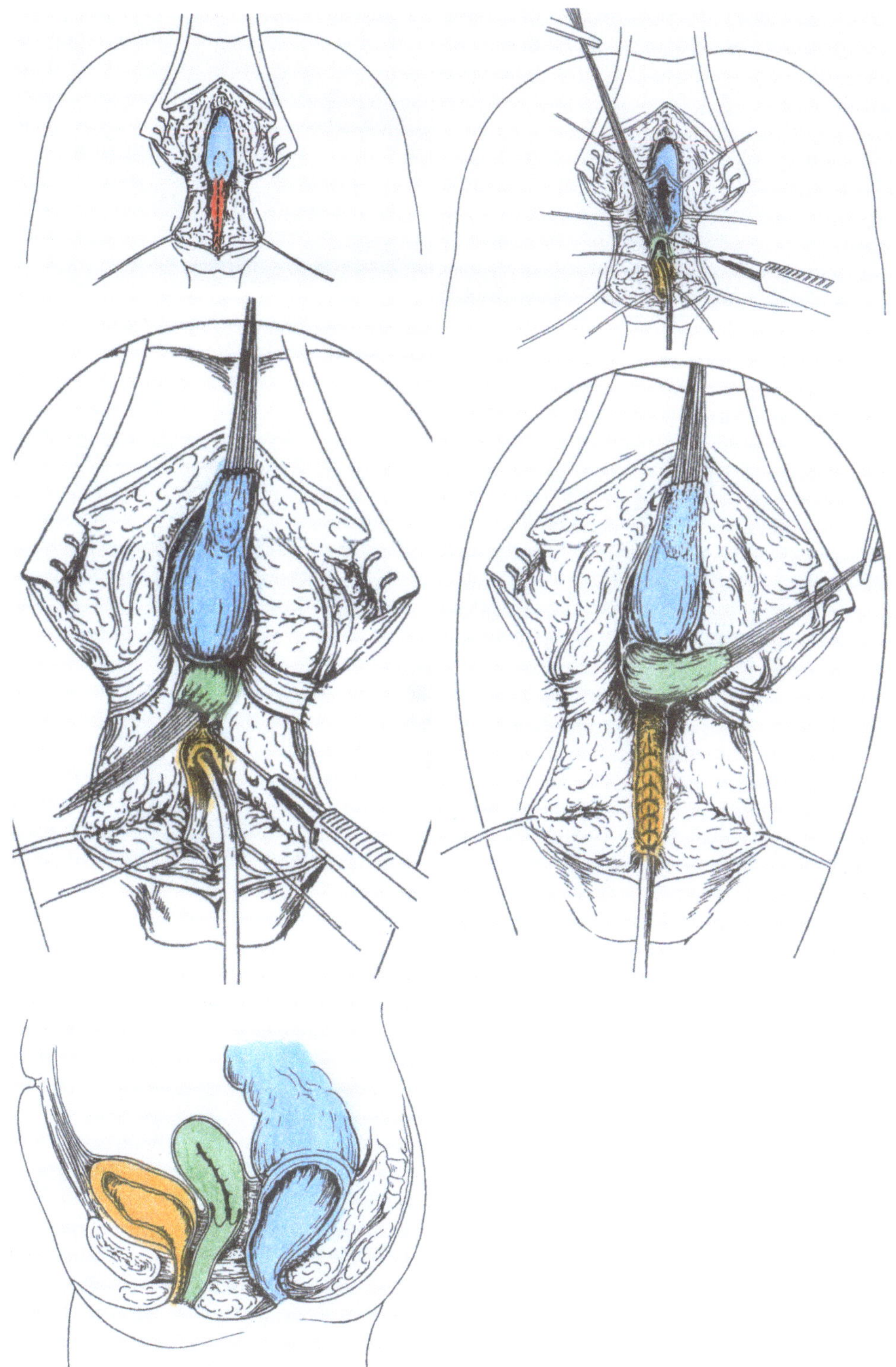

Fig. 14.8 PSARVUP for cloaca correction. The cloaca is opened in the midline. The anterior rectal wall is separated from the posterior vaginal wall (*upper right*). The anterior vaginal wall is separated from the common wall with the urethra (*center, left*). The urethra is reconstructed with the sinus (*center right*). Final aspect (*down*)

is then separated from the rectum. Since there is no cleavage plane, the dissection is carried out in the rectal submucosa for 2–3 cm and then full thickness. Then the vagina is separated from the urethra with the rectum retracted posteriorly. This dissection is very delicate because the common wall is very thin and less elastic. It is important to be close to the vagina because the opening of the urethra and bladder neck may lead to incontinence or fistula. In case of vaginal opening, you can twist the vagina 90° to avoid the overlap of the suture lines and the formation of vesicovaginal fistulas. The urethra is reconstructed using cloacal walls. The mobilized vagina is sutured to the skin, near the urethra. If necessary the rectum is tapered and, along with the anus, it is placed in the middle of the external sphincter, identified with an electrostimulator. During the maneuver the intestinal wall is secured to the muscles in order to avoid future prolapses. Neo-anus is sutured to the skin. Dilatations start 2 weeks later and last for 6 months. Colostomy is closed after 2–3 months.

Total mobilization of the UG sinus was devised and described by Peña in 1997 to overcome some of the complications of PSARVUP and consists of performing an "en bloc" mobilization of the urogenital sinus that is brought down to the perineum as a unit. Total urogenital mobilization (TUM) is adequate if the urethra is long enough (>1.5 cm) or the channel is short (less than 3 cm). Otherwise, a vaginal pull-through is preferred [19]. The urethral length and the position of the entrance of the vagina are relevant elements for choosing the surgical management. If the urethra is very short or the vaginal insertion is very high, you cannot lower the bladder neck all the way down to the perineum. TUM consists of dissection of all the attachments of the cloacal channel through a posterior sagittal approach. When the urethra and the vagina are identified, they are brought down to the perineum instead of being separated. Dissection is thus performed in a precise cleavage plane behind the pubis, ventral to the UGS, and then circumferentially around the lateral and posterior vaginal walls and the anterior urethral and vesical wall. In the past the lower redundant tissue that was exposed after the dissection was discarded, but now it can be used for vaginoplasty and introitoplasty.

Complex cloacae can pose extreme difficulties to correction, especially in cases of vaginal hypoplasia. In these cases it is essential to understand maneuvers for vaginal mobilization and augmentation. A combined abdominoperineal approach is often necessary (Fig. 14.9).

You should be prepared to change the position of the infant. The first thing to do is to free the vaginostomy, if present. A piece of gut is prepared in case of short or hypoplastic vaginas, after their disconnection, to bridge larger gaps performing a *sigmoid (ileum) vaginoplasty*. Care should be paid with ureters (usually entering the bladder very close to the vaginas). Some authors suggest placing a ureteral catheter during cystoscopy. In case of large and duplex vaginas, a *vaginal switch* (hemihysterectomy and mobilization of a hemipart of the vagina) should be prepared to bring the vagina to the perineum [20].

14.3.3 Outcomes

14.3.3.1 Postoperative Complications and Long-Term Outcomes

Complications include urethrovaginal fistula (7–11 %), vaginal stenosis (10 %), and acquired vaginal atresia (2 %). The reconstructed urethra may be difficult to catheterize making impossible the CIC.

- *Urinary incontinence*
  Urinary incontinence seems to occur in approximately one third of patients and it is usually secondary to a neuropathic bladder. Incontinence can be traumatic or primary. The status of the sacrum is relevant as in case of abnormalities; continence (urinary and fecal) will be found in only 29 % of cases [21]. In case of long channels (>3 cm), two thirds of patients need CIC to empty their bladders [18, 22]. These patients may benefit a Mitrofanoff and Malone – MACE performed during laparotomy.
- *Neurogenic bladder and ARM*
  Ninety percent of patients with cloaca have abnormal urodynamics at baseline [23]. Neurogenic bladders have specific urodynamic pattern with hyperreflexic bladder (upper motor lesion). Atonic bladder (lower

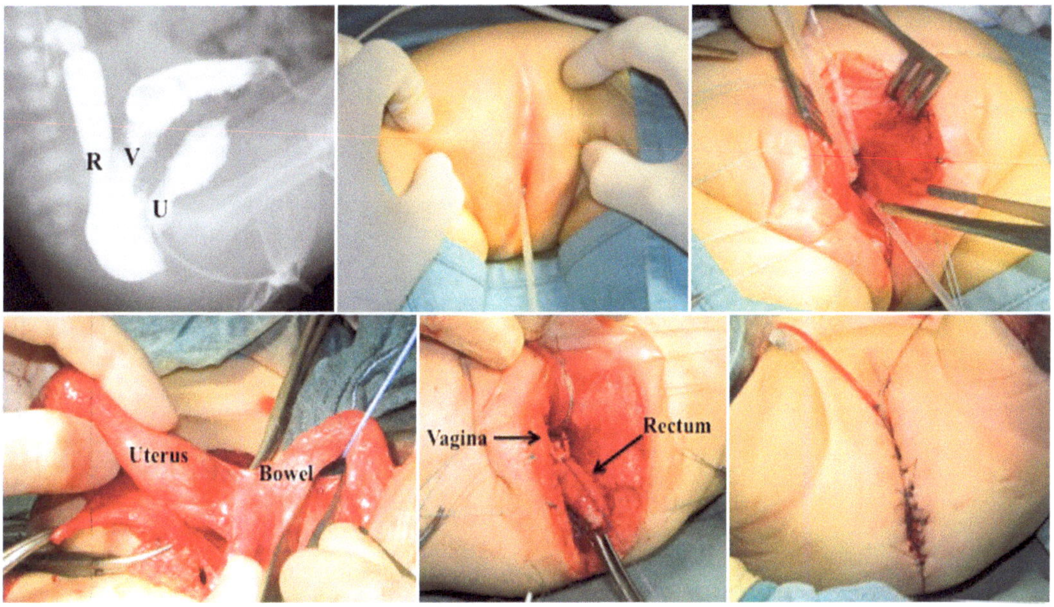

Fig. 14.9 Radiological preoperative evaluation (*upper left*). The correction of the cloaca started with the perineal approach (*upper center* and *right*). The confluence of the vagina in the cloaca was too high and we had to change the position of the baby. We performed a laparotomy and we identified the uterus and the bowel (*down, left*). These structures were isolated and pulled through the perineum (*down, center*). Final aspect (*down, right*)

motor lesion) on urodynamic evaluation is usually associated with surgical injury. You have to be careful not to do too extensive retrovesical dissection looking for the rectum with the help of a good cysto-vagino-cologram to avoid nerve lesions. Bladder nerve lesions are more common after combined abdomino-perineal pull-through.

14.3.3.2 Long-Term Outcomes

Predictable of favorable outcomes are short cloacal channel, good bladder neck, normal sacrum (without spinal cord anomalies), and two normal kidneys.

Urinary continence with voiding is present in about 54 % of patients while 46 % require CIC to stay dry (most with long channel). Continence rate is higher with low cloaca (72 %) and it is related to an abnormal sacrum [24]. The group of Great Ormond Street had similar results. Eighty percent of children seem to have urinary continence, but only 22 % void (12 % of CIC alone and 46 % of CIC after reconstructive surgery). Patients with short channel (<3 cm) do much better than those with long channels and sacral abnormalities worsen continence [23]. This has been also referred by Rink in his experience: 78 % of patients with channels >3 cm need CIC versus 28 % <3 cm [18]. Chronic renal failure accounts for 55 % of cases, some of them are related to dysplasia but many of them by mismanagement of the early hydrocolpos. Concerns have been expressed regarding the circumferential dissection of TUM over peripheral pelvic plexus nerves and this point is not so clear. The experience of Leclair who shows that after TUM 47 % of patients void and 53 % need CIC is interesting [25]. Gynecological outcomes are important since there are so many Müllerian abnormalities. The group of Hendren showed that 17/24 adults had intercourse and six had children [26] However, the group of Peña looked at 22 pubertal girls and nine of them had some palpable mass with or without cyclic pain (atresia of Müllerian ducts) [27]. During abdominal exploration, one should always be sure of the permeability of Müllerian structures, a way of doing that is to use a fallopian tube catheter and irrigate with normal saline. The group of Great Ormond Street [28] found functioning uterine tissue in 68 % at puberty.

References

1. Domini R, Rossi F (1998) Chirurgia del seno urogenitale. In: Domini R (ed) Chirurgia delle malformazioni urinarie e genitali. Piccin, Padova, pp 689–714
2. Yerkes EB, Rink RC (2010) Surgical management of female genital anomalies, disorders of sexual development, urogenital sinus, and cloacal anomalies. In: Gearhart JP, Rink RC, Mouriquand PDE (eds) Pediatric urology. Saunders Elsevier, Philadelphia, pp 476–499
3. Karlin G, Brock W, Rich M et al (1989) Persistent cloaca and phallic urethra. J Urol 142(4):1056–1059
4. Fleming SE, Hall R, Gysler M et al (1986) Imperforate anus in females: frequency of genital tract involvement, incidence of associated anomalies, and functional outcome. J Pediatr Surg 21(2):146–150
5. Kluth D (2010) Embryology of anorectal malformations. Semin Pediatr Surg 19(3):201–208
6. Rink RC, Cain MP (2008) Urogenital mobilization for urogenital sinus repair. BJU Int 102(9):1182–1197
7. Lima M, Ruggeri G, Randi B et al (2010) Vaginal replacement in the pediatric age group: a 34-year experience of intestinal vaginoplasty in children and young girls. J Pediatr Surg 45(10):2087–2091
8. Kim KS, Kim J (2012) Disorders of sex development. Korean J Urol 53(1):1–8
9. Öçal G (2011) Current concepts in disorders of sexual development. J Clin Res Pediatr Endocrinol 3(3):105–114
10. Hendren WH, Crawford JD (1969) Adrenogenital syndrome: the anatomy of the anomaly and its repair. Some new concepts. J Pediatr Surg 4:49
11. Jones HW, Wilkins L (1961) Gynecological operations in 94 patients with intersexuality. Am J Obstet Gynecol 82:1142
12. Gonzalez R, Fernandes ET (1990) Single-stage feminization genitoplasty. J Urol 143:776
13. Paserini-Glazel G (1989) A new one-stage procedure for clitorovaginoplasty in severely masculinized female pseudohermaphrodites. J Urol 142:565
14. Levitt MA, Peña A (2010) Cloacal malformations: lessons learned from 490 cases. Semin Pediatr Surg 19(2):128–138
15. Salle JL, Lorenzo AJ, Jesus LE et al (2012) Surgical treatment of high urogenital sinuses using the anterior sagittal transrectal approach: a useful strategy to optimize exposure and outcomes. J Urol 187(3):1024–1031
16. Peña A (1997) Total urogenital mobilization – an easier way to repair cloacas. J Pediatr Surg 32(2):263–267
17. Warne SA, Hiorns MP, Curry J et al (2011) Understanding cloacal anomalies. Arch Dis Child 96(11):1072–1076
18. Rink RC, Herndon CD, Cain MP, Kaefer M et al (2005) Upper and lower urinary tract outcome after surgical repair of cloacal malformations: a three-decade experience. BJU Int 96(1):131–134
19. Peña A, Levitt M (2003) Surgical management of cloacal malformations. Semin Neonatol 8(3):249–257
20. Bischoff A, Levitt MA, Breech L et al (2013) Vaginal switch – a useful technical alternative to vaginal replacement for select cases of cloaca and urogenital sinus. J Pediatr Surg 48(2):363–366
21. Peña A (1989) The surgical management of persistent cloaca: results in 54 patients treated with a posterior sagittal approach. J Pediatr Surg 24(6):590–598
22. Braga LH, Lorenzo AJ, Dave S et al (2007) Long-term renal function and continence status in patients with cloacal malformation. Can Urol Assoc J 1(4):371–376
23. Warne SA, Wilcox DT, Ransley PG (2002) Long-term urological outcome of patients presenting with persistent cloaca. J Urol 168(4 Pt 2):1859–1862
24. Peña A, Levitt MA, Hong A et al (2004) Surgical management of cloacal malformations: a review of 339 patients. J Pediatr Surg 39(3):470–479
25. Leclair MD, Gundetti M, Kiely EM et al (2007) The surgical outcome of total urogenital mobilization for cloacal repair. J Urol 177(4):1492–1495
26. Hendren WH (1998) Cloaca, the most severe degree of imperforate anus: experience with 195 cases. Ann Surg 228(3):331–346
27. Levitt MA, Stein DM, Peña A (1998) Gynecologic concerns in the treatment of teenagers with cloaca. J Pediatr Surg 33(2):188–193
28. Warne SA, Wilcox DT, Creighton S et al (2003) Long-term gynecological outcome of patients with persistent cloaca. J Urol 170(4 Pt 2):1493–1496

Neurogenic Bladder

15

Mario De Gennaro and Giovanni Mosiello

Acronyms

BTX	Botox
CNS	Central nervous system
DLPP	Detrusor leak point pressure
DO	Detrusor overactivity
DSD	Detrusor sphincter dyssynergia
EMG	Electromyography
LPP	Leak point pressure
LUT	Lower urinary tract
LUTD	Lower urinary tract dysfunction
MRI	Magnetic resonance imaging
NBD	Neurogenic bladder dysfunction
NDSD	Neurogenic detrusor sphincter dysfunction
QoL	Quality of life
RNC	Renal nuclear cystography
UDS	Urodynamics
UTI	Urinary tract infection
VCUG	Voiding cystourethrography
VUR	Vesicoureteral reflux

M. De Gennaro (✉) • G. Mosiello
Department Nephrology–Urology,
Robotic Surgery and Urodynamic Division,
Children's Hospital Bambino Gesù,
Piazza Sant'Onofrio, 4, Rome 00165, Italy
e-mail: mario.degennaro@opbg.net;
giovanni.mosiello@opbg.net

15.1 Introduction

Neuropathic bladder dysfunction (NBD) in children is an ever-evolving condition. This condition contributes to various forms of lower urinary tract dysfunction which may lead to incontinence, urinary tract infections (UTIs), vesicoureteral reflux (VUR), and renal scarring. Conservative treatment is nowadays preferred, but surgery may be required. Neurogenic detrusor sphincter dysfunction (NDSD), if not managed properly, can cause renal failure, requiring dialysis or transplantation.

Management of NDSD in children has undergone major changes over the years. In the mid-1950s, there were few insights and minimal alternatives to being in diapers or wearing an appliance over an abdominal wall stoma. Initially long-term renal preservation was the only aim of therapy, and early diversion had the best long-term results for preserving renal function.

Starting with the development of adequate X-ray assessment and reliable urodynamic investigation (UDS), the advent of clean intermittent catheterization (CIC), artificial sphincter implantation, continent urinary conduits, a plethora of drug therapies that modulate lower urinary tract function, and a multitude of rehabilitative surgical techniques, we have learned a great deal about the pathophysiology, pathogenesis, and treatment of these disorders and the evidence-based ways to manage them [1].

M. Lima, G. Manzoni (eds.), *Pediatric Urology: Contemporary Strategies from Fetal Life to Adolescence*,
DOI 10.1007/978-88-470-5693-0_15, © Springer-Verlag Italia 2015

First of all, the introduction of clean (self)-intermittent catheterization revolutionized the management of children with NBD. It not only made conservative management a very successful treatment option but also made surgical creation of continent reservoirs a very effective alternative with a good quality of life [2].

Myelodysplasia, the most common cause of NBD in children, is the best example to explain how the recognition of "at-risk" patterns and CIC had dramatically changed the outcome. About 15 % of neonates with myelodysplasia have no signs of lower urinary tract dysfunction (LUTD) when initially studied [3]. Nearly 60 % of them may develop upper tract deterioration due to increased detrusor filling pressures and infections, with or without reflux [4].

Children do not develop upper tract deterioration when managed early with CIC and antimuscarinic medication [5, 6].

For neurogenic bladder dysfunction, urodynamic studies allow to understand the nature and severity of the problems and administer management in a rational manner according to the functional characteristics of the bladder. The main goals of treatment remain the prevention of urinary tract deterioration and the achievement of continence.

15.2 Definition of Neurogenic Bladder

Neurogenic detrusor sphincter dysfunction (NDSD) can develop as a result of a lesion at any level in the nervous system, including the cerebral cortex, spinal cord, or the peripheral nervous system.

15.3 Causes

The most common cause of NBD in children and the most detrimental is *neurospinal dysraphism*. This condition presents with various patterns of detrusor–sphincter dysfunction within a wide range of severity. Traumatic and neoplastic spinal lesions of the cord are less frequent in children (Table 15.1).

Table 15.1 The principal causes of neurogenic bladder in children

Spinal dysraphism	
Open – myelodysplasia	85 %
Closed – occult dysraphism	8 %
Sacral agenesis	1 %
Imperforate anus (~40 % incidence)	1 %
Central nervous system insults	
Cerebral palsy	3 %
Spinal cord injury	1 %
Tumors – brain, spinal cord (primary, metastatic)	n.s.
Infection	n.s.

15.3.1 Spinal Dysraphism

The failure of mesodermal ingrowth over the developing spinal canal results in an open lesion most commonly seen in the lumbosacral area. The degree of this closure deficiency contributes to a variable presentation of neural injury with varying degrees of LUTD and lower extremity problems.

Developmental anomalies that result from defects in neural tube closure are generically termed as *myelodysplasia*. This term includes a group of lesions like spina bifida occulta, meningocele, lipomyelomeningocele, or myelomeningocele, which is by far the most common defect. The neurologic lesions produced by myelodysplasia are variably contingent on the neural elements that protrude within the meningocele sac. The bony vertebral level correlates poorly with the neurologic lesions produced.

The deterioration is an acquired phenomenon secondary to the development or progression of various LUT hostility factors such as neurogenic DO, poor bladder compliance, detrusor–sphincter dyssynergia, and/or high LPP from denervation fibrosis [8, 9]. Urodynamic studies corroborated their reliability by reporting that the prediction of upper urinary tract deterioration on the basis of urodynamic testing is possible with 90 % accuracy.

In *closed myelodysplasia* the lesions are not overt and often with no obvious signs of neurologic lesion (*occult dysraphism*). The diagnosis of this condition has increased since the advent of spinal ultrasonography and magnetic resonance imaging. In nearly 90 % of patients, a cutaneous abnormality overlies the lower spine, and this condition can easily be suspected by simple inspection of the lower back. These cutaneous lesions can vary from a dimple or a skin tag to a tuft of hair, a dermal vascular malformation, or an obvious subdermal lipoma. Back pain and an absence of perineal sensation are common symptoms in older children. Incidence of abnormal lower urinary tract function in patients with spina bifida occulta is as high as 40 %.

15.3.2 Sacral Agenesis

It is a rare congenital anomaly that involves absence of part or all of one or more sacral vertebrae. Perineal sensation is usually intact, lower extremity function is usually normal, and the diagnosis is made when a flattened buttock and a short gluteal cleft are seen on physical examination. This lesion may produce variable degrees and patterns of LUTD.

The lesion can be missed in infancy because of its subtle clinical manifestations, with generally no loss of lower extremity motor and sensory function, and the nonprogressive nature of its pathophysiology [10]. Urinary and fecal incontinence usually manifest themselves at an older age when the child fails to toilet train on time. A careful physical examination noting flattened buttocks and a short gluteal crease is pathognomonic for the diagnosis: 30 and 40 % of these patients have an upper-motor-neuron-type lesion with DO and an intact but dyssynergic sphincter, while 25–50 % have signs of a lower motor neuron deficit with acontractile detrusor and denervation in the sphincter, and 15–20 % have normal LUT function [11].

15.3.3 Imperforate Anus

This rare anomaly with a closed rectum may present with accompanying spinal cord pathology.

The timing of investigational studies is critical. Spinal ultrasound in the newborn period is needed due to the likelihood of an intraspinal abnormality. The incidence of NBD approaches 40 % but varies from 10 to 50 % [12] depending on the height of the rectal lesion (positive correlation) and how thorough the investigation [13]. If a suspected neuropathic bladder is confirmed by UDS, then spinal MRI is indicated [14, 15]. UDS determines the presence of DO, the degree of denervation in the external urethral and rectal sphincters, and DSD in the first few months of life, after an initial colostomy or definitive pull-through surgery is performed, serving as a baseline for patients with an occult dysraphism [16].

Persistent urinary and bowel incontinence suggest unrecognized NBD from an occult spinal dysraphism. Some infants with normal lower urinary and bowel function in the first year of life suffer from tethering of the spinal cord with increasing age. This leads to permanent damage if not detected early. Thus, baseline and surveillance UDS help determine the current or changing neurologic lesion that warrants MRI imaging and possibly spinal cord untethering, if an operable lesion is found. It is extremely rare for these children to exhibit lower extremity neurologic impairment or a cutaneous manifestation of this associated condition.

15.3.4 Spinal Cord Injury

The scarcity and variability of spinal cord injuries in children makes it difficult to propose any one treatment program unless the specific type of LUT function is known on the basis of urodynamic testing [17, 18]. Even if the individual regains the ability to void spontaneously and empty his/her bladder, it is imperative to know the detrusor filling and emptying (detrusor) pressures, in order to determine the potential risk for VUR and hydroureteronephrosis [19]. Effective voiding with pressures below 40 cm H_2O in the absence of detrusor–sphincter dyssynergia ensures a stable upper urinary tract. A cauda equina injury usually leads to a lower motor neuron type of deficit of the striated sphincter that may not require any treatment to prevent upper tract damage because the bladder empties readily at low pressure, but it probably necessitates medical and/or surgical therapy to achieve continence.

Urodynamic monitoring has demonstrated to be relevant in the follow-up and prevention of upper tract deterioration in a retrospective cohort study [17]. Further urodynamic follow-up is "standard" alike in adult patients [20].

15.3.5 Cerebral Palsy

Patients may also present with varying degrees of LUTD usually in the form of overactive detrusor and wetting. The vast majority of the children with cerebral palsy tend to toilet train completely, but often at an age that is later than expected for normal individuals [21].

It has been suggested on the basis of expert opinion that cystometry and sphincter EMG are to be considered only when frequent toileting or anticholinergic therapy fails to control incontinent episodes, the child develops urinary infection from ineffective voiding, or when ultrasonography reveals hydronephrosis. A conservative approach is the choice in most of the cases [22].

15.3.6 Tumors (Either Primary or Metastatic)

Tumors of the central nervous system in children are rare and the symptom complexes; they produce quite varied; the workup should be individualized and tailored to the specific location of the disease. LUT dysfunction occurs after sacrococcygeal teratoma resection, and urodynamic evaluation is necessary during follow-up of those children [23, 24]. A recent study showed that children with central nervous tumors can have urodynamic abnormalities, whether the tumor is in the spinal cord or not. A child with a CNS tumor regardless of location needs urological and urodynamic testing [25].

15.4 Classification of Neurogenic Bladder

There are various systems of classification of the neurogenic bladder. Most systems are based on the localization of the neurologic lesion and findings of the neurourologic examination and have been of more value in adults with spinal cord injury. In children the spinal level and extent of congenital lesion are poorly correlated with the clinical outcome.

15.4.1 Pathophysiology

The detrusor and sphincter are two units working in harmony to make a single functional unit. Determined by the nature of the neurologic deficit, they may be either in an overactive or in an inactive state. The detrusor may be overactive with increased contractions, with a diminished bladder capacity and compliance, or be inactive with no effective contractions; the bladder outlet (urethra and sphincter) may be independently overactive causing functional obstruction or paralysis with no resistance to urinary flow leading to stress incontinence. These conditions may exist in any combination. Four major types are usually used to describe the detrusor–sphincter dysfunction:

1. Detrusor overactivity with sphincter overactivity (dyssynergia)
2. Detrusor overactivity with normal or underactive sphincter
3. Detrusor underactivity with sphincter overactivity
4. Detrusor underactivity with sphincter underactivity

15.5 Patient Evaluation

The first evaluation is based on several factors depending on when the child presents and/or is diagnosed (Fig. 15.1).

In the first years of life, the kidneys are highly susceptible to back pressure and infection, documentation on UDS pattern is required [26, 27]. Ultrasound studies and a VCUG or video urodynamics to exclude reflux has to be performed soon after birth. These studies provide a baseline for the appearance of the upper and lower urinary tracts. A urodynamic evaluation needs to be repeated at regular intervals, in combination with evaluation of the upper tracts [28].

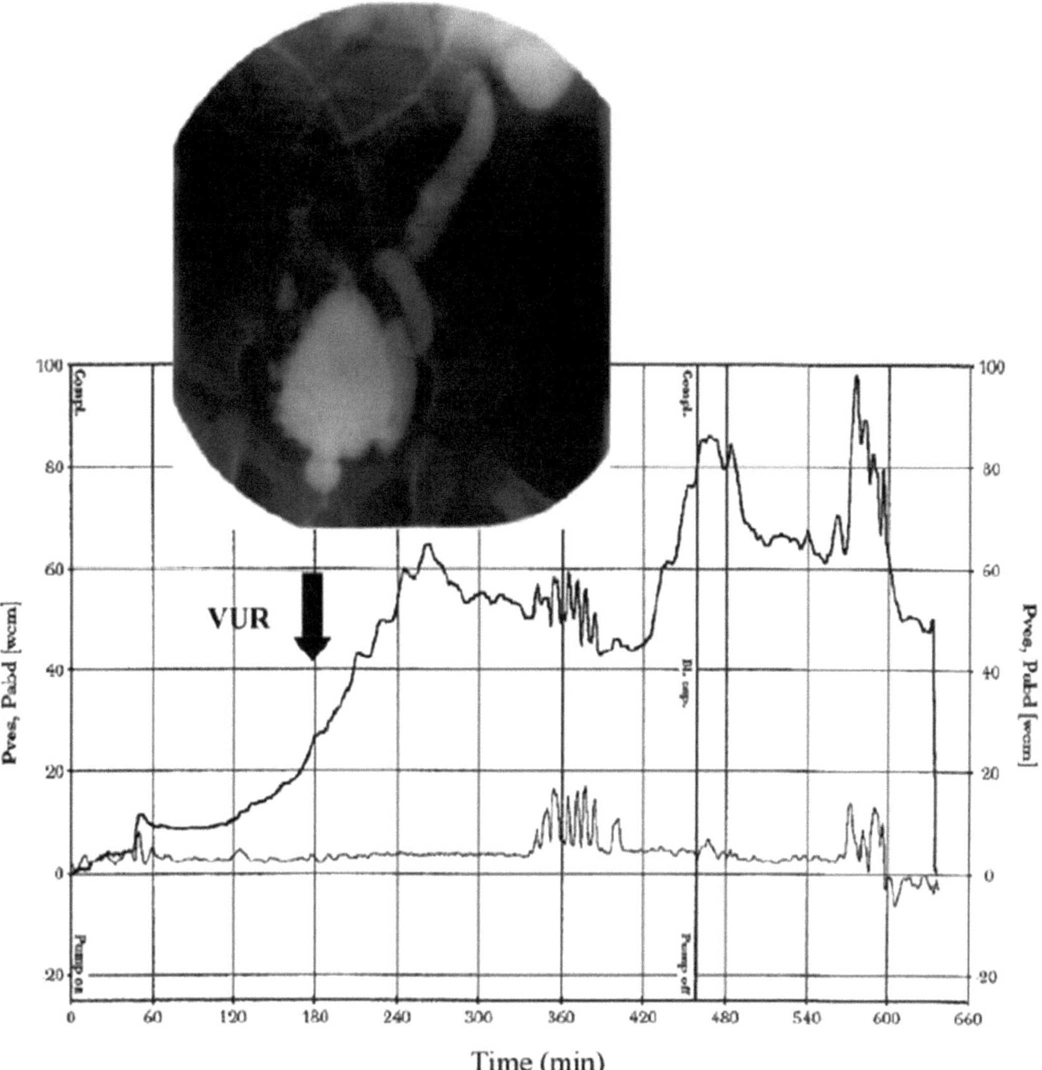

Fig. 15.1 Video urodynamic study (*VUD*) of a 3-month-old girl with recurrent urinary tract infection (*UTI*), incontinence, and sacral myelomeningocele showing neurogenic bladder dysfunction, high bladder pressure, and overactive detrusor contractions (*arrow*). At the same time vesicoureteral reflux (*VUR*) of grade IV was demonstrated with an irregular bladder wall and a wide bladder neck. The filling rate was 10 ml/min (Reproduced with permission from [7])

Approximately 90 % of children born with meningomyelocele will have a normal upper urinary tract at birth. Over time, many children who have not received proactive urological care develop upper and/or LUT deterioration: a urodynamic risk score including a DLPP of >40 cmH_2O was calculated. The grades of renal dilatation are compatible with increases in relative unsafe cystometric capacity and the calculated urodynamic risk score [9]. Prevention of high bladder filling pressure (before upper tract dilatation is observed) is necessary and feasible even before any urodynamic diagnosis [29].

When incontinence develops in spite of strict adherence to bladder and bowel continence programs, or when changes occur in leg function or sensation, or when the child experiences back pain or increasing scoliosis, a change in neurological impairment might be expected. A number of myelodysplastic children have progressive neurological deficits as they grow up and reach puberty [30].

Regarding *occult spinal dysraphism*, the preoperative urodynamic evaluation has documented abnormalities in striated urethral sphincter function (denervation and/or detrusor–sphincter dyssynergia) in 20–35 % of babies under 2 years of age with normal neurological examinations, thus emphasizing the need for urodynamic testing in these children [31]. A close urological follow-up is essential in children with OSD because of possible upper urinary tract and renal function deterioration, in those with urodynamic at-risk conditions [32]. An efficacious response in EMG activity, with stabilization or improvement in up to 60 %, was shown on postoperative urodynamic assessment when the dysraphic state was corrected before 2 years of age [33].

It was observed that children with meningomyelocele, as compared to closed dysraphism, tended to have more bladder dysfunction as exemplified on clinical history and urodynamic assessment. Evaluation after operation tended to show better outcome in children with closed dysraphism.

15.5.1 Urodynamic Testing

For the last 20 years initial urodynamic studies very early in the neonatal period have been recommended for children with myelodysplasia, to help identify children at risk for subsequent urinary tract deterioration or a changing neurological picture [34]. In an exhaustive review of the efficacy and reliability of urodynamic studies in newborns with myelodysplasia [35], of 24 studies analyzed, 21 studies were at level of evidence 4, 2 were at level 3, and 1 was at level 1, the urodynamic patterns of normal detrusor function (66 %), acontractile detrusor (33 %), DO (57 %), and detrusor compliance, as well as detrusor–sphincter synergia (21 %) and dyssynergia (37 %) and sphincter denervation (60 %), were similar, with little variability across comparable studies.

Technique, reliability, and reproducibility of tests. Differences in urodynamic parameters exist from one study to another. Chou et al. provided reference ranges for "normal" variability in urodynamic parameters that can be considered as "no real change" [36]. A reduced rate of filling, e.g., 10 % of the expected bladder volume per minute, has been recommended in children to accurately determine detrusor compliance and bladder volume [37]. The temperature of the instillate (25° versus 37.5 °C) does not significantly affect detrusor pressures [38].

For very young infants it may be better to insert a suprapubic catheter under anesthesia the day before the test to be more accurate. Most children can undergo urodynamic studies without premedication, some requiring some sedation. In the 5th International Consultation on Incontinence - ICI 2012, the recommendation was made that children should receive comprehensive urodynamic testing in a laboratory that is specialized in pediatrics, with appropriately trained personnel [39].

15.6 Follow-Up of Congenital Neurogenic Bladder in Children

Newborn to childhood. Once UDS has been performed, a decision can be made as to whether the child is a candidate for continuing CIC or allowed to void freely. It is advisable to repeat UDS (cystometry) 2–3 months later to confirm that therapy is adequately reducing bladder pressures. Indications for repeating a VCUG or RNC include a change in upper urinary tract dilation, poor renal growth, loss of parenchyma, or symptomatic pyelonephritis. It would be wise to consider a baseline DMSA study if reflux is noted at the primary examination, for later comparison. During this time a yearly or biannual ultrasound is recommended to follow the child, looking at residual urine or changes in the degree of hydronephrosis or bladder wall thickening. If any one of these is noted, UDS should be reconsidered.

Adolescents and transitional care to adulthoods. It is during the rapid growth that tethering can occur, so careful monitoring of signs is mandatory. New-onset wetting and recurrent UTI are indicators of potential changes in lower urinary tract function: UDS and upper tract evaluation are in general for patients who have completed their growth and are not likely to develop any further changes in the spinal cord that would precipitate tethering. It is imperative that these young adults be followed closely to ensure they are maintaining good CIC routines and are periodically being checked for unrecognized UTI or stone formation.

Sexuality becomes progressively more important as the patient gets older. This issue has historically been overlooked in individuals with myelodysplasia. Patients with myelodysplasia have sexual encounters, and studies indicate that at least 15–20 % of males are capable of fathering children and 70 % of females can conceive and carry a pregnancy to term. Therefore counseling patients on CIC regarding sexual development is important in early adolescence.

Maternity. When reconstructing girls it is essential to have a future pregnancy in mind: the reservoir and pedicles should be fixed on one side to allow enlargement of the uterus on the other. Pregnancy may be complicated and requires the joint care of obstetrician and urologist: chronic urinary infection is almost inevitable and occasionally an indwelling catheter is needed in the third trimester.

15.6.1 Management of the Neuropathic Bladder

The main aim in management of NBD in children is to ensure and maintain a reservoir with normal age-matched capacity and good compliance that can be emptied completely at low pressures and at regular intervals. While continence is usually addressed as the child reaches school age, issues such as elevated detrusor pressure, hydronephrosis and/or reflux, and chronic UTIs are treated at any time (Fig. 15.2).

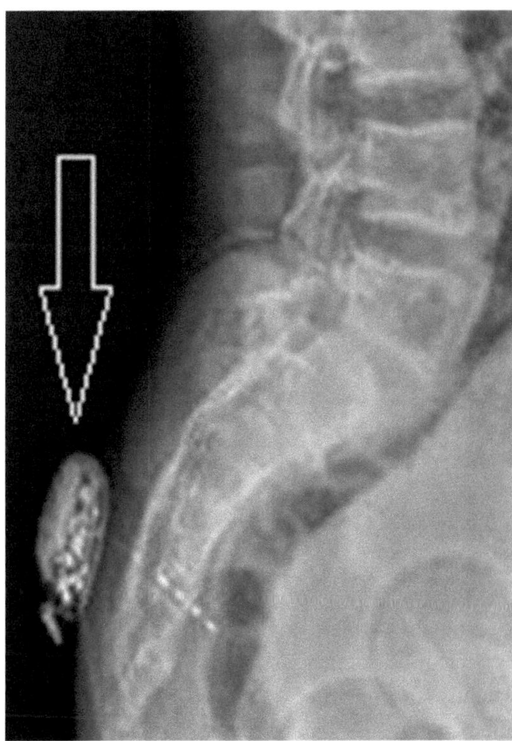

Fig. 15.2 Sacral neuromodulation. An 11-year-old boy, with previous incomplete spinal cord injury and neurogenic dysfunction with detrusor overactivity. Management of the bladder by antimuscarinic drugs to prevent urinary incontinence and intermittent catheterization to empty completely after partial spontaneous voiding. Neuromodulation implant allowed to stop drugs and CIC. Rx shows the intraspinal electrode and battery implanted (*arrow*)

15.6.2 Conservative Treatment

There are multiple conservative modalities of intervention for infants and children with NBD, which should be promoted before undertaking surgical interventions. These treatment modalities include pharmacologic agents, medical devices, and neuromodulation. Indications for these nonsurgical treatments depend on issues related to intravesical pressures, upper urinary status, prevalence of UTI, and degree of incontinence.

15.6.2.1 Pharmacotherapy

Anticholinergics/antimuscarinics are the mainstay of medical treatment for NBD. They are used to diminish DO and intravesical storage pressures when children have low detrusor compliance that places them at risk for renal compromise. There is excellent level 1 evidence for the efficacy of anticholinergics to reduce bladder storage pressure and DO [40].

Oxybutynin is the first modern anticholinergic agent; it has undergone extensive examination in children with NBD. It is the only FDA-approved anticholinergic in the United States for pediatric use in NBD. The dosing of oral and intravesical oxybutynin is 0.2 mg/kg/dose every 8 h. The incidence of side effects of oral oxybutynin ranges from 6 to 57 %, whereas side effects from intravesical oxybutynin are approximately 9 % [8]. Besides oxybutynin, there has been an emergence of new selective anticholinergic medications that are designed to diminish side effects by either targeting specific muscarinic receptor subtypes or by altering the structural compounds so that they are less likely to cross organ barriers. Tertiary amines (oxybutynin, tolterodine, darifenacin, solifenacin, and propiverine) are more likely to cross the blood–brain barrier than the quaternary amines propantheline and trospium.

Botulinum-A toxin (BTX-A). BTX-A is an attractive treatment for NBD because it inhibits acetylcholine neurotransmitter release at the neuromuscular junction. Intravesical BTX-A is considered an alternative to improving continence and urodynamic parameters of NBD in children. A recent review using BTX-A was conducted that provided a current summary of the efficacy and safety profile of BTX-A in children with NBD [41]. Collectively, these small, uncontrolled studies demonstrate a significant improvement in clinical and urodynamic parameters as evidenced by complete continence in approximately 65–87 % of children and a reduction in maximum detrusor pressure and an increase in detrusor compliance in the majority of those treated [42, 43].

The dose of BTX-A is 10 U/kg up to a maximal dose of 300 U involving 30 injections of 10 U/kg/ml in the detrusor. BTX-A appears to reach efficacy levels at 2 weeks and maximum effects within 4–6 weeks. Duration of the BTX-A effect ranges from 3 to 8 months depending on short-term versus long-term repeated injections [41].

15.6.2.2 Catheters

As mentioned in the Introduction, clean intermittent catheterization has had a profound impact on the management of NBD in children. Given the high prevalence of latex sensitivity in the NBD population, non-latex catheters are employed exclusively.

The early initiation of intermittent catheterization in the newborn period makes it easier for parents to master it and for children to accept it as they grow older [44, 45]. Hydrophilic-coated catheters are helpful in the setting of painful catheterization or in the presence of urethral strictures and/or false passages in boys. In two recent randomized trials comparing hydrophilic-coated catheters to uncoated catheters, there was a reduction in microscopic hematuria and better overall satisfaction with the hydrophilic-coated catheters [7]. One concern expressed by families and primary care providers is the risk of reusing the same catheter for CIC and the incidence of bacteriuria. A Cochrane review examined sterile versus clean catheterization technique, coated (pre-lubricated) versus uncoated (separate lubricant) catheters, single (sterile) or multiple use (clean) catheters, self-catheterization versus catheterization by others, and any other strategies designed to reduce UTIs. This review found a lack of evidence to state that the incidence of UTI is affected by using sterile or clean technique [46]. Thus, modification of catheters and catheter regimens should be made on an individual basis for children with NBD.

15.6.2.3 Neuromodulation Treatments

Intravesical Electrical Stimulation

Intravesical electrical stimulation of the bladder has been introduced more than four decades ago, and it has been tested in some open clinical trials in children since 1984. Its practice is limited to a few centers who have reported varying results. It is labor intensive, time consuming, and controversial in the only reported randomized, placebo-controlled trial; there was no efficacy demonstrated [47].

Sacral Nerve Stimulation

Sacral nerve stimulation has primarily been reported in the treatment of patients with a non-neuropathic bladder [48]. The safety and effectiveness have not been established for children <16 years of age or for patients with neurological disease. The only report of sacral nerve modulation, by intraspinal implantation, conducted in children with NBD had mixed results and the study design was limited [49]. At our institution

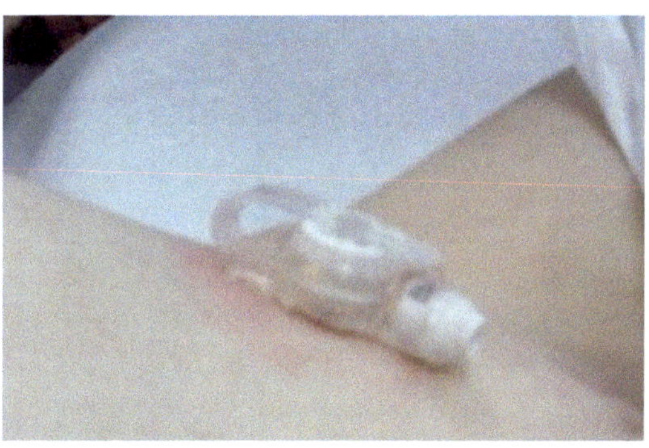

Fig. 15.3 Cystostomy button. Girl 3 years old, with at-risk neurogenic detrusor dysfunction (detrusor overactivity and detrusor–sphincter dyssynergia), following surgery for pelvic neuroblastoma. Clean intermittent catheterization was not accepted, by parents, and a cystostomy button allowed to empty the bladder regularly and lower intravesical pressure, waiting for further treatment

we experienced sacral implantation in a number of children and adolescent with NB, with very good results on improvement of bladder sensation of fullness and number of catheterisms needed per day and very satisfactory response from patients and families. Other modalities of nerve electrical stimulation have been considered in children, i.e., percutaneous posterior tibial nerve stimulation, but with little experience in neurogenic bladders [50] (Fig. 15.3).

15.7 Surgical Treatment

Intermittent catheterization and drug therapy are usually sufficient in the majority of cases for maintaining continence and preserving upper tracts. Surgical procedures should be considered if conservative measures fail to achieve continence between catheterizations or preserve upper tracts. Surgical management has to be tailored to each individual case, based on careful consideration of urodynamic findings, medical history, age, and presence of other disabilities. Urologists should identify that limited group that may require surgery. Surgical procedures develop gradually and often are tested without rigorous statistics. Efforts to promote bladder healing and protecting and achieving normal bladder function should be supported. Research may lead to earlier and more aggressive treatment of many of the complex anomalies now treated by the surgical procedures.

15.7.1 To Manage Continence

15.7.1.1 Gastrostomy Button

A modified technique of vesicostomy is described using a gastrostomy button, which could be used as a continent urinary stoma in children with incomplete voiding. Button vesicostomy is a useful addition to the options available for a catheterizable continent urinary stoma in children in the short or medium term.

15.7.1.2 The Mitrofanoff Principle

In the long term it is necessary to have a catheterizable channel. Mitrofanoff's name is given to the principle of burying a narrow tube within the wall of the bladder or urinary reservoir whose distal end is brought to the abdominal wall to form a catheterizable stoma suitable for intermittent catheterization. The technique is simple and familiar to all urologists who are accustomed to reimplanting ureters. Several narrow tubes are available for the Mitrofanoff conduit. In the original description, the appendix was used. The system achieves reliable continence (90–100 %) which is maintained in long-term follow-up, for a high proportion of patients.

15.7.2 To Augment Bladder Storage

15.7.2.1 Enterocystoplasty

The indication for bladder augmentation, replacement of the bladder, or the creation of a continent urinary diversion is either the morphological or functional loss of normal bladder function. The main goal of this surgery is to relieve high pressure and low capacity of the urinary bladder and create a new reservoir with low storage pressures that can be emptied periodically. It is particularly important that the patients understand that spontaneous voiding will not be possible after such surgery and lifelong intermittent catheterization will be required.

There are several important principles for bladder augmentation and replacement that should be respected:

- Use the minimal amount of bowel.
- A low-pressure large capacity reservoir is essential (this requires detubularization of any intestinal segment used).
- A reliable continence mechanism (continent urinary outlet) must be assured.
- Because of the only resorbable sutures and staples that should be used (risk of stone formation).

The invasiveness of enterocystoplasty, and its long-term severe complication rate, has greatly reduced its indication. Recently, it is gaining more attention, in relation to the availability of mini-invasive procedures, i.e., the robotic-assisted laparoscopy [51].

15.7.2.2 Autoaugmentation

The principle of autoaugmentation of the bladder is the excision of a great portion of the detrusor while leaving the urothelium intact, creating a large diverticulum for the storage of urine at lower pressures. This urine stored at a low pressure can be drained by intermittent catheterization. The theoretical advantages of this procedure are the low complication rates of the surgery, reduced operative morbidity with shorter stay in the hospital, absence of urine salt resorption, less mucous production in the urine, and possibly absence of carcinogenic potential [52].

More recently, some authors have proposed the laparoscopic autoaugmentation as a minimally invasive procedure for the treatment of low capacity/low compliance bladder [53].

15.7.3 To Increase Outlet Resistances

15.7.3.1 Bulking Agents

The injection of bulking substances in the tissues around the urethra and bladder neck to increase outlet resistance in children dates back to at least 1985. The search for safer, biocompatible substances to create periurethral compression has first led to the use of cross-linked bovine collagen, with initially reported success in about 20–50 % of children [54, 55].

Usually the substance is injected endoscopically in the bladder neck area (finding the best spot is often the most difficult part of the procedure): more than one procedure may be necessary. On average 2.8–3.9 ml is injected.

15.7.3.2 Fascial Sling

The technique involves suspension of the bladder neck with an autologous fascial strip or artificial material secured to the rectus fascia or the pubic symphysis. It is believed that the mechanism of action involves coaptation of the bladder neck due to traction and/or elevation of the urethra to an intra-abdominal position, which increases tension on the bladder neck with abdominal straining. Complication rates are modest and include difficult catheterization and rectal injury, while in long-term erosions or persistent incontinence may occur.

15.7.3.3 Bladder Neck Closure/Reconstruction

In “desperate” cases the bladder neck may be closed, the indication being persistent leakage despite several attempts to enhance outlet resistance. Long-term results are usually disappointing: persistent urinary leakage, stomal stenosis and leakage, or stone formation.

The optimal bladder neck procedure should increase bladder outlet resistance at minimal cost of decreasing bladder capacity, maintaining easy catheterization, and still allowing some leakage at high pressure in order to protect the upper urinary tract. Different operative techniques with the aforementioned aims have been used with varying outcomes.

15.7.3.4 Artificial Urinary Sphincters (AUS)

Many surgeons are reluctant to implant an AUS as it consigns patients to further revision surgery and the potential risk of deterioration in bladder function and a concomitant deleterious effect on upper urinary tract drainage. However, with improved durability of newer models that have an average life span of about 8 years, revision rates have become less [56]. The ideal patients for AUS implantation are postpubertal males or females, who can void volitionally and empty the bladder completely [57]. On the contrary, a common problem is the development of reduced bladder compliance with time. Overall, 40–50 % of neurogenic patients require a bladder augmentation concomitantly or subsequently to the AUS implantation.

15.7.3.5 Evaluation of Outcome

Our prejudice is that reconstruction does, indeed, improve the lives of children. Quality of life does not mean absence of disease or a level of complications acceptable to the reviewing clinician. It is a difficult concept to measure because of lack of validated instruments, difficulties in translating from one culture or language to another, the difficulties in selecting control groups, and variations in clinical situations.

The main justification for performing a bladder reconstruction or continent diversion is to improve the individual's quality of life (QoL). It would seem logical that continent urinary diversion would be better than a bag. This is not always the case, and in adults the only sure advantage is cosmetic. Validated QoL surveys in children have not been reported, primarily because of the lack of suitable instruments.

References

1. Bauer SB (2003) The management of the myelodysplastic child: a paradigm shift. BJU Int 92:23–28
2. Lapides J, Diokno AC, Silber SJ et al (1972) Clean intermittent self-catheterization in the treatment of urinary tract disease. J Urol 107:458–462
3. Bauer SB (1985) The management of spina bifida from birth onwards. In: Whitaker RH, Woodard JR (eds) Paediatric urology. Butterworths, London, pp 87–112
4. Hunt GM, Whitaker RH (1987) The pattern of congenital renal anomalies associated with neural tube defects. Dev Med Child Neurol 29:91–95
5. Kasabian NG et al (1992) The prophylactic value of clean intermittent catheterization and anticholinergic medication in newborns and infants with myelodysplasia at risk of developing urinary tract deterioration. Am J Dis Child 146:480–487
6. Wang SC et al (1989) Urethral dilatation in the management of urological complications of myelodysplasia. J Urol 142:1054–1055
7. Szabó L, Lombay B, Borbás E, Bajusz I (2004) Videourodynamics in the diagnosis of urinary tract abnormalities in a single center. J Pediatr Nephrol 19(3):326–331. doi:10.1007/s00467-003-1341-8
8. McGuire EJ et al (1981) Prognostic value of urodynamic testing in myelodysplastic patients. J Urol 126(2):205–209
9. Wang QW, Wen JG, Song DK et al (2006) Is it possible to use urodynamic variables to predict upper urinary tract dilatation in children with neurogenic bladder-sphincter dysfunction? BJU Int 98(6):1295–300
10. Guzman L et al (1983) Evaluation and management of children with sacral agenesis. Urology 22(5):506–510
11. Abokson H, Holm-Bentzen M, Hald T (1985) The evaluation and management of children with sacral agenesis and dysgenesis. Neurourol Urodyn 4:99
12. De Gennaro M, Rivosecchi M, Lucchetti MC et al (1994) The incidence of occult spinal dysraphism and the onset of neurovesical dysfunction in children with anorectal anomalies. Eur J Pediatr Surg 4(Suppl 1):12–14
13. Mosiello G, Capitanucci ML, Gatti C et al (2003) How to investigate neurovesical dysfunction in children with anorectal malformations. J Urol 170(4 Pt 2):1610–1613
14. Capitanucci ML, Rivosecchi M, Silveri M et al (1996) Neurovesical dysfunction due to spinal dysraphism in anorectal anomalies. Eur J Pediatr Surg 6(3):159–162
15. Taskinen S, Valanne L, Rintala R (2002) Effect of spinal cord abnormalities on the function of the lower urinary tract in patients with anorectal malformations. J Urol 168:1147–1149
16. Boemers TM, Beek FJ, van de Gool JD et al (1996) Urologic problems in anorectal malformations. Part 1: urodynamic findings and significance of sacral anomalies. J Pediatr Surg 31:407–410
17. Generao SE et al (2004) Spinal cord injury in children: long-term urodynamic and urological outcomes. J Urol 172(3):1092–1094; discussion 1094
18. Silveri M, Salsano L et al (2006) Pediatric spinal cord injury: approach for urological rehabilitation and treatment. J Pediatr Urol 2(1):10–15
19. Pannek J, Diederichs W, Botel U (1997) Urodynamically controlled management of spinal cord injury in children. Neurourol Urodyn 16(4):285–292
20. Nosseir M, Hinkel A, Pannek J (2007) Clinical usefulness of urodynamic assessment for maintenance of bladder function in patients with spinal cord injury. Neurourol Urodyn 26(2):228–233
21. Decter RM et al (1987) Urodynamic assessment of children with cerebral palsy. J Urol 138(4 Pt 2):1110–1112
22. Ersoz M, Kaya K, Erol SK et al (2009) Non invasive evaluation of lower urinary tract function in children with cerebral palsy. Am J Phys Med Rehabil 88(9):735–741
23. Mosiello G, Gatti C, De Gennaro M et al (2003) Neurovesical dysfunction in children after treating pelvic neoplasms. BJU Int 92(3):289–292
24. Ozkan KU, Bauer SB, Khoshbin S et al (2006) Neurogenic bladder dysfunction after sacrococcygeal teratoma resection. J Urol 175(1):292–296; discussion 296
25. Nguyen HT, Sencan A, Silva A et al (2010) Urodynamic studies are recommended in children

with central nervous system tumors regardless of location. J Urol 184(6):2516–2520
26. Bauer SB (2008) Neurogenic bladder: etiology and assessment. Pediatr Nephrol 23:541–551
27. Meyrat BJ, Tercier S, Lutz N et al (2003) Introduction of a urodynamic score to detect pre- and postoperative neurological deficits in children with a primary tethered cord. Childs Nerv Syst 19:716–721
28. Satar N, Bauer SB, Scott RM et al (1997) Late effects of early surgery on lipoma and lipomeningocele in children less than 1 year old. J Urol 157:1434–1437
29. Dik P, Klijn AJ, van Gool JD et al (2006) Early start to therapy preserves kidney function in spina bifida patients. Eur Urol 49(5):908–913
30. Lais A, Kasabian NG, Dyro FM et al (1993) The neurosurgical implications of continuous neurourological surveillance of children with myelodysplasia. J Urol 150(6):1879–1883
31. Kumar R, Singhal N, Gupta M et al (2008) Evaluation of clinico-urodynamic outcome of bladder dysfunction after surgery in children with spinal dysraphism – a prospective study. Acta Neurochir (Wien) 150(2):129–137
32. Capitanucci ML, Iacobelli BD, Silveri M et al (1996) Long-term urological follow-up of occult spinal dysraphism in children. Eur J Pediatr Surg 6(Suppl 1):25–26
33. Keating MA, Rink RC, Bauer SB et al (1988) Neurourological implications of the changing approach in management of occult spinal lesions. J Urol 140(5 Pt 2):1299–1301
34. Sidi AA, Dykstra DD, Gonzalez R (1986) The value of urodynamic testing in the management of neonates with myelodysplasia: a prospective study. J Urol 135(1):90–93
35. McLellan D, Bauer SB (2003) In section on urology, American Academy of Pediatrics, New Orleans
36. Chou FH et al (2006) Normal ranges of variability for urodynamic studies of neurogenic bladders in spinal cord injury. J Spinal Cord Med 29(1):26–31
37. Hoebeke P et al (1998) Urodynamics in children: what and how to do it? Acta Urol Belg 66(2):23–30
38. Van Meel TD, de Wachter S, Wyndaele JJ (2007) Repeated ice water tests and electrical perception threshold determination to detect a neurologic cause of detrusor overactivity. Urology 70(4):772–776
39. Rosier PFWM, Huo HC, De Gennaro M et al (2013) Urodynamic Testing Patient evaluation: Children. In: Abrams P, Cardozo L, Khoury S, Wein A (eds) Incontinence. pp 472–488
40. Andersson KE, Chapple CR, Cardozo L et al (2009) Pharmacological treatment of overactive bladder: report from the International Consultation on Incontinence. Curr Opin Urol 19:380–384
41. Game X, Mouracade P, Chartier-Kastler E et al (2009) Botulinum toxin-A (Botox) intradetrusor injections in children with neurogenic detrusor overactivity/neurogenic overactive bladder: a systematic literature review. J Pediatr Urol 5:156–164
42. Pascali MP, Mosiello M, Marciano A, Capitanucci et al (2011) A simplified technique for Botulinum toxin injections in children with neurogenic bladder. J Urol 185:2558–2562
43. Pascali MP, Mosiello G, Boldrini R et al (2011) Effects of Botulinum toxin type a in the bladder wall of children with neurogenic bladder dysfunction: a comparison of histological features before and after injections. J Urol 185:2552–2557
44. Lindehall B, Moller A, Hjalmas K et al (1994) Long-term intermittent catheterization: the experience of teenagers and young adults with myelomeningocele. J Urol 152:187–189
45. Joseph DB, Bauer SB, Colodny AH et al (1989) Clean intermittent catheterization in infants with neurogenic bladder. Pediatrics 84:78–83
46. Moore KN, Fader M, Getliffe K (2007) Long-term bladder management by intermittentcatheterisation in adults and children. Cochrane Database Syst Rev (2):CD006008
47. Boone TB, Roehrborn CG, Hurt G (1992) Transurethral intravesical electrotherapy for neurogenic bladder dysfunction in children with myelodysplasia: a prospective, randomized clinical trial. J Urol 148:550–554
48. De Gennaro M, Capitanucci ML, Mosiello G et al (2011) Current state of nerve stimulation technique for lower urinary tract dysfunction in children. J Urol 185:1571–1577
49. Guys JM, Haddad M, Planche D et al (2004) Sacral neuromodulation for neurogenic bladder dysfunction in children. J Urol 172:1673–1676
50. Capitanucci ML, Camanni D, Demelas F et al (2009) Long-term efficacy of percutaneous tibial nerve stimulation for different types of lower urinary tract dysfunction in children. J Urol 182:2056–2061
51. Razmaria AA, Marchetti PE, Prasad SM et al (2013) Does robot-assisted laparoscopic ileocystoplasty (RALI) reduce peritoneal adhesions compared with open surgery? BJU Int. doi:10.1111/bju.12284
52. Lindley RM, Mackinnon AE, Shipstone D et al (2003) Long-term outcome in bladder detrusorectomy augmentation. Eur J Pediatr Surg 7–1
53. Chung SY, Meldrum K, Docimo SG (2004) Laparoscopic assisted reconstructive surgery: a 7-year experience. J Urol 171:372–375
54. Capozza N, Caione P, DeGennaro M et al (1995) Endoscopic treatment of vesicoureteral reflux and urinary incontinence. Technical problems in the pediatric patient. Br J Urol 75:538–542
55. Guys JM, Simeoni-Alias J, Fakhro A et al (1999) Use of polydimethylsiloxane for endoscopic treatment of urinary incontinence in children. J Urol 162:2133–2135
56. Gonzalez R, Merino FG, Vaughn M (1995) Long-term results of the artificial urinary sphincter in male patients with neurogenic bladder. J Urol 154:769–770
57. Catti M, Lortat-Jacob S, Morineau M et al (2008) Artificial urinary sphincter in children—voiding or emptying? An evaluation of functional results in 44 patients. J Urol 180:690–693

16 Surgery for Incontinence

Emilio Merlini

16.1 Definition

Urinary incontinence is defined by the International Children's Continence Society (ICCS) [1] as an "uncontrollable leakage of urine. It can be continuous or intermittent."

Continuous incontinence means constant leakage of urine, and it is almost always associated with a malformation of the urinary tract like bladder or cloacal exstrophy, epispadias, neuropathic bladder, ectopic ureters, and urogenital sinus or with an iatrogenic or traumatic damage to the sphincter mechanisms. Intermittent incontinence means leakage in discrete amounts that can occur during daytime and/or nighttime and, in most cases, represents a functional phenomenon that doesn't require surgical repair.

Pseudoincontinence is a continuous urinary leakage associated with normal micturition and a normal bladder development; it is found only in females and it is due to an ectopic ureter draining outside the domain of the urinary sphincter. In most cases the ureter belongs to the upper pole of a complete duplex kidney and drains either in the genital tract or in the urethra, distal to the sphincteric area.

E. Merlini
Division of Pediatric Urology, Regina Margherita Children's Hospital, Citta' Della Salute e Della Scienza Di Torino, Torino 10100, Italy
e-mail: emilio.vittorio.merlini@gmail.com

16.2 Pathophysiology

Urinary continence is generally attained between 2 and 3 years of age in normal children, and it consists in the capability of voluntary controlling micturition, both postponing and starting it under cortical control [2].

Normal micturition requires intact neural pathways linking the central and peripheral nervous system with the bladder/sphincter complex and a bladder of adequate capacity, contractility, and compliance and a functioning sphincter.

Voluntary micturition is under neural control by several cortical areas and by the pontine micturition center that coordinates the sensitive afferences from the bladder and proximal urethra and the efferent output to the motoneurons in the sacral portion of the spinal cord.

Disruption of these fine neural control mechanisms is responsible for urinary incontinence observed in congenital and acquired neuropathic bladder [3].

The bladder is meant to store and expel urine at low pressure and at proper time and place; to obtain this result the bladder must have an adequate compliance and capacity for age, without overactive contractions.

In a newborn, the bladder, capacity is approximately 30 ml and it increases to approximately 300 ml in teenagers. A practical rule to estimate normal bladder capacity for age is 30 ml X (age in years +1). Compliance is rather complicated to calculate in children as no reliable normal values

M. Lima, G. Manzoni (eds.), *Pediatric Urology: Contemporary Strategies from Fetal Life to Adolescence*, DOI 10.1007/978-88-470-5693-0_16, © Springer-Verlag Italia 2015

are available in literature. A rule of thumb is that detrusor pressure should not exceed 10 cm H_2O at bladder capacity.

Normal bladder capacity and compliance and the absence of involuntary phasic contractions during filling are necessary conditions to obtain continence, while a small, fibrotic, low-compliance, or overactive bladder will never allow storing enough urine at low pressure.

An intact bladder outlet is the second necessary condition for continence; bladder outlet includes the bladder neck and proximal urethra that, together, may be regarded as a single unit acting as a sphincter. There is no anatomically distinct striated and smooth sphincter, but, rather, a mixture of smooth and striated muscle with elastic fibers extending from the bladder neck to the membranous urethra in males and to mid-urethra in females and creating a high-pressure zone that has sphincteric function [4].

Several factors contribute to the maintenance of a normal pressure in the sphincteric area: Intrinsic factors include smooth and striated muscle tone and contractility and elastic fibers of the bladder neck and urethral wall.

Extrinsic factors comprise the transmission of abdominal pressure to an adequately long portion of the urethra located within the abdomen and structural support of the posterior urethra and bladder neck by the perineal diaphragm and muscles. An intact perineal diaphragm counteracts the tendency of bladder and urethra to slip outside the abdominal cavity because of the abdominal pressure and provides a sound structure against which the urethra is compressed with increasing abdominal pressure.

In many conditions causing incontinence in children, most of the factors promoting continence are inadequate or absent.

16.3 Clinical Conditions Associated with Structural Incontinence

The conditions associated with structural incontinence, i.e., caused by anatomical factors, can be classified as:

1. Conditions characterized by a congenital anomaly of the bladder and/or urinary sphincter:
   - Exstrophy complex (epispadias, bladder exstrophy, cloacal exstrophy, and exstrophic variants)
   - Bilateral ectopic single ureters
   - Congenitally short urethra, generally associated with a urogenital sinus malformation
   - Anomalies of the urethra and bladder, mainly incontinent duplication of the bladder and/or urethra
   - Incontinent ureterocele
2. Conditions with deficient neural supply to the bladder and sphincters:
   - Congenital or acquired neurogenic bladder
3. Acquired conditions:
   - Iatrogenic injury to the urethral sphincter
   - Posterior urethra trauma and stenosis

The treatment of these conditions differs according to the various causes; this chapter will deal only with the procedures required to reinforce the bladder outlet when this is defective.

16.4 Preoperative Evaluation

A thorough preoperative evaluation is necessary, and both upper and lower urinary tract must be assessed together with renal function and average daily urinary output.

Incontinence can be multifactorial and be caused by insufficient bladder neck and/or by insufficient bladder capacity and/or compliance; therefore, the main diagnostic problem is to evaluate the responsibility of every single structure involved in the process of keeping a child dry. In other words, it is necessary to understand if incontinence is purely an effect of a weak bladder outlet or if a concomitant bladder dysfunction is a cofactor. In such case, a concomitant bladder augmentation is needed at the time of bladder outlet surgery.

Clinical evaluation with a voiding diary, a 4 h observation protocol together with a video urodynamic test, is generally sufficient to evaluate the lower urinary tract. Video urodynamic in particular is an indispensable tool, showing, at the same time, the anatomy of the bladder, bladder neck, and urethra and the pressure at which urine leaks together with the dynamics of the posterior urethra.

To perform a correct and useful video urodynamic investigation, because of leakage around standard urodynamic catheters, occlusion of the bladder outlet with a balloon catheter is needed to judge bladder capacity, contractility, and compliance, while leak point pressure is evaluated with the balloon deflated.

Inadequate bladder outlet resistance can be assumed if the leak point pressure is under 30–40 cm H_2O and the bladder neck is open on fluoroscopy, while if bladder capacity is less than 50–60 % than expected for age and compliance less than 2 cm H_2O per ml, most probably the bladder needs to be augmented at the time of bladder outlet surgery [5].

16.5 Principles of Surgical Treatment of Incontinence

No single procedure, with the exception of artificial sphincters, is able to recreate a sphincteric mechanism working exactly in the same manner as native sphincters, that is to assure continence and volitional voiding to completion at will. Most of the procedures can provide either "continence" for a limited period of time, generally 3 h (the so-called social continence), coupled with volitional voiding or "dryness," which means that children are dry for a limited period of time but require clean intermittent catheterization (CIC) to empty their bladder. Preoperative evaluation and the choice of the surgical procedures must take into account factors influencing the ultimate outcome of the procedure: need for CIC, intellectual capabilities of the patient, manual dexterity, and availability of a motivated caregiver to assist the patient in CIC. In general, most neuropathic bladders are already being treated with CIC and they continue after continence procedure, while patients with exstrophy or epispadias generally are not on CIC preoperatively, and they and their parents need a very clear explanation that after the procedure, especially if associated with bladder augmentation, patients may need to empty their bladder with CIC, most likely through an appendicovesicostomy.

16.6 Surgical Procedures

Procedures aiming at increasing bladder outlet resistance can be divided into:

1. Urethral lengthening and tightening procedures, aiming at creating a long and narrow tube out of the trigone (Young–Dees–Leadbetter, Mitchell procedure, and modifications)
2. Construction of a flap mechanism that progressively increases its resistance as the bladder fills
3. Suspension and external compression of the urethra (slings, artificial sphincter)
4. Injection of bulking substance within or around the urethral wall
5. Closure of the bladder neck

16.6.1 Urethral Lengthening Procedures

The first procedure for "bladder neck reconstruction" was initially described by Young in 1922 and later modified by Dees in 1949 and Leadbetter in 1964 [6] who added ureteral reimplantation moving the ureters in a more cranial position. It is popular for treatment of incontinence in exstrophy-epispadias population where continence rates between 70 and 86 % have been reported in large series [7], while its use in neuropathic bladder has not gained a vast popularity, and only few reports of its success rate in this subset of incontinent population are available in the literature [8].

The procedure starts (Fig. 16.1) with the patient lying supine with his back hyperextended to facilitate bladder exposure. The bladder wall can be reached through a midline incision or a modified Pfannenstiel with midline longitudinal opening of the abdominal fascia and rectus muscles.

The anterior bladder wall is incised in the midline starting at the beginning of the urethra.

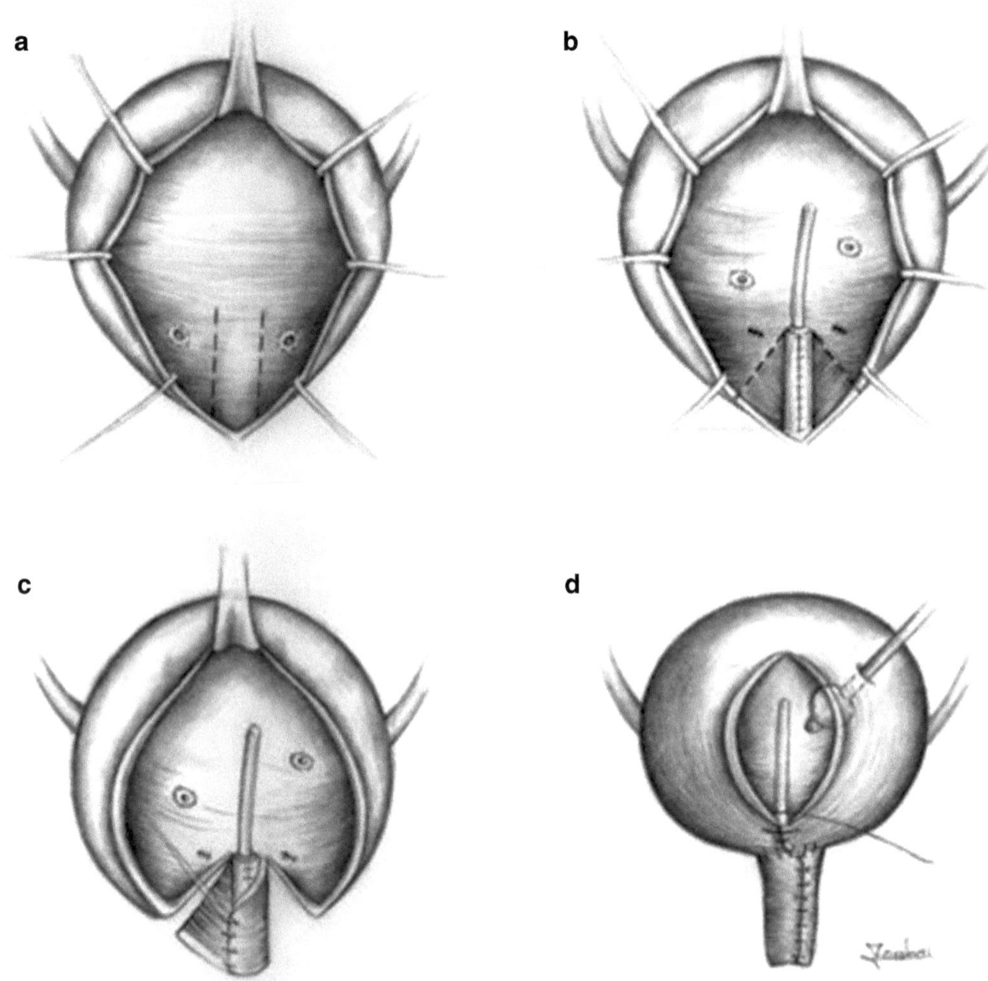

Fig. 16.1 Bladder neck repair according the Young-Dees Leadbetter procedure . The bladder is open vertically (**a**) and a longitudinal strip is outlined on the trigone, in continuity with the posterior wall of the urethra . (**b**) Ureters are reimplanted, cephalad, in a cross trigonal fashion. The mucosal strip is tubularized around a soft multiperforated stent (8 or 10 Fr.) and the mucosa lateral to the tubularized strip is removed, leaving two detrusor triangles. (**c**) A horizontal incision is carried out at the junction between the denuded detrusor flaps and intact bladder wall. The two muscular flaps are wrapped around the mucosal tube in a "pants over vest" fashion, to create the new posterior urethra and bladder neck. (**d**) a suprapubic catheter is inserted and the bladder is closed vertically.

A longitudinal strip 12–14 mm wide and 3–4 cm long is outlined in the trigone, in continuity with the posterior wall of the urethra, reaching the level of the ureteric orifices. It is of utmost importance that the longitudinal strip starts as far as possible in the proximal urethra to avoid the hourglass deformity responsible for many failures of YDL technique. The ureters are dissected and reimplanted cephalad in a cross-trigonal fashion. The mucosal strip is then tubularized in the midline, over an 8 or a 10 Fr. catheter with reabsorbable sutures to create a long and narrow mucosal tube. The mucosa lateral to the tubularized strip is then removed, creating two denuded detrusor triangles. In the original technique, a horizontal incision is carried at the junction between denuded and intact detrusor, creating a muscular flap that is wrapped around to cover and reinforce the new urethra. A similar maneuver is carried on the other side, creating a second flap that is sutured to the first one, covering the urethra in a pants-over-vest fashion. Some

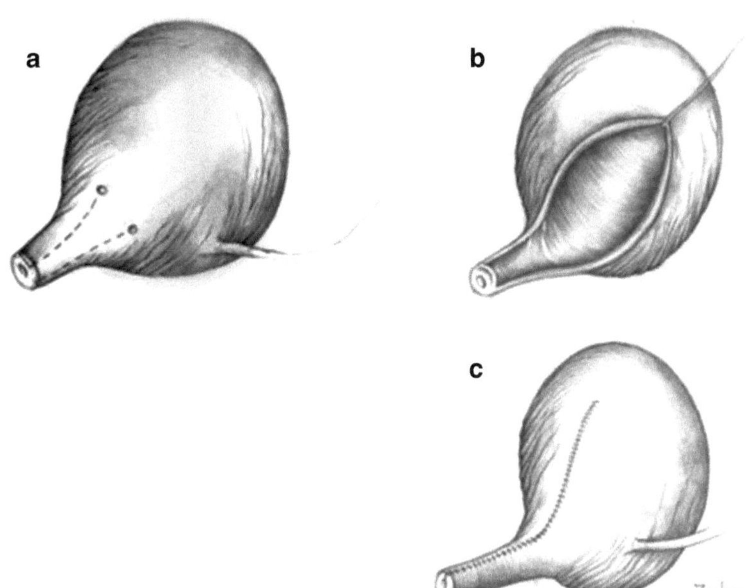

Fig. 16.2 Mitchell's bladder neck repair. (**a**) A transverse incision is carried out on the anterior aspect of posterior urethra and is extended cranially along the posterior lateral wall of the urethra and bladder, creating a (**b**) triangular flap of anterior urethral and bladder that is incorporated in the bladder. (**c**) The urethral strip is tubularized around an 8 or 10 Fr. catheter, creating a long and narrow urethra.

modifications of this step have been described: Gearhart does not cut horizontally the muscle and he wraps the two muscular flaps around the urethra, making only multiple limited incisions in the free edge of the muscle, in order to elongate the flaps [9]. The bladder is then closed in two layers; the outer muscular layer and the bladder neck are suspended to the undersurface of the pubic symphysis to maintain the bladder neck and proximal urethra in an intra-abdominal position buttressing it against the pubic bones to improve continence. We leave a short and soft stent in the reconstructed posterior urethra for a week, while urine is drained by a suprapubic Foley catheter that is kept open for 10–12 days and then clamped and released until normal voiding habits are resumed. Generally some months after surgery are necessary to achieve social continence and day continence precedes nighttime continence.

This procedure has been modified by some authors, Mollard and Koff [10, 11] among them, keeping the basic principle of elongating the posterior urethra and adding fixed resistance at the bladder outlet.

In 1993 Jones and Mitchell returned to Young's original concept of creating a long and narrow tube using the trigone muscle, without adding additional muscular support [12].

The procedure (Fig. 16.2) starts with a transverse incision on the anterior aspect of the posterior urethra, as distal as possible, extending approximately for half of the circumference; the incision is extended proximally on both sides of the urethra and bladder up to the ureteric orifices, outlining a posterior strip of muscle and mucosa, 1.5 cm large. The ureters are reimplanted. Then the strip is tubularized around an 8 or a 10 Fr catheter with a running reabsorbable suture, creating a long and narrow tube. The bladder is closed vertically in the midline. The main advantage of this procedure is that it provides excellent continence rate, sacrificing only a minimal portion of bladder capacity. Recently, Mitchell has described a further improvement in continence rate after bladder neck repair, using a demucosalized muscular flap and wrapping it around the reconstructed urethra.

These procedures are mainly used in the exstrophy–epispadias group, and the reported success rate, that means dry night and day for at least 3 h and voiding normally through the urethra, goes from 60 to 70 % in most series[13]; another 25 % may become continent after bladder augmentation. The YDL and variations have their main role in creating continence, allowing, in many cases, spontaneous voiding; if voiding is not an issue, like in most neuropathic bladders, already on CIC to empty the bladder, other continence procedures may be chosen. Nevertheless, even if the child is voiding before treatment, clinical experience and urodynamic evidence tend to show that creation of a fixed resistance at the bladder outlet, coupled with transection of nerves running around the bladder neck, a densely innervated area, in few years causes progressive detrusor insufficiency with increasing postvoiding residuals, making CIC, often coupled with bladder augmentation, inevitable.

16.6.2 Construction of Flap Mechanism

Another philosophy for obtaining continence is the use of a flap valve mechanism; the Kropp and Pippi Salle procedures belong to this group, where continence is obtained at the expense of the capacity of spontaneous voiding.

The Kropp procedure has been described by Kropp and Angwafo in 1986 [14]. The operation consists in tubularizing an anterior bladder wall flap and reimplanting it submucosally in the posterior trigonal area, creating a one-way valve mechanism, following the principles of the antireflux procedures for the ureters. In the original procedure, the tubularized bladder together with the urethra was completely detached from the bladder, which made CIC very difficult in the majority of patients; later the procedure was modified leaving the posterior wall of the urethra in continuity with the trigone, in part obviating the difficulties in catheterization. This procedure requires CIC for emptying the bladder because the continence mechanism increases with the intravesical pressure; therefore, spontaneous micturition is impossible.

The anterior bladder wall and proximal urethra are exposed, and a vertically oriented rectangular strip, 5–7 cm long and 2–2.5 cm large, is outlined on the anterior bladder wall. The base of the strip coincides with the bladder neck. The bladder is opened and both ureteric orifices are catheterized. The junction between the trigone and the bladder neck is identified, and the mucosa and superficial muscle are incised carrying this incision upward to join the two longitudinal incisions. If needed, the ureters are reimplanted in a more cephalad and lateral position to give space in the midline, and the anterior bladder wall strip is tubularized in one layer, starting precisely at the bladder neck and continuing upward. A 6 cm. long submucosal tunnel is then developed in the trigone staying exactly in the midline; the tunnel must be large enough to accommodate easily the bulky detrusor tube that is pulled through the submucosal tube, carefully, not to tear the fragile trigonal mucosa.

The opening of the new urethra is secured to the bladder wall with interrupted sutures, and the anterior bladder is closed around the new bladder neck at the base of the neourethra.

The Kropp procedure gives good results in terms of dryness, approximately over 80 %, but, unfortunately, most of the patients experience severe problems with catheterization of the new urethra. Moreover, the tubularized anterior wall is quite bulky and difficult to reimplant in the posterior bladder wall.

The majority of these patients require bladder augmentation at the time of the Kropp procedure or later because of the loss of bladder volume due to the use of the anterior bladder wall.

Pippi Salle developed a bladder outlet repair for incontinence, creating a new urethra, composed of both anterior and posterior bladder flaps [15].

The procedure (Fig. 16.3) starts with exposure of the anterior bladder wall, then a wide-based, full-thickness, 5 cm long, longitudinal anterior bladder wall flap is developed with a tongue of mucosa extending beyond the distal border of the full-thickness flap. A narrow (1 mm) strip of mucosa is then removed from the lateral margins of the flap, leaving a denuded area of detrusor muscle. After catheterization of the ureters, two longitudinal parallel incisions, 1 cm apart, are carried out in the posterior wall mucosa. The anterior strip is sutured in two layers to the posterior one. The redundant bladder mucosa in continuity with the anterior strip is folded back to cover the intravesical neourethra, facilitating bladder closure. Lastly, the bladder wall is closed in the midline, paying attention not to exert too much compression over the anterior wall flap.

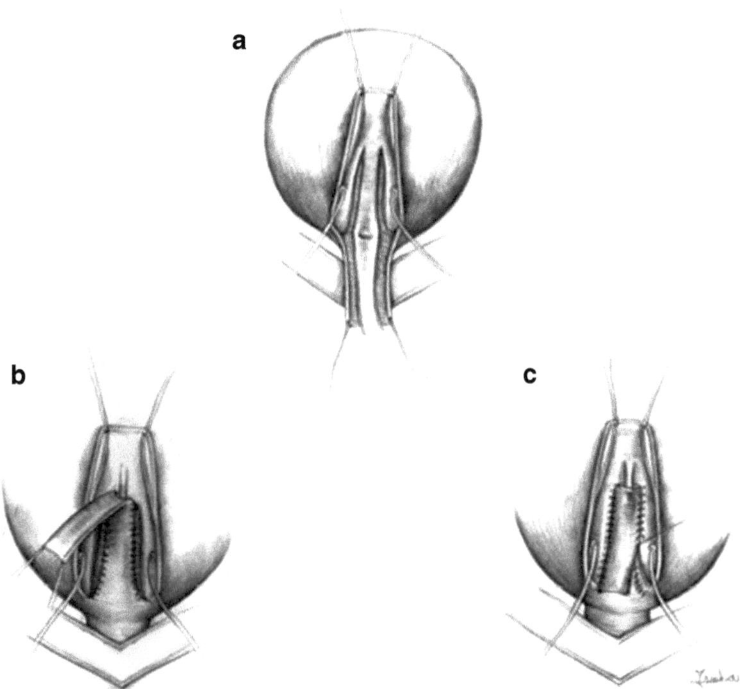

Fig. 16.3 Pippi Salle anterior bladder wall flap. (**a**) A 5 cm. long longitudinal flap of anterior bladder wall is developed; a narrow lateral strip of mucosa is removed from the flap and two vertical, parallel incisions are carried out on the trigonal mucosa. (**b**) The anterior flap is sutured in two layers to the posterior one, creating an intravesical "tube", (**c**) that is covered with the bladder mucosa. The anterior bladder wall is then closed in the midline.

The success rate of this procedure ranges from 72 to 94 %; combining all the reported patients, the success rate in achieving continence is 80 % (44 out of 55) with 16 % experiencing difficulties in catheterization.

16.6.3 Suspension and External Compression of the Urethra

16.6.3.1 Suspension

In the past, bladder neck suspensions have been very popular for the treatment of female incontinence. Marshall–Marchetti–Krantz or Burch suspension [16, 17] in association with bladder augmentation has obtained an immediate success rate around 70–80 %, but this success rate seems not durable in time, and, therefore, these procedures have been mostly abandoned in favor of periurethral slings.

McGuire and Lytton [18] popularized the concept of using a strip of isolated rectus fascia, passed beneath the bladder neck and sutured to the anterior rectal fascia at the insertion of the muscles on the pubic bones.

The slings obtain the result of elevating the bladder neck and compressing it on the posterior and lateral portions of its circumference; they find their main indication in the treatment of incontinence in neuropathic bladders, and the best results are obtained in females, even if their use is popular also in males. Children with bladder exstrophy and epispadias are best served by alternative procedures because slings may erode into the urethra, probably because the quality of tissue is poor in this group of patients.

Children with neuropathic bladder who are unable to stay dry with CIC and maximal medical management of bladder dysfunction are good candidates for sling; other good candidates are those who are incontinent after posterior urethra injury or iatrogenic injury to the sphincteric mechanism.

The evaluation of the candidates to a sling procedure must be very careful, taking into account several aspects: the detrusor responsibility in causing incontinence, the planned method of bladder drainage after surgery, the need for a continent stoma, and, finally, whether a bladder augmentation may be necessary.

It's unusual that the detrusor of a neuropathic bladder is completely normal; even in patient with apparent areflexic detrusor, it may show hyperreflexia after having increased the bladder outlet resistance; therefore, detrusor function must be assessed with careful urodynamics, in order to evaluate the need for a bladder augmentation at the time of the sling.

In general, patients undergoing a sling procedure are already catheterizing themselves, but after positioning of the sling, and especially in males, catheterization may become more difficult or even impossible, so providing a catheterizable abdominal channel may be a sensible adjunct to the procedure, mainly in wheelchair-bound children who, generally, prefer to catheterize through an abdominal continent stoma.

The sling may be constructed with rectus fascia or sometimes in fat children; it can be harvested from the fascia lata, making abdominal closure easier [19]. Decellularized porcine submucosa, SIS, has shown long-term good efficacy, while synthetic materials tend to erode into the urethra [20].

Also allografts, using cadaveric fascia lata, have given good results, favorably comparing with autologous rectus fascia.

The periurethral space may be developed transvaginally in adult women or in adolescents, while in male and young girls an anterior retropubic approach is more adequate. The procedure starts with incising the endopelvic fascia, close to the bladder neck, and developing a plane between the urethra and the vagina in female and seminal vesicles in males, cautiously spreading the blades of a right angle clamp. Great care should be used not to damage the bladder neck anteriorly or the rectum or vagina posteriorly. Once the space is obtained, an umbilical tape is threaded around the bladder neck, and when an adequate space is created, the sling is positioned, avoiding compression of the ureters. Because the sling tends to curl, it is stabilized with few stitches that keep it flat and adherent to the bladder neck. If the child is on CIC through an abdominal stoma, the sling can be tightened as much as possible to obtain a good continence, but if the child needs to catheterize himself through his urethra, it is necessary to check repeatedly the ease of catheterization during the positioning of the sling.

Lottman et al. [21] has described a midline retrovesical approach to the bladder neck that is useful mainly in neuropathic bladder. After careful detachment of the peritoneum from the bladder dome, the space between the posterior wall of the bladder and the anterior wall of the vagina in females or seminal vesicles in males is cautiously developed, remaining strictly in the midline and leaving the ureters laterally. Once the bladder neck is identified, a right angle is passed laterally on each side, so creating a space around the bladder neck, where the sling can be pulled through in the same way as described before.

The sling can also be crisscrossed in the midline, thereby exerting 360° compression on the bladder neck; this modality seems to be more effective in males. Even more effective is the tapering of the bladder neck associated with placement of a crisscrossed periurethral sling [22] (Fig. 16.4).

16.6.3.2 External Compression of the Bladder Neck

External compression of the bladder neck or urethra can be fixed or variable; fixed compression is obtained by means of fascial or synthetic wraps placed around the bladder neck, while variable compression is achieved using the artificial urinary sphincter.

Fixed External Compression

Walker et al. [23] described a procedure to wrap and compress the bladder neck using a strip of rectus fascia, with good results; Bugg and Joseph [24] added the suspension of the wrap to the pubic bone. A vascularized myofascial flap made of rectus muscle and fascia, wrapped around the bladder neck and suspended to the pubic bone, has been reported by Kolligian and Firlit [25] with good results in a small series of patients.

The use of synthetic material to create a wrap around the bladder neck has been generally fraught with a high complication rate due to the erosion of the cuff into the urethra, and the overall experience is limited in children. Some devices have given good results like the urethral constrictor described by Lima et al. [26] who reported 100 % continence rate in 42 patients.

Recently, a new device for the treatment of urinary incontinence in males has been proposed;,

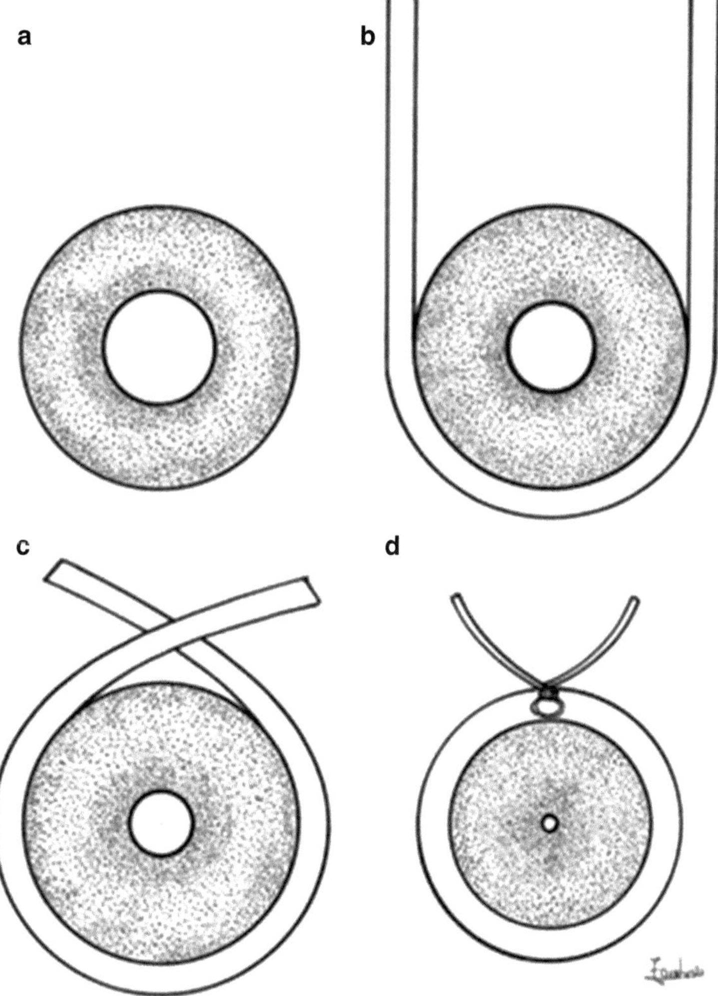

Fig. 16.4 Suspension and external compression of bladder neck (**a**, **b**) The sling compresses the posterior and lateral walls of the bladder neck. (**c**, **d**) The sling can be crisscrossed in the midline, exerting a 360° compression over the bladder neck (cinch) and can be suspended to the undersurface of pubic bones increasing its efficacy

it is a polypropylene male perineal sling, called "InVance®" (American Medical Systems Inc., Minnetonka, MN), that has been used successfully in adults to treat postprostatectomy incontinence, with low morbidity and a low complication rate [27]. The device consists of a polypropylene mesh that is secured to the descending pubic ramus bilaterally with titanium screws; the sling tension is adjusted to exert maximal pressure over the bulbar urethra. The experience in pediatric age is still limited.

The AdVance® (American Medical Systems Inc., Minnetonka, Mn) transobturator male sling has been recently employed to treat adolescent males affected by neuropathic incontinence with a 65 % success rate [28].

Variable External Compression: Artificial Urinary Sphincter

Variable compression over the bladder neck or urethra is provided by the artificial urinary sphincter, described by Scott in 1972 [29], and repeatedly modified and made more reliable in order to obviate the once frequent mechanical problems. The newest model (AMS 800) has a mechanical failure rate of 7.6 % and a nonmechanical failure rate of 9 % in a series of 184 adults with a mean follow-up of 40.8 months [30]. In children the long-term (7–10 years) survival rate is approximately 80 % in most reported series [31].

The sphincter is a mechanical device comprised of three components: an inflatable cuff that can be positioned around the bladder neck

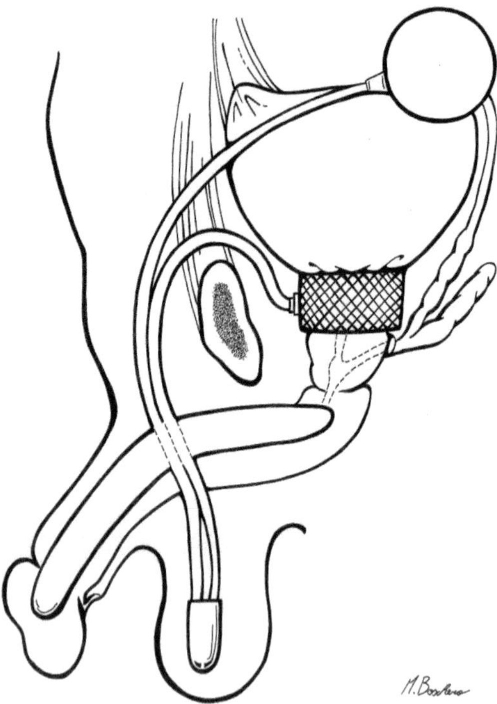

Fig. 16.5 AMS 800 Artificial urinary Sphincter. See text for description

or posterior urethra or around the bulbar urethra, a pressure-regulating reservoir balloon, and a control pump. In children the bladder neck is the preferred site of placement of the cuff; usual minimal age for placement is 6 years in boys and 8–9 years for girls. After placement the sphincter should be kept deactivated for approximately 1 month to prevent erosion.

The pressure-regulating balloon maintains the cuff inflated, exerting a constant pressure around the urethra, generally between 61 and 70 cm H_2O; the pump, located within the scrotum in boys and in the labia majora in girls, can be squeezed manually; this maneuver empties the cuff and the patient can void or catheterize himself or herself. Then the cuff fills again in approximately 3 min. The sphincter can be deactivated pressing a button located in the pump (Fig. 16.5).

The main indication for artificial sphincter placement is neurogenic incontinence in a patient with a stable and compliant bladder who can void spontaneously; in the past it was feared that intermittent catheterization could cause erosion of the urethra, but now it is clear that CIC can be performed safely even in these patients, provided that the cuff is deflated. Ability to void spontaneously can deteriorate with time, and Gonzales has reported that 74 % of patients, followed for a mean of 8 years after sphincter placement, ultimately required CIC [32].

Selection of the patients is extremely important because patients who had previous bladder neck surgery are poor candidates for artificial sphincter, and patient with a hyperreflexic, hypocompliant bladder is at risk of deterioration of the upper tract and persisting incontinence. A careful video urodynamic evaluation with bladder neck occlusion is needed before a child is selected for an implant. Unfortunately at least 20 % of patients will undergo progressive detrusor dysfunction after sphincter placement, and, currently, no test can predict who will undergo these changes. Approximately 30 % of patients require bladder augmentation with the bowel either as a simultaneous or later procedure [33]. Bladder augmentation, especially if performed simultaneously with sphincter placement, may increase the risk of infection of the device.

The most frequent complications requiring sphincter removal or substitution are mechanical malfunction, erosion of the urethra, and infection of the device. The last two complications generally preclude the possibility of implanting a new sphincter.

16.6.4 Injection of Bulking Substances

Several substances both organic and synthetic have been injected under the mucosa of the bladder neck or around the bladder neck to improve continence. Politano et al. popularized the injection of Teflon paste in adults and children with an 86 % success rate [34]; the use of this substance was later abandoned because of concerns about its safety and migration to other organs.

Organic material like autologous fat or chondrocytes was proposed but early abandoned because of their inefficacy, probably due to reabsorption. More successful was the use of X-linked bovine collagen that gave variable results, better in the exstrophy–epispadias group than in neuropathic bladders. Bomalski et al. reported a 22 % cure rate of incontinence with another 54 % improved in 40 children followed for a mean of 4.5 years [35]. Concern exists about long-term degradation of collagen with progressive worsening of continence.

Synthetic materials in use nowadays include polydimethylsiloxane (Macroplastique®) and dextranomer/hyaluronic acid copolymer (Deflux®). Macroplastique is composed of particulate silicone; Guys et al. [36] have reported a continence rate of 33 % and improvement of 14 % after one or more injections of this substance in 49 children affected by neurogenic bladder. Some concerns have been recently raised because of possible migration of smaller particles [37].

Deflux is widely used for treatment of vesicoureteral reflux; Lottman et al. [38] have reported a 50 % success rate (cure or substantial improvement) in children affected by severe urinary incontinence.

Injection is generally performed transurethrally, using a cystoscope with a 5 Fr. working channel; the bulking substance is administered in two or more sites at the bladder neck until a good mucosal apposition is observed. Any further instrumentation or catheterization of the urethra should be avoided in the following days in order to avoid dislocation or extrusion of the injected substance.

The injection can be performed also in an antegrade fashion; this is particularly useful when the bladder neck has already undergone prior surgery and identification of the proper injection site is difficult. Antegrade vision of the bladder neck helps in a more accurate placement of bulking material.

In our experience the use of injectable material for continence has proved helpful to gain additional continence after a partially successful urethral lengthening procedure, but it has proven useless as a single procedure in case of structural bladder neck incompetence.

Conclusions

Treatment of structural urinary incontinence in children remains very challenging, and surgery should be offered to the patients only if all the available medical options have failed. Patients and their families must be very motivated and psychologically ready to face less than perfect results. The percentage of failures, reoperations, and complications must be stated clearly and honestly to give the patient and family the possibility of giving a really informed consent. If augmentation is planned together with a continence procedure, it must be explained very clearly that the patient will never void normally in the future and he or she will be bound to intermittent catheterization for the rest of his/her life. These patients and their families need a long-lasting emotional support.

Once patients and family consent to perform a continence procedure, the patient needs to be studied thoroughly and, if necessary, repeatedly until a very clear anatomical and functional picture of the situation is obtained, and then the most appropriate procedure for that particular patient can be chosen. Despite accurate preoperative evaluation, after increasing the bladder neck resistance, the detrusor will deteriorate in a high percentage of cases, causing a less efficient micturition with increasing postvoiding residuals, upper urinary tract changes, and recurrent incontinence. These cases need to be identified early because they need further surgery to create a bladder reservoir at low pressure that can be emptied with intermittent catheterization. Therefore, patients need an accurate lifelong follow-up. The field of incontinence surgery is evolving with the introduction of new injectable substances and artificial devices that will contribute in making this surgery less invasive; anyhow the principles for obtaining continence remain always the same: a low-pressure reservoir of adequate capacity, enough resistance at the bladder outlet, and the possibility of emptying the bladder easily and reliably.

Acknowledgments The author wants to thank Prof. Paolo Belgioioso, Professor of Artistic Anatomy at Accademia Albertina di Belle Arti, and Turin and his students Elena Zanonato, Maria Boschero, and Laura Dosio for their invaluable help in preparing the original drawings for this chapter.

References

1. Neveus T, Von Gontard A, Hoebeke P et al (2006) The standardization of terminology of lower urinary tract function in children and adolescents: report from the standardization Committee of the International Children's Continence Society. J Urol 176:314–324
2. Neveus T, Sillen U (2013) Lower urinary tract function in childhood; normal development and common functional disturbances. Acta Physiol 207:85–92
3. Yoshimura N, De Groat WC (1997) Neural control of the lower urinary tract. Int J Urol 4:111–125
4. Blaivas J, Romanzi L, Heritz D (1998) Urinary incontinence: pathophysiology, evaluation, treatment overview and nonsurgical management. In: Walsh P, Retik A, Vaughn E, Wein A (eds) Campbell's urology. W. B. Saunders, Philadelphia, pp 1007–1036
5. De Badiola F, Castro-Diaz D, Hart-Austin C et al (1992) Influence of preoperative bladder capacity on the outcome of artificial sphincter implantation in patients with neurogenic sphincter incompetence. J Urol 148:1493–1495
6. Leadbetter GW (1964) Surgical correction of total urinary incontinence. J Urol 91:261–264
7. McMahon DR, Cain MP, Husmann DA et al (1996) Vesical neck reconstruction in patients with the exstrophy-epispadias complex. J Urol 155:1411–1413
8. Donnahoo K, Rink R, Cain M et al (1999) The use of the Young-Dees-Leadbetter bladder neck repair in patients with neurogenic incontinence. J Urol 155:1411–1413
9. Geahrart J, Jeffs RD (1998) Exstrophy-epispadias complex and bladder anomalies. In: Walsh P, Retik A, Vaughn E, Wein A (eds) Campbell's urology. W.B. Saunders, Philadelphia, pp 1939–1990
10. Mollard P (1980) Bladder reconstruction. J Urol 124:525–529
11. Koff SA (1990) A technique for bladder neck reconstruction in exstrophy: the cinch. J Urol 144:546–549
12. Jones J, Mitchell M, Rink R (1993) Improved results using a modification of the Young-Dees-Leadbetter bladder neck repair. Be J Urol 71:555–561
13. Chan DY, Jeffs RD, Gearhart JP (2001) Determinants of continence in the bladder exstrophy population after bladder neck reconstruction. Urology 57:774–777
14. Kropp K, Angwafo F (1986) Urethral lengthening and reimplantation for neurogenic incontinence in children. J Urol 135:533–536
15. Salle J, De Fraga J, Amarante A et al (1994) Urethral lengthening with anterior bladder wall flap for urinary incontinence: a new approach. J Urol 152:803–804
16. Marshall V, Marchetti A, Krantz K (1949) Correction of stress continence by simple vesicourethral suspension. Surg Gyn Obstet 88:509–518
17. Burch J (1961) Urethrovaginal fixation to Cooper's ligament for correction of stress incontinence, cystocele and prolapse. Am J Obstet Gynecol 81:281–290
18. Mc Guire E, Lytton B (1978) Pubovaginal sling for stress incontinence. J Urol 119:82–84
19. Govier FE, Gibbons RP, Correa RJ et al (1997) Pubovaginal sling using fascia lata for the treatment of intrinsic sphincter deficiency. J Urol 157:117
20. Kobashi KC, Dmochowski R, Mee L et al (1999) Erosion of woven polyester pubovaginal sling. J Urol 162:2070
21. Lottmann H, Traxer O, Aigrain Y, Melin Y (1999) Posterior approach to the bladder for implantation of the 800 AMS artificial sphincter in children and adolescents: technique and results in eight patients. Ann Urol 33:357–363
22. Herschorn S, Radomski S (1992) Fascial slings and bladder neck tapering in the treatment of male urologic incontinence. J Urol 147:1073–1075
23. Walker D III, Flack CE, Hawkins-Lee B et al (1995) Rectus fascial wrap: early results of a modification of the rectus fascial sling. J Urol 154:771
24. Bugg CE, Joseph DB (2003) Bladder neck cinch for pediatric neurogenic outlet deficiency. J Urol 170:1501–1503
25. Kolligian ME, Palmer LS, Cheng EY, Firlit CF (1998) Myofascial wrap to treat intractable urinary incontinence in children. Urology 52:1122–1127
26. Lima SV, Araujo LA, Vilar FO (1997) Further experience with the periurethral expander : a new type of artificial sphincter. Br J Urol 80:460
27. Athanasopulos A, Kostantinopoulos A, Mc Guire E (2010) Efficacy of the InVance male sling in treating stress urinary incontinence: a three year experience from a single centre. Urol Int 85:436–442
28. Groen LA, Spinoit AF, Hoebeke P et al (2012) The advance male sling as a minimally invasive treatment for intrinsic sphincter deficiency in patients with neurogenic bladder sphincter dysfunction: a pilot study. Neurourol Urodyn 31:1284–1287
29. Scott FB, Timm GW (1974) Treatment of incontinence by an implantable prosthetic urinary sphincter. J Urol 112:75
30. Elliott D, Barrett D (1998) Mayo Clinic long term analysis of the functional durability of the AMS 800 artificial urinary sphincter: a review of 323 cases. J Urol 159:1206–1208
31. Hafez A, McLorie G, Bagli D, Khoury A (2002) A single-center long-term outcome analysis of artificial urinary sphincter placement in children. BJU Int 83:1120–1131
32. Gonzalez R, Merino F, Vaughn M (1995) Long term results of the artificial urinary sphincter in male patients with neurogenic bladder. J Urol 154:769–770
33. Barrett D, Parulkar B, Kramer S (1993) Experience with AS 800 artificial sphincter in pediatric and young adult patients. Urology 42:431–436

34. Vorstman B, Lockhard J, Kaufman M, Politano V (1985) Polytetrafluoroethylene injection for urinary incontinence in children. J Urol 133:248–250
35. Bomalski M, Bloom D, Mc Guire E et al (1996) Glutaraldehyde cross-linked collagen in the treatment of urinary incontinence in children. J Urol 155:699–702
36. Guys JM, Breaud J, Hery G et al (2006) Endoscopic injection with polydimethylsiloxane for the treatment of pediatric urinary incontinence in the neurogenic bladder: long term results. J Urol 175:1106–1110
37. Henly DR, Barrett DM, Wieland TL et al (1995) Particulate silicone for use in periurethral injections: local tissue effects and search for migration. J Urol 153:2039–2043
38. Alova I, Margaryan M, Bernuy M et al (2012) Long term effects of endoscopic injection of dextranomer/hyaluronic acid based implants for treatment of urinary incontinence in children with neurogenic bladder. J Urol 188:1905–1909

17 Lower Urinary Tract Dysfunction

Mario De Gennaro and Maria Luisa Capitanucci

17.1 Pathophysiology

Since different types of lower urinary tract dysfunction (LUTD) commonly overlap, knowledge of pathophysiology is mandatory to distinguish the prevalent type and start a correct program of therapy.

The predominant pathophysiological theory to explain idiopathic overactive bladder (OAB) in children is that OAB is due to delayed maturation of reticulospinal pathways and inhibitory center in the midbrain and cerebral cortex [3]. Cortical control is normally established between ages 3 and 5. Delay in bladder–sphincter coordination during voiding causes uninhibited detrusor contractions, to be met with voluntary external sphincter contractions. Consequent increase in intravesical pressure is recognized by children as sense of urgency and may lead to development of vesicoureteral reflux (VUR). It has been known that OAB is associated with high incidence of VUR and that successful treatment of OAB significantly improves the rate of reflux resolution as compared to controls [4, 5].

Since voluntary external sphincter and pelvic floor contraction may induce temporary reflex relaxation of the detrusor, holding maneuvers, such as leg crossing, penile grabbing, and squatting, can be implemented by children to get momentary relief from urgency. The mechanisms of bladder inhibition via these maneuvers could rely on sympathetic activation through the pudendal nerve, suppressing detrusor contraction by stimulation of β-adrenergic receptors. Despite holding maneuvers, children may experience urge incontinence, mostly when tired or when the focus is on activity that requires concentration. Recurrent isometric detrusor contraction against a closed or incompletely relaxed sphincter/pelvic floor can induce progressive detrusor hypertrophy. Hypertrophy may lead to decreased functional bladder capacity and increased detrusor overactivity, creating a vicious circle in which OAB can only get worse [3].

The pathophysiology of dysfunctional voiding (DV) remains unclear. It has been hypothesized that detrusor overactivity eventually leads to overactivity of the pelvic floor with subsequent insufficient relaxation during voiding [6]. Another theory suggests that poor relaxation of the pelvic floor muscles during voiding is a learned condition during the toilet training

M. De Gennaro (✉) • M.L. Capitanucci
Department Nephrology–Urology,
Robotic Surgery and Urodynamic Division,
Children's Hospital Bambino Gesù,
Piazza Sant'Onofrio, 4, Rome 00165, Italy
e-mail: mario.degennaro@opbg.net;
mluisa.capitanucci@opbg.net

M. Lima, G. Manzoni (eds.), *Pediatric Urology: Contemporary Strategies from Fetal Life to Adolescence*,
DOI 10.1007/978-88-470-5693-0_17, © Springer-Verlag Italia 2015

years, adopted following episodes of urinary tract infection or constipation or occurring after sexual abuse [7]. Moreover, toilet conditions and privacy issues can trigger or exacerbate voiding disturbances [8]. In some girls DV may be associated with anatomical anomalies of the external urethral meatus: the urine stream may be deflected anteriorly and cause stimulation of the clitoris with reflex activity of the bulbocavernosus muscle, causing intermittent voiding [9]. In these cases, no structural transurethral obstruction can be identified and staccato or intermittent voiding is termed as functional disturbances. Long-standing overactivity of the pelvic floor may lead in some children to detrusor decompensation due to detrusor hypocontractility; however, no data are available to support this theory.

Dysfunctional disturbances of the LUT and bowel (constipation) describe the dysfunctional elimination syndrome (DES) [4]. Children in early stage of defecation disorders show an incomplete and infrequent bowel emptying. With progression of the disorder, the rectum and descending colon are distended with decrease in normal sensation; children develop constipation which may be associated with fecal retentive incontinence [10]. Abnormal recruitment of the external anal sphincter during defecation may elicit concomitant urethral sphincter and pelvic floor co-contractions, leading to functional obstruction in both systems. Consequently, high pressure generated by the detrusor to overcome functional obstruction can stimulate detrusor hypertrophy and detrusor overactivity and lead to incompetence of the vesicoureteral junction [1].

17.2 ICCS Definition of Lower Urinary Tract Symptoms and Conditions [1, 2]

Since the final steps of lower urinary tract (LUT) control development are usually achieved at the age of 3 or 4 years, definitions of LUT symptoms (LUTS) and conditions are relevant from the age of 5 years.

17.2.1 Lower Urinary Tract Symptoms (LUTS)

LUTS are classified according to their relation with storage or voiding phase of bladder function.

17.2.1.1 Storage Symptoms

- *Increased or decreased voiding frequency*: The normal range is 3–7 voiding per day. Therefore, the observation that a child voids eight or more times daily denoted increased daytime frequency, whereas three or fewer voiding daily indicates decreased voiding frequency. Clearly, fluid intake must be considered in evaluating voiding frequency.
- *Urinary incontinence* (*UI*): It is an uncontrollable leakage of urine. When UI is continuous, it is almost exclusively associated with congenital anomalies or iatrogenic damage of the external urethral sphincter. Differently, intermittent UI is due to functional problems and can occur in daytime, in nighttime (enuresis), or in both. When associated with urgency, intermittent UI is called urge incontinence.
- *Urgency*: It means the sudden and unexpected experience of an immediate need to void.
- *Nocturia*: The child must awaken at night to void.

17.2.1.2 Voiding Symptoms

- *Hesitancy*: It denotes that the child has difficulty in the initiation of micturition or must wait a considerable period of time before voiding starts.
- *Straining*: The child applies abdominal pressure to initiate and maintain voiding.
- *Weak stream*: It is the observed ejection of urine with a weak force.
- *Intermittency*: Micturition occurs in several discrete spurts.

17.2.1.3 Other Symptoms

- *Voiding postponement*: Children with incontinence who habitually postpone micturition, often in specific situation, using holding maneuvers. This is often associated with low micturition frequency and feeling of urgency due to a full bladder. Psychological comorbidity or behavioral disturbances are often associated.

- *Holding maneuvers*: They are observable strategies to postpone micturition as well as squatting, standing on tiptoe, and forcefully crossing the legs.
- *Feeling of incomplete bladder emptying.*
- *Post-micturition dribble*: It is an involuntary urine leakage which occurs immediately after voiding has finished.

17.2.2 LUT Conditions

They include nighttime, daytime, and symptom-specific conditions:

17.2.2.1 Nighttime Condition

Enuresis

The term defines a form of intermittent nocturnal incontinence. That means that the term of enuresis is not synonymous with incontinence. Enuresis is an involuntary voiding during sleep, at least three times a week, in children over 5 years of age in the absence of congenital or acquired defects of the central nervous system. The new ICCS classification distinguishes *monosymptomatic* (bed-wetting without daytime symptoms) from *non-monosymptomatic* (bed-wetting with daytime symptoms) enuresis and *primary* (children who have never been free of bed-wetting for 6 months) from *secondary* (reemergence of bed-wetting after a dry period of at least 6 months) enuresis. The classification in monosymptomatic (MNE) and non-monosymptomatic (NMNE) nocturnal enuresis is very important when we consider treatment strategies. NMNE is not an isolated phenomenon but a part of symptom complex which is expression of a LUT dysfunction (LUTD). Therefore, children with NMNE are more appropriately managed in the context of LUTD. NME is an isolated phenomenon due to delayed in maturation in one or more of the following systems: stability of bladder function, arginine vasopressin release, or response and ability to wake from sleep to full bladder sensations. Combinations of all three problems may be present in the same children.

17.2.2.2 Daytime Conditions/Lower Urinary Tract Dysfunction (LUTD)

Overactive Bladder (OAB)

OAB defines the symptom complex of urgency, which may or may not be associated with urge incontinence and is not a direct result of known neurological damage. The term urgency refers to a sudden compelling desire to void that is often difficult to defer. Urge incontinence means incontinence concomitant with urgency. Increased voiding frequency is often present; however, this symptom is not a necessary prerequisite to define OAB, especially when fluid intake and post-voiding residuum are not evaluated. The hallmark symptom, urgency, arises from detrusor overactivity (detrusor contractions during filling phase). During invasive urodynamic study, detrusor contractions during filling phase are countered by voluntary contraction of the pelvic floor to postpone voiding and minimize urge incontinence.

Dysfunctional Voiding (DV)

Children with DV are not able to fully relax the sphincter or pelvic floor muscles during voiding. Children with DV usually present with low voiding frequency, incontinence, and urinary tract infections. However, this condition cannot be defined unless repeated flowmetries show curve with staccato or interrupted pattern. The term *staccato voiding* indicates a continuous urine flow with periodic reductions in flow rate precipitated by bursts of pelvic floor activity; voiding is commonly prolonged and incomplete. *Interrupted voiding* is represented by micturition in separate fractions due to unsustained voiding contractions; voided volume is usually larger than age-expected capacity and relevant residual urine is often present.

Underactive Bladder (UB)

The term UB replaces the old entity of lazy bladder. This term is reserved for children with a need to increase abdominal pressure to initiate and maintain or complete voiding. The children with UB show an inability to void using detrusor pressure alone; they often produce an interrupted or plateau pattern with relevant post-voiding residual urine. In these cases, invasive urodynamics is mandatory to define the presence of detrusor underactivity during voiding.

17.2.2.3 Symptom-Specific Conditions

Voiding Postponement (VP)

Children with urinary incontinence who habitually and voluntary postpone micturition. VP is often associated with low voiding frequency and a feeling of urgency due to a full bladder. Some children restrict fluid intake to increase intervals between micturitions and to decrease incontinence. These children often present with psychological comorbidity or behavioral disturbances.

Vaginal Reflux (VR)

To prepubertal girls with moderate incontinence which occurs within 10 min after normal voiding. This is not associated with other LUTS.

Giggle Incontinence

It is a rare syndrome in which complete voiding occurs specifically during or immediately after laughing. Bladder function is normal when children are not laughing.

Extraordinary Daytime Urinary Frequency

Children who void often and with small volumes during the daytime only. Daytime voiding frequency is at least once hourly and mean voided volume is less than 50 % of expected bladder capacity for age.

Dysfunctional Elimination Syndrome (DES)

This term is used to describe dysfunctional emptying of bowel and bladder. ES is seen more frequently in girls than in boys and is significantly associated with the presence of both vesicoureteral reflux (VUR) and urinary tract infection (UTI). Children with ES commonly present with incontinence, non-monosymptomatic nocturnal enuresis, urgency, infrequent voiding recurrent UTI and VUR, constipation, and fecal incontinence.

17.3 Assessment

A standardization document for diagnostic evaluation of children with UI and LUTS has been recently published by the International Children's Continence Society [11]. A noninvasive approach is recommended in these children by means of detailed and structured history (developmental, voiding, and medical), physical examination, and bladder diary. Urinalysis, uroflowmetry with pelvic floor electromyography, and pre- and post-voiding bladder ultrasound can be added. These tools enable to make differential diagnosis between different types of LUTD (Table 17.1) and to select patients who will need further urodynamic (cystometry, pressure-flow studies, videourodynamics) and imaging studies (upper urinary tract ultrasound, micturition cystography). With the same instruments, children with neurogenic bladder or structural anomalies of the lower urinary tract should be identified.

17.3.1 Medical History

Obstetrical history (fetal distress, anoxia, birth trauma, prenatal hydronephrosis, and oligohydramnios), age appropriateness of developmental milestones, and age at toilet training should be evaluated. LUTS should be collected by children and successively matched and completed with information reported by parents. Urgency and reactions to urge, voiding frequency, urinary tract infections, and frequency and amount of possible urine loss during day and/or night should be assessed. When urine loss is present, it is important to distinguish between continuous (anatomical causes) and intermittent (idiopathic LUTS) incontinence. As previously mentioned, urgency is the subjective hallmark of OAB. Urgency must be clearly explained to children and parents such as sudden and unexpected experience of an immediate need to void. It is always necessary to clarify the difference between urgency and the strong desire to void after a period of voiding postponement. Urgency may be associated with increased voiding frequency and urine loss of different amount. Since pelvic floor overactivity

Table 17.1 Diagnostic work-up in children with lower urinary tract dysfunction

Diagnostic tools	Overactive bladder	Dysfunctional voiding
Medical history	Urgency	
	Holding manoeuvres to contrast urgency	Holding manoeuvres to postpone micturition
	±Increased void. frequency[a]	Increased/decreased void. frequency[a]
	±Urge Incontinence	±Intermittent incontinence
	±Urinary tract infection	±Urinary tract infection
	±Constipation	±Constipation
Bladder diary	Episodes of urgency	
	Increased number of voiding[a]	Abnormal number of voiding[a]
	Low voided volume[b]	Normal/high voided volume[b]
	Episodes of incontinence + urge	Episodes of incontinence without urge
	Amount of urine loss	Amount of urine loss
	Bowel movements	Bowel movements
Uroflowmetry	Tower-shaped curve	Staccato or Interrupted curve
	Low voided volume[b]	Normal/high voided volume[b]
Pelvic-floor EMG	Relaxed pelvic floor	Overactive pelvic floor
Pre-voiding US	Low bladder capacity[b]	Normal/increased bladder capacity[b]
	Bladder wall	Bladder wall
	Normal or thickened	Normal or thickened
Post-voiding US	No post-voiding residuum	±Post-voiding residuum

[a]Normal voiding frequency in children: 5–7/day [2]
[b]Expected bladder capacity for age [30+ (age in years ×30)] in ml [2]

could be present, information on toilet behavior and subjective quantification of urinary stream should be collected. Finally, constipation and soiling should be assessed always. Validated questionnaires for LUTS [12] and bowel chart [13] are available also in children. However, it is recommended that questionnaires not to be used as a single investigation: they should be combined with a more objective examination such as bladder diary and uroflowmetry [11].

17.3.2 Clinical Examination

Besides abdominal palpation to assess bladder distension and fecal impaction, neurological and genital examinations must be done. Neurological evaluation includes accurate inspection of the back in order to identify cutaneous manifestation (deep sacral dimple, lipoma, skin discoloration, hair tuft) of an underlying occult spinal dysraphism, examination of the lower extremities (muscle atrophy, foot deformities, and any buttock and lower extremity asymmetry), and evaluation of perianal and perineal sensation and anal sphincter tone and reflex. Labia fusion, abnormal position of urethral meatus, and lesions of hymen and phimosis, hypospadias, and recurvatum should be excluded in girls and boys, respectively.

17.3.3 Bladder Diary

Recording of symptoms under normal condition is crucial for the assessment of both lower urinary tract and bowel function [2]. Bladder diary records fluid intake, micturition frequency, voided volume, episode of urgency, and urine loss. For diagnostic purpose, it should cover at least 3 days of registration [1]. A bowel movement chart and Bristol stool chart [13] are also important, either separate from or in conjunction with bladder diary.

17.3.4 Urinalysis

It may provide information about urinary tract infection, possible associated diabetes, and renal

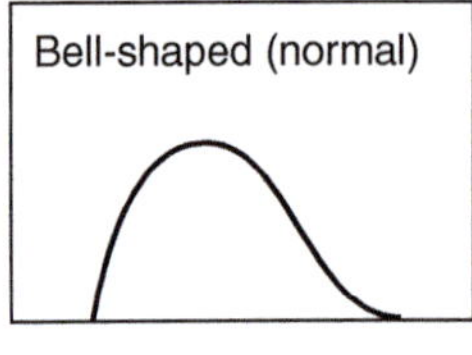

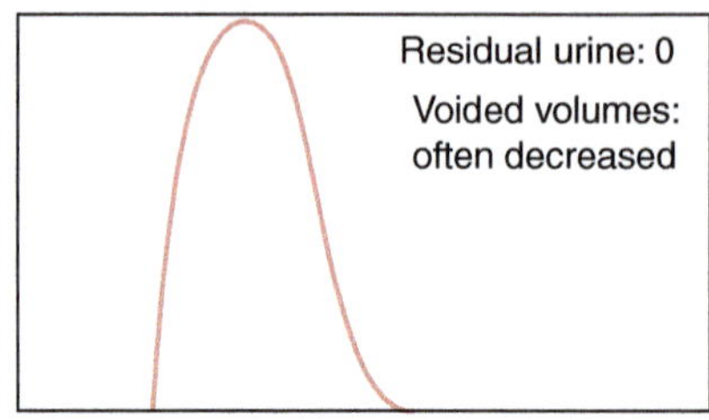

Tower shaped curve: overactive bladder

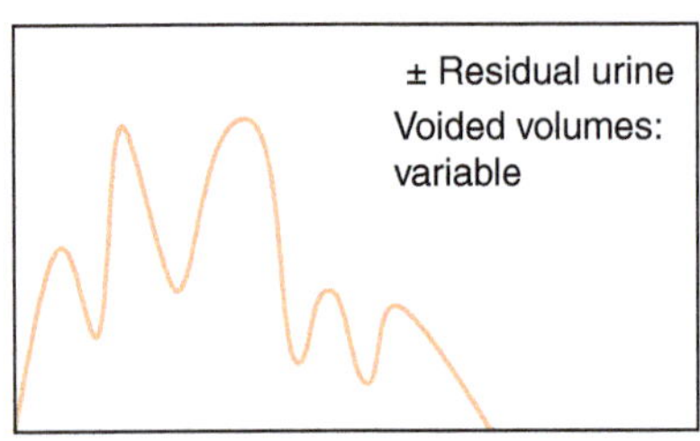

Staccato curve: dysfunctional Voiding

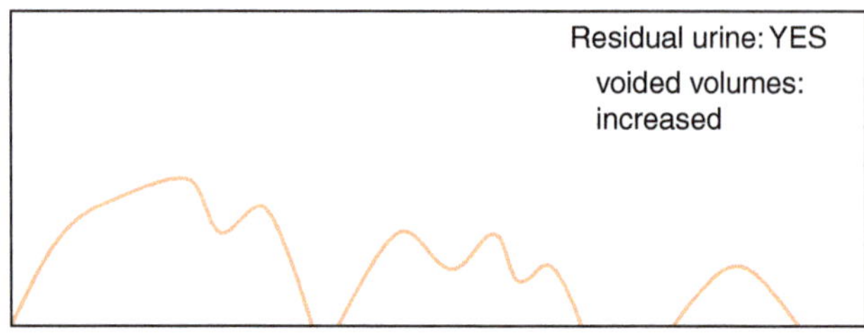

Interrupted curve: dysfunctional voiding or underactive bladder

Fig. 17.1 Uroflowmetry pattern in children with lower urinary tract dysfunction

damage or disease-causing proteinuria. Dipstick may be useful in clinical practice to achieve quickly these informations [14].

17.3.5 Uroflowmetry

It is the least invasive of all urodynamic studies and, therefore, is perfect for pediatric patients [15]. Moreover, results of uroflowmetry combined with those of history, bladder diary, and pre- and post-voiding residual (PVR) urine evaluation seem to be more effective than standard urodynamic study in detecting both OAB and dysfunctional voiding. In children, more than one uroflowmetry recording should be obtained in the same session before drawing conclusions, and three evaluations are advised [1, 2]. Pelvic floor EMG and ultrasound evaluation of post-voiding residual urine are recommended, increasing the value of uroflowmetry measurement. The shape of the flow curve is the most important factor to analyze in pediatric patients [2]. In normal voiding the curve is bell shaped (Fig. 17.1). OAB may produce an explosive voiding contraction that appears as a high-amplitude flow curve of short duration, namely, a *tower-shaped curve* (Fig. 17.1). Sphincter overactivity during voiding is seen as sharp peaks and troughs in flow curve that is an irregular or *staccato flow curve* (Fig. 17.1). In case of underactive or acontractile detrusor, when abdominal contraction is the main force to empty the bladder, flow curve shows discrete peaks corresponding to abdominal strain, separated by segments with zero flow, the so-called interrupted or fractionated curve (Fig. 17.1). Anatomical obstruction often has a low amplitude and rather even flow curve that is a *plateau curve* (Fig. 17.1). Generally, in children with OAB voided volume is lower than expected bladder capacity for age (EBC). On the contrary, in children with DV, voided volume can be higher than EBC. EBC for age is estimated by the formula [30 + (age in years × 30)] in ml [1]. Evaluating uroflowmetry, EBC is of great importance because it has been shown that uroflow curve changes when the voided volume is less than 50 % of EBC [16]. In children, poor correlation exists between Qmax and outflow resistance. Therefore, Qmax is of minor importance than in adult age.

17.3.6 Ultrasound

In all children with proven LUTD, bladder ultrasound is indicated. It should be performed with the bladder full, before and after voiding. Pre-void

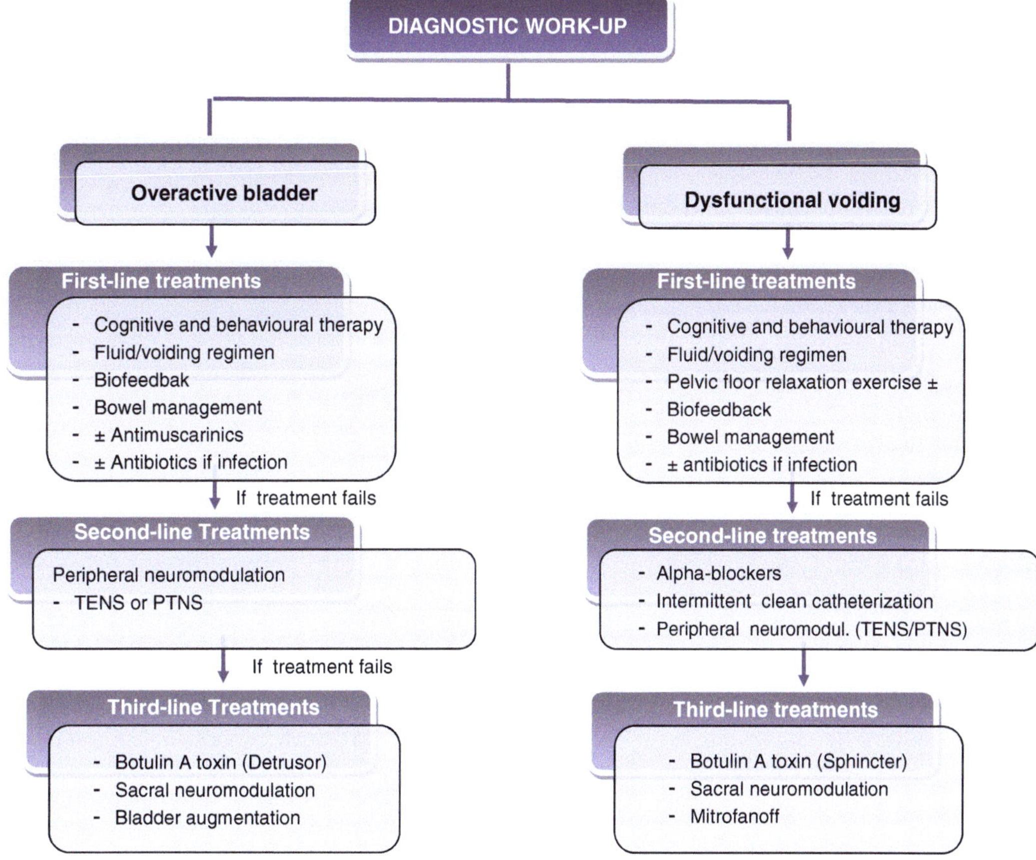

Fig. 17.2 Treatment of children with lower urinary tract dysfunction

examination contributes to the overall assessment of bladder capacity, bladder wall, lower ureteral dilatation, and bladder neck appearance. Since bladder wall thickness depends on the degree of bladder filling and from age of children, it is of great variability in pediatric age and normal value are not disposable. However, correlations have been demonstrated in children with LUTD between bladder wall thickness, urodynamic pattern, and treatment outcome, with good specificity [17, 25]. Therefore, a thickened bladder wall may alert clinician on the presence of a longstanding LUTD, leading to detrusor hypertrophy. Ultrasound evaluation of the bladder immediately after voiding can demonstrate residual urine. A post-voiding residual ≥10 % of EBC or ≥20 ml is considered significant [1, 2]. Portable ultrasound instruments such as BladderScan can be used also in children to easily evaluate post-voiding residual urine [18]. Even if rectal ultrasound and advanced dynamic ultrasound are not part of the standard assessment, they can give information on the presence and severity of constipation and ability of children to contract and relax the pelvic floor, respectively [19, 20]. Particularly, a ≥30 mm ultrasound transverse diameter of the rectum in the absence of urge to pass stool is a strong signal for constipation [20], with a good sensitivity and specificity compared to proctoscopy and colonic transit [21].

17.3.7 Invasive Examinations

Following noninvasive procedures, in selected cases, urodynamics, or videourodynamics, is indicated. Every physician, prior to proceeding with invasive examinations in a child with non-neurogenic lower urinary tract symptoms, has to answer to the question “whether these diagnostic procedures are necessary." In general urodynamic studies will only be done if the outcome will alter the management. The diagnostic information needed is that which is necessary to find the correct treatment.

At present there are no studies indicating that a voiding cystourethrogram (VCUG) is useful in children with incontinence, but without urinary tract infections. Indicators include straining or manual expression during voiding, a weak urinary stream, previous febrile urinary tract infection, continuous dribbling incontinence or pronounced apparent stress incontinence, or previously identified dilating vesicoureteral reflux.

The finding of genitourinary abnormalities or signs of occult spinal dysraphism at physical examination also indicates the need for further diagnostics, as urodynamics and/or VCUG.

Invasive urodynamic study may be necessary to clarify diagnosis in those children with uroflowmetric patterns of obstruction (plateau-shaped curve) or detrusor–sphincter–pelvic floor dyscoordination (intermittent curve).

In conclusion, invasive studies in the majority of cases do not provide significant additional information to justify this type of investigation as a routine procedure in children with non-neurogenic LUT dysfunction.

17.4 Treatment

The treatment of LUTD involves a multimodal approach (Fig. 17.1), involving strategies such as urotherapy and drugs [1]. Underlying and potentially complicating conditions such as constipation and urinary tract infection should be managed prior to intervention.

17.4.1 Urotherapy

Initial intervention in LUTD is non-pharmacologic, nonsurgical, and termed as *urotherapy* [1]. It is synonymous of lower urinary tract rehabilitation. The aim of urotherapy is to normalize the micturition pattern and to prevent further functional disturbances. This is achieved through a combination of patient education and physical therapy. In particular, urotherapy can be divided into *standard urotherapy* and *specific interventions* [2].

17.4.1.1 Standard urotherapy

Standard urotherapy includes:

- *Information* about normal lower urinary tract function and malfunction
- *Instruction* on regular voiding habits, voiding posture, and avoiding holding maneuvers
- *Lifestyle advice* regarding fluid intake and prevention of constipation
- *Documentation* of LUTS and voiding habits using frequency–volume chart or bladder diary; *support and encouragement*

17.4.1.2 Specific interventions

Specific interventions include:

- *Pelvic floor training* [22]: There are no standardized protocols for pelvic floor training in children. Several centers adopt an escalating approach in which the initial step is standard urotherapy, followed by teaching position, action, and interaction of the abdominal and pelvic floor muscle. Exercises of pelvic floor contraction and relaxation teach children to exert and feel pelvic muscle relaxation during voiding. This pelvic floor awareness and control may be enhanced by uroflow pattern and biofeedback.
- *Biofeedback* (*BFB*): BFB is a technique in which physiological activity is monitored, amplified, and conveyed to the patient as visual or acoustic signal, providing the patient with information about unconscious physiological processes. It can help children to identify how to relax their pelvic floor muscles (DV and OAB) or recognize involuntary detrusor contraction (OAB). In children with OAB, BFB may be performed by cystometrogram during which children learn to recognize and inhibit involuntary detrusor contractions by watching the pressure curve during cystometry. Since cystometric BFB is invasive and time consuming, it has limited application as a routine treatment [1]. In both children with DV and OAB, two main types of BFB

can be performed: programs that teach muscle isolation using EMG surface electrode feedback and programs that improve urine flow by having patients view the flowmetry curve when they void. Interactive computer games are commonly used to make BFB training more attractive to children [22].

- *Clean intermittent catheterization (CIC)*: If children with underactive bladder do not achieve complete bladder emptying with timed or double voiding, clean intermittent catheterization may be instituted. Frequency of CIC depends on the severity of the problem and may vary between four times a days and once a day, preferably before going to bed.
- *Neuromodulation*: Various techniques of electrostimulation have been used in adult and pediatric urology to treat refractory LUTD such as anogenital and intravesical electrical stimulation and sacral neuromodulation [23]. However, invasiveness of all of these techniques hinders their applicability in children. Other modalities have been considered to bridge the gap between noninvasive and urorehabilitative procedures and invasive treatment in pediatric patients: *transcutaneous electrical nerve stimulation* (TENS), via surface electrodes stimulating the sacral root S3, and *percutaneous posterior tibial nerve stimulation* (PTNS), via a 34 gauge needle inserted two fingers cephalad to the medial malleolus. Both TENS and PTNS have proved useful adjunctive therapies in children with OAB and DV [24]. In 2008, Roth et al. published the first report on *sacral neuromodulation* in 20 children with DES LUTS and constipation improved in 88 % of cases and complications were seen in 20 % of patients [24].

17.4.2 Drugs

17.4.2.1 Antimuscarinics

Treatment of pediatric OAB has been based on anticholinergics for many years. However, the majority of children with OAB can be successfully treated combining cognitive and behavioral therapy (explanation of bladder function, teaching children to recognize and suppress sensation of urgency) with timed voiding regimen, biofeedback, and bowel management program for constipation (Fig. 17.1). Nowadays, antimuscarinics should be considered only in children refractory to these therapies [25, 26].

- *Oxybutynin*: Traditionally the drug of choice is oxybutynin. However, side effects are present four times more frequently than in adults and cause discontinuation of therapy in more than 10 % of children [27, 28]. Moreover, constipation may be worsened during oxybutynin administration. More recently, a long-acting formulation, oxybutynin XL, with a more favorable tolerability profile, has been approved by the FDA for use in children [1].
- *Tolterodine tartrate* has been tested in pediatric trials, showing a side effect profile superior to that of oxybutynin [25]. However, tolterodine has not been approved for use in children.
- *New bladder-selective anticholinergics* [1] such as *darifenacin*, *solifenacin*, *terodiline*, *propiverine*, and *trospium* are expected to possess more favorable safety and tolerability profiles and might have a greater role in the future management of pediatric OAB [29, 30].

17.4.2.2 Alpha-Adrenergic Blockade

Treatment of overactive pelvic floor with alpha-adrenergic blockade seems promising, but from the present studies it is difficult to draw firm conclusions [1]. Moreover, use of alpha-blockers in children with LUTD is currently off-label and not approved by global regulatory boards [22].

17.4.2.3 Botulinum-A Toxin

Botulinum-A toxin inhibits the acetylcholine release at the presynaptic neuromuscular junction and results in flaccid muscular paralysis. Clinically, it has been used safely to treat focal dystonia, muscle spasm, and spasticity. Even if botulinum-A toxin is not registered for injection in the detrusor or in the sphincter in children, it has been applied to treat refractory LUTD [1]. Results of endoscopic injection of botulinum-A toxin in children with OAB and DV are encouraging [1, 22].

References

1. Abrams P, Cardozo L, Khoury S, Wein A (2013): Incontinence. 5th Edition ICUD-EAU eds. Layout: SMART-DOT marketing & web consultants, www.smart-dot.com
2. Neveus T, von Gontard A, Hoebeke P, Hjalmas K, Bauer S, Bower W, Jorgensen TM, Rittig S, Vanda Walle J, Yeung CK, Djurhuus JC (2006) The Standardization of terminology of lower urinary tract function in children and adolescents: report from the standardization committee of the International Children's Continence Society. J Urol 176:314–324
3. Franco I (2007) Overactive bladder in children. Part 1: pathophysiology. J Urol 178:761–768
4. Koff SA, Lapides J, Piazza DH (1979) Association of urinary tract infection and reflux with uninhibited bladder contractions and voluntary sphincteric obstruction. J Urol 122:373–376
5. Koff SA, Murtagh D (1983) The uninhibited bladder in children: effect of treatment on recurrence of urinary tract infection and on vesico-ureteral reflux resolution. J Urol 130:1138–1141
6. Abidari JM, Shortliffe LM (2002) Urinary incontinence in girls. Urol Clin N Am 29:661–675
7. Ellsworth PI, Merguerian PA, Copening ME (1995) Sexual abuse: another causative factor in dysfunctional voiding. J Urol 153:773–776
8. Cooper CS et al (2003) Do public school teach voiding dysfunction? Results of an elementary school teacher survey. J Urol 170:956–958
9. Hoebeke P et al (1999) Anomalies of the external urethral meatus in girls with non-neurogenic bladder-sphincter dysfunction. BJU Int 83:294–298
10. Chase JW et al (2004) Functional constipation in children. J Urol 171:2641–2643
11. Hoebeke P, Bower W, Combs A, De Jong T, Yang S (2010) Diagnostic evaluation of children with daytime incontinence. J Urol 183:699–703
12. De Gennaro M, Niero M, Capitanucci ML et al (2010) Validity of the International Consultation on Incontinence questionnaire-pediatric lower urinary tract symptoms: a screening questionnaire for children. J Urol 194:1662–1667
13. Heaton KW, Radvan J, Cripps H et al (1992) Defecation frequency and timing and stool form in the general population: a prospective study. Gut 33:818–824
14. Mori R, Yonemoto N, Fitzgerald A et al (2010) Diagnostic performance of urine dipstick testing in children with suspected UTI: a systematic review of relationship with age and comparison with microscopy. Acta Paediatr 99(4):581–584
15. Griffiths DJ, Scholtmeijer RJ (1984) Place of the free flow curve in the urodynamic investigation of children. Br J Urol 56:474–477
16. Yang SS, Wang CC, Chen YT (2003) Home uroflowmetry for the evaluation of boys with urinary incontinence. J Urol 169:1505–1507
17. Sreedar B, Yeung CK, Leung VYF, Chu CW (2008) Ultrasound bladder measurements in children with severe primary nocturnal enuresis: pretreatment and posttreatment evaluation and its correlation with treatment outcome. J Urol 179:1568–1572
18. De Gennaro M, Capitanucci ML, Di Ciommo V et al (2006) Reliability of bladder volume measurements with bladderscan in paediatric age. Scand J Urol Nephrol 40(5):370–375
19. Klijn AJ, Asselman M, Vijverberg MS et al (2004) The diameter of the rectum on ultrasonography as a diagnostic tool for constipation in children with dysfunctional voiding. J Urol 172:1986–1988
20. de Jong TPVM, Klijn AJ, Vijverberg MA et al (2006) Ultrasound imaging of sacral reflexes. Urology 68:652–654
21. Bijos A, Czerwionka-Szaflarska M, Mazur A, Romanczuk W (2007) The usefulness of ultrasound examination of the bowel as method of assessment of functional chronic constipation in children. Pediatr Radiol 37(12):1247–1252
22. Chase J, Austin P, Hoebeke P, Mckenna P (2010) The management of dysfunctional voiding in children: a report from the standardization committee of the International Children's Continence Society. J Urol 183:1296–1302
23. De Gennaro M, Capitanucci ML, Mosiello G, Zaccara A (2011) Current state of nerve stimulation technique for lower urinary tract dysfunction in children. J Urol 185(5):1571–1577
24. Roth TJ et al (2008) Sacral Neuromodulation for the dysfunctional elimination syndrome: a single center experience with 20 children. J Urol 180:306–311
25. Nijman RJ (2004) Role of antimuscarinics in the treatment of nonneurogenic daytime urinary incontinence in children. Urology 65(Suppl 3A):45–50
26. Franco I (2007) Overactive bladder in children. Part 2: management. J Urol 178:769–774
27. Jonville AP, Duetertre JP, Barbellion M et al (1993) Adverse effect of oxybutynin chloride in pediatrics. Arch Fr Pediatr 50:27–29
28. Nijman RJ (2000) Classification and treatment of functional incontinence in children. BJU Int 85((suppl3):37–42
29. Hoebeke P, De Pooter J, De Caestecker K et al (2009) Solifenacin for therapy resistant overactive bladder. J Urol 182:2040–2044
30. Alloussi S, Murtz G, Braun R et al (2009) Efficacy, tolerability and safety of propiverine hydrochloride in comparison to oxybutynin in children with urge incontinence due to overactive bladder: results of a multicentre observational cohort study. BJU Int 106:550–556

Part IV

Urethra

18 Posterior Urethral Valves

Alaa El Ghoneimi and Matthieu Peycelon

18.1 Definition/Introduction

Posterior urethral valves (PUVs) represent the most severe obstructive uropathy in children detected by prenatal ultrasonography (US) [1] with an incidence ranging from 1 per 3,000 to 8,000 male births [2]. Despite advances in medical and surgical management of PUVs in the last few decades, 13–64 % of children still have chronic renal failure (CRF) or end-stage renal disease (ESRD) at long-term follow-up [3]. Prenatal diagnosis of PUVs has not yet improved this rate [4].

Many factors have been associated with the final outcome of such children, and the search to improve their long-term renal function has steadily improved the quality of management and treatment [5]. Age at diagnosis, nadir serum creatinine during the first year of life, vesicoureteral reflux (VUR), bladder dysfunction, and urinary tract infection have been identified as predictive of future renal function [6, 7].

Several options of surgical management of infants with PUVs are available, and the mainstay of treatment is primary valve ablation [8–10]. Many studies documented that urinary diversion does not have an advantage over valve ablation in terms of renal and bladder functions [9–11].

Since the advent of fiber optic lighting and Hopkins rod lens system in pediatric endoscopes, endoscopic ablation of PUVs using various modalities under direct vision has become widely accepted and practiced all over the world [8, 10–19]. The incidence of complications after valve ablation has been reported to be between 5 and 25 % [4, 20, 21].

18.2 Prenatal Diagnosis

18.2.1 Diagnosis and Prognosis Parameters

The prenatal parameters taken in account during the last two decades are mainly: gestational age at diagnosis, renal parenchyma on US, amniotic fluid volume, and urine and fetal blood biochemical markers.

Long-term renal function remains the most important determinant of quality of life outcome in boys with PUVs [22]. In recent decades, there has been continuous improvement in the survival of these patients, while the impact of prenatal diagnosis in reducing the morbidity is still controversial. According to many published series, the postnatal outcome of these patients is variable [23–25].

Prenatal detection was initially thought to improve the outcome, but, in fact, earlier studies

A. El Ghoneimi, MD, PhD, FEBPS, FEAPU (✉)
M. Peycelon
Department of Pediatric Urology,
University Children Hospital Robert Debré, APHP,
University of Paris Diderot,
48 Boulvard Serurier, 75019 Paris Cedex 19, France
e-mail: alaa.elghoneimi@rdb.aphp.fr;
matthieu.peycelon@yahoo.fr

M. Lima, G. Manzoni (eds.), *Pediatric Urology: Contemporary Strategies from Fetal Life to Adolescence*,
DOI 10.1007/978-88-470-5693-0_18, © Springer-Verlag Italia 2015

failed to demonstrate that long-term outcome of boys with prenatally detected PUVS is better than that of symptomatic boys with postnatally detected PUVs [23, 24]. Moreover, in one study the outcome of prenatally detected cases was worse than that of postnatally detected cases [25]. One possible explanation is that in the more obstructive and, thus, more severe cases, hydronephrosis is already more distinct before birth, leading to the discovery of PUVs on prenatal US. Furthermore, of the postnatally diagnosed cases, the most obstructive probably are detected early, whereas cases detected later are less obstructed and, therefore, more rarely progress to permanent CRF and ESRD.

We have reported the experience of our center in 2008 with a total of 79 cases of PUVs prenatally detected between 1987 and 2004 [7]. Of these cases 65 were managed postnatally, while pregnancy was terminated in 14. Primary valve ablation was done in all cases except two. Median follow-up was 6.8 years [range 1–14.3]. At the end of follow-up, there were 11 cases of renal failure [17 %] with 5 detected before 24 weeks of gestation, 6 cases of oligohydramnios, and 9 cases of abnormal parenchyma. Gestational age at diagnosis and oligohydramnios were statistically significant predictors of final renal outcome ($p=0.003$ and $p=0.02$, respectively). When fetal urinalysis detected good prognosis (12 cases), renal failure was developed in none, compared to two of the three cases with a bad prognosis. Continence was achieved in 42 of 55 toilet-trained children (76 %), 3 had nocturnal enuresis, and 10 (18 %) were incontinent.

Data from our team were also published in 1999, in which any significant improvement in the final outcome of these patients or a predictive value of our studied prenatal parameters was found [23]. Our more recent results have revealed significant value of some of prenatal parameters that were not significant in our first study. The discrepancy between the findings in this series and our initial report in 1999 has strengthened the need for such reevaluation with larger numbers of patients and longer follow-up.

Surgical management in our series consisted of primary valve ablation and surveillance. Urinary diversion was indicated in cases of anuria before or after valve ablation. This approach seemed reasonable when one considers that the proportion of boys with renal failure at follow-up was similar to the results achieved in those with PUVs detected postnatally [3, 26] and lower than that reported in another series of patients with prenatally diagnosed PUVs [24]. Prenatal diagnosis allowed us to treat most of the patients within the first 48 h after birth, and, thus, bladder recycling was not interrupted.

It is difficult to compare the results of different published series because of wide variation in regard to availability of obstetrical service to account for in utero mortality, routine practice of early prenatal US in all pregnant women, postnatal indicators of renal function, duration of follow-up, type of surgical procedure, and patient age at treatment. In our series the inherent bias of in utero mortality was markedly reduced by review of all department files on PUVs during the study period, including data on prenatal diagnosis, pediatric nephrology, pediatric urology, and fetopathology. Actually, if we consider pregnancy termination as a poor outcome and we add the 14 terminations to the 11 cases of renal failure, the poor outcome changes from 17 to 32 % for the global outcome of our series.

Hutton et al. reported a series of 31 boys with prenatally detected PUVs [27]. Of the 17 cases diagnosed at or before 24 weeks of gestation, nine (53 %) had a poor outcome at follow-up, while only 1 of 14 cases (7 %) diagnosed after 24 weeks had a poor outcome ($p=0.05$). Of our 11 cases diagnosed before 24 weeks of gestation, 5 (45 %) had a poor outcome, compared to 6 of 54 cases (11 %) diagnosed after 24 weeks. Our results appear statistically significant, similar to those of Hutton et al. and allow us to be equally optimistic regarding prediction of a good outcome when the diagnosis is made after 24 weeks of gestation. Recently the same bad prognosis of early prenatal diagnosis was confirmed by our study of 709 cases of prenatally detected megacystis (PUVs included) [28].

Different studies have shown that oligohydramnios predicts poor outcome in more than 80 % of cases [3, 29, 30]. Our results, in which 6 of our 11 patients (55 %) with oligohydramnios had a poor outcome, are in accordance with these series.

Initial US may be useful for identifying patients at higher risk for deterioration of renal function. Hulbert et al. in 1992 stated that the appearance of the initial renal US can be considered as a possible predictor of renal function at follow-up [31]. In a report by Muller et al. of 40 boys with prenatally detected obstructive uropathy, 8 of 10 patients (80 %) with an abnormal appearance of the renal parenchyma on US had a poor prognosis, compared to 7 of 30 (23 %) with normal parenchyma [29]. Duel et al. in 1998 found that normal renal echogenicity and corticomedullary differentiation (CMD) are useful for predicting a good outcome, while loss of CMD and increased echogenicity are relatively insensitive and poorly specific [22]. The finding of at least one kidney with good CMD on US has been associated with a good prognosis.

In our long-term study, we have observed that initial renal US was abnormal in all patients in whom renal failure developed but was also abnormal in 77 % of those with normal renal function [7]. Thus, abnormal parenchyma on US was not specific. Furthermore, normal parenchyma could not predict a good outcome. This finding may be biased by the fact that it is a retrospective study and the absence of abnormal parenchyma on US could not strictly exclude the presence of these anomalies, since they may be missed during the US examination.

Long-term results of prenatally detected PUVs confirm that early valve ablation can be considered as the primary management in the majority of cases, without the need for preoperative drainage or diversion [7]. Gestational age at diagnosis and volume of amniotic fluid are significant predictors of long-term renal function. Nevertheless, other parameters need to be also considered [7, 23].

Our current prenatal management of PUVs includes: detailed serial US study of renal parenchyma, anteroposterior diameter of the renal pelvis and calices, amniotic fluid volume, bladder size and wall thickness, and ureteral dilatation. A detailed morphological examination of all other extra-urinary system is done with the help of fetal MRI if needed. The case is discussed in the multidisciplinary weekly meeting, and then decision is taken whether there is a need for further invasive investigations as urine or blood biochemical markers analysis (beta-2 microglobulin, calcium, sodium, phosphorus). Fetal blood analysis is feasible in cases after 22 weeks of gestation. The prognosis is based on the combined results of all the investigations and adapted to the age of gestation.

18.2.2 Prenatal Treatment and Fetal Surgery

PubMed, Medline, and Embase database included 22 articles about fetal surgery for PUVs. The last review article published in 2011 by Casella et al. describes fetal surgery as case reports, small series with poor outcomes [32]. Research on vesico-amniotic shunt on fetal lamb models showed that the possibility of relieving the obstruction could improve the amniotic fluid, prevent pulmonary hypoplasia and bladder and renal damage, and recover nephrogenesis with an affordable loss of nephrons (5 % versus 20 % with persistent obstruction) [33–36]. Historically the first prenatal procedure consisted of fetal ureterostomies and cutaneous vesicotomies [37]. Because of high risk of open fetal surgery on maternal morbidity and future reproductive function, minimally invasive procedures as in utero vesico-amniotic shunt by a percutaneous approach under US guidance have been developed [38–42].

Vesicocentesis (puncturing the bladder and aspirating the urine) has to be performed several times and has disappeared nowadays [43]. A trocar was introduced into the fetal bladder in which a double-j catheter was placed to drain the fetal urine into the amniotic cavity. Fetal mortality and complication rates including preterm labor, preterm rupture of the membranes, and infections were 4.6 and 44 %, respectively, in the first 5-year review [44] and were considered too high to let vesico-amniotic shunt as a daily procedure. In 1997, Coplen et al. reported a survival rate of

47 % for 169 vesico-amniotic shunts, but 40 % of newborn infants presented an ESRD [45]. Mc Lorie et al. reduced obstetric complication rate by placing the catheter between 20 and 28 weeks of gestation [46]. Several meta-analysis showed a higher survival rate but a stable postnatal ESRD rate [47, 48].

Another procedure is fetal cystoscopy through an abdominal trocar. It has been first described in 1995 [49]. A valve ablation was performed in a few cases [50] without any difference on survival rate between vesico-amniotic shunt and cystoscopy [51]. Survival rates for shunting and cystoscopy are 40 and 75 %, respectively, whereas postnatal renal function rates are 50 and 65 %, respectively [34].

Even if fetal surgery for PUVs has been developed since 25 years, series are small without any randomized controlled trials, and outcomes need to be analyzed carefully. Morris et al. reported 20 studies in the last two decades with 261 interventions on 369 fetuses including vesico-amniotic shunt and fetal cystoscopy [48]. Prenatal surgery seems to be more effective than no intervention on survival rate but postnatal renal function is worst in the fetal surgery group. To summarize, results after vesico-amniotic shunting are poor because of poor patient selection, technical complications, US misdiagnosis (between 58 and 67 %) [43, 52, 53], and lack of good renal function predictors. Technical complications are quite high between 40 and 48 % [38, 45, 54], and fetal mortality rate is close to 50 %.

Long-term outcomes have not been improved by fetal surgery. Prenatal intervention may not change the prognosis of renal function or may not be a predictor for possible urinary diversion [55]. Despite all of these patients having favorable urinary electrolytes, this did not seem to have any implication postnatally. When counseling families about fetal intervention, efforts should be focused on that intervention may assist in delivering the fetus to term and that the sequelae of PUVs may not be preventable. Fetal surgery for obstructive uropathy should be performed only for the carefully selected patient who has severe oligohydramnios and "normal"-appearing kidneys [55]. There is clinical evidence that relief of obstruction may improve postnatal pulmonary function, but there is no evidence that it improves renal function [34].

In consequence pediatric urologists expected soon to read outcomes of PLUTO (percutaneous shunting in lower urinary tract obstruction) trial which began in 2008. This study design is to compare 150 fetuses with LUTO undergoing vesico-amniotic shunting or observation. It could lead finally to standardize fetal surgery with appropriate indications [56]. But PLUTO randomized controlled trial stopped prematurely because of poor recruitment. Conclusions are hard to be defined: the relative effectiveness of vesico-amniotic shunting is uncertain with poor prognosis at 1 year. Normal liquid volume and age at diagnosis seem to be good predictor factors. For the time being, patients who are selected for fetal surgery are fetuses with a normal karyotype and with severe LUTO (dilated bladder with key-hole sign and bilateral hydronephrosis), oligohydramnios, or any hydramnios and favorable fetal urinalysis [29, 34, 57].

18.3 Postnatal Management

A multidisciplinary approach is necessary to improve short- and long-term outcomes for patients born with PUVs. Metabolic disorders have to be managed by pediatric nephrologists to avoid any added damage to the renal function. Micturating cystourethrogram (MCUG) remains today the most reliable tool to confirm the diagnosis of PUVs and to study the morphology of the bladder and the bladder neck (Fig. 18.1). MCUG can be done either retrograde through urethral catheter or by suprapubic puncture (Fig. 18.2). Our preference goes to suprapubic puncture. We believe that the urethra should be kept intact without any trauma till valve ablation. In fact there is no evidence to advocate for one or another method. As most of the patients with PUVs are managed in our center after prenatal referral, it is feasible for us to manage the newborn in the first 24 h without the need for urinary drainage. Suprapubic insertion of intravenous catheter is done under US guidance. If the diagnosis is con-

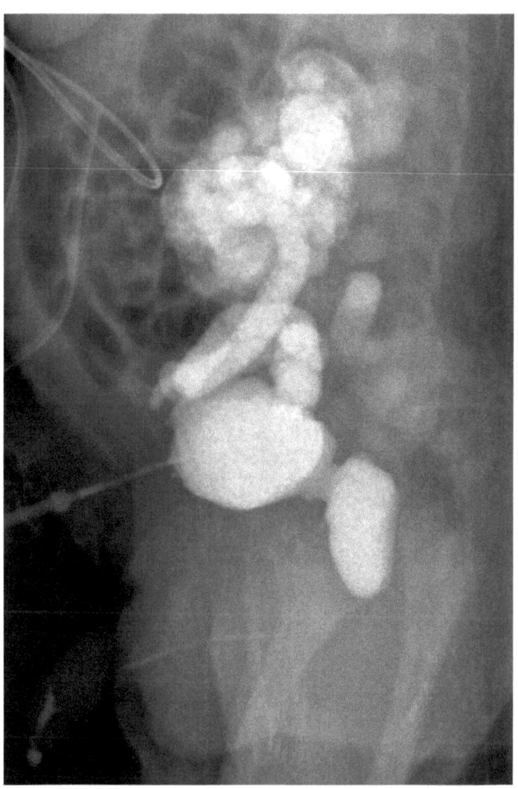

Fig. 18.1 Micturating cystourethrogram: posterior urethral valves with posterior urethral dilatation, bladder neck hypertrophy, and bilateral high-grade vesicoureteral reflux

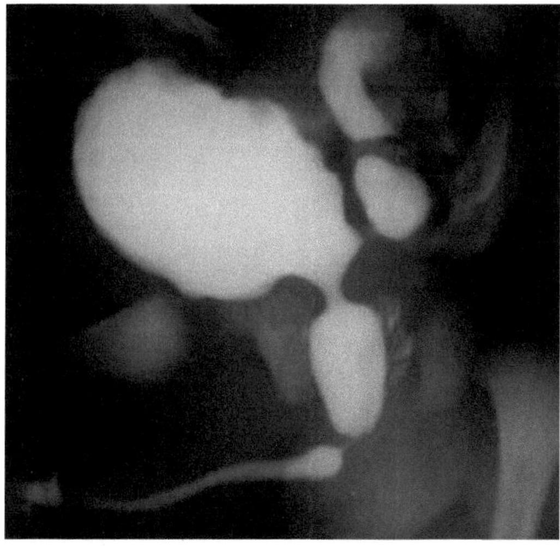

Fig. 18.2 Micturating cystourethrogram by suprapubic puncture. Note the reflux in the ejaculatory ducts associated with typical aspect of posterior urethral valves, urethra, and bladder neck

firmed, the newborn is managed in few hours at the operating room for valve ablation.

Surgical treatment aims at relieving obstruction. It could be done by urinary diversion or valve ablation (Fig. 18.3) under general anesthesia. Low diversion includes vesicostomy or bladder catheterization [58–60]. Complications of catheter drainage are more frequent with infection, bladder contraction, and ureterovesical obstruction. Vesicostomy reproduces bladder filling and contraction and eases bladder reconstruction in comparison to supravesical diversion. In our current practice, it is used for children less than 2 kg. High drainage as pyelostomy or ureterostomy did not improve renal function outcomes and decreased bladder cycling function [61, 62]. In some instance, a refluxing unilateral lateral ureterostomy can be an option to relieve the obstruction in severely sick children.

Different options of ablation have been described. Blind methods have disappeared and must be kept as historic, because of poor results and severe complications [63, 64]. The development of pediatric endoscopes since 1970 and Hopkins and Storz has been the best technical progress. Valve ablation could be done by a Bugbee, a cold knife (Fig. 18.4), or a laser [13]. These techniques need experienced pediatric urologists to minimize urethral trauma, operative time, and irrigation. Cold knife is preferred than resectoscope with diathermy loop to reduce postoperative retention and strictures. No routine preoperative and postoperative drainage is needed in our experience.

Several studies have investigated the best timing and approach in treatment of patients with PUVs [4, 9, 11]. Smith et al. stated that PUVs should be treated with primary valve ablation, and vesicostomy should be reserved for patients in whom valve ablation is not technically possible [10]. Regardless of whether a vesicostomy or a high urinary diversion is performed, eventually the valves have to be resected or incised.

Currently, with the advance in endoscopes and fiber optics, better instruments have allowed surgeons to treat valves endoscopically using different modalities under direct vision with minimal incidence of complications [4].

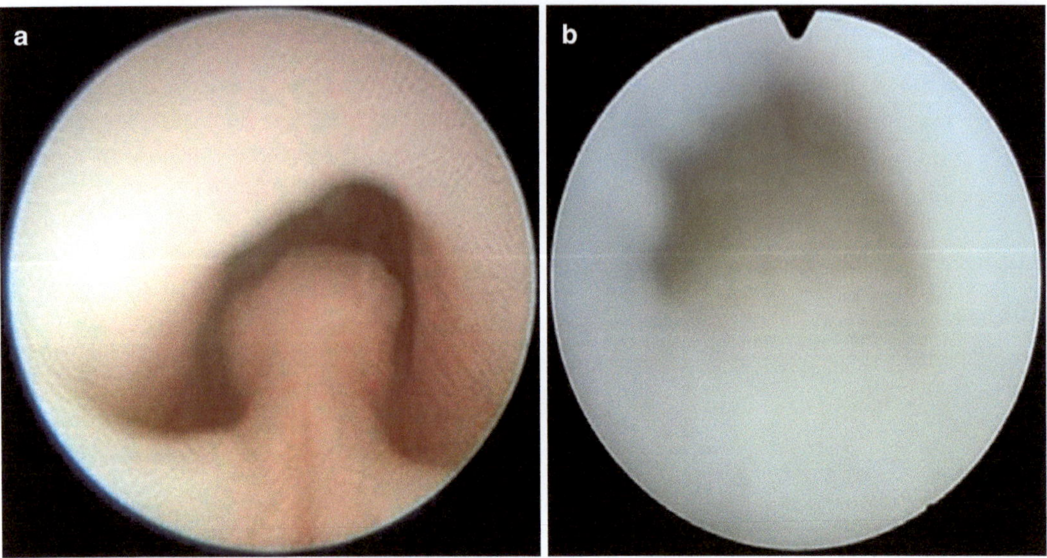

Fig. 18.3 (**a**) Endoscopy view of posterior urethral valves. (**b**) Endoscopic view of neonatal aspect of PUV, before any endoscopic or catheter introduction, notice the verumontanum visible in the background

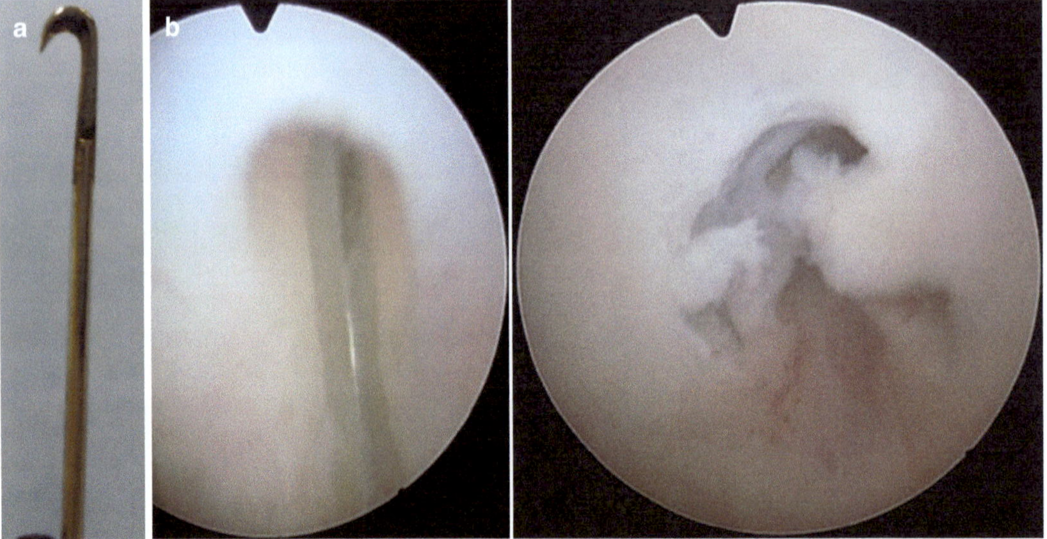

Fig. 18.4 (**a**) Cold knife hook used to perform valves ablation under cystoscopy. (**b**) The hook localizes the first point of section at 12 o'clock, followed by 5 and 7 o'clock

Complications after valve ablation have been reported to be between 5 and 25 % [18, 65]. Sarhan et al. published an incidence of complications of 7.5 % which is nearly similar to that reported by Nijman et al. in 1991 who reported an incidence of only 5 % complication rate in a group of 85 boys undergoing electroincision of urethral valves [19, 20].

Stricture formation after valve ablation occurs infrequently ranging from 0 to 25 % [4, 18, 19, 21, 65, 66]. Urethral strictures were reported after fulguration in 7 of 28 patients (25 %) by Myers et al. in 1981 [18], 3 of 36 patients (8 %) by Crooks et al. in 1981 [21], 4 of 30 patients (13 %) by Bruce et al. in 1987 [66], and 3 of 82 (3.6 %) by Lal et al. in 1999 [65]. On the other hand, Nijman et al. in his series of 85 patients including newborn and infants reported no incidence of urethral stricture [19].

Prevention of urethral stricture after valve ablation depends on many factors. These are gentleness in surgical technique, avoidance of oversized instrumentation in a small caliber urethra especially since patients with PUVs are usually small for age, minimizing fulguration time, avoiding excessive and deep fulguration, fulguration under direct vision, and shortening the duration of preoperative catheterization and use of nonreactive small-sized catheters [20, 65].

Sarhan et al. retrospectively reviewed database of 291 patients with PUVs treated by primary valve ablation from two separate centers between 1987 and 2006 [20]. Primary valve ablation was performed in all patients regardless of serum creatinine level or upper tract configuration. A hot loop resectoscope was used in 122 patients, cold knife urethrotome in 108, a hook diathermy electrode in 18, and a diathermy coagulation Bugbee in 20, while stripping using Fogarty catheter was performed in 23. The follow-up duration ranged from 1.5 to 20 years (median = 6.5). Early postoperative complications occurred in 22 patients (7.5 %). The most common complication was urine retention in 16 patients (5.5 %). Urinary extravasations occurred in three cases, significant hematuria from urethral bleeding occurred in two, and obstructive anuria developed in one patient. The majority of cases were treated conservatively. Urethral strictures developed in six patients (2 %) mainly after endoscopic loop resection (four of six). All were treated by visual internal urethrotomy and urethral dilatation with successful results without the need of open urethroplasty.

Risk factors for the development of postoperative complications were studied by a univariate analysis by Sarhan et al. in 2010 [20]. The incidence of complications was significantly related to preoperative catheter drainage. Postoperative complications developed in 16 out of 130 patients (12.3 %) in whom preoperative draining catheter was fixed, while it occurred in only 6 out of the 161 patients (3.7 %) with no preoperative drainage ($p < 0.05$). This may be due to the fact that patients who needed preoperative drainage were actually of poor general condition with uremia that make them at risk of development of postoperative complications. None of the 41 patients who did not have postoperative catheter developed any complications, while all the 22 patients who developed complications had postoperative drainage ($p < 0.05$). Patient age at valve ablation had no significant relation with the occurrence of postoperative complications. Also, technique of valve ablation had no statistically significant impact on complications although the incidence was more with resection group (12.3 %) than other groups, but the difference was not statistically significant ($p = 0.08$). Multivariate analysis showed that preoperative catheter drainage was the independent risk factor for the development of postoperative complications. On the univariate analysis, stricture formation does not have statistically significant relation with either age at ablation, technique of valve ablation, or presence or absence of pre- or postoperative drainage. Although four out of the six cases with stricture urethra developed after electroresection, the difference from other techniques was not statistically significant. The same finding was noted with preoperative catheter drainage which was associated with more incidence of stricture formation (four out of six) especially when the suprapubic catheter drainage was maintained after endoscopic incision.

18.4 Outcomes

18.4.1 Bladder Function

It has been documented that there is a window for bladder healing that is limited to the first few months of life [23]. Primary valve ablation allows bladder cycling without obstruction, thus setting up the milieu for resumption of bladder function. Urinary incontinence has been a common problem in boys after valve ablation [65, 67]. Although numerous related causes exist, post-obstructive bladder dysfunction has gained recognition as the principal factor in the etiology of incontinence after valve surgery [67]. The reported incidence of significant voiding dysfunction in boys after valve surgery varies from 13 to 38 % [65, 67]. Sarhan et al. evaluated the incidence of voiding dysfunction at 41 % in toilet-trained children [7]. Using their criteria, bladder dysfunction could be overestimated because all children who had symptoms of voiding dysfunction were included. The most severe cases requiring clean intermittent catheterization (CIC) or bladder augmentation comprised only 4.6 % of the study population.

Others advocate for routine drainage of the bladder before valve ablation [5], which may add morbidity to the treatment of these children [prolonged hospital stay, risk of nosocomial infection]. Sarhan et al. rarely had to divert the urine before or after valve ablation, and initial serum creatinine level was not a parameter to drain or to start valve ablation [7]. These results are overall comparable to others and may indicate that routine urine drainage should be reconsidered.

Early management of children born with PUVs is to reduce the rate of "valve bladder syndrome" first described by Hoover et al. in 1982 [68]. The most frequent urodynamic patterns found in these dysfunctional bladders are bladder overactivity, poor compliance, and myogenic failure. The incidence of these three types of bladder dysfunction varies markedly among authors and may be related to the patient's age at time of urodynamic study. It has become apparent that bladder function is a dynamic process and puberty has specific effects on these bladders [69]. High pressure in a noncompliant bladder alters upper urinary tract, increases hydronephrosis, reduces glomerular filtration rate, and leads to polyuria and tubulopathy. To avoid bladder dysfunction, bladder surgery and indwelling catheters should be avoided. Bladder has to be evaluated by MCUG, US, and post-voiding residual and video-urodynamics studies (Fig. 18.5a–c). For children with not toilet-trained bladder, 4-h observation will give an idea about post-void residual (PVR) and the average bladder capacity. For toilet-trained children, urodynamics and voiding diary are mandatory. Voiding diary includes amount of liquid intake, frequency of voiding, amount of voiding, and quantification of urinary leaks. Urodynamics is composed of flowmetry associated with electromyogram and PVR and video-urodynamics. Video-imaging is interesting in valves bladder specially if there is VUR. This exam will define if the reflux is either a low-pressure or a high-pressure reflux. Bladder capacity at the onset of the VUR will be also evaluated. Urodynamics is mandatory to distinguish the two categories of valves bladder: the poor compliant overactive bladder with high risk for the upper urinary tract and the compliant large capacity bladder with detrusor myogenic insufficiency (Figs. 18.5a–c). The last group is synonym of urinary incontinence and urinary tract infections, treated usually by either regular voluntary voiding and if insufficient CIC either by the urethra or through a Mitrofanoff channel.

The first-line treatment is anticholinergic medications with progressive increasing dose. This treatment is monitored by evaluation of PVR and upper tract dilatation then urodynamics studies. This can be associated with alpha-blocker treatment to decrease the outlet pressure. If these treatments are insufficient and the child had high-pressure voiding, CIC is added to the management. Night drainage can be an option to avoid overdistention of the bladder during the long hours of night. There are a few sets of data that suggest overnight bladder drainage can bring about profound improvements in the degree of upper-tract hydronephrosis, renal function, or bladder function [70].

Bladder augmentation is an option that needs to be discussed as an ultimate treatment and only if all other measures had failed. In our experience with over 200 patients with PUVs, only two children needed bladder augmentation, and these children were born with severe damage of the bladder and ESRD at birth. Ureterocystoplasty should be considered when augmentation is needed and one of the kidneys is not functioning [71]. Indications for augmentation is limited to few cases of extremely small low compliance bladder with no response to anticholinergic and CIC and with upper urinary tract deterioration.

18.4.2 Renal Transplantation

In children with ESRD secondary to PUVs, bladder evaluation before renal transplantation remains a challenging task to avoid the risk of graft deterioration secondary to bladder dysfunction. In our recent study on long-term evaluation of bladder function in patients with PUVs after renal transplantation, we found an improvement of bladder dysfunction. This is probably the result of reduction of pretransplantation polyuria. Fifteen children aged between 3 and 15 years were transplanted with PUVs between 1989 and 2006 at Robert Debré Children University Hospital. Three children were excluded from the study: one had bladder augmentation before transplantation, and two were lost of follow-up. Mean follow-up after transplantation was 13.1 years [5–20]. The evolution was favorable in these children with a graft survival of 63 % at 10 years. Patients were divided into three groups: (1) group I with no

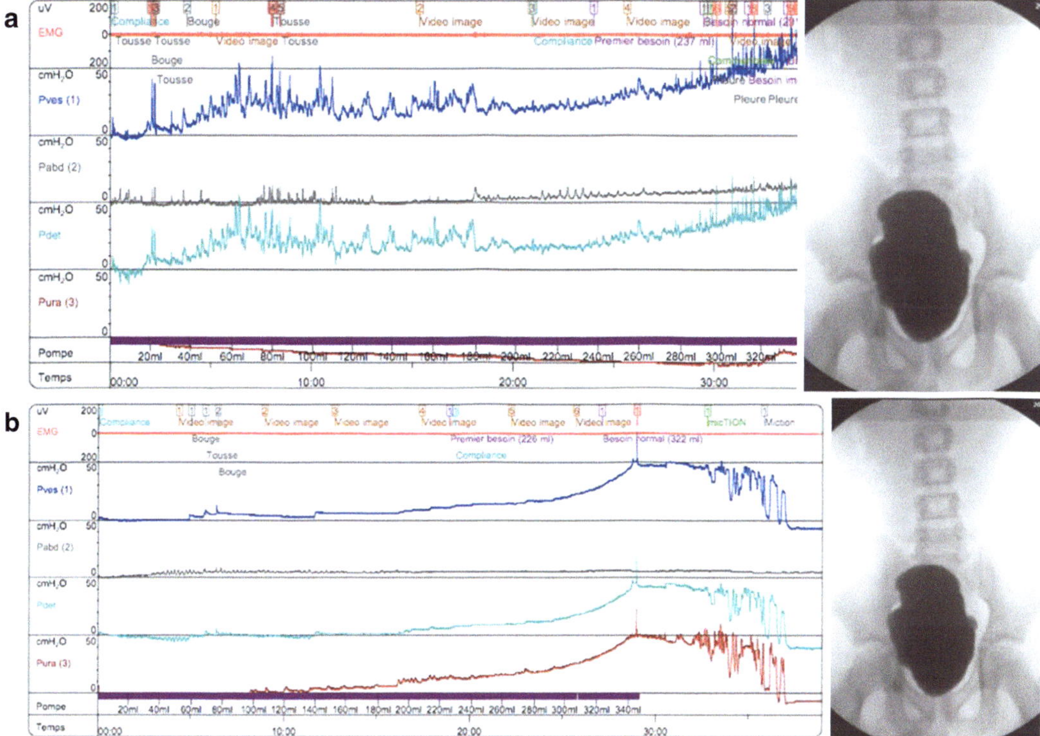

Fig. 18.5 (**a**) Ten-year-old boy treated in infancy for posterior urethral valves. Current symptoms: increasing hydronephrosis, incontinence, and recurrent febrile urinary tract infection. The video-urodynamics study showed bladder capacity at 320 mL, overactive bladder, and poor compliance. Parents and the child were advised bladder management by clean intermittent catheterization and anticholinergics. (**b**) The family did not come back, and they did not follow the advised management; 20 months later, they came for follow-up. The child had no febrile urinary tract infection and became dry between voiding. The ultrasonography showed improvement of the hydronephrosis. Video-urodynamics showed significant improvement with a normoactive low-pressure bladder (10 cmH_2O/300 mL) with a voiding detrusor pressure at 50 cmH_2O and without post-voiding residual. Management was advised by voiding diary every 3 h and to avoid over distended bladder. (**c**) Eighteen months after the last video-urodynamics, his clinical status was stable with regular voiding, dryness, and stable normal renal function at 50 μmol/L and without any anticholinergics. Urodynamics showed a bladder capacity of 400 mL, hyposensitive bladder, and efficient voiding without residual. Note that the morphology of the bladder and the bladder neck did not change over this period of puberty; meanwhile a significant improvement was achieved in bladder function

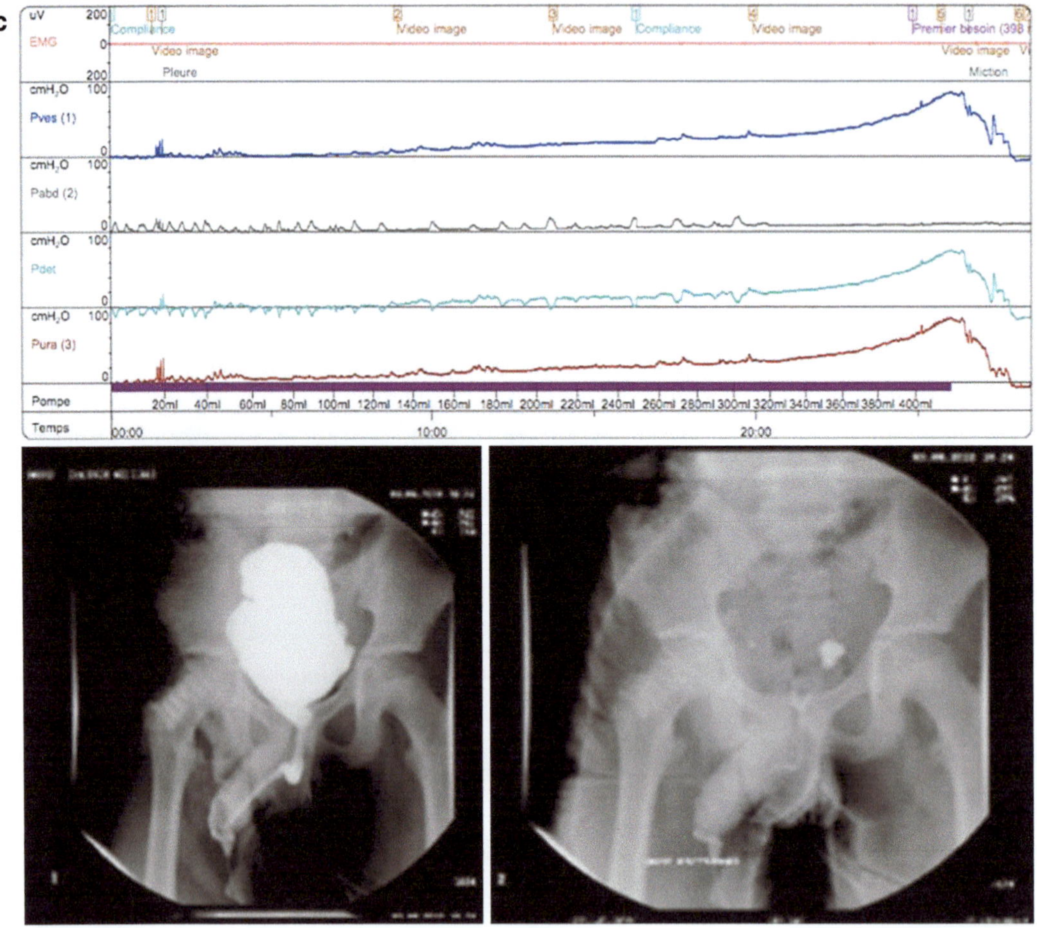

Fig. 18.5 (continued)

voiding disorders ($n=3$), (2) group II with voiding disorders who received pharmacological treatment ($n=6$, three hyperreflexic bladders, two myogenic failures, one poor compliant bladder), and (3) group III with severe bladder dysfunction requiring intermittent catheterization ($n=3$), all had small overactive poor compliant bladders. After transplantation, in group II, five of six patients had improved their voiding disorders, and bladder treatment was stopped. In group III, two of three patients had improved their bladder function, and CIC was no more needed (Fig. 18.6). In borderline cases, bladder augmentation before transplantation must be reconsidered under condition of having prudent post-transplantation follow-up [72].

18.4.3 Renal Function

Prenatal diagnosis has allowed categorizing newborns with high risk of renal failure. When negative parameters were absent and fetal urine biochemistry predicted good outcome, there were no cases of ESRD in early infancy [23]. Gestational age at diagnosis and volume of amniotic fluid are significant predictors of long-term renal function [7]. But other parameters like renal parenchyma or presence of renal cysts need to be also considered. Fetal urine includes sodium and beta-2 microglobulin measurements [7, 23, 29]. It is difficult to compare the results of different published series because of wide variation in regard to the availability of obstetrical service to

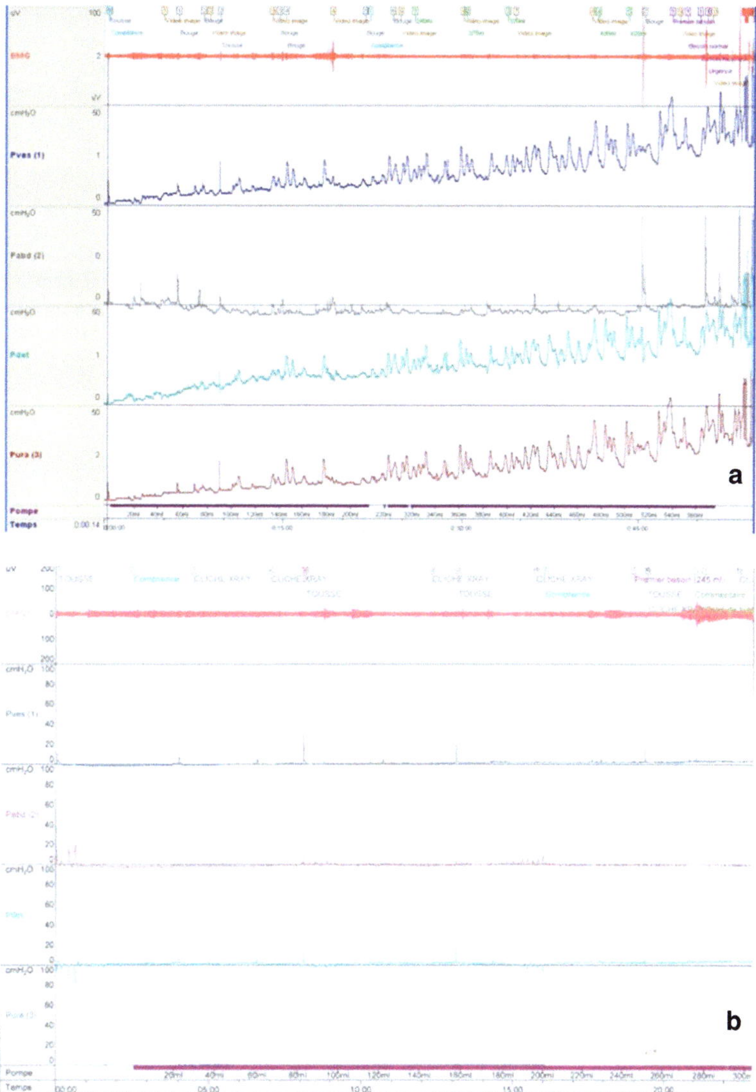

Fig. 18.6 Case of a boy included in group III. (**a**) Before transplantation, he had a small overactive poor compliant bladder. (**b**) Eight years after transplantation, he had a normocompliant bladder with normal capacity and without overactivity

account for in utero mortality, the routine practice of early prenatal US in all pregnant women, postnatal indicators of renal function, duration of follow-up, type of surgical procedure, and patient age at treatment. Mortality has dropped from 50 to 3 % thanks to medical management and the reduction of urinary sepsis and electrolyte complications. Renal failure ranged from 10 to 60 % in the literature. Serum creatinine above 80 μmol/L 7 days after valves ablation and at 1 year is predictive of ESRD [73, 74]. Renal transplantation is possible for boys with PUVs and ESRD. Good allograft survival is good if valve bladder is well managed before and after transplantation in using adequately anticholinergic and CIC thanks to video-urodynamics data.

18.4.4 Fertility

Different factors may contribute to the impairment of fertility in adolescents with treated PUVs. Libido and potency can be already affected by the renal failure in PUVs patients. Sexual function and fertility remain a matter of speculation and require further investigation owing to the scarcity of studies on these issues and the discrepancies in some of the results of semen analysis observed in the published series with small number of patients [69]. However, in the recent review by Lopez-Pereira et al., it would seem that these patients have normal sexual function (some with slow ejaculation). They have normal semen counts, but viscosity, pH, and liquefaction time can be increased, and there may also be abnormal sperm agglutination. The ability to father children appears to be more dependent on renal failure than on PUVs.

Conclusion

Prenatal diagnosis of PUVs has been a major factor of postnatal management of these children with this congenital bladder outlet obstruction. Gestational age at diagnosis and volume of amniotic fluid are significant predictors of long-term renal function. Nevertheless, other parameters need to be also considered. Early valve ablation can be considered as the primary treatment in the majority of cases without the need of preoperative drainage or diversion. Endoscopic treatment is feasible safely in the neonatal period if experienced surgeons use specific minimally sized pediatric cystoscopies. Early bladder management is the best option even if bladder prognosis seems unpredictable but could be possibly improved in a long-term period. Any early bladder surgery should be avoided. In fact the surgical management of PUVs became minimally interventional but intensively focused on bladder evaluation and closed follow-up. In conclusion, multidisciplinary approach is advocated for the long-term management of patients with PUVs.

References

1. Jee LD, Rickwood AM, Turnock RR (1993) Posterior urethral valves. Does prenatal diagnosis influence prognosis? Br J Urol 72(5 Pt 2):830–833
2. Casale AJ (1990) Early ureteral surgery for posterior urethral valves. Urol Clin North Am 17(2): 361–372
3. Merguerian PA, McLorie GA, Churchill BM, McKenna PH, Khoury AE (1992) Radiographic and serologic correlates of azotemia in patients with posterior urethral valves. J Urol 148(5):1499–1503
4. Yohannes P, Hanna M (2002) Current trends in the management of posterior urethral valves in the pediatric population. Urology 60(6):947–953
5. López Pereira P, Martinez Urrutia MJ, Jaureguizar E (2004) Initial and long-term management of posterior urethral valves. World J Urol 22(6):418–424
6. Denes ED, Barthold JS, González R (1997) Early prognostic value of serum creatinine levels in children with posterior urethral valves. J Urol 157(4):1441–1443
7. Sarhan O, Zaccaria I, Macher M-A, Muller F, Vuillard E, Delezoide A-L et al (2008) Long-term outcome of prenatally detected posterior urethral valves: single center study of 65 cases managed by primary valve ablation. J Urol 179(1):307–312; discussion 312–313
8. Chertin B, Cozzi D, Puri P (2002) Long-term results of primary avulsion of posterior urethral valves using a Fogarty balloon catheter. J Urol 168(4 Pt 2):1841–1843
9. Farhat W, McLorie G, Capolicchio G, Khoury A, Bägli D, Merguerian PA (2000) Outcomes of primary valve ablation versus urinary tract diversion in patients with posterior urethral valves. Urology 56(4):653–657
10. Smith GH, Canning DA, Schulman SL, Snyder HM 3rd, Duckett JW (1996) The long-term outcome of posterior urethral valves treated with primary valve ablation and observation. J Urol 155(5):1730–1734
11. Walker RD, Padron M (1990) The management of posterior urethral valves by initial vesicostomy and delayed valve ablation. J Urol 144(5):1212–1214
12. Bolduc S, Upadhyay J, Sherman C, Farhat W, Bagli DJ, McLorie GA et al (2002) Histology of upper pole is unaffected by prenatal diagnosis in duplex system ureteroceles. J Urol 168(3):1123–1126
13. Hendren WH (1971) Posterior urethral valves in boys. A broad clinical spectrum. J Urol 106(2):298–307
14. Bhatnagar V, Agarwala S, Lal R, Mitra DK (2000) Fulguration of posterior urethral valves using the Nd: YAG laser. Pediatr Surg Int 16(1–2):69–71
15. Diamond DA, Ransley PG (1987) Fogarty balloon catheter ablation of neonatal posterior urethral valves. J Urol 137(6):1209–1211
16. Tank ES (1986) Experience with endoscopic incision and open unroofing of ureteroceles. J Urol 136(1 Pt 2):241–242
17. Duckett JW Jr (1974) Current management of posterior urethral valves. Urol Clin North Am 1(3):471–483
18. Myers DA, Walker RD 3rd (1981) Prevention of urethral strictures in the management of posterior urethral valves. J Urol 126(5):655–657
19. Nijman RJ, Scholtmeijer RJ (1991) Complications of transurethral electro-incision of posterior urethral valves. Br J Urol 67(3):324–326
20. Sarhan O, El-Ghoneimi A, Hafez A, Dawaba M, Ghali A, Ibrahiem E-H (2010) Surgical complications of posterior urethral valve ablation: 20 years experience. J Pediatr Surg 45(11):2222–2226
21. Crooks KK (1982) Urethral strictures following transurethral resection of posterior urethral valves. J Urol 127(6):1153–1154

22. Duel BP, Mogbo K, Barthold JS, Gonzalez R (1998) Prognostic value of initial renal ultrasound in patients with posterior urethral valves. J Urol 160(3 Pt 2):1198–1200; discussion 1216
23. El-Ghoneimi A, Desgrippes A, Luton D, Macher MA, Guibourdenche J, Garel C et al (1999) Outcome of posterior urethral valves: to what extent is it improved by prenatal diagnosis? J Urol 162(3 Pt 1):849–853
24. Reinberg Y, de Castano I, Gonzalez R (1992) Prognosis for patients with prenatally diagnosed posterior urethral valves. J Urol 148(1):125–126
25. Dinneen MD, Dhillon HK, Ward HC, Duffy PG, Ransley PG (1993) Antenatal diagnosis of posterior urethral valves. Br J Urol 72(3):364–369
26. Connor JP, Burbige KA (1990) Long-term urinary continence and renal function in neonates with posterior urethral valves. J Urol 144(5):1209–1211
27. Hutton KA, Thomas DF, Arthur RJ, Irving HC, Smith SE (1994) Prenatally detected posterior urethral valves: is gestational age at detection a predictor of outcome? J Urol 152(2 Pt 2):698–701
28. Al-Hazmi H, Dreux S, Delezoide A-L, Dommergues M, Lortat-Jacob S, Oury J-F et al (2012) Outcome of prenatally detected bilateral higher urinary tract obstruction or megacystis: sex-related study on a series of 709 cases. Prenat Diagn 32(7):649–654
29. Muller F, Dommergues M, Mandelbrot L, Aubry MC, Nihoul-Fekete C, Dumez Y (1993) Fetal urinary biochemistry predicts postnatal renal function in children with bilateral obstructive uropathies. Obstet Gynecol 82(5):813–820
30. Elder JS, O'Grady JP, Ashmead G, Duckett JW, Philipson E (1990) Evaluation of fetal renal function: unreliability of fetal urinary electrolytes. J Urol 144(2 Pt 2):574–578; discussion 593–594
31. Hulbert WC, Rosenberg HK, Cartwright PC, Duckett JW, Snyder HM (1992) The predictive value of ultrasonography in evaluation of infants with posterior urethral valves. J Urol 148(1):122–124
32. Casella DP, Tomaszewski JJ, Ost MC (2012) Posterior urethral valves: renal failure and prenatal treatment. Int J Nephrol 2012:351067
33. Kitagawa H, Pringle KC, Koike J, Zuccollo J, Sato Y, Sato H et al (2004) The early effects of urinary tract obstruction on glomerulogenesis. J Pediatr Surg 39(12):1845–1848
34. Ruano R (2011) Fetal surgery for severe lower urinary tract obstruction. Prenat Diagn 31(7):667–674
35. Kitagawa H, Pringle KC, Koike J, Nagae H, Zuccollo J, Sato Y et al (2006) Early bladder wall changes after creation of obstructive uropathy in the fetal lamb. Pediatr Surg Int 22(11):875–879
36. Nagae H, Kitagawa H, Pringle KC, Koike J, Zuccollo J, Sato Y et al (2006) Pressure-limited vesicoamniotic shunt tube for fetal obstructive uropathy. J Pediatr Surg 41(12):2086–2089
37. Harrison MR, Golbus MS, Filly RA, Callen PW, Katz M, de Lorimier AA et al (1982) Fetal surgery for congenital hydronephrosis. N Engl J Med 306(10):591–593
38. Biard J-M, Johnson MP, Carr MC, Wilson RD, Hedrick HL, Pavlock C et al (2005) Long-term outcomes in children treated by prenatal vesicoamniotic shunting for lower urinary tract obstruction. Obstet Gynecol 106(3):503–508
39. Kim SK, Won HS, Shim JY, Kim KS, Lee PR, Kim A (2005) Successful vesicoamniotic shunting of posterior urethral valves in the first trimester of pregnancy. Ultrasound Obstet Gynecol 26(6):666–668
40. Springer A, Fartacek R, Reck CA, Horcher E, Bettelheim D (2010) Major complication after intrauterine vesico-amniotic shunting. Afr J Paediatr Surg AJPS 7(3):200–202
41. Won H-S, Kim S-K, Shim J-Y, Lee PR, Kim A (2006) Vesicoamniotic shunting using a double-basket catheter appears effective in treating fetal bladder outlet obstruction. Acta Obstet Gynecol Scand 85(7):879–884
42. Brown C, Morris RK, Daniels J, Khan KS, Lilford RJ, Kilby MD (2010) Effectiveness of percutaneous vesico-amniotic shunting in congenital lower urinary tract obstruction: divergence in prior beliefs among specialist groups. Eur J Obstet Gynecol Reprod Biol 152(1):25
43. Jouannic J-M, Hyett JA, Pandya PP, Gulbis B, Rodeck CH, Jauniaux E (2003) Perinatal outcome in fetuses with megacystis in the first half of pregnancy. Prenat Diagn 23(4):340–344
44. Elder JS, Duckett JW Jr, Snyder HM (1987) Intervention for fetal obstructive uropathy: has it been effective? Lancet 2(8566):1007–1010
45. Coplen DE (1997) Prenatal intervention for hydronephrosis. J Urol 157(6):2270–2277
46. McLorie G, Farhat W, Khoury A, Geary D, Ryan G (2001) Outcome analysis of vesicoamniotic shunting in a comprehensive population. J Urol 166(3):1036–1040
47. Clark TJ, Martin WL, Divakaran TG, Whittle MJ, Kilby MD, Khan KS (2003) Prenatal bladder drainage in the management of fetal lower urinary tract obstruction: a systematic review and meta-analysis. Obstet Gynecol 102(2):367–382
48. Morris RK, Malin GL, Khan KS, Kilby MD (2010) Systematic review of the effectiveness of antenatal intervention for the treatment of congenital lower urinary tract obstruction. BJOG Int J Obstet Gynaecol 117(4):382–390
49. Quintero RA, Johnson MP, Romero R, Smith C, Arias F, Guevara-Zuloaga F et al (1995) In-utero percutaneous cystoscopy in the management of fetal lower obstructive uropathy. Lancet 346(8974):537–540
50. Quintero RA, Shukla AR, Homsy YL, Bukkapatnam R (2000) Successful in utero endoscopic ablation of posterior urethral valves: a new dimension in fetal urology. Urology 55(5):774
51. Morris RK, Ruano R, Kilby MD (2011) Effectiveness of fetal cystoscopy as a diagnostic and therapeutic intervention for lower urinary tract obstruction: a systematic review. Ultrasound Obstet Gynecol 37(6):629–637

52. Abbott JF, Levine D, Wapner R (1998) Posterior urethral valves: inaccuracy of prenatal diagnosis. Fetal Diagn Ther 13(3):179–183
53. Robyr R, Benachi A, Daikha-Dahmane F, Martinovich J, Dumez Y, Ville Y (2005) Correlation between ultrasound and anatomical findings in fetuses with lower urinary tract obstruction in the first half of pregnancy. Ultrasound Obstet Gynecol 25(5):478–482
54. Lewis KM, Pinckert TL, Cain MP, Ghidini A (1998) Complications of intrauterine placement of a vesicoamniotic shunt. Obstet Gynecol 91(5 Pt 2):825–827
55. Holmes N, Harrison MR, Baskin LS (2001) Fetal surgery for posterior urethral valves: long-term postnatal outcomes. Pediatrics 108(1):E7
56. Morris RK, Kilby MD (2009) An overview of the literature on congenital lower urinary tract obstruction and introduction to the PLUTO trial: percutaneous shunting in lower urinary tract obstruction. Aust N Z J Obstet Gynaecol 49(1):6–10
57. Nicolini U, Spelzini F (2001) Invasive assessment of fetal renal abnormalities: urinalysis, fetal blood sampling and biopsy. Prenat Diagn 21(11):964–969
58. Duckett JW Jr (1974) Cutaneous vesicostomy in childhood. The Blocksom technique. Urol Clin North Am 1(3):485–495
59. RICKHAM PP (1962) Advanced lower urinary obstruction in childhood. Arch Dis Child 37:122–131
60. Cendron J, Deburge JP, Karlaftis C (1969) Valvulae of the posterior urethra. J Urol Néphrologie 75(1):15–38
61. Reinberg Y, de Castano I, Gonzalez R (1992) Influence of initial therapy on progression of renal failure and body growth in children with posterior urethral valves. J Urol 148(2 Pt 2):532–533
62. Close CE, Carr MC, Burns MW, Mitchell ME (1997) Lower urinary tract changes after early valve ablation in neonates and infants: is early diversion warranted? J Urol 157(3):984–988
63. Whitaker RH, Sherwood T (1986) An improved hook for destroying posterior urethral valves. J Urol 135(3):531–532
64. Levard G, Aigrain Y, Politi B, Weisgerber G, Boureau M (1986) Rupturing of valves of the posterior urethra in the newborn using a balloon catheter. Results of the technic apropos of a series of 10 children. Chir Pédiatrique 27(4):196–200
65. Lal R, Bhatnagar V, Mitra DK (1999) Urinary continence following posterior urethral valves treatment. Indian J Pediatr 66(1):49–54
66. Bruce J, Stannard V, Small PG, Mayell MJ, Kapila L (1987) The operative management of posterior urethral valves. J Pediatr Surg 22(12):1081–1086
67. Churchill BM, Krueger RP, Fleisher MH, Hardy BE (1983) Complications of posterior urethral valve surgery and their prevention. Urol Clin North Am 10(3):519–530
68. Hoover DL, Duckett JW Jr (1982) Posterior urethral valves, unilateral reflux and renal dysplasia: a syndrome. J Urol 128(5):994–997
69. Lopez Pereira P, Martinez Urrutia MJ, Espinosa L, Jaureguizar E (2013) Long-term consequences of posterior urethral valves. J Pediatr Urol 9(5):590–596
70. Fumo MJ, McLorie GA (2006) Management of the valve-bladder syndrome and congenital bladder obstruction: the role of nocturnal bladder drainage. Nat Clin Pract Urol 3(6):323–326
71. Youssif M, Badawy H, Saad A, Hanno A, Mokhless I (2007) Augmentation ureterocystoplasty in boys with valve bladder syndrome. J Pediatr Urol 3(6):433–437
72. Botto N, Paye-Jaouen A, El Ghoneimi A (2012) Long-term evaluation of bladder function in patient with PUVs after renal transplantation. In: ESPU Annual Meeting. Zurich
73. Bajpai M, Dave S, Gupta DK (2001) Factors affecting outcome in the management of posterior urethral valves. Pediatr Surg Int 17(1):11–15
74. Oliveira EA, Diniz JS, Cabral AC, Leite HV, Colosimo EA, Oliveira RB et al (1999) Prognostic factors in fetal hydronephrosis: a multivariate analysis. Pediatr Nephrol Berl Ger 13(9):859–864

Urethral Abnormalities

19

Paolo Caione, Michele Guidotti,
and Federico Scottoni

19.1 Introduction

The urethra is very often presenting acquired or congenital abnormalities, the latter being more frequent in newborn and pediatric age, especially in males [1, 2]. Hypospadias, with a prevalence evaluated as 1:300–700 live male newborns, and posterior urethral valves (PUV), which are found in 1: 1,000–2,000 male newborns [3], are the most frequent urethral abnormalities and are described in different chapters.

Although we exclude PUV and the hypospadias-epispadias complex, congenital anomalies of the male and female urethra are most common and present a wide spectrum of anatomical variants. *Urethral congenital abnormalities* are often associated with complex or multiple malformations and often could present diagnostic and therapeutic difficulties for the pediatric urologist.

To better define urethral abnormalities, a short reminder of the embryology and anatomy of the urethra could be welcomed. A classification is proposed, to allow an organic view of this group of congenital diseases of the urinary tract, not infrequently observed in pediatric urology (Fig. 19.1).

P. Caione (✉) • M. Guidotti • F. Scottoni
Department of Nephrology-Urology,
Children's Hospital Bambino Gesù,
Piazza S. Onofrio, 4, Rome 00165, Italy
e-mail: paolo.caione@opbg.net

19.2 Embryology

During the sixth week of gestation, the *urogenital sinus* cavity extends onto the surface of the genital tubercle and gives rise to urethral development. This *endodermal derived groove* becomes a solid plate of cells, which eventually tubularizes in proximal-to-distal fashion to form the phallic urethra. This developing process happens after the ninth week of gestation until when there exist no differences between male and female urethral buds.

Four distinct regions have been identified in male mature urethra: *prostatic and membranous urethras*, derived from the urogenital sinus, proximally, and *bulbar and pendulous urethras*, derived from the urethral plate, distally [4].

The two proximal regions are totally composed of delicate transitional epithelium changing to simple squamous epithelium in the context of the two distal portions. These proximal regions are not completely androgen dependent, as they are responsible for the development of the female urethra. However, the bulbar and pendulous urethras are completely androgen dependent and are only present in males [5].

Unlike its proximal counterpart, the urethra which forms within the glans is lined by a stratified squamous epithelium and has a more controversial development. Some authors argue that an ectodermal ingrowth of epidermis canalizes the glandular urethra [6]; however, recent papers suggested, with immunohistochemical support, that the entire urethra, including the glans portion, was formed by

M. Lima, G. Manzoni (eds.), *Pediatric Urology: Contemporary Strategies from Fetal Life to Adolescence*,
DOI 10.1007/978-88-470-5693-0_19, © Springer-Verlag Italia 2015

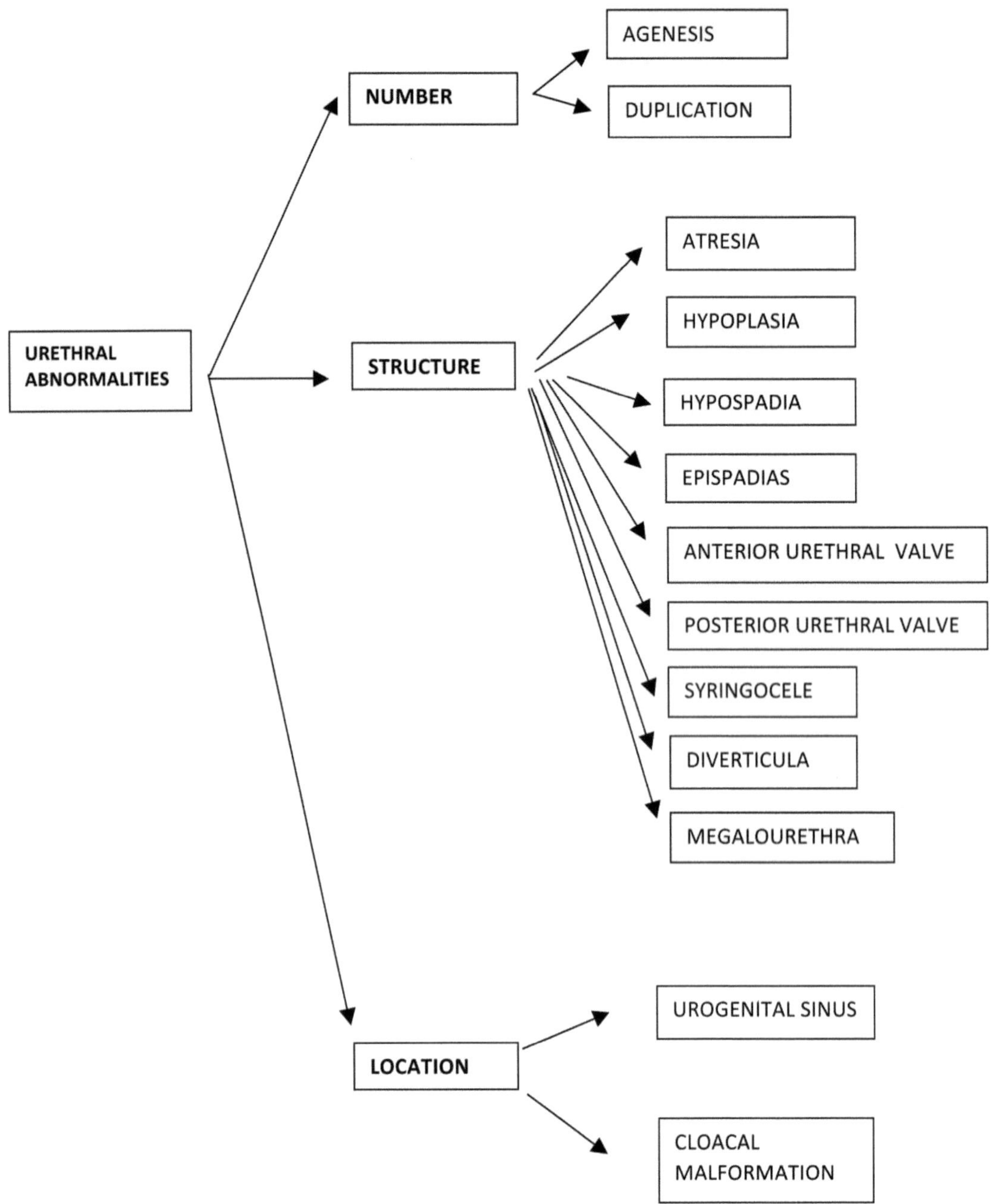

Fig. 19.1 Classification of congenital urethral abnormalities

dorsal extension and disintegration of the urethral plate combined with ventral growth and fusion of the urethral folds [7]. All these different hypotheses on the structural anomalies of the urethra may be related to the complexity of its embryology and may represent the reasons for the number and frequency of urethral abnormalities in children.

19.3 Atresia

A very severe and very uncommon malformation, atresia occurs early in the embryonic fetal life, and it is due to a flawed canalization of the endodermic groove around the ninth week of gestation.

As a result of the developmental defect, the kidney does not continue to mature. This condition is often not compatible with life. The kidney maturation is possible only if an alternative communication with the bladder, such as a patent urachus, exists [8]. The few living newborns show dysplastic kidneys, renal cystic malformations, and prune-belly syndrome.

19.4 Anterior Urethral Valve

Anterior urethral valve (AUV) is a rare entity, with the largest series reporting 17 patients [9]; it is reported to be seven times less common than posterior urethral valve (PUV); however, it can be equally devastating [10]. AUV may occur in every portion of the anterior urethra. It seems to have a unique pathophysiologic spectrum from valvular diseases to anterior urethral diverticula according to the degree of dilation due to the obstruction, so a urethral diverticulum should be considered in every case of AUV.

The etiology of these anomalies is still not completely clear. Williams and Retik suggested that they may arise from congenital cystic dilation of normal or accessory periurethral glands that communicate with the urethra, resulting in a flaplike valve [9]. Firlit referred AUV as consequence of an incomplete development of the corpus spongiosum [10]; recently Kajbafzadeh proposed that they seem to represent an incomplete fusion of a segment of urethral plate [11].

Clinical presentation of patients with AUV is similar to those with PUV. The spectrum ranges from *mild urethral dilation* to *severe bilateral hydronephrosis* with renal failure, according to the degree of urinary obstruction; luckily only fewer than 5 % of patients with AUV progress to chronic renal failure [12]. In 2010, JC Routh et al. asserted that congenital anterior urethral obstruction in children has a generally good prognosis but may occasionally result in a poor renal outcome. The combination of pretreatment azotemia, vesicoureteral reflux, and urinary tract infection is highly predictive of a poor renal outcome [13].

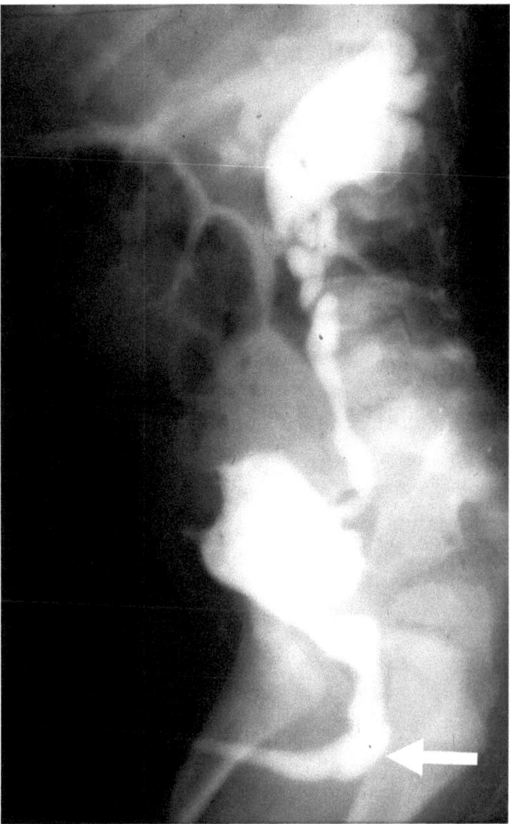

Fig. 19.2 Voiding cystourethrogram in a 3-year-old boy with vesicoureteral reflux and trabeculated bladder, wide bladder neck secondary to anterior urethral valve (*arrow*)

An anterograde cystourethrogram has to be performed when anterior urethral obstruction is suspected; cystoscopy or retrograde urethrography may fail to detect the valve as it remains open with retrograde flow. Renal sonography and serum creatinine complete the diagnostic process evaluating the presence and degree of renal impairment (Fig. 19.2).

Management of AUV may be endoscopic or open. Endoscopic procedure consists in electrocauterization of valve tissue. When performing this procedure, the surgeon must be careful not to injure the urethral wall: it can be very thin and terminal injury may result in urethral strictures and urethrocutaneous fistula. A urethroplasty and open resection of the valve are recommended in patients with massive urethral diverticula to pack an adequate urethral caliber.

19.5 Congenital Anterior Urethra Diverticula

Congenital *anterior diverticula of the urethra* are not frequent in the male. The wide-mouthed (saccular) diverticulum and the small-mouthed peduncolate (globular) diverticulum are two well-recognized varieties of the lesion [9]. Diagnoses of these conditions are usually performed in patients with lower urinary tract symptoms such as dysuria, frequency, and postvoid dribbling.

The most common congenital anterior diverticula are syringoceles that arise from cystic dilation of the Cowper's gland duct on the ventral midline and *lacuna magna*, a dorsal urethral diverticulum of the fossa navicularis.

19.6 Syringoceles

These anomalies consist in dilation of *Cowper's gland duct* within the bulbous urethra. Maizels et al. divided these conditions in four groups depending on their radiographic appearance [14]: (1) *simple syringocele*, only a minimally dilated duct; (2) *perforate syringocele*, a spatulous duct that drains into the bulbous urethra and appears as a diverticulum; (3) *imperforate syringocele*, a submucosal cyst, stocked by the duct, appearing as a radiolucent mass protruding into the urethra at voiding cystourethrogram; and (4) *ruptured syringocele*, a membrane remaining after the rupture of dilated duct [14]. Based on building luminal pressures within the ducts, syringoceles may follow a standard maturation from simple to imperforate to either perforated or ruptured, but more data is needed to confirm this hypothesis [15].

More recently Bevers et al. proposed a simplified classification dividing the diverticula in *open syringoceles* and *closed syringocele*; the first can cause postvoid incontinence, and the second, infravescical obstruction [16].

Usually types 2 and 4 have the urethroscopic appearance of a diverticulum. Their typical presentations are urethral infections, hematuria, dysuria, and urinary dribbling. Types 1 and 3 cause urethral obstruction resulting in voiding difficulties. More rarely, it is possible to observe in these patients a perineal mass or hydronephrosis.

The initial evaluation of Cowper's syringocele typically involves a thorough voiding history. A high index of suspicion justifies noninvasive imaging. Ultrasonography (US) sometimes visualizes closed cystic lesions in the anatomic region of Cowper's gland. Final diagnosis can be gained by cystourethroscopy or by retrograde urethrography (Fig. 19.3a, b).

Cystic dilations of Cowper' gland ducts are frequently asymptomatic in children; they may be more common than currently realized [16]. Although many symptomatic ones eventually require *surgical intervention*, a period of *conservative management* seems prudent, as spontaneous resolution of symptoms over time is not uncommon. Bevers et al. described several cases of confirmed both open and closed syringoceles whose symptoms resolved on their own: one case resolved after successful treatment for a UTI; others resolved with no intervention [16]. Treatments have to be considered in cases of repeated infection or severe obstruction. Careful clinical, radiologic, endoscopic, and urodynamic evaluations are mandatory before treatment to avoid unnecessary surgery.

The treatment of choice, when necessary, is *endoscopic unroofing of the diverticulum* by transurethral incision, thereby marsupializing it into the urethra. However, current opinion recommends open intervention for certain populations, such as children with large diverticula and inadequate spongiosum. In such cases, diverticulectomy should be considered [17–19].

19.7 Lacuna Magna or Sinus of Guerin

This entity, initially described by Morgagni in 1719, consists in a septum that persists between the canalized glandular ingrowth of ectodermal tissue and the distally advancing urethra [20], giving origin to a diverticulum in fossa navicularis. Sommer and Stephens reported its association with urological symptoms for the first time,

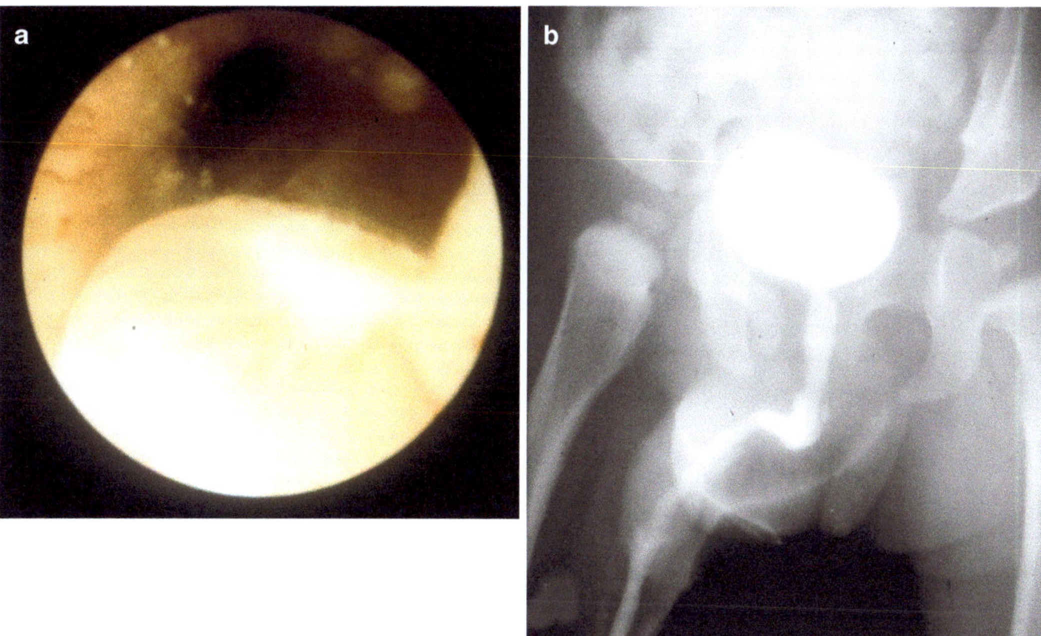

Fig. 19.3 Syringocele. (**a**) Endoscopic view of a closed syringocele. (**b**) Voiding cystogram: the urethral lesion is observed at the bulbous urethra

in 1980 [20]. Since then, only few cases of lacuna magna have been reported in the literature. It may be present in a considerable number of boys, Bellinger et al. described a prevalence of 30 % [21]; however, only a few become symptomatic due to a valvelike effect of the septum.

The diagnosis of *lacuna magna* can be accurately made if this condition, though less common, is kept at the back of the mind. Diagnosis may be gained by voiding cystourethrography and cystoscopy.

The main goals in the treatment of lacuna magna are relief of symptoms, control of infection, and elimination of any obstruction. Most pediatric urologists now agree that treatment of choice consists in endoscopic incision with cutting current of the septum and fulguration of the base of the diverticulum [21–23].

19.8 Cobb's Collar

Congenital stricture of the urethral bulb has become a controversial issue and may in fact represent what may be more accurately termed a perforate congenital urethral membrane or diaphragm [2].

Cobb et al. described in 1968 26 cases of proximal urethral bulb strictures in patients without history of urethritis, urethral or perineal trauma, previous urethroscopy, or urethral surgery [24]. This congenital stricture differs from acquired types of stricture in that there is a distinct lack of periurethral fibrosis or any abnormal tissue surrounding the urethra (Fig. 19.4). It is important to differentiate *Cobb's collar*, also called *Moormann's ring* [25], from type III posterior urethral valve as described by Young et al. [3]: in some cases the posterior urethral membrane may prolapse until the bulbar urethra, making these two conditions similar; however, the fold is attached to the verumontanum in all cases of posterior urethral valve.

Three different types of Cobb's collar have been identified. All these forms of obstruction are located just below the external sphincter. Type I appears as a ridge of tissue; type II represents a well-defined stricture of the bulbar urethra, while type III is a very tight pinhole [26].

The clinical presentation is related to various degrees of urinary obstruction; other described symptoms are enuresis, urinary tract infection, hematuria, and failure to thrive [24, 25]. In adulthood, these patients may manifest poor ejaculation [27].

Ultrasound showed a *thickened bladder* wall with a significant postvoiding residual. Voiding cystourethrography may detect the stricture, but definitive diagnosis is available by cystoscopy. Treatment of choice is endoscopic dilation or, in case of ineffectiveness, incision of the stricture walls. A cold knife is preferable to electrocautery for incising this fine anterior lesion.

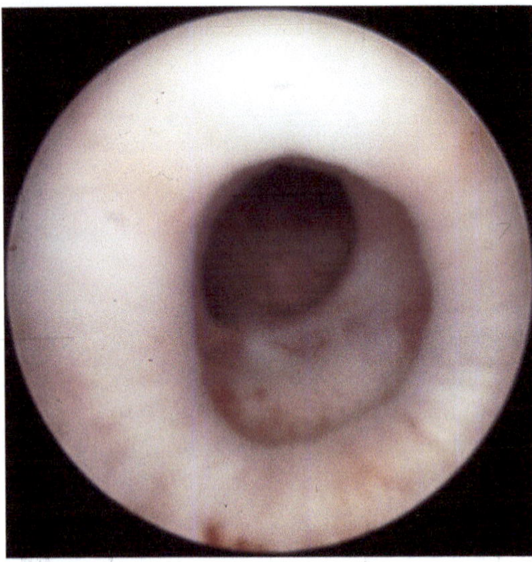

Fig. 19.4 Cobb's collar or Moormann's ring: a ring is observed by urethroscopy at bulbar urethra level. External sphincter is observed proximally to the ring, without periurethral fibrosis

19.9 Megalourethra

The term "*megalourethra*" was suggested originally by Nesbitt to describe a very rare congenital malformation characterized by diffuse dilation of the penile urethra [28]. It consists of a urogenital malformation of the anterior urethra secondary to a mesodermal defect.

Megalourethra is characterized by dilation and elongation of the penile urethra, associated with *absence or severe hypoplasia of the corpora spongiosa and cavernosa*. Postnatal complications include voiding and erectile dysfunction as well as renal insufficiency and pulmonary hypoplasia. Congenital megalourethra is caused by abnormal development or hypoplasia of the penile erectile tissue which has been related to distal urethral obstruction in the prenatal period. In fact, it is often responsible for a serious outflow obstruction during fetal life which can lead to oligo- or anhydramnios, bilateral renal failure, and Potter syndrome-like manifestations in the newborn.

Megalourethra can be subdivided into two different types: *fusiform* megalourethra and *scaphoid* megalourethra. In the fusiform variety, the corpora cavernosa and the corpus spongiosum are absent; in the scaphoid type, only the corpus spongiosum is absent (Fig. 19.5a–c). Fusiform dilation of the megalourethra may result from underdevelopment of the corpus spongiosum and support structures of the urethra. This condition has been related commonly to *prune-belly syndrome*. The characteristic association of deficient abdominal muscles, undescended testes, and

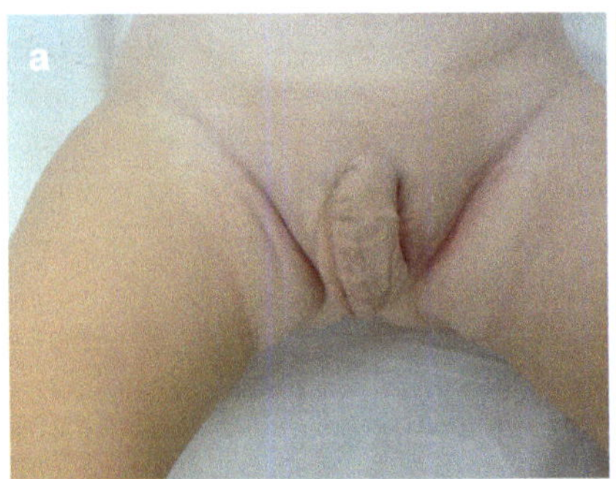

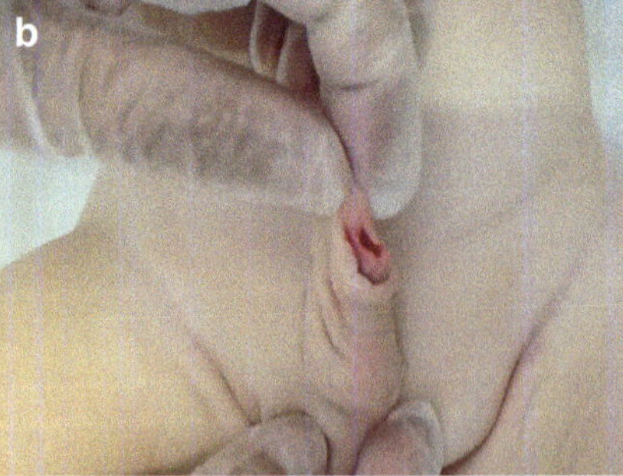

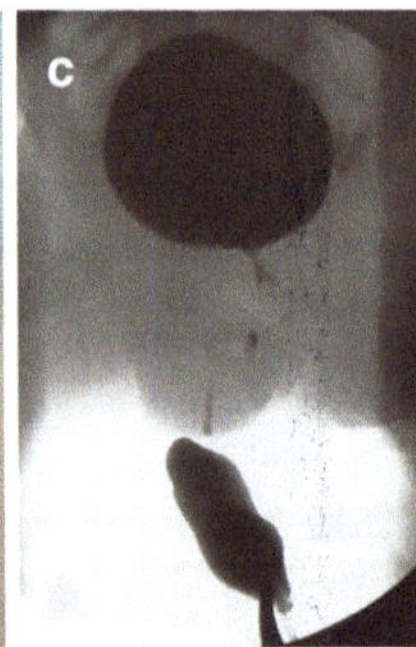

Fig. 19.5 (**a**, **b**) Morphological appearance of the fusiform type of megalourethra. (**c**) Radiological appearance at voiding cystogram

urinary tract abnormalities probably results from severe urethral obstruction in fetal life [29].

If the amniotic fluid volume is normal during prenatal ultrasound, survival is possible. However, all live-born infants manifest voiding and renal dysfunction as well as sexual disorders. Megalourethra should be considered in all male fetuses presenting prenatally with megacystis. A detailed fetal ultrasound scan should show an elongated and/or distended phallic structure as well as any associated anomalies.

Diagnosis is by voiding cystourethrography (Fig. 19.5c). Early bladder outlet obstruction removal is necessary soon after birth. Reconstructive surgery is required. Surgical treatment of scaphoid type of megalourethra consists of a Nesbitt's urethroplasty. The operative technique for fusiform megalourethra with genital malformation has to be tailored to each individual case, depending on the intraoperative and endoscopic findings [28, 29].

19.10 Congenital Urethral Polyps

Urethral polyps are rare congenital lesions; they usually arise from the verumontanum; anterior ones are extremely rare and may be piping out into the bladder neck, causing bladder outlet obstruction (Fig. 19.6a, b).

Urethral polyps are benign lesions, not to be confused with protuberant polypoid mass of sarcoma botryoides. The histologic examination reveals a fibroepithelial core with transitional epithelium; sometimes squamous metaplasia is found (Fig. 19.6c).

Possible etiologies include abnormal protrusion of the urethral wall and metaplastic changes secondary to maternal estrogens [2, 12].

Urethral polyps in children occur exclusively in boys; average age is 5.2 years. Clinical presentation is related to variable degrees of obstruction: dysuria, incontinence, diminished stream, incomplete emptying, and hematuria are the typical presenting symptoms.

Physical examination is usually not helpful for diagnosis except for larger lesions that can be felt at rectal examination. Definitive diagnosis can be gained with cystourethrography or endoscopy.

Treatment of choice is endoscopic resection with fulguration of the base of the lesion; in case of displacement of the polyp into the bladder, a transvesical approach could be an acceptable alternative.

19.11 Urethral Meatal Stenosis

Congenital *stenosis of the distal urethral meatus* is a rare condition compared with acquired ones. Meatal stenosis could be suspected in boys less than 4 years of age if the meatus measured less than 8 F and in boys over ten if the meatus calibrated to less than 10 F [2].

Daily meatal dilation by parents, using a lubricant for 2 weeks, sometimes helps to assure a satisfactory result [1]. In refractory cases, surgical meatotomy has to be considered the treatment of choice [12].

19.12 Urethral Duplication

Urethral duplication is an extremely rare congenital disease which mostly afflicts male population. It is often associated with genitourinary and gastrointestinal anomalies including hypospadias, epispadias, imperforate anus, congenital heart disease, etc. Less than 300 cases have been reported in literature. Clinical presentation varies because of the different anatomical patterns of this abnormality. Typical manifestations include deformed penis, twin stream, urinary tract infection, urinary incontinence, outflow obstruction, and symptoms related to the associated anomalies [30, 31].

The embryonic origin of urethral duplication is uncertain and various hypotheses exist. It can be caused by abnormal *Mullerian duct* termination and growth arrest of the urogenital sinus or misalignment of the termination of the cloaca membrane with the genital tubercle. The male urethra develops mostly or completely from the endoderm except the distal most glandular part which is of ectodermal origin.

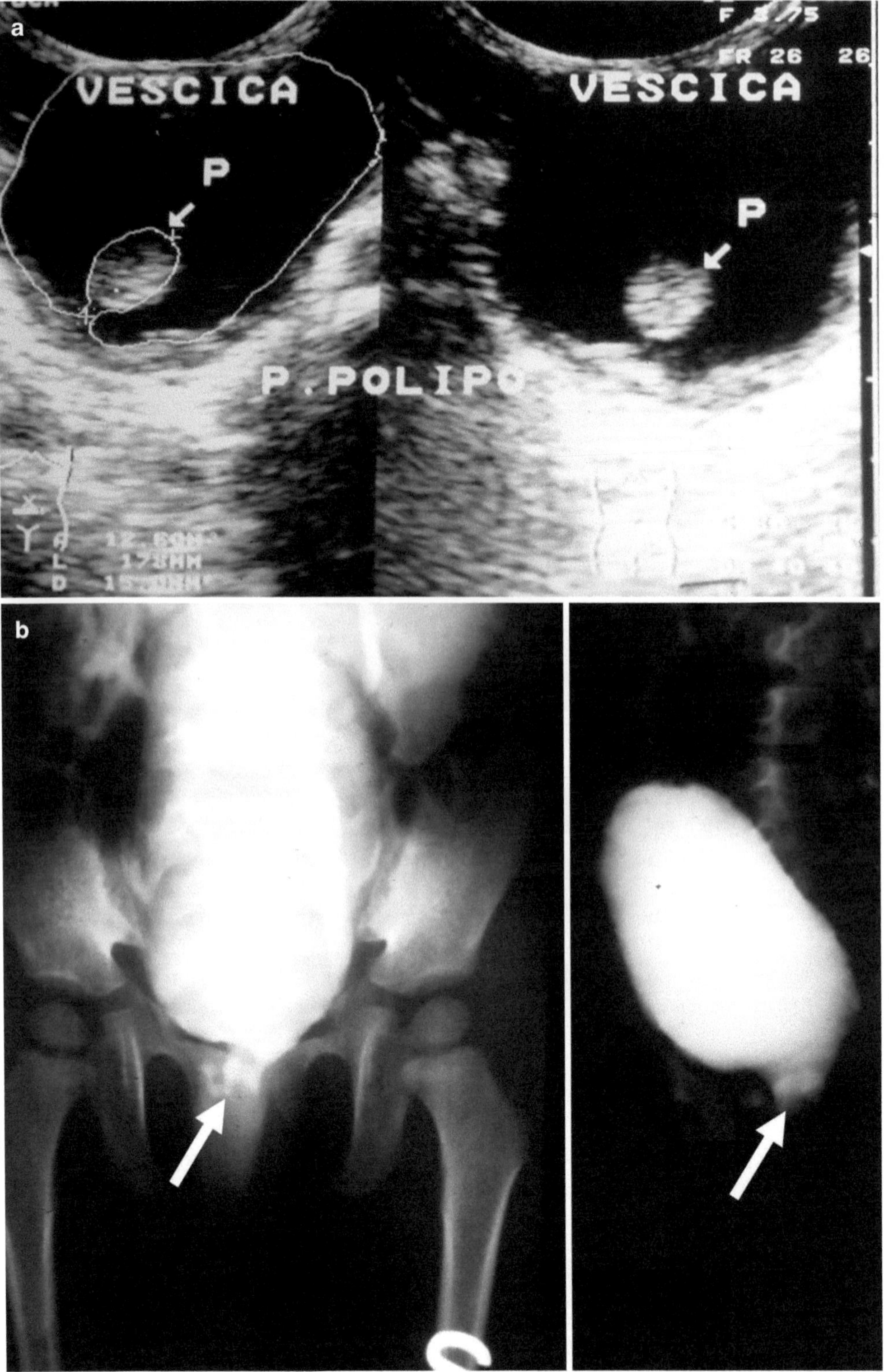

Fig. 19.6 (**a**) Ultrasonographic appearance of a congenital urethral polyp, plongeant into the bladder. (**b**) Voiding cystourethrogram of the same case: wide and not emptying bladder with obstruction under the bladder neck (*arrow*). (**c**) Macroscopic specimen of the lesion, after transurethral resection

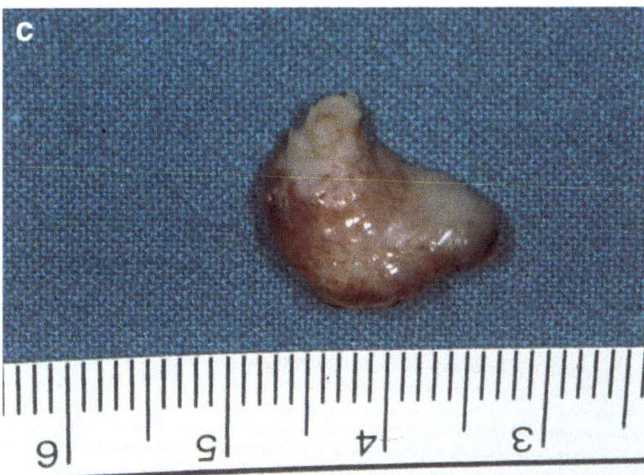

Fig. 19.6 (continued)

The forms of urethral duplications are completely different in males and females.

In males, urethral duplication is classified into three types (*Effman's classification*) [30]:

Type I: blind-ending accessory urethra (incomplete urethral duplication):

- *IA*Distal—duplicated urethras opening on the dorsal or ventral surface of the penis but not communicating with the urethra or bladder (the most common type)
- *IIB* Proximal—accessory urethra opening from the urethral channel but ending blindly in the periurethral tissues (rare)

Type II: completely patent accessory urethra. It is divided into two parts—A (two meatuses) and B (one meatus):

- *IIA*—two noncommunicating urethras arising independently from the bladder
- *IIB*—second channel arising from the first and coursing independently into a second meatus (Y-type)
- *IIIC*wo urethras arising from the bladder or posterior urethra and uniting into a common channel distally

Type III: accessory urethras arising from duplicated or septated bladders:

In females, urethral duplication is classified into the following types [31]:

I. Double urethra and double bladder
II. Double urethra, single bladder
III. Accessory urethra posterior to the normal channel
IV. Double proximal urethra and single distal urethra
V. Single proximal urethra and duplicated distal urethra

Onofre et al. [31] describe two types of urethral duplication based on the presentation: sagittal and coronal. Each group, sagittal or coronal, has a few similarities that may be helpful in their management.

MRI should be preferred to voiding cystourethrography due to the superior contrast resolution and multiplanar capability. MRI delineates the exact urethral anatomy much better. Effectively, voiding cystourethrography can diagnose whether there is a duplication or not but cannot diagnose the precise relation of the duplicated urethras with other pelvic structures [32].

The first purpose is to identify the *orthotopic urethra*. It can be identified because the main urethra shows the presence of verumontanum; it is related to the sphincter and it maintains contact with the prostate bundle. Furthermore, the main urethra is often dysplastic and hypoplastic and can be found in association with genitourinary anomalies like *bifid scrotum or diphallus.* Even bladder duplications have been described, but never a duplication of the prostate has been observed (Fig. 19.7a, b).

Once identified, the main urethra is often treated with the *PADUA technique*, which consists in a procedure for the treatment of severe urethral hypoplasia. The PADUA acronym means *progressive augmentation by dilating the urethra anterior* [33].

The ancillary urethra can be removed or not. This is a choice made by the surgeon based on the individual clinical presentation of each patient, taking into consideration the procedure's advantages and disadvantages, the coexistence of incontinence, or the presence of urinary tract infections.

Skin grafts and urethroplasty usually complete the process.

Urethral duplication is a complex anomaly and the different manifestations probably have different embryological origins. Every diagnosed case presents a unique anatomy, and surgical treatment must be individualized depending of the structural and functional context.

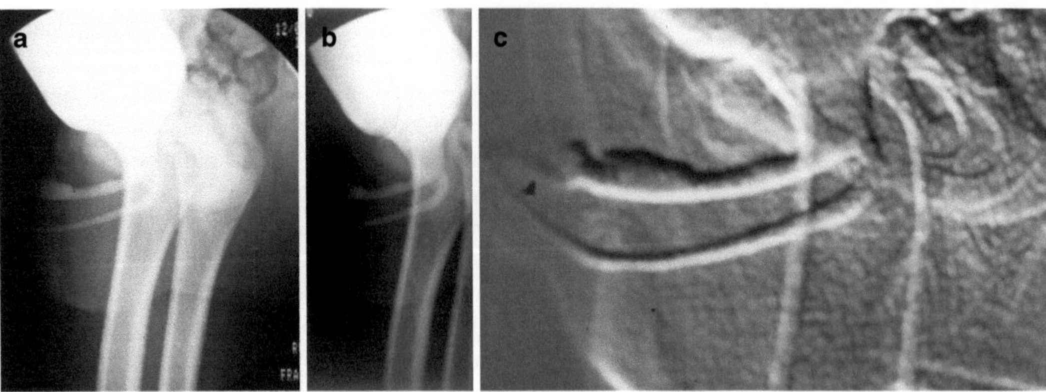

Fig. 19.7 (**a**–**c**) Voiding cystourethrogram of a 6-year-old boy with complete urethral duplication; both urethras arise from a wide bladder neck. The orthotopic urethral is smaller, is posterior placed, and is related to the prostatic bundle

References

1. Firlit CF (1978) Urethral abnormalities. Urol Clin North Am 5:31–55
2. King LR (1985) Posterior urethra. In: Kelalis PP, King LR, Belman AB (eds) Clinical pediatric urology. W.B. Saunders Company, Philadelphia, pp 527–558
3. Young HH, Frontz WA, Baldwin JC (1919) Congenital obstruction of the posterior urethra. J Urol 3:289–365
4. Hynes PJ, Fraher JP (2004) The development of the male genitourinary system: III. The formation of the spongiose and glandar urethra. Br J Plast Surg 57:203–214
5. Hynes PJ, Fraher JP (2004) The development of the male genitourinary system: II. The origin and formation of the urethral plate. Br J Plast Surg 57:112–121
6. Krishnan A, de Souza A, Konijeti R et al (2006) The anatomy and embryology of posterior urethral valves. J Urol 175:1214–1220
7. Kurzrock EA, Baskin LS, Cunha GR (1999) Ontogeny of the male urethra: theory of endodermal differentiation. Differentiation 64(2):115–122
8. Gonzales R, De Filippo R, Jednak R, Barthold JS (2001) Urethral atresia: long-term outcome in 6 children who survived neonatal period. J Urol 165:2241–2244
9. Williams DI, Retik AB (1969) Congenital valves and diverticula of the anterior urethra. Br J Urol 41:228–234
10. Firlit RS, Firlit CF, King LP (1978) Obstructing anterior urethral valves in children. J Urol 119:819–822
11. Kajbafzadeh A (2005) Congenital urethral anomalies in boys. Part II. Urol J 2(3):125–131
12. Glassberg KI, Horowitz M (2002) Urethral valve and other anomalies of the male urethra. In: Belman AB, King LR, Kramer SA (eds) Clinical pediatric urology, 4th edn. Martin Dunitz Ltd, London, pp 899–945
13. Routh JC, McGee SM, Ashley RA, Reinberg Y, Vandersteen DR (2010) Predicting renal outcomes in children with anterior urethral valves: a systematic review. J Urol 184(5):1615–1619
14. Maizels M, Stephens FD, King LR, Firlit CF (1983) Cowper's syringocele: a classification of dilatations of Cowper's gland duct based upon clinical characteristics of 8 boys. J Urol 129(1):111–114
15. Melquist J et al (2010) Current diagnosis and management of syringocele: a review. Int Braz J Urol 36(1):3–9
16. Bevers RF, Abbekerk EM, Boon TA (2000) Cowper's syringocele: symptoms, classification and treatment of an unappreciated problem. J Urol 163(3):782–784
17. Campobasso P, Schieven E, Fernandes EC (1996) Cowper's syringocele: an analysis of 15 consecutive cases. Arch Dis Child 75:71–73
18. Oesch I, Kummer M, Bettex M (1983) Congenital urethral diverticula in boys. Eur Urol 9:139–141
19. McLellan DL, Gaston MV, Diamond DA, Lebowitz RL, Mandell J, Atala A et al (2004) Anterior urethral valves and diverticula in children: a result of ruptured Cowper's duct cyst? BJU Int 94:375–378
20. Sommer JT, Stephens FD (1980) Dorsal urethral diverticulum of the fossa navicularis: symptoms, diagnosis and treatment. J Urol 124:94–97
21. Bellinger MF, Purohit GS, Duckett JW, Cromie WJ (1983) Lacuna magna: a hidden cause of dysuria and bloody spotting in boys. J Pediatr Surg 18(2):163–166
22. Seskin FE, Glassberg KI (1994) Lacuna magna in 6 boys with post-void bleeding and dysuria: alternative approach to treatment. J Urol 152:980–982
23. Friedman RM, King LR (1993) Valve of Guerin as a cause of dysuria and hematuria in young boys: presentation and difficulties in diagnosis. J Urol 150:159–161
24. Cobb BG, Wolf JA, Ansell JS (1968) Congenital stricture of the proximal urethral bulb. J Urol 99:629
25. Moormann JG (1972) Congenital bulbar urethral stenosis as a cause of disease of the urogenital junction. Urologe 11:157–160

26. Adorisio O, Bassani F, Silveri M (2013) Cobb's collar: a rare cause of urinary retention. BMJ Case Rep. Jan 22; pii: bcr2012008137 doi: 10.1136/bcr-2012-008137
27. Cranston D, Davies AH, Smith JC (1990) Cobb's collar: a forgotten entity. Br J Urol 66(3):294–296
28. Nesbitt TE (1955) Congenital megalourethra. J Urol 73:839–842
29. Zugor V, Schrott KM, Schott GE (2006) A complex case of megalourethra and its repair. J Pediatr Urol 6:592–595
30. Effman EL, Lebowitz RL, Colodny AH (1976) Duplication of the urethra. Radiology 1:179–185
31. Onofre LS, Leao JQ, Gomes AL, Heinisch AC, Leao FG, Carnevale J (2011) Urethral duplication: a wide spectrum of anomalies. J Pediatr Urol 7(3):349–355
32. Bhaduri S, Parashari UC, Singh R, Kohli N (2009) MRI in congenital duplication of urethra. Indian J Radiol Imaging 19(3):232–234
33. Passerini-Glazel G, Aragona F, Chiazza L, Artibani W, Rabinowitz R, Firlit CF (1988) The P.A.D.U.A. (progressive augmentation by dilatation of the urethra anterior) procedure for treatment of severe urethral hypoplasia. J Urol 140:1247–1249

Part V

Genitalia

Disorders of Sex Development: A Clinical Guide

20

Christopher R.J. Woodhouse

20.1 Introduction

The term "disorder of sex development" (DSD) was introduced at a consensus meeting in Chicago in 2006 [1]. It replaces titles such as "hermaphrodite" and "intersex" which were thought to be pejorative to patients. At the same time, the classification of the disorders was altered so that the diagnostic labels reflected the molecular genetic abnormality rather than the clinical appearance. The Chicago proposals are shown in Table 20.1. Although they have been generally accepted by specialists in the field, modifications are still being made. For the nonspecialist and for those attempting to review past literature, DSD remains a most confusing field. Indeed, students and postgraduates may well find the subject so difficult that they pass it by altogether. Medical exams seldom have questions on DSD, and patients are not common in general urologic clinics.

Although there are advantages in the new nomenclature, some older terms are still commonly used. For example, the commonest DSD is still called *congenital adrenal hyperplasia* (CAH) which, in females, would be classified as 46XX DSD. While the nomenclature is in a state of flux, it is important to avoid the older terms, particularly "hermaphrodite" and the very imprecise diagnoses such as *male pseudohermaphrodite*.

C.R.J. Woodhouse
Emeritus Professor of Adolescent Urology,
Department of Urology, University College,
31, Eustace Building, 372, Queenstown Road,
London SW8 4NT, UK
e-mail: Christopher@crjwoodhouse.fsnet.co.uk

20.2 Fetal Development

To understand the clinical syndromes that are seen, it is helpful to have an outline of the way in which the fetus develops.

The default development for the fetus is female. Although this statement is not strictly true, it is accurate enough for a starting point. In the absence of some positive developmental influence, a fetus will be born with a substantially female phenotype. Conversely, with androgenic influence, a 46XX fetus will be born with a substantially male phenotype.

The *Y chromosome* encodes a testis determining factor, the *gene SR-Y*. A genetic abnormality may produce the wrong gonad, a mixed gonad, or a different gonad on each side.

Testes produce testosterone, *anti-Mullerian hormone* (AMH) [also known as Mullerian inhibiting substance (MIS)], and Insulin-like growth factor.

Testosterone acts on receptors to produce most aspects of male development. But, there is a *masculinizing programming window* between 8 and 12 weeks of fetal life. Failure of testosterone action at this time will, therefore, lead to some feminization of an otherwise male individual.

Some testosterone is converted to *dihydrotestosterone* by the action of *5-alpha reductase*

M. Lima, G. Manzoni (eds.), *Pediatric Urology: Contemporary Strategies from Fetal Life to Adolescence*,
DOI 10.1007/978-88-470-5693-0_20, © Springer-Verlag Italia 2015

Table 20.1 Proposed nomenclature from Chicago consensus meeting [1]

Previous	New
Intersex	Disorder of sex development
Male pseudohermaphrodite	–
Undervirilization of XY male	46 XY DSD
Undermasculinization of an XY male	–
Female pseudohermaphrodite	–
Overvirilization of an XX female	46 XX DSD
Masculinization of an XX female	–
True hermaphrodite	Ovotesticular DSD
XX male or XX sex reversal	Ovotesticular DSD
XY sex reversal	46 XY complete gonadal dysgenesis

(5-AR). Five-AR is needed for testicular descent and phallic and *prostatic growth.*

AMH is secreted by *Sertoli cells* of testis. It causes regression of the uterus, Fallopian tubes, the lining of ovaries, and the upper third of vagina. Its highest concentration is at birth, and its function stops completely at puberty. It acts unilaterally so it is possible for the genitalia in the two sides of the pelvis to be different.

Insulin-like growth factor is secreted by *Leydig cells* and acts bilaterally. It is required for development of the *penis* and for general fetal growth. Absence will cause *microphallus*, but no other genital anomalies, and possibly *growth hormone*-resistant maldevelopment.

Although these are the most important influences on the fetus, there are other factors that contribute.

SR-Y and other sex determining genes (not all on the sex chromosomes, e.g., *WT1*, *SOX9*, *SF1*) contribute to regression of *Mullerian* structures, general male development, and, perhaps most importantly, brain sexual differentiation. In particular, the *Gadd45g gene* has been identified as an important determinant of testis and male sex development and fertility [2]. Their absence in a 46XY fetus will push development towards a female pathway, and the gonads will be little streaks or dysgenetic. Because the gonad is not a testis, it does not produce MIS, and so female genitalia develop.

Hormones unrelated to the genital system are also relevant. *Congenital adrenal hyperplasia* is due to blocks in the development of steroids in the adrenal. This leads to the accumulation of steroid precursors that are androgenic in action. They cause masculinization of androgen-sensitive structures including the brain and retention of *Mullerian* structures. In a 46XY fetus, the effect may pass unnoticed except in severe cases with salt wasting. In the 46XX fetus, there is genital ambiguity (another term to be avoided) due to androgenization of the *clitoris* and the *brain*.

Androgens are only able to exert their effect if they are bound to receptors in the target organs. Complete or partial failure of the receptors prevents the androgens working. This means that the target will maintain its default, female appearance and function. This produces the *androgen insensitivity syndromes* – complete (CAIS) and partial (PAIS).

If the androgens are bound to the receptors, male development and function occur. The vas deferens, seminal vesicles, and epididymes develop from the *Wolffian duct*. In the brain, androgens first undergo aromatization to the estrogen 17-β-oestrodiol and then bind to estrogen receptors.

20.3 Clinical Effects of DSD

20.3.1 The Penis

The penis is the most obvious manifestation of maleness in the neonate. In the past, a *small phallus*, regardless of other factors, sometimes mandated a female sex. Such an assignment was based on the view that gender development could be directed by administration of appropriate hormones and external influences and that it was easier to create a vagina than a penis by surgery.

It has now become clear that the most important influence on gender-specific thoughts and behavior is the hormone milieu in the brain during fetal development. An androgenized brain is difficult to divert from male-type function.

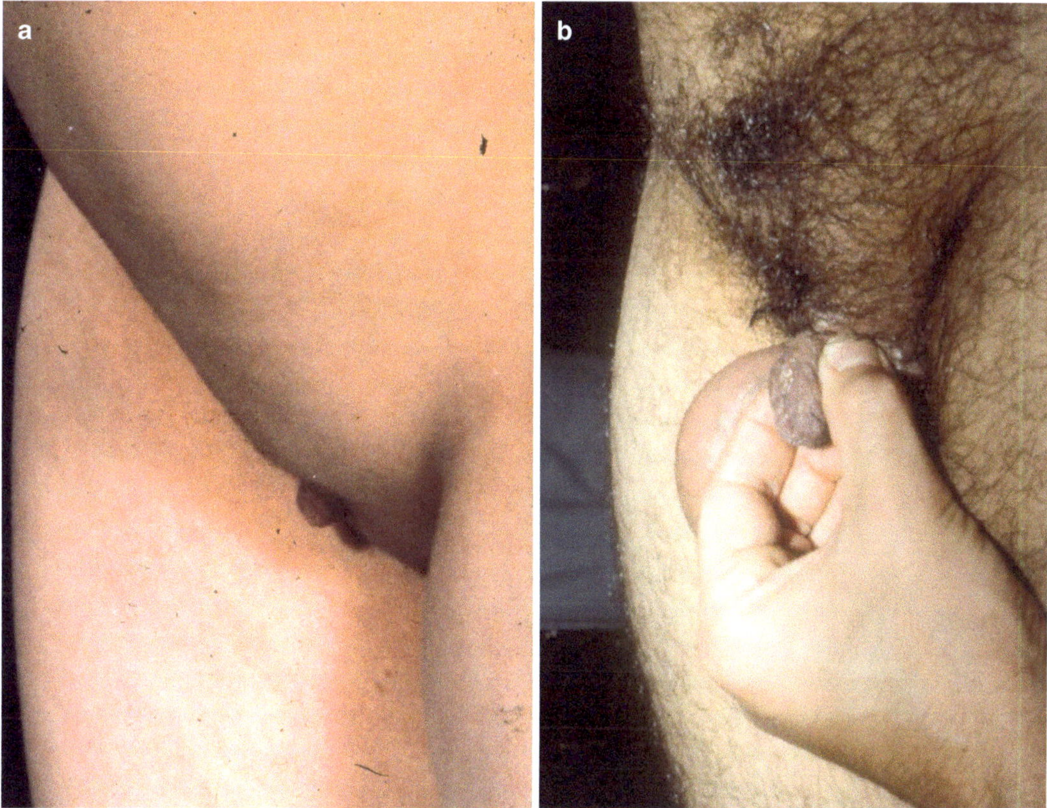

Fig. 20.1 (**a**) Clinical photograph of prepubertal micropenis. (**b**) Clinical photograph of an adult with micropenis

The penis grows at puberty under the influence of *testosterone*. Testosterone given before puberty produces some growth, but probably no more than would occur at puberty anyway. *Dihydrotestosterone cream* may give some penile development after puberty. However, in practice, a baby born with a *small penis* (more than two standard deviations below the mean stretched length) will grow up with a small penis (Fig. 20.1). There are few data on the sexual function of a small penis. However, that which is available indicates that it is satisfactory, at least to the man (Table 20.2). The attitude of sexual partners is unknown.

In practice, it may be difficult to convince an adolescent that his small penis is compatible with normal *sexual function*. There are so many images on the *Internet* and so much public discussion that those who feel their penis is inadequate may seek reconstructive surgery. They are also aware that such surgery is possible, especially using the techniques available for female to male gender reassignment [3]. It is possible to incorporate the small natural penis in the reconstructed one so that some of the original sexual function is preserved. Although sexual sensation is reported in the reconstructed phallus, there are no long-term data in patients with DSD.

20.3.2 The Clitoris

The clitoris has no known function other than to provide sexual pleasure. If exposed to androgens in utero it will enlarge. This is most commonly seen in *CAH*. Even the most precise endocrine control does not make the clitoris shrink, though it may prevent further hypertrophy.

Surgery to reduce the size of the clitoris, bury it or even to amputate it, has been used exten-

Table 20.2 Literature review of sexual function in men with micropenis

Reference	[29]	[30]	[31]	[32]	[33]	[34]	[35]	Total
Patients	20	19	9	20	13	8	3	92
GID	0	–	2	0	0	0	0	2
Erections	20	15	9	20	13	–	3	80 (95 %)
Heterosexual	20	–	6	19	10	–	3	58
Homosexual	0	–	3	–	1	–	–	4
Bisexual	0	–	–	1	2	–	–	3
Regular SI	15	6	–	12	–	6	3	42

GID gender identity disorder, *SI* sexual intercourse

sively in CAH in the past. Burial of the clitoris is no longer practiced because it results in painful erections with sexual arousal. Amputation of the clitoris is now recognized as a crime in most countries.

Clitoral reduction may be requested by the parents of a CAH neonate. They perceive a problem in child care by nonfamily members. It is also felt that school-age children may be embarrassed by a visible clitoris. Unfortunately, clitoral surgery both in infancy and in adults reduces, or may even abolish, *sexual sensation* and *orgasm* [4, 5]. In a study of the fine clitoral sensation in women with CAH who had or had not had *clitoral reduction*, only 22 % of the operated patients were normal compared to 80 % of the unoperated ones [4].

Furthermore, women who have had clitoral reduction in infancy, obviously without their consent, often feel that they have been mutilated and have considerable psychological problems as a result [6]. It is, of course, possible that women who did not have surgery and grew up with a conspicuous clitoris may also have psychological issues, but data are lacking. The *Chicago consensus* recommended that *clitoral reduction* should only be performed for gross enlargement [1]. However, some support groups advocate that such surgery should not be performed until the woman can give informed consent [7].

20.3.3 The Vagina

In *CAH* with a 46XX genotype, the vagina and *urethra* form a single *urogenital sinus*. The level of confluence is variable but always below the bladder neck so they are continent.

The timing of *vaginal reconstruction* appears to have been a matter of contention for at least 25 years. It would seem that only a minority of children are reconstructed in a single operation in infancy or early childhood [8]. In looking at the long-term follow-up of 16 women (of an original 32 children), Lattimer's group concluded in 1976 that the results of *vaginoplasty* were so poor that the operation should not be done before puberty [9].

There is some conflict about the wisdom of routine *dilatation of the vagina* after *genitoplasty* in infancy. Krege et al. suggest that it should not be a routine if only because of the *psychological problems* that it may cause (though they offer no evidence for this fear) [10]. Gearhart and, even more strongly, Hendren recommend dilatation to prevent postoperative stenosis [11]. In spite of this, all of Hendren's patients required further, albeit minor, surgery at puberty to allow *intercourse*. Nonetheless, *feminizing vaginoplasty* is commonly done in infancy though there continues to be pressure to delay it.

More complex vaginal reconstructions may use self-dilatation or surgical reconstruction with skin, bowel, or grafted tissues (Figs. 20.2 and 20.3). There is general agreement that such surgery should be reserved for the time of puberty or later.

Follow-up of complex *vaginoplasties* is limited and often has been confined to establishing that *intercourse* takes place without undue difficulty (Table 20.3). For example, up to 70 % of women who had an *intestinal vagina* formed report the ability to have intercourse with a

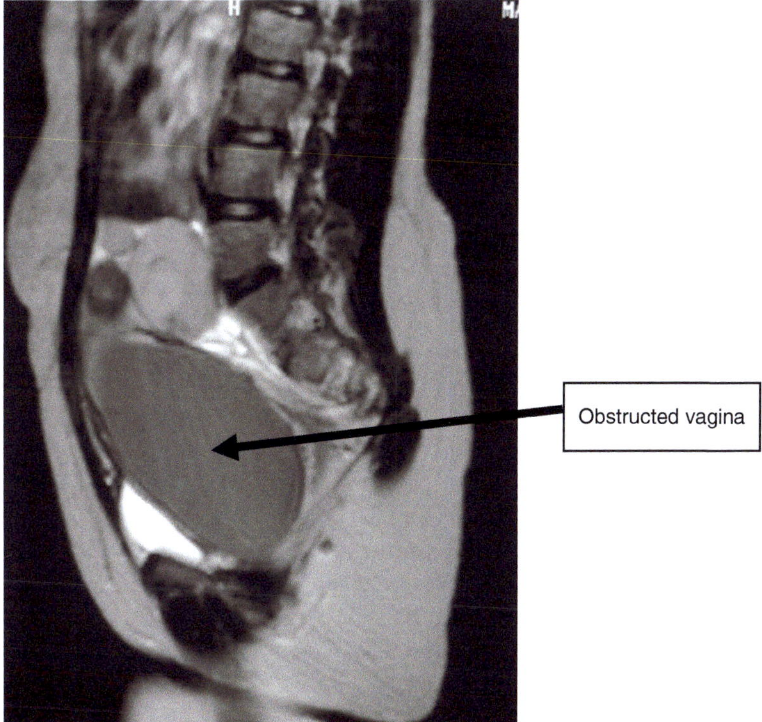

Fig. 20.2 Sagittal view of an MRI of the pelvis showing an obstructed vagina that has been dilated by repeated menstruation

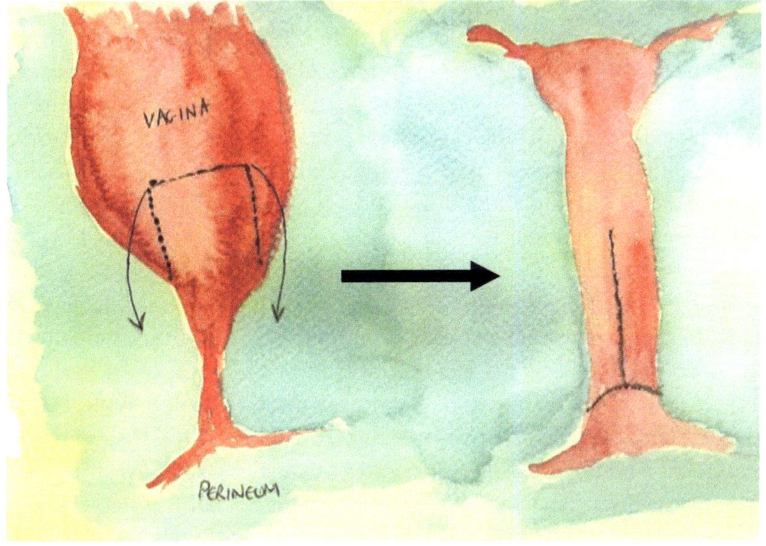

Fig. 20.3 Diagram to show how the obstructed upper vagina can be opened with an inferiorly based flap which is folded down to reach the perineum (Courtesy of D.N.Wood)

10 % incidence of *dyspareunia* [12]. Schober, in an extensive review of the literature, found that follow-up assessment was usually confined to the observation that penetrative *intercourse* was possible with no attempt to measure its quality [7]. There was little critical evaluation of *female sexuality*.

Although it is correct to evaluate the quality of intercourse as well as possible to decide which technique is the best, it must be remembered that such surgery is only done to enable penetrative intercourse to take place – it might be said that poor intercourse may be better than none at all.

Table 20.3 The table shows the number of women who have a patent vagina after primary surgery (1 year patency) and the additional number patent after revision surgery (2 year patency)

Reference	[8]	[11]	[36]	[10]
Number	42	28	13	27
1-year patency	5	6	0	14
2-year patency	33	18	2	8
Intercourse	33	11	0	6 of 15[a]

In the paper by Alizai et al.[36], the mean age of the patients was 13.1; although all were postpubertal, all were thought to be too young for intercourse to be considered. In Krege et al.'s [10] paper, intercourse was only considered in 15[a] patients over 15 years who completed a questionnaire

20.3.4 The Gonads

The gonads can be the most difficult part of DSD conditions to understand, especially as they may be different on each side. In females with *CAH*, the gonads are *ovaries* which are structurally normal though with reduced function [13]. Conversely, patients with complete *androgen insensitivity*, by definition 46XY, have gonads that are testicular with *Sertoli cells* but very few germ cells and are usually undescended. In PAIS, up to 64 % may have one descended *testis* [14].

As a *Y chromosome* is necessary to form a *testis*, syndromes in which it is absent will have gonads that are ovarian-like in structure with very variable function. Even if there is a Y chromosome present, absence or defect of the testis determining genes may lead to a *dysgenetic gonad*, a mixed gonad, or a different one on each side. In some, germ cells may be present.

Abnormal gonads are at increased risk of *neoplasia,* and this has an impact on the management. The majority are *germ cell neoplasms,* and so some germ cells must be present in the gonad, even though primitive and small in number. The more dysplastic the germ cells, the higher the risk of neoplasia.

The highest risk is with *dysgenetic gonads* in individuals who are 46XY. The commonest example of this rare group has *Swire's syndrome*. The babies are phenotypically female without genital ambiguity with normal internal female structures. With *mixed gonadal dysgenesis,* the genitalia are ambiguous, and there is usually some fairly normal testicular tissue on one side. The gonads are either streaks or contain some testicular tissue and may be different on each side.

The usual tumor is a *gonadoblastoma*. This is a mixed tumor of *Sertoli cells* and *germ cells*, with occasional *Leydig cells*. The gonadoblastoma never metastasizes and may even regress, but in a third of cases, the germ cell portion becomes malignant. The endocrine cells may secrete active hormones, especially *testosterone* [15]. The tumors may occur, though rarely, in utero or childhood [16]. The incidence rises rapidly after puberty and is highest at the usual age for germ cell tumors in the second and third decades [15, 17].

Primary, *malignant dysgerminoma* may occur occasionally in dysgenetic gonads. This is the name given to a *seminoma* in a gonad thought to be an *ovary* or of indeterminate type.

In androgen insensitivity, especially in its complete form seminomas occur. They are rare in childhood but commoner in the second and third decades.

On testicular biopsy, abnormal cells can be seen which precede the development of *carcinoma in situ* which has been taken as an indication for gonadectomy [18]. However, some patients wish the gonads to remain in situ as *aromatization* of the *androgens* produced are thought to give more normal femininity than the synthetic replacement estrogen that would be given after gonadectomy [19]. The problem then is in determining when the gonads are becoming malignant. *Carcinoma in situ* has been identified in gonads that by MRI criteria look benign [20] (Fig. 20.4).

46XX individuals are at relatively low risk of germ cell neoplasia. This is particularly true of the commonest condition – *CAH*.

It is also important to note that 46XY patients with CAH may develop scrotal masses. They may be large and bilateral. They are not neoplasms but due to *hypertrophy of adrenal rests*. They will resolve with proper adrenal suppression. The testes should not be removed [21].

20.3.5 Internal Genitalia

The female internal genitalia will be present to some extent if there is a failure of the *Mullerian*

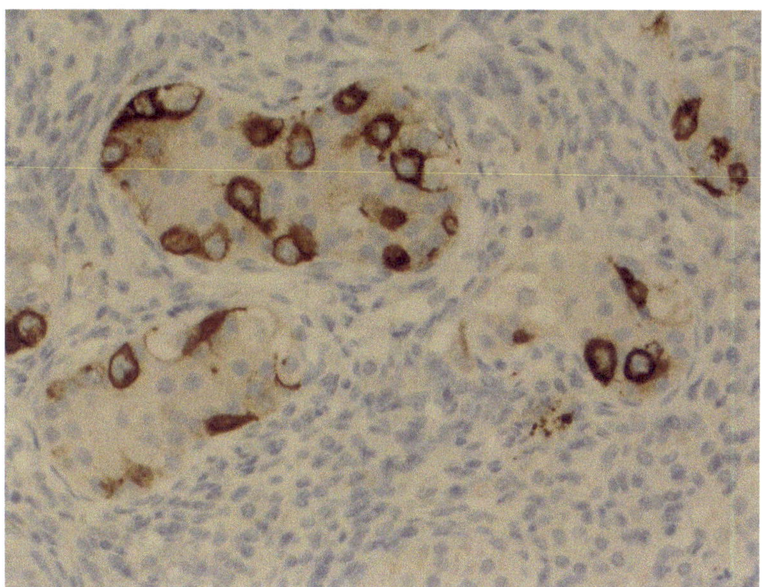

Fig. 20.4 Photomicrograph showing intratubular germ cell neoplasia in a Sertoli cell nodule which had benign characteristics on MRI scan. The dark brown cells are stained with antibody against placental alkaline phosphatase confirming their malignant nature (Courtesy of Dr Alex Freeman)

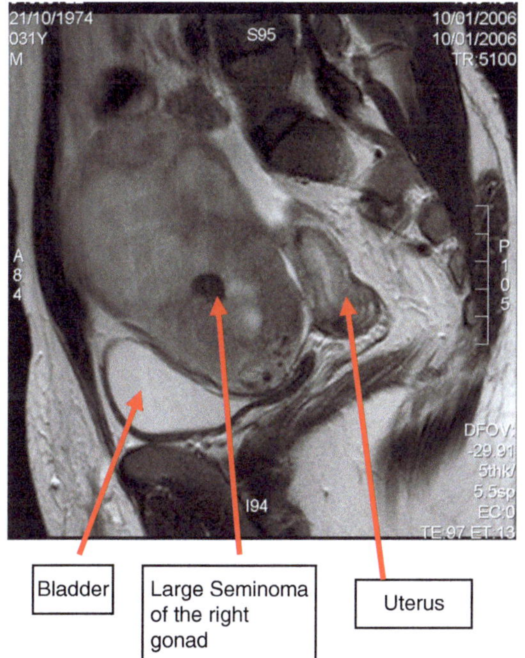

Fig. 20.5 MRI scan, sagittal view of a 46XY male with failure of Mullerian regression. He presented with an abdominal mass which was found to be a gonadal seminoma. A uterus is seen to be present attached to the *top* of the prostate

inhibiting substance, regardless of the genotype. This is illustrated in Fig. 20.5. The structures are usually small and nonfunctional. Cystic or tubular structures on the back of the prostate in otherwise normal men are reasonably common. They are not usually functional and are found by chance. They do not have to be removed unless a symptomatic complication arises.

20.4 Gender

In the past, the birth of a baby with indeterminate gender was considered to be an emergency. A gender of rearing was quickly decided on the best evidence then available and maintained. Current practice is to postpone a decision until a complete diagnosis can be made. Some clinicians advocate leaving a decision until sufficient social development of the child occurs to give a clue to internal gender identity. Although such practice has obvious advantages, it is very difficult for most families to cope with a child who is neither boy nor girl.

The major influences in the decision are the genotype, the likely hormonal environment of the brain in fetal life, and the prospects for fertility. The appearance of the genitalia is less influential. However, it is recognized that election to change gender or even to live in an in-between state may well occur in later life.

This means that the decision in the commonest diagnosis is relatively easy. Babies with *CAH* will almost always be raised in gender of their genotype unless the diagnosis is delayed. The brain in 46XX CAH individuals is androgenized in utero which leads to some "male-type" imprinting.

Undervirilized babies with 46XY genotype but some functioning testes will usually be raised male. The former view that an inadequate penis was an indication for female assignment is no longer accepted. Most will continue to live as males.

On the other hand, babies found to have CAIS are always raised female and continue to live as such. In partially affected babies (PAIS), the decision is based on the degree of virilization, and the long-term outcome is unpredictable.

20.5 Fertility

20.5.1 Congenital Adrenal Hyperplasia

Fertility is diminished in CAH patients of both sexes. In males, providing the steroid control is meticulous, the problem is much less.

Women with 21-hydroxylase deficiency, 11-beta-hydroxylase deficiency, and 3-beta-hydroxylase deficiency are potentially fertile. However, infrequent ovulation compounded by poor compliance with steroid replacement therapy reduces the likelihood of *pregnancy*. The ovulation rate per cycle is only about 40 % with a good correlation between plasma testosterone and 17-hydroxyprogesterone levels [22].

Up until the 1980s, although the fertility rate was known to be about 60 % reports of successful pregnancy in salt losers were uncommon [23]. In a relatively large and unselected series of 80 women (half being salt losers), 40 were having heterosexual *intercourse*. Fifteen of twenty-five with simple virilization had 25 pregnancies producing 20 normal children. In contrast, only 1 of 15 salt losers became pregnant, and she had an elective termination [24].

It would seem that better steroid management has improved prospects for salt losers. In a more recent series, three of five with salt wasting CAH and two of three with simple virilizing CAH who were sexually active had eight successful pregnancies [22].

20.5.2 Other Female Conditions

In the rarer conditions, pregnancies have been reported. Unfortunately, even if there are useful ova, the uterus may be so hypoplastic that a pregnancy cannot be supported. Nonetheless, "*reproductive technology*" is becoming progressively more sophisticated which, combined with greater acceptance of surrogacy, is improving the prospects. Pregnancies have been reported in *Swire's syndrome* and in some 46XX/46XY mosaics.

20.5.3 Males

The techniques that have been developed to allow the direct injection of a single sperm into an ovum (ICSI) have revolutionized the prognosis of difficult male factor infertility. Most countries allow the use of *sperm* retrieved from ejaculate, *epididymis,* or testis. The use of sperm precursors is more controversial both because of poor results and for ethical considerations.

In *Klinefelter's syndrome* (47XXY) and in *5-alpha reductase deficiency,* occasional paternity has been reported [25, 26].

20.6 Impact of Adult Outcomes on Future Management of Infants

The observation that adult outcomes of babies born with DSD are not uniformly satisfactory does not, in any way, imply that earlier management was wrong, let alone malevolent. Medical protocols are based on the best evidence available at the time. They are adapted, slowly, as more information becomes available from science and from the patients themselves. It is always difficult to predict the future and particularly so when a "right answer" appears to be so elusive.

It should also be remembered that it is only recently that children born with intersex were informed of their diagnosis. There may be many adults living perfectly fulfilled lives, unaware that they had an intersex condition.

In some intersex conditions, *intercourse* may be impossible without surgery. If the outcome of surgery allows intercourse to take place but is unsatisfactory, it might be that it is better than no intercourse at all.

At one end of the spectrum, there is the view that babies could be raised in an indeterminate gender until they are old enough to make their own decision. In a limited way, such a policy is followed in *Papua New Guinea* where babies with *5-alpha reductase deficiency* are recognized as a third gender. In most countries, especially where DSD babies are very rare, society may not be sophisticated enough to cope with an indeterminate gender. Indeed, anecdotally, families in whom there has been a reassignment of gender of a baby have had difficulty in coping – often having to relocate to a new neighborhood.

Individuals cannot be divorced from the culture in which they live. In some countries male children are economically more valuable than female; in others, the prospects for sexual *intercourse* are influential. *Gender assignment* may be governed by factors that impress the parents and doctors but might be rejected by the child when an adult. It would be virtually impossible to escape from the views of the parents and the wider society in deciding on the management of infants. Nonetheless, it would be hoped that interests of the child could be put above all others. The patient pressure group, the *Intersex Society of North America* advocates, at the very least, withholding of genital surgery until the children are old enough to identify their own sexuality. Such a view seems even more correct when the possibilities for fertility are considered.

It would seem prudent to manage children on the basis that *fertility* will be possible so that gonadal tissue and the reproductive organs should be preserved.

In girls with poor development of the *uterus* or absent *Fallopian tubes*, the uterus should be preserved. There have even been anecdotal cases of pregnancy running to term outside a uterus [27, 28]. In future, a uterus may not be a prerequisite for a pregnancy.

In some cases the initial management might involve the removal of germinal tissue. It is now possible to store this material in case the decision is later reversed. The practicalities are experimental, and the ethical aspects are unresolved. Nonetheless, if storage is not undertaken, the present generation of patients will lose any possibility of parenthood.

Testicular tissue can be preserved from prepubertal boys but should only be done as part of an approved research project at present. *Spermarche* is at a mean age of 13.4. At present, it is not known to what use the tissues could be put, and there are considerable ethical dilemmas both in raising expectations which may not be fulfilled and in predicting the outcome of research yet to be done.

References

1. Hughes IA, Houk C, Ahmed SF, Lee PA (2006) Consensus statement on the management of intersex disorders. Arch Dis Child 91:554–563
2. Johnen H, Gonzalez-Silva L, Carramolino L, Flores JM, Torres M, Salvador JM (2013) Gadd45g is essential for primary sex determination, male fertility and testis development. PLoS One 8(3):e58751
3. Vardi Y, Gruenwald I (2009) The status of penile enhancement procedures. Curr Opin Urol 19:601–605
4. Minto CL, Liao L-M, Woodhouse CRJ, Ransley PG, Creighton SM (2003) The effect of clitoral surgery on sexual outcome in individuals who have intersex conditions with ambiguous genitalia: a cross sectional study. Lancet 361:1252–1257
5. Schober JM (2001) Sexual behaviours, sexual orientation and gender identity in adult intersexuals: a pilot study. J Urol 165:2350–2353
6. Zucker KJ, Bradley SJ, Oliver G, Blake J, Fleming S, Hood J (1996) Psychosexual behaviour of women with congenital adrenal hyperplasia. Horm Behav 30:300–318
7. Schober JM (1999) Feminising genitoplasty for intersex. In: Stringer MD, Oldham KT, Mouriquand PDE, Howard ER (eds) Paediatric surgery and urology: long term outcomes. W.B.Saunders, London, pp 549–558
8. Azziz R, Mulaikal RM, Migeon CG, Jones HW, Rock JA (1986) Congenital adrenal hyperplasia: long term results following vaginal reconstruction. Fertil Steril 46:1011–1014

9. Sotiropoulos A, Morishima A, Homsy Y, Lattimer JK (1976) Long term assessment of genital reconstruction in female pseudohermaphrodites. J Urol 115:599–601
10. Krege S, Walz KH, Hauffa BP, Körner I, Rübben H (2000) Long term follow up of female patients with congenital adrenal hyperplasia from 21-hydroxylase deficiency, with special emphasis on the results of vaginoplasty. Br J Urol Int 86:253–259
11. Bailez MM, Gearhart JP, Migeon CG, Rock JA (1992) Vaginal reconstruction after initial construction of the external genitalia in girls with salt wasting adrenal hyperplasia. J Urol 148:680–684
12. Hensle TW, Dean GE (1992) Vaginal replacement in children. J Urol 148:677–679
13. Gastaud F, Buvattier C, Duranteau L (2007) Impaired sexual and reproductive outcomes in women with classical forms of congenital adrenal hyperplasia. J Clin Endocrinol Metab 92:1391–1396
14. Morel Y, Teinturier C, Nicolino M, Michel-Calemard L, Mowszowicz I, Jaubert F et al (2002) Aetiological diagnosis of male sexual ambiguity: a collaborative study. Eur J Pediatr 161:49–59
15. Savage MO, Lowe DG (1990) Gonadal neoplasia and abnormal sexual differentiation. Clin Endocrinol 32:519–533
16. Manuel M, Katayama KP, Jones HW (1976) The age of occurrence of gonadal tumours in intersex patients with a Y chromosome. Am J Obstet Gynecol 124:293–300
17. Ramani P, Yeung CK, Habeebu SSM (1993) Testicular intratubular germ cell neoplasia in children and adolescents with intersex. Am J Surg Pathol 17:1124–1133
18. Muller J, Skakkebaek NE, Neilson OH, Graem N (1984) Cryptorchidism and testis cancer: atypical germ cells followed by carcinoma in situ in adult age. Cancer 54:629–634
19. Crouch NS, Creighton SM, Woodhouse CRJ (2003) Changing attitudes to intersex management. Eur Urol Today 14(2):1–5
20. Nakhal RS, Hall-Craggs M, Freeman A, Kirkham A, Conway GS, Arora R et al (2013) Evaluation of retained testes in adolescent girls and women with complete androgen insensitivity syndrome. Radiology 268(1):153–160
21. Cutfield RG, Bateman JM, Odell DD (1983) Infertility caused by bilateral testicular masses secondary to congenital adrenal hyperplasia (21-hydroxylase deficiency). Fertil Steril 40:809–814
22. Premawardhana LD, Hughes IA, Read GF, Scanlon MF (1997) Longer term outcome in females with congenital adrenal hyperplasia (CAH): the Cardiff experience. Clin Endocrinol 20(11):690–694
23. Klingensmith GJ, Garcia SC, Jones HW, Migeon CG, Blizzard RM (1977) Glucocorticoid treatment of girls with congenital adrenal hyperplasia: effects on height, sexual maturation and fertility. J Pediatr 90:996–1004
24. Mulaikal RM, Migeon CG, Rock JA (1987) Fertility rates in female patients with congenital adrenal hyperplasia due to 21-hydroxylase deficiency. N Engl J Med 316:178–182
25. Katz MD, Kligman I, Cai L-Q, Zhu Y-S, Fratianni CM, Zervoudakis I et al (1997) Paternity by intrauterine insemination with sperm from a man with 5-alpha reductase deficiency. N Engl J Med 336:994–998
26. Tournaye H, Staessen C, Liebaers I, van Assche E, Devroey P, Bonduelle M (1996) Testicular sperm recovery in nine 47XXY Klinefelter patients. Hum Reprod 11:1644–1649
27. Sinha RK (1970) Primary abdominal pregnancy: review of the literature and a report of three cases. Med J Malaya 25:108–112
28. Dahniya MH, Shoukry IF, Balami WI, Fatukasi JI (1990) Simultaneous advanced extra uterine and intra uterine pregnancy. Int J Gynaecol Obstet 31:61–65
29. Reilly JM, Woodhouse CRJ (1989) Small penis and the male sexual role. J Urol 142:569–571
30. Miller MAW, Grant DB (1997) Severe hypospadias with genital ambibuity: adult outcome after staged hypospadias repair. Br J Urol 80:485–488
31. Money J, Lehne GK, Pirerre-Jerome F (1985) Micropenis: gender, heterosexual coping strategy and behavioural health in nine pediatric cases followed into adulthood. Comp Psychiatr 26:29–42
32. Husmann DA (2004) The androgen insensitive micropenis: longterm follow-up into adulthood. J Pediatr Endocrinol Metab 17(8):1037–1041
33. Wisniewski AB, Migeon CG, Gearhart JP, Rock JA, Berkowitz DG, Plotnick LP et al (2001) Congenital micropenis: long term medical, surgical and psychosexual follow-up of individuals raised male or female. Horm Res 56:3–11
34. Bin-Abbas B, Conte FA, Grumbach MM, Kaplan SL (1999) Congenital hypogonadotrophic hypogonadism and micropenis: effect of testosterone treatment on adult penile size why sex reversal is not indicated. J Pediatr 134:579–583
35. van Seters AP, Slob AK (1988) Mutually gratifying heterosexual relationship with micropenis of husband. J Sex Marital Ther 14:98–107
36. Alizai N, Thomas DFM, Lilford RJ, Batchelor AGG, Johnson N (1999) Feminizing genitoplasty for congenital adrenal hyperplasia: what happens at puberty? J Urol 161:1588–1591

Disorders of Sexual Development: Surgical Management

21

Richard C. Rink and Konrad M. Szymanski

21.1 Introduction

There is no topic in pediatric urology/surgery that generates as much controversy as surgery for *disorders of sexual development* (DSD). Furthermore it is one of the most complex surgical problems this specialty will encounter. While there is less disagreement in the treatment of children with *congenital adrenal hyperplasia* (CAH) than with other forms of DSD, it certainly has its own share of controversies. Historically most parents have elected early surgery (infancy) to "normalize" their child's ambiguous genitalia. This has been thought to be of psychological benefit to the child, parents, and caregivers, but there is little data to support this. Both Lloyd et al. [1] and Akbiyik and Kutlu [2] have now shown there to be tremendous variability in genital proportions of "normal" adults and children who do not have a DSD. Advocacy groups and some physicians have challenged the wisdom of early surgery with some even calling for a moratorium on any DSD genital surgery until the patient is old enough to decide for themselves whether or not they want surgery [3]. Creighton et al. have noted that the thought of "doing nothing" can be stressful for families [4]. The ethical considerations of parental versus child rights to make decisions about surgery remain unresolved in the United States. This is an extraordinarily difficult time for young parents who give birth to a child with DSD. We feel strongly that the parent should know of all pros and cons of both having surgery and not having surgery. No parent should ever be talked into having surgery. The parents should also be an integral part of the gender assignment team and participate in all decisions. Families should be supported regardless of decision for or against surgery. Advocacy groups can be of great help to the families, and we would recommend that the families have access to the CARES Foundation (caresfoundation.org), Accord Alliance (accordalliance.org), and the Magic Foundation (magicfoundation.org) prior to ever seeing the surgeon.

The overwhelmingly most common cause of genital ambiguity occurs secondary to CAH, and therefore the vast majority of those undergoing feminizing genitoplasty do so for CAH. We therefore will concentrate our discussion on CAH, but the principles described herein are applicable to all DSD patients undergoing surgery to feminize the genitalia regardless of their age. For the purposes of this chapter, we will address the management and surgical options of these anomalies under the assumption that everyone involved in the decision-making process, including the patient, family, and the multidisciplinary medical team, agree that surgery is appropriate. If surgery

R.C. Rink, MD, FAAP, FACS (✉)
K.M. Szymanski, MD, MPH
Department of Pediatric Urology,
Riley Hospital for Children, Indiana University
School of Medicine, 705 Riley Hospital Drive
ROC #4230, Indianapolis, IN 46202, USA
e-mail: rrink@iupui.edu; szymanko@iupui.edu

M. Lima, G. Manzoni (eds.), *Pediatric Urology: Contemporary Strategies from Fetal Life to Adolescence*,
DOI 10.1007/978-88-470-5693-0_21, © Springer-Verlag Italia 2015

is elected, options for the precise timing of surgery and their particular advantages and disadvantages need to be discussed.

21.2 Anatomy

With virilization found in CAH, there is almost always some degree of clitoral hypertrophy, varying degrees of a *urogenital sinus* (UGS), and the labia majora tend to have varying amounts of fusion and are anteriorly displaced. The labia minora are absent. The urethra and vagina normally exit the pelvis separately between the labia. This does not happen in cases of persistent UGS, where a communication persists between the urinary tract and the vagina and the common channel exits on the perineum (Fig. 21.1). UGS anomalies generally occur in two main forms, those with ambiguous genitalia and those with pure UGS abnormalities. It is our belief that a pure UGS is forme fruste of a cloacal anomaly and much different from those with CAH. In the CAH group, the Prader scale is useful for assessing external genitalia, but external appearance does not always correlate with internal appearance [5].

Although the *confluence of the vagina with the urethra* is usually described as "low" (near the perineum) or "high" (near the bladder neck), it actually occurs in a spectrum of presentation [6–8]. We are in agreement with Ganesan that the distance from the bladder neck to the vagina is relatively constant in CAH [9]. Overall, three elements contribute to an appearance of a higher confluence: (1) a longer distance from the vagina to the UGS meatus; (2) the virilization of the UGS gives an appearance of a male-like external sphincter, verumontanum, and prostatic-like tissue [10]; and (3) a more compact, android pelvis. While it may be unclear if a true high confluence exists in patients with CAH, patients with a longer UGS certainly appear to be more virilized and are much more difficult to repair.

21.3 Evaluation

Management of patients with CAH begins with medical stabilization, making the appropriate diagnosis and assembling the multidisciplinary *gender assignment team*. The team consists of specialists in neonatology, genetics, endocrinology, pediatric urology/surgery, and psychiatry [11]. Making the correct diagnosis is mandatory, but once done, the anatomy needs to be defined. Historically, this has been done by genitography and endoscopy. In certain situations, pelvic and abdominal ultrasound and, rarely, MRI may be beneficial. At a high-volume tertiary institution like ours, routine genitography for patients with CAH may not be beneficial [12], but it remains helpful in patients with cloacal anomalies and other forms of DSD.

One of the critical, and often missed, parts of the evaluation of patients with DSD and UGS anomalies is a thorough assessment and appropriate management of any *associated anomalies*. This is particularly true in the setting of cloacal anomalies that have genital ambiguity. Associated abnormalities include upper urinary tract, cardiac, spinal cord, limb, and lumbosacral spine anomalies [13–17].

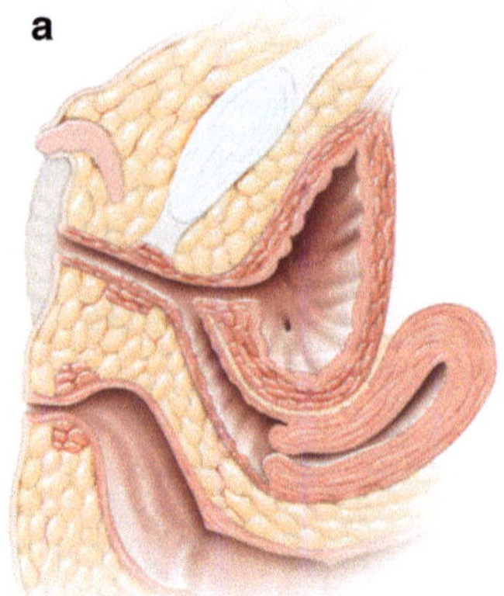

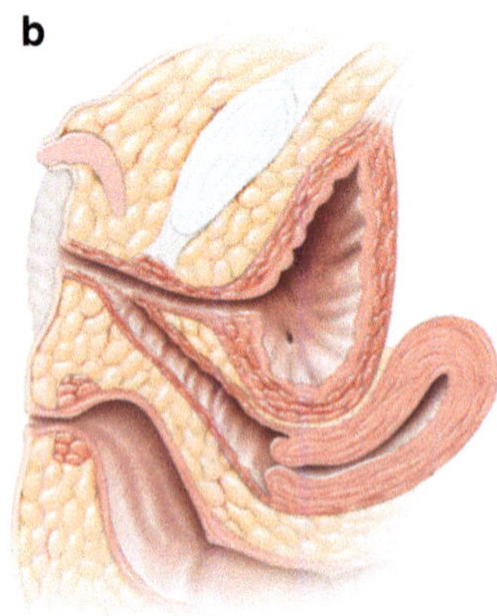

Fig. 21.1 High (**a**) and low (**b**) UGS

21.4 Surgical Approach

The surgical issues in the setting of CAH, as noted above, typically include (1) clitoromegaly, (2) labial abnormalities, and (3) the common UGS and how to manage the vagina. Consequently, surgical management involves (1) clitoroplasty, (2) labioplasty, and (3) vaginoplasty. Without question, the most controversial aspect regarding surgery for DSD is the timing of surgery. These *controversies* have been well covered in other publications but revolve around whether the parents have the right to make the decision for surgery or should these decisions always be made by the patient when they are old enough to do so. Another controversy revolves around whether the results are better in infancy or at puberty, particularly when considering the potential for postoperative vaginal stenosis. It is important to remember the differences between gender assignment, gender role, and gender identity. In general, the options are doing all three surgical components in infancy, which has been the norm in the United States, or waiting until puberty. There is a hybrid of these two approaches, which has many proponents around the world, where the clitoroplasty and labioplasty are performed in infancy and the vaginoplasty is delayed until puberty. We, and others, believe that surgery after puberty is more difficult [4]. For now, the controversy will continue, as unfortunately, there is no clear evidence to help us determine whether infantile or pubertal surgery has better long-term results.

21.5 Operative Technique

Preoperatively, the patient should be metabolically stable, particularly if the child has CAH. All children receive preoperative broad-spectrum antibiotics. Most children with CAH require only an enema, but a complete bowel preparation with a polyethylene glycol-electrolyte solution (GoLYTELY) may be warranted in a setting of a high confluence. Children with CAH should receive "stress dose" steroid replacement at the time of surgery.

After general anesthesia, endoscopy is performed. We initially place a Fogarty catheter into the vagina; its balloon is inflated, and the catheter is clamped and left indwelling. A Foley catheter is then anchored in the bladder (Fig. 21.2). Although some prefer to place the child in a lithotomy position, we find that this position limits vision to only the surgeon, hinders teaching, and prevents repositioning if a prone or abdominal approach is required. We prepare the lower body, from the nipples to the feet, with povidone-iodine, wrap the legs in stockinette, and pass the lower part of the body through the aperture in the drapes (Fig. 21.3). This allows the surgeon access to the abdomen and genitalia, as well as permit exposure in the supine or prone position. In postpubertal patients, total body preparation may be difficult, and the lithotomy position may be necessary.

a

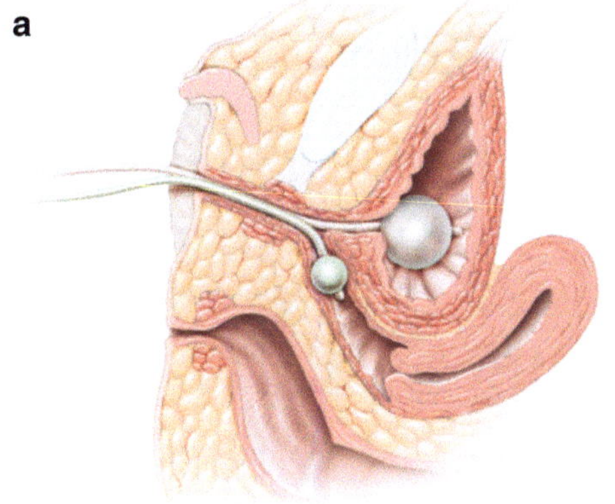

b

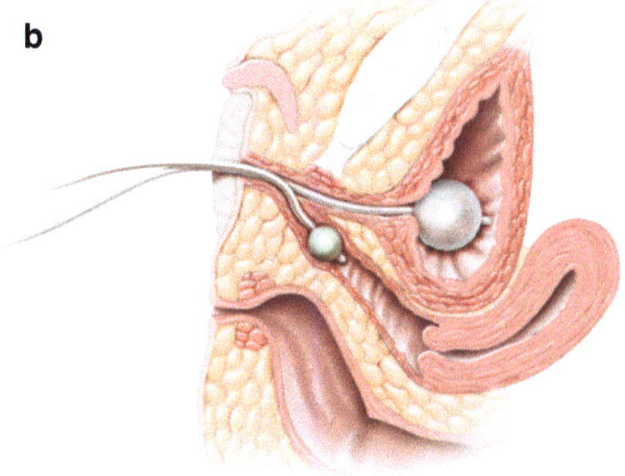

Fig. 21.2 A Fogarty catheter is placed into the vagina and a Foley catheter into the bladder (**a**) high UGS, (**b**) low UGS

21.6 Clitoroplasty

Historically, patients with clitoromegaly underwent clitoral amputations [18, 19]. Later, clitoral recession was used [20], but the procedure was

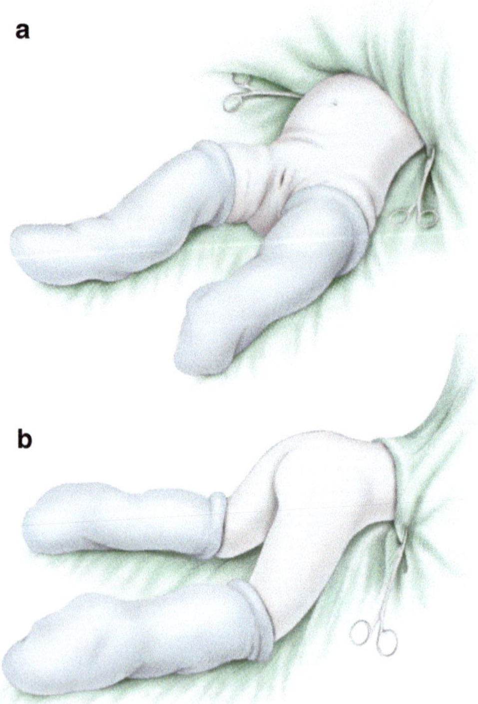

Fig. 21.3 Patient's preparation: front (**a**) and back (**b**)

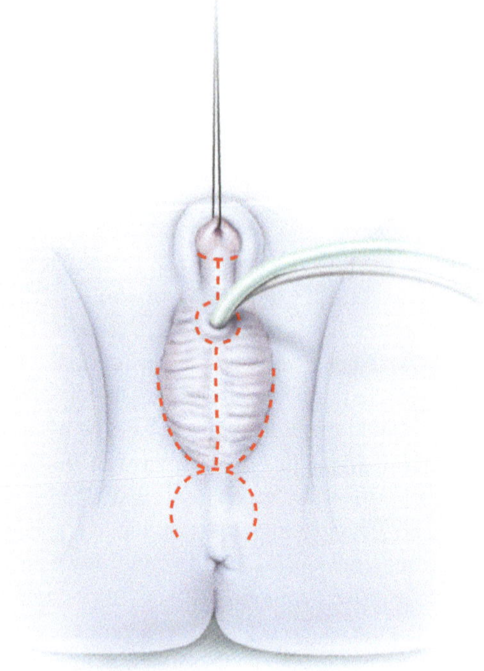

Fig. 21.4 Preposed incisions

associated with painful erections. Subsequent approaches were developed to expose the neurovascular bundles and amputate the corporal bodies, techniques which are still in use [21–25]. We believe a better approach involves excising erectile tissue alone [26]. Based on the work by Baskin and coworkers [27], we have modified the original lateral incisions described by Kogan to bilateral ventral incisions in order to prevent any injury to the neurovascular bundles [8]. We now preserve all of the preputial skin, which has been shown to be the second most sensitive area on the female perineum [28], to use in the construction of a clitoral hood.

The operation begins with placement of a traction suture in the glans clitoris. Proposed incisions are outlined with a skin scribe and injected with 0.5 % lidocaine with 1:200,000 epinephrine subcutaneously (Fig. 21.4). The initial incision is carried out dorsally at the junction of the inner preputial surface with the outer clitoral skin. The entire clitoris is degloved along the plane between the Buck fascia and the Dartos circumferentially. Ventrally, the incision is carried around the UGS meatus. The omega-shaped perineal flap should extend to near the meatus [29]. Parallel incisions on either side of the UGS plate will allow for the sinus to be preserved for later use in the reconstruction.

The perineal flap is elevated with its underlying subcutaneous and adipose tissue to expose the UGS. The bifurcation of the corporal bodies is exposed ventrally. A vertical ventral midline incision is made along the entire length of each corporal body from near the glans to near the bifurcation of the corporal bodies (Fig. 21.5). The erectile tissue is exposed and excised. Care must be taken not to injure the Buck fascia, the tunica albuginea, the *neurovascular bundle,* or glans. The proximal end of each bundle of erectile tissue is oversewn with 5-0 polyglycolic acid sutures. Buck's fascia is then folded, and the glans is secured to the corporal stumps with 5-0 polydioxanone sutures. Suturing the glans to the pubis prevents the glans from being appropriately concealed. In situations where the glans is quite large, one should resist aggressive glans reduction. If any reduction of the glans is done, it

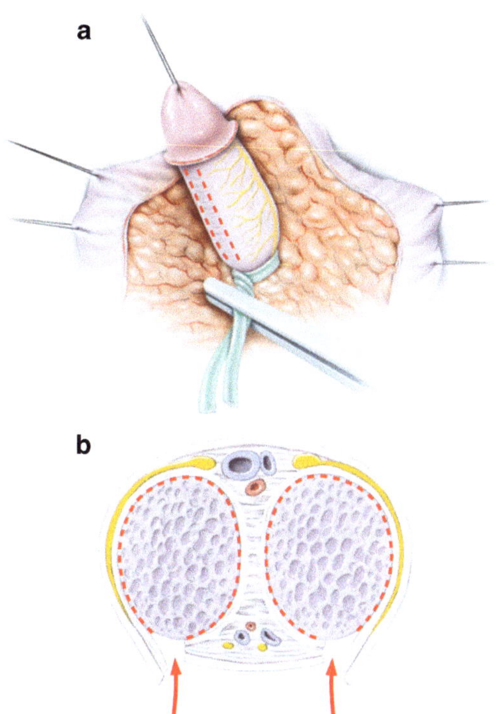

Fig. 21.5 Vertical ventral midline incision made along the entire lenght of each corporal body (**a**, **b**)

should only occur on its ventral aspect in order to prevent loss of sensation, as has been shown by Baskin [11, 27]. It is of note that no paper has shown that having a large clitoral glans is a medical problem. Salle's clitoroplasty involves a separation of the erectile bodies, concealing them in the labia [30]. This approach allows for a possible reassembly in the event of gender dysphoria. In conclusion, we only excise the erectile tissue, remain ventrally away from the neurovascular bundle, preserve all tunics, and avoid an aggressive glansplasty. It must be remembered that the clitoris is a sexual organ so every effort is made to preserve clitoral sensation and function, but even with modern techniques, some authors have concerns of sensory loss [31–33].

21.7 Vaginoplasty

The vaginoplasty is the most complex surgical component in feminizing genitoplasty. Adequate exposure is of utmost importance. The vagina can be accessed through the perineum, abdomen, or rectum. Importantly, any surgical dissection should avoid the area of the urethral sphincter and aims to preserve sensation and function. The multitude of vaginoplasties which have been described can be divided into four types: (1) cutback vaginoplasty, (2) flap vaginoplasty, (3) pull-through vaginoplasty, and (4) complete vaginal replacement. The choice of approach is guided by the level of the confluence between the UGS and the vagina. We believe that the distance between the bladder and the vagina is the most critical aspect of choosing management [34, 35].

While *cutback vaginoplasty* has recently been reported to have successful outcomes [36], we have significant concerns with this technique. Simply "cutting back" to the level of the confluence does not allow the surgeon to enter into the normal caliber of the proximal vagina, past the distal stenotic segment. Failure to do so results in apparent vaginal stenosis. The technique involves a midline vertical incision that is closed transversely in a Heineke-Mikulicz fashion. We use this only for simple *labial fusion*.

The flap vaginoplasty is used in cases of low vaginal confluence. Originally, the U-shaped flap was wide based, from one ischial tuberosity to the other. It has been shown that an omega-shaped flap with a narrower base avoids the appearance of a triangular introitus without compromising cosmesis [29]. In a flap vaginoplasty, the perineal flap is inserted into the opened ventral wall of the urogenital sinus and posterior vagina. It is imperative that the incision be carried through the narrowed distal vagina into the normal caliber proximal vagina in order to prevent later *vaginal stenosis*. Avoiding any dissection of the anterior and lateral aspects of the vagina decreases the risk of vaginal ischemia, thus avoiding stenosis.

It must be noted that the flap vaginoplasty simply opens the introitus to expose the vagina. It will always leave a somewhat hypospadiac urethra, and the posterior vaginal wall will be made of skin. The flap vaginoplasty is by far the most common procedure for UGS anomalies and has the least risks. In general, if the flap reaches into the normal caliber of the proximal vagina in a tension-free fashion, the risk of vaginal stenosis should be significantly lessened over historical vaginoplasty reports. Importantly, redundancy of the flap should be avoided, as it will create a lip or mound of tissue at the introitus.

The flap vaginoplasty technique is contraindicated in patients with a high vaginal confluence, since it will result in a short, severely hypospadiac urethra, potential injury to the continence mechanism and add to vaginal pooling of urine. Hendren and Crawford [6] realized this problem and proposed the *pull-through vaginoplasty*, where the vagina is taken off the UGS and moved to the perineum. The initial portion of this procedure is identical to the flap vaginoplasty. It is critical to divide the bulbospongiosus muscle and sweep the rectum posteriorly in order to expose the entire posterior wall of the vagina. The vagina is opened in the midline, exposing the Fogarty balloon. At this point, we find it helpful to rotate the patient to the prone position and elevate the posterior wall of the vagina with a malleable retractor, providing excellent exposure of the anterior vaginal wall and its confluence with the urethra, although others have not found this to be necessary [37]. The dissection of the anterior wall of the vagina from the urethra and bladder neck is the most difficult part of the procedure. If not performed with excellent exposure and care, the urethra or sphincteric mechanism can be injured. With the vagina separated from the urethra and sinus, the opened UGS is closed in layers over a Foley catheter to create a urethra. The catheter remains in the urethra, and a Penrose drain is left in the vagina.

In reality, the pull-through vaginoplasty is a misnomer, since in most cases the vagina does not reach the perineum despite complete circumferential vaginal mobilization. Historically, this has required perineal skin flaps posteriorly and preputial or labial flaps anteriorly. Hendren's original work was a monumental contribution but represented a difficult surgical approach, which left an isolated perineal vaginal opening and reliance on multiple skin flaps. A number of articles addressed the complexity of exposure of this approach. In 1997, three groups reported on ways to improve exposure to aid in complex pull-through vaginoplasties. Our group reported the posterior prone approach as noted above [37].

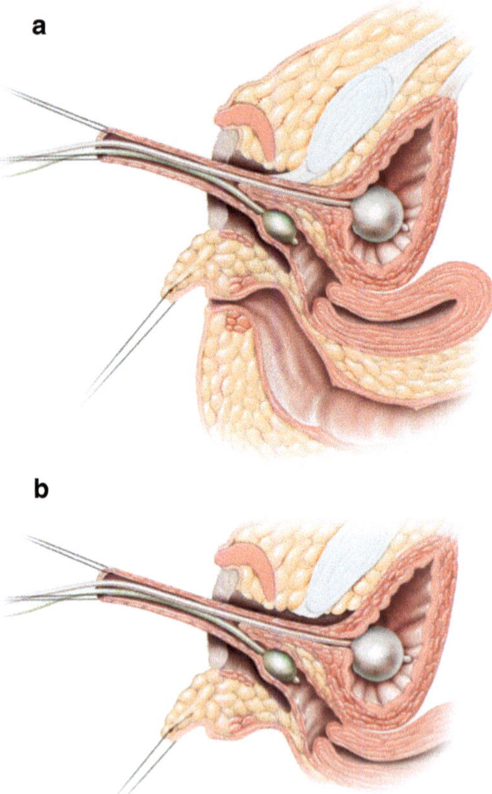

Fig. 21.6 Sagittal illustration of total urogenital mobilization – TUM (**a**) and partial urogenital mobilization – PUM with the dissection stopping at the pubourethral ligament (**b**)

Domini et al. reported an even more aggressive anterior sagittal approach splitting the anterior rectal wall (known as ASTRA) [38]. This technique of opening the rectal wall is very helpful in improving exposure in patients with a very high vaginal confluence. In that same year, Peña et al. described total UGS mobilization [39].

Total urogenital mobilization (TUM) involves a complete circumferential dissection of the intact UGS, urethra, and vagina from the pubis (Fig. 21.6). While this approach was originally proposed for cloacal anomalies, it has been successfully used in patients with UGS. TUM allows a midlevel vagina to be moved to the perineum easily, avoiding a pull-through vaginoplasty. Even in situations where the high confluence vagina may still require a pull-through vaginoplasty, TUM allows for the separation of the vagina from the urinary tract to be performed more easily.

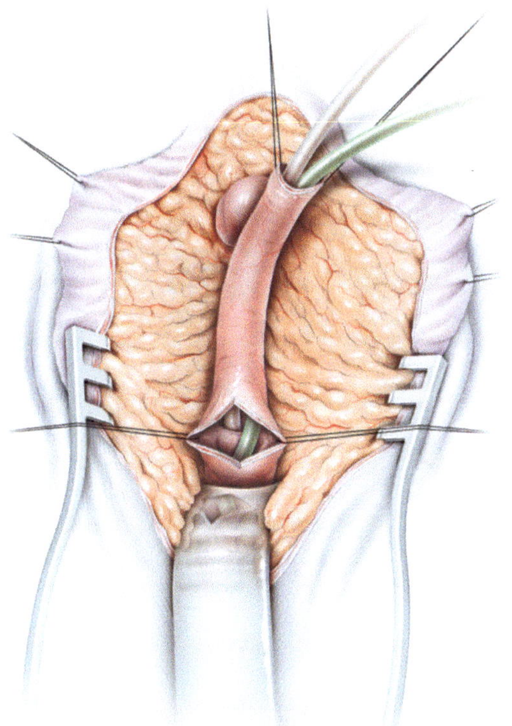

Fig. 21.7 The vagina is opened near the confluence

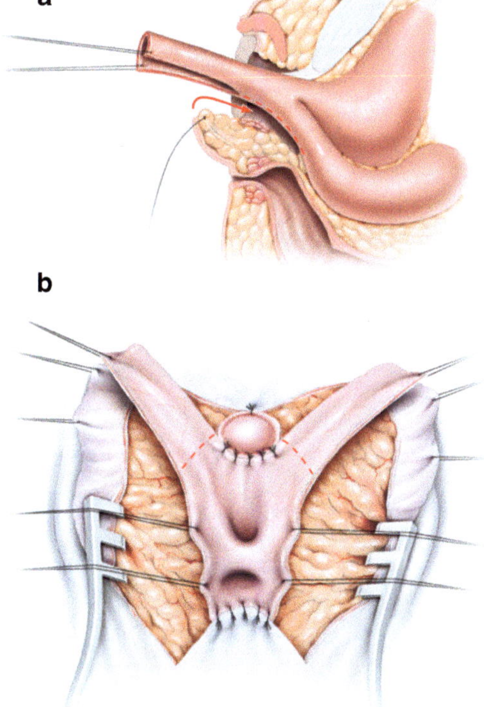

Fig. 21.8 Vaginoplasty in case of insufficient vaginal length to reach the perineum. The excess of the sinus is used after TUM or PUM. Sinus may be split ventrally (**a**) to create a mucosa-lined vestibule (**b**)

TUM is a means of exposure but is not, in and of itself, a vaginoplasty. The above techniques can be used in conjunction with the TUM. The initial incisions in TUM are similar to those described above, with the exception that the UGS is mobilized intact from the corporal bodies. The anterior dissection is carried out between their bifurcation, through the pubourethral ligament, to above the pubis. The dissection is continued posteriorly in the midline, separating the rectum from the posterior wall of the vagina. After palpating the Fogarty balloon within the vagina, an incision is made into the vaginal wall posteriorly near the confluence (Fig. 21.7). If the vagina reaches the perineum at this point, it is sewn to the to the perineum. We believe it is beneficial to use a perineal flap to prevent later stenosis.

In the event that the vagina does not reach the perineum, it can be separated from the sinus as described for a pull-through vaginoplasty (Figs. 21.8 and 21.9). We find this separation is more easily accomplished by placing the patient prone.

Peña originally described simply amputating mobilized sinus tissue [39]. Our group has shown that this important tissue can be used for further reconstruction. The sinus tissue can be split ventrally to make a mucosa-lined vestibule [40–42] (Fig. 21.10), dorsally for an anterior vaginal wall, similar to the Passerini technique [43], or laterally for a posterior vaginal wall [42, 44] (Figs. 21.11 and 21.12). In this latter technique, the sinus acts as the "flap" for the vaginoplasty, thus avoiding a skin flap, which is potentially hair bearing.

While recent reports state there has been no incontinence with TUM [35, 45], we have been concerned that this aggressive retropubic dissection raises the potential for later stress urinary incontinence or injury to clitoral innervation. For this reason, Rink et al. [41] described *partial urogenital mobilization* (PUM), where the anterior dissection stops at the pubourethral ligament. We believe this procedure reduces potential risks while preserving

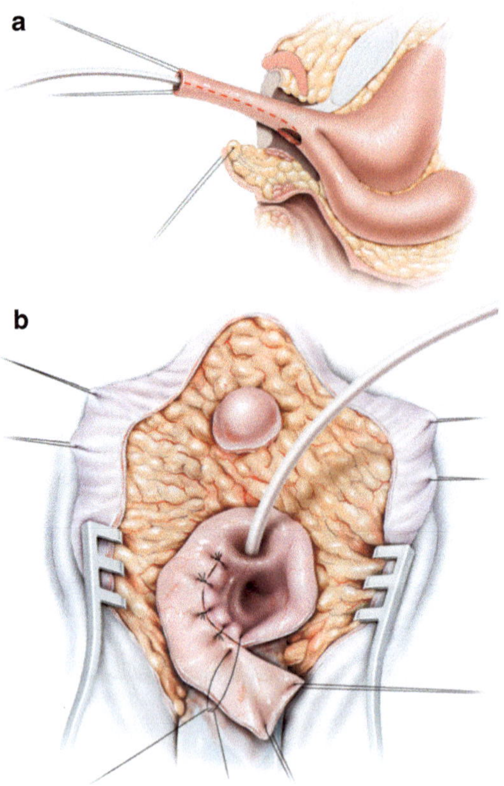

Fig. 21.9 Vaginoplasty in case of insufficient vaginal length to reach the perineum. A lateral incision helps completing the vaginoplasty (**a**). The incised sinus is then rotated in a spiral fashion to extend the vagina (**b**)

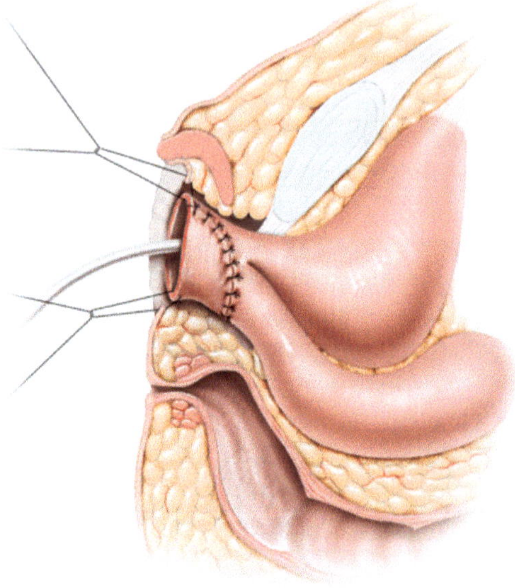

Fig. 21.10 The vestibule is obtained by ventral sinus tissue split

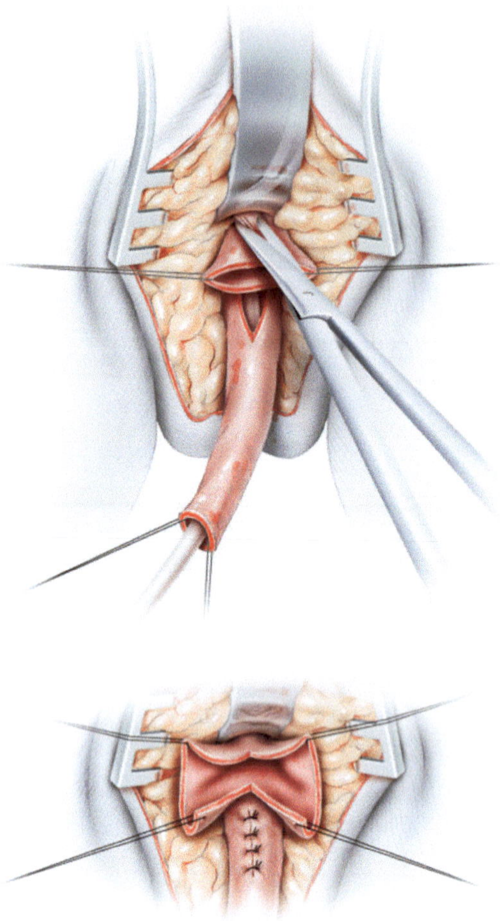

Fig. 21.11 The vestibule is obtained by dorsal sinus tissue split

the ability to use mobilized tissue for improved function and cosmesis similar to the TUM. In most CAH children, PUM adequately exteriorizes the vagina when combined with a flap vaginoplasty. For a high UGS, PUM does not prevent proceeding with a more extensive TUM. Reviewing our own experience with 50 patients who underwent vaginoplasties, 44 had some UGS mobilization technique: either PUM (n=26) or TUM (n=18) (unpublished data). Patients after PUM were all dry and voiding. Of the patients who underwent TUM, 44 % were dry and voiding spontaneously, while the rest required intermittent catheterizations to be continent. Preoperatively, this latter group had neurologic impairment. The most important predictor of spontaneous voiding was not the surgical technique but rather preoperative neurological status.

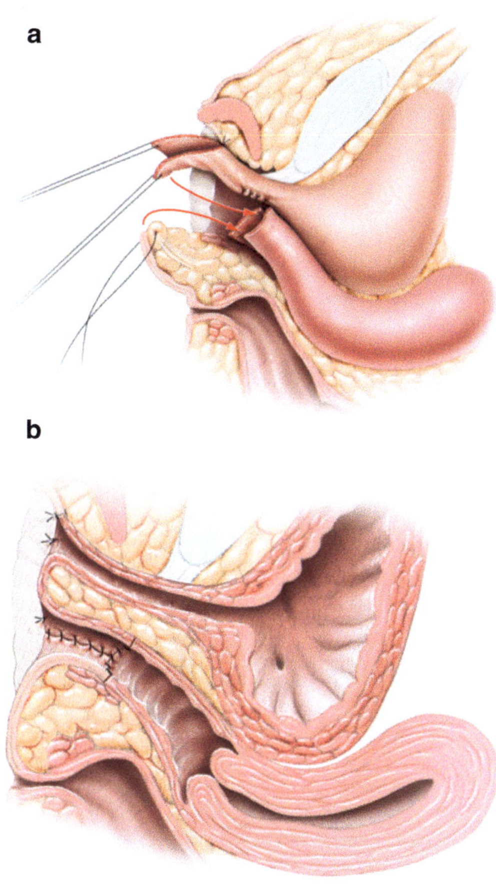

Fig. 21.12 The sinus is split ventrally (**a**) in order to create a vestibule and to complete the vaginoplasty (**b**)

Patients with normal neurological status prior to the TUM did well, while patients with a neuropathic bladder prior to the procedure continued to have one afterwards, possibly requiring clean intermittent catheterizations.

21.8 Labioplasty

In the setting of CAH, the labia minora are missing, and the labia majora are often fused and anteriorly displaced. The goal of surgery is to create labia minora and move the labia majora inferiorly, allowing the vagina to come out between them. Bilateral Y-V-plasties dramatically help in the appearance of the labia majora.

The clitoroplasty and vaginoplasty are followed by labial reconstruction. The phallic skin is unfurled and divided in the midline longitudinally, similar to Byar flaps. The incision should stop short of the base to allow creation of a clitoral hood. We then create a clitoral hood by securing the split clitoral skin to the preserved preputial skin. For improved cosmesis, we find it helpful to plicate the clitoral skin in the midline prior to suturing it to the inner prepuce. These preputial skin flaps are then sutured in place inferiorly along either side of the vagina to create labia minora. Incisions in a Y-V fashion are used to mobilize the anteriorly displaced labia majora posteriorly (Fig. 21.13). The mobilized labia majora are sutured to the labia minora medially and to the perineal skin laterally.

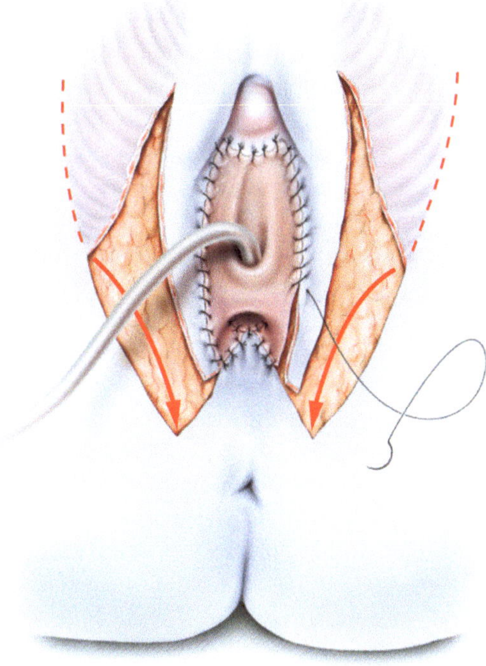

Fig. 21.13 Y-V incisions used to create the labia majora

21.9 Challenges and Future Direction

All parents want their child to be normal, including children born with disorders of sexual development [28]. In an excellent paper looking at premenopausal women without urological problems, it appears that there is a wide range of normal external female anatomy, including clitoral length and width, labial length, width, and rugations as well as vaginal length [1]. Recently, a report from Turkey has shown a similar range of phenotypes in healthy children [2].

Little long-term data exists, and the published experience is typically assessed from the surgeon's viewpoint, which has significant limitations. Surgeons focus on cosmetics, vaginal size, and continence, while patients center on sexual sensation, orgasm, and pain-free intercourse. There is a need to move toward patient-reported outcomes when assessing the results in feminizing genitoplasty. No data exists that surgery improves psychological outcomes. However, there is also no data on psychological outcome of raising a child with ambiguity [46]. Furthermore, no papers discuss long-term endocrine control, which is critical.

Published data on feminizing genitoplasty is limited, nearly always retrospective with small numbers of patients, reviewed from the surgeon's view point and often reviews outdated or unreported surgical techniques. We will not have meaningful data until long-term, multi-institutional reports that include the degree of virilization, level of confluence, type of procedure, and the hormonal control are carried out. In fact, our current data is so poor that Braga and Salle noted that it was "scientifically pointless" to try to make sense of the current available literature [47]. Because of the above, we will not review all of this data as one can find reports to justify the bias of either early or late surgery. It is, however, important for the reader to know that published results are often poor. Vaginal stenosis following vaginoplasty has been reported in up to 98 % of patients. Further surgery on the clitoris after clitoroplasty has been noted in up to 40 % with reports of decreased thermal and vibratory sensation. Cosmetic outcomes have also been variable, but some have reported poor results in up to 40 %. While there has been tremendous progress in this field surgically, we still have to do better.

In the future, not only do we have to continue to seek new techniques but also continue to improve the results of the techniques we currently have. One exciting area of study is the impact of estrogens on healing. We must also understand the impact of not correcting genital ambiguity. Surgical outcomes must focus on issues important to the patient. We still need to define the ethical issues involved, who has the right to decide on surgery, the parents or the child [48], acknowledging that surgery does not "cure" intersexuality.

Conclusions

Given the complexity of field of surgical management of DSD, certain general conclusions can be drawn. We believe that endoscopy is better than genitography at reliably assessing internal anatomy. We believe that the vaginal confluence in CAH is nearly always the same location. The "high vagina" appearance in CAH is due to elongated common UGS channel surrounded by "prostatic-like" tissue and the appearance of an external sphincter in a narrow pelvis. Most CAH children do not need a TUM and will do well with PUM. There is virtually never a need to skeletonize the neurovascular bundles. One should never talk a family into surgery. Genital appearance varies greatly, even in healthy children. Parents should be provided with all the advantages and disadvantages of surgery versus no surgery [49]. While we have generally performed clitoroplasty, labioplasty, and vaginoplasty during infancy, vaginoplasty in the child with a very small vagina is probably best left until puberty. Cloacal anomalies are often easier to repair than a high UGS, because the rectum is completely moved out of the area, greatly improving exposure. Lastly, we strongly believe that one should never dilate the vagina in prepubertal children and examinations of the genitalia should only rarely be done following surgery. In the rare situation where examination is required, child life specialists should be used to alleviate the child's anxiety whenever possible.

References

1. Lloyd J, Crouch NS, Minto CL et al (2005) Female genital appearance: "normality" unfolds. BJOG 112:643–646
2. Akbiyik F, Kutlu AO (2010) External genital proportions in prepubertal girls: a morphometric reference for female genitoplasty. J Urol 184:1476–1481
3. Diamond M, Garland J (2014) Evidence regarding cosmetic and medically unnecessary surgery on infants. J Pediatr Urol 10:2–6

4. Creighton S, Chernausek SD, Romao R et al (2012) Timing and nature of reconstructive surgery for disorders of sex development – introduction. J Pediatr Urol 8:602–610
5. Rink RC, Adams MC, Misseri R (2005) A new classification for genital ambiguity and urogenital sinus anomalies. BJU Int 95:638–642
6. Hendren WH, Crawford JD (1969) Adrenogenital syndrome: the anatomy of the anomaly and its repair. Some new concepts. J Pediatr Surg 4:49–58
7. Powell DM, Newman KD, Randolph J (1995) A proposed classification of vaginal anomalies and their surgical correction. J Pediatr Surg 30:271–275; discussion 275–276
8. Rink RC, Kaefer M (2002) Surgical management of intersexuality, cloacal malformation and other abnormalities of the genitalia in girls. In: Walsh P, Retik AB, Vaugh EP, Wein AJ (eds) Campell's urology. W.B. Saunders, Philadelphia, pp 2428–2467
9. Ganesan A, Smith GH, Broome K et al (2002) Congenital adrenal hyperplasia: preliminary observations of the urethra in 9 cases. J Urol 167:275–278; discussion 278–279
10. Rink RC Surgical management of disorders of sexual development and cloacal and anorectal malformations. In Walsh P RAB, Vaugh EP, Wein AJ (eds) Campell's urology. W.B. Saunders, Philadelphia (in press)
11. Rink RC, Adams MC (1998) Feminizing genitoplasty: state of the art. World J Urol 16:212–218
12. Vanderbrink BA, Rink RC, Cain MP et al (2010) Does preoperative genitography in congenital adrenal hyperplasia cases affect surgical approach to feminizing genitoplasty? J Urol 184:1793–1798
13. Pena A (1989) The surgical management of persistent cloaca: results in 54 patients treated with a posterior sagittal approach. J Pediatr Surg 24:590–598
14. Jaramillo D, Lebowitz RL, Hendren WH (1990) The cloacal malformation: radiologic findings and imaging recommendations. Radiology 177: 441–448
15. De Filippo RE, Shaul DB, Harrison EA et al (1999) Neurogenic bladder in infants born with anorectal malformations: comparison with spinal and urologic status. J Pediatr Surg 34:825–827; discussion 828
16. Morimoto K, Takemoto O, Wakayama A (2003) Tethered cord associated with anorectal malformation. Pediatr Neurosurg 38:79–82
17. Hendren WH (1998) Cloaca, the most severe degree of imperforate anus: experience with 195 cases. Ann Surg 228:331–346
18. Hampson JG (1955) Hermaphroditic genital appearance, rearing and eroticism in hyperadrenocorticism. Bull Johns Hopkins Hosp 96:265–273
19. Money J, Hampson JG, Hampson JL (1955) Hermaphroditism: recommendations concerning assignment of sex, change of sex and psychologic management. Bull Johns Hopkins Hosp 97:284–300
20. Lattimer JK (1961) Relocation and recession of the enlarged clitoris with preservation of the glans: an alternative to amputation. J Urol 86:113–116
21. Shaw A (1977) Subcutaneous reduction clitoroplasty. J Pediatr Surg 12:331–338
22. Barrett TM, Gonzales ET Jr (1980) Reconstruction of the female external genitalia. Urol Clin North Am 7:455–463
23. Glassberg KI, Laungani G (1981) Reduction clitoroplasty. Urology 17:604–605
24. Mollard P, Juskiewenski S, Sarkissian J (1981) Clitoroplasty in intersex: a new technique. Br J Urol 53:371–373
25. Rajfer J, Ehrlich RM, Goodwin WE (1982) Reduction clitoroplasty via ventral approach. J Urol 128: 341–343
26. Kogan SJ, Smey P, Levitt SB (1983) Subtunical total reduction clitoroplasty: a safe modification of existing techniques. J Urol 130:746–748
27. Baskin LS, Erol A, Li YW et al (1999) Anatomical studies of the human clitoris. J Urol 162:1015–1020
28. Schober JM, Meyer-Bahlburg HF, Ransley PG (2004) Self-assessment of genital anatomy, sexual sensitivity and function in women: implications for genitoplasty. BJU Int 94:589–594
29. Freitas Filho LG, Carnevale J, Melo CE et al (2003) A posterior-based omega-shaped flap vaginoplasty in girls with congenital adrenal hyperplasia caused by 21-hydroxylase deficiency. BJU Int 91:263–267
30. Pippi Salle JL, Braga LP, Macedo N et al (2007) Corporeal sparing dismembered clitoroplasty: an alternative technique for feminizing genitoplasty. J Urol 178:1796–1800; discussion 1801
31. Creighton SM, Minto CL, Steele SJ (2001) Objective cosmetic and anatomical outcomes at adolescence of feminising surgery for ambiguous genitalia done in childhood. Lancet 358:124–125
32. Minto CL, Liao LM, Woodhouse CR et al (2003) The effect of clitoral surgery on sexual outcome in individuals who have intersex conditions with ambiguous genitalia: a cross-sectional study. Lancet 361:1252–1257
33. Crouch NS, Minto CL, Laio LM et al (2004) Genital sensation after feminizing genitoplasty for congenital adrenal hyperplasia: a pilot study. BJU Int 93:135–138
34. Rink RC, Herndon CD, Cain MP et al (2005) Upper and lower urinary tract outcome after surgical repair of cloacal malformations: a three-decade experience. BJU Int 96:131–134
35. Ludwikowski BM, Gonzalez R (2013) The surgical correction of urogenital sinus in patients with DSD: 15 years after description of total urogenital mobilization in children. Front Pediatr 1:41
36. Escala Aguirre JM, Cadena Y, Lopez PJ et al (2009) Feminizing genitoplasty in adrenal congenital hyperplasia: one or two surgical steps? Arch Esp Urol 62:724–730
37. Rink RC, Pope JC, Kropp BP et al (1997) Reconstruction of the high urogenital sinus: early perineal prone approach without division of the rectum. J Urol 158:1293–1297
38. Domini R, Rossi F, Ceccarelli PL et al (1997) Anterior sagittal transanorectal approach to the urogenital sinus in adrenogenital syndrome: preliminary report. J Pediatr Surg 32:714–716

39. Pena A (1997) Total urogenital mobilization–an easier way to repair cloacas. J Pediatr Surg 32:263–267; discussion 267–268
40. Rink RC, Cain MP (2008) Urogenital mobilization for urogenital sinus repair. BJU Int 102:1182–1197
41. Rink RC, Metcalfe PD, Kaefer MA et al (2006) Partial urogenital mobilization: a limited proximal dissection. J Pediatr Urol 2:351–356
42. Yerkes EB, Rink RC (2001) Surgical management of female genital anomalies, intersex (urogenital sinus) disorders and cloacal anomalies. In: Gearhart JP, Rink RC, Mouriquand PDE (eds) Pediatric urology. W.B. Saunders, Philadelphia
43. Passerini-Glazel G (1989) A new 1-stage procedure for clitorovaginoplasty in severely masculinized female pseudohermaphrodites. J Urol 142:565–568; discussion 572
44. Rink RC, Metcalfe PD, Cain MP et al (2006) Use of the mobilized sinus with total urogenital mobilization. J Urol 176:2205–2211
45. Palmer BW, Trojan B, Griffin K et al (2012) Total and partial urogenital mobilization: focus on urinary continence. J Urol 187:1422–1426
46. Rangecroft L, British Association of Paediatric Surgeons Working Party on the Surgical Management of Children Born With Ambiguous G (2003) Surgical management of ambiguous genitalia. Arch Dis Child 88:799–801
47. Braga LH, Pippi Salle JL (2009) Congenital adrenal hyperplasia: a critical appraisal of the evolution of feminizing genitoplasty and the controversies surrounding gender reassignment. Eur J Pediatr Surg 19:203–210
48. Lee PA, Witchel SF (2002) Genital surgery among females with congenital adrenal hyperplasia: changes over the past five decades. J Pediatr Endocrinol Metab 15:1473–1477
49. Creighton SM, Liao LM (2004) Changing attitudes to sex assignment in intersex. BJU Int 93: 659–664

22 Hypospadias Repair: The Ongoing Challenge

Santiago Vallasciani, Dario G. Minoli, and Gianantonio Manzoni

22.1 Introduction

The wide spectrum of hypospadias anomalies and the many options available for hypospadias reconstruction continue to challenge the urological, pediatric surgical, and plastic surgical skills of the pediatric urologist. Since the beginning of the modern era of hypospadiology in the 1980s, there have been many scientific studies reporting on the causes of hypospadias, but the assessment and management of this condition have remained quite subject to bias and preference. Although new information from evidence-based outcomes has made us look more critically at our decision-making process for choice of repairs, controversies in nearly every aspect of hypospadias management still exist. It is the aim of this chapter to review the areas of ongoing controversy, to provide a simple and reliable algorithm for choice of procedure that we have found useful, and to create a keener awareness about the need to base the choice of technique on intraoperative anatomical findings rather than on the preoperative location of the meatus. Finally, the need of long-term follow-up into the postadolescent years and the importance of outcomes studies from the patient's point of view are emphasized.

S. Vallasciani, MD (✉) • D.G. Minoli, MD
G. Manzoni, FEAPU, FRCS
Pediatric Urology Unit, Fondazione IRCCS Ca' Granda – Ospedale Maggiore Policlinico, Via della Commenda, 10, Milan 20122, Italy
e-mail: santiago.vallasciani@gmail.com; darioguido.minoli@policlinico.mi.it; gianantonio.manzoni@policlinico.mi.it

22.2 Incidence, Prevalence, and Cause

In the early 1990s, Paoluzzi et al. reported an increase in the incidence of hypospadias from the commonly quoted 1:500 live male births to 1:250 male live births in the period 1968–1993 in the United States. An environmental factor (contamination) was proposed [1]. Further studies emphasized the increase in incidence [2] while a multicenter European paper showed that the positive trend had stopped in the last years [3]. Two further papers from the United States reported an increase in penile anomalies, but the incidence of true hypospadias remained stable [4, 5].

There is growing evidence of environmental factors contributing to the onset of hypospadias. Of 37 papers that discussed the etiology of hypospadias written during 2007–2012, 25 confirmed the etiological role of environmental factors: nutrition, hormones, and chemicals (endocrine-disrupting chemicals, valproic acid, and organochlorine pesticides) which represent the vast majority [6]. The complex mechanisms by which these environmental interactions cause hypospadias are thought to be controlled by several factors rather than a single process (i.e. environmental factors can result in hypospadias in an individual with predisposing genetic factors).

M. Lima, G. Manzoni (eds.), *Pediatric Urology: Contemporary Strategies from Fetal Life to Adolescence*, DOI 10.1007/978-88-470-5693-0_22, © Springer-Verlag Italia 2015

Recent attention has been focused on the ventral aspect of the hypospadic penis indicating that this tissue may be lacking in specific growth factors that may be required for normal development. Kojima et al. reported how a cascade of several factors both in early (androgen-independent) and late (androgen-dependent) gestational age is related to the formation of a complete virilized penis. The authors conclude that there is no single factor that can be identified for causing hypospadias [7]. Kalfa et al. highlighted the relationship between the environmental and the genetic factors and proposed a model of how they may interact in cases of hypospadias and disorders of sexual development [8].

22.3 Preoperative Assessment and Management

22.3.1 Adjuvant Hormonal Therapy

Preoperative androgen stimulation is commonly used in proximal hypospadias to obtain an increase in penile size, reduce ventral curvature, and improve vascularity of the preputial and penile skin, though no standardized protocol is presently available.

The only randomized trial compared patients with both distal and proximal hypospadias receiving preoperative topical dihydrotestosterone cream (2.5 %) versus no treatment. The authors found fewer urethroplasty complications in the treated group [9].

More recent studies, based on dermatological literature, showed a potential negative effect on the wound healing process and an increase in surgical complications in patients hormonally treated [10]. In a multivariable analysis, Bush and Snodgrass examined outcomes in patients who received preoperative testosterone (glans diameter increased from mean of 11 to 15.7 mm) versus untreated patients whose glans width was already ≥14 mm. They found that testosterone treatment was an independent factor for developing glans dehiscence [11]. Accordingly, these authors have completely stopped the use of testosterone for preoperative penile stimulation.

A very recent and excellent systematic review and meta-analysis by Braga has evaluated the effect of preoperative hormonal stimulation on operative outcomes after posterior hypospadias repair. He concluded that the published literature is of low quality and lacking standardized reporting, making it impossible at the present time to draw any strong conclusions about the value of hormonal stimulation. Clear documentation of the agent and dose and timing of stimulation, along with rigid criteria in patient selection, are needed for future randomized studies [12].

We recently analyzed the correlation between hormonal stimulation and hypospadias complications at our medical center. Although we found no statistical difference in the complication rate between treated and untreated patients, a difference was found in the number of complications in relationship to the timing of the stimulation. Among patients who received hormonal stimulation within 3 months of surgery, we had a much higher rate of dehiscence (seven dehiscences and three fistulas), compared to those stimulated earlier (one dehiscence and four fistulas) [13].

22.3.2 Timing of Surgery

There has been a progressive reduction in age at surgery over the years. The principal factors to consider include anesthetic risk, psychosexual factors, and potential risk of urethroplasty complications at different ages.

From an anesthetic point of view, only the first month of life has an increased risk for elective surgery in healthy children [14]. It has been reported that hypospadias repair can be safely performed in the ambulatory surgical setting, in otherwise healthy full-term babies, starting from the age of 3 months [15].

Recently, an additional factor has been highlighted that might encourage surgical correction at an early age. The levels of cytokines present in the foreskin are different according to age with lower levels in the first months of life. This may explain why wound healing in younger children seems to be associated with less scar formation and better cosmetic results [16].

The ideal age for genital surgery from the psychological point of view has been clearly highlighted by Schultz and later by the American Academy of Pediatrics [17–19] with the window between 6 and 18 months of age being reported as the best period. Others, who challenged these conclusions, using questionnaires and standardized interview, did not find significant differences in health-related quality of life (HRQoL), psychological adjustment, gender role behavior, or penile self-perception in patients who had genital surgery before or after 18 months of age [20]. It seems therefore that guidelines for surgical treatment are based on psychological assertions that have not been empirically confirmed. The assumption that a surgical correction of a hypospadias at the earliest age in order to minimize the adverse effects on the boys development deserves particular attention.

Penile dimensions can have some impact on surgical timing only before the age of 6 months, the crucial period where penile growth can be observed. As stated in Aaronson's nomogram [21], further significant growth is seen only at puberty.

Although studies have tried to correlate the impact of age on urethroplasty complications, different conclusions were reached, and it is therefore difficult to determine if age is an independent variable predicting the final outcome [22–25].

22.4 Intraoperative Assessment and Management

22.4.1 Spectrum of Anatomical Defects

The surgeon facing with a hypospadias repair must pay particular attention to all the anatomical elements involved into the defect. A careful analysis of each individual component (skin, urethral plate and degree of ventral curvature) is of paramount importance for the subsequent surgical strategy.

The old concept of classifying a hypospadias based on the position of the meatus is, in fact, obsolete, since it is evident that the true severity of the defect can be only defined *intraoperatively* after complete degloving of all tethering layers (skin, dartos, and Buck's fascia) and careful examination for the location of diverging corpus spongiosum. The quality of the urethra and of the spongiosum will also determine the severity of the anatomical defect and the surgical strategy (Fig. 22.1). An apparently distal form may become an obvious more proximal defect in which case the original surgical reconstruction plan would have to be modified accordingly.

The term "*chordee*" is a nonspecific word for bending of the penis during an erection. It has been used in a clinical sense to describe ventral penile curvature associated with hypospadias implying that there is abnormal tissue present, variously described as "fibrous," "dysplastic," or "dysgenetic" that causes the ventral curvature. The term "*chordee*" is used quite interchangeably with ventral penile curvature, but it also suggests that abnormal tissue formation is responsible for curvature. Its etiology is unknown, and only theories have been proposed. Some authors reported that chordee is a normal state of penile development at the 16th week of gestation but that the curvature resolves spontaneously by the 25th week. According to this theory, the presence of curvature could be explained as an arrest in the normal penile development [26, 27].

Patients with a nearly normally positioned meatus who have ventral curvature and often other features common in hypospadias are said to have "chordee without hypospadias." We believe that this term should be eliminated, and these cases should more appropriately be referred to as "hypospadias variants." These patients present at an early age and usually have some "stigmata of concealed hypospadias" such as an incomplete foreskin, a deficient and poorly developed ventral shaft skin, and in some cases, a dysplastic urethra.

The evaluation of both the penile and preputial skin for quality and quantity will help to determine the options of surgical reconstruction and the complexity of the repair. Occasionally, the urethral reconstruction may be the easiest part of the procedure compared to the much more

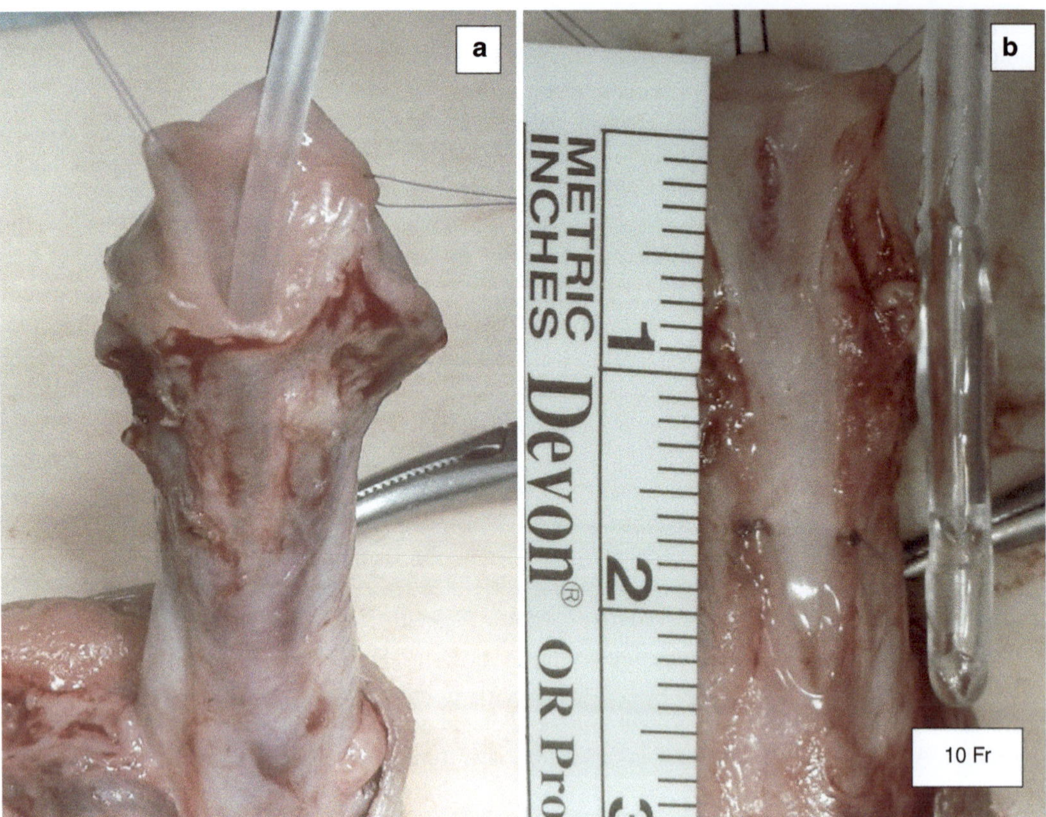

Fig. 22.1 Urethral true assessment after complete degloving. (**a**) Note absent spongiosum in distal urethra. (**b**) Urethra opened up to the point of normal spongiosum (note abnormal plate)

demanding penile skin resurfacing where plastic surgical imagination and creativity become necessary (Figs. 22.2 and 22.3).

We are all indebted to John Duckett and the Philadelphia school for the concept of the "urethral plate" which some argue defines the origin of modern *hypospadiology*. He taught the plate should be preserved whenever possible [28].

The width and quality of the urethral plate must be assessed to determine if it can be preserved and used for the reconstruction. The optimal width has been proposed by Orkiszewski et al. [29] but remains a subjective issue since many papers do not provide exact measures. Some authors use terms as "soft" or "elastic," while others describe the diameter of the catheter around which the urethral plate should be rolled [30].

A similar concept may apply to the glans configuration and to the glans width measured at its widest point. Snodgrass has recently provided convincing data comparing measurements of glans width in normal (circumcised) boys with those boys who have distal and proximal hypospadias. He confirmed that the smallest size glans occurred in patients with proximal hypospadias [15].

The approach to the preoperative anatomical assessment is one of the most controversial aspects of the hypospadias discipline in which we are still relying on subjective evaluations and decisions rather than on a more scientific and standardized methodology for our choice of surgical procedures.

22.4.2 Glanular ("Minimal") Hypospadias

Glanular hypospadias, where there is some glans tissue between the meatus and the coronal margin, involves mainly cosmetic implications compared to coronal, middle and proximal forms

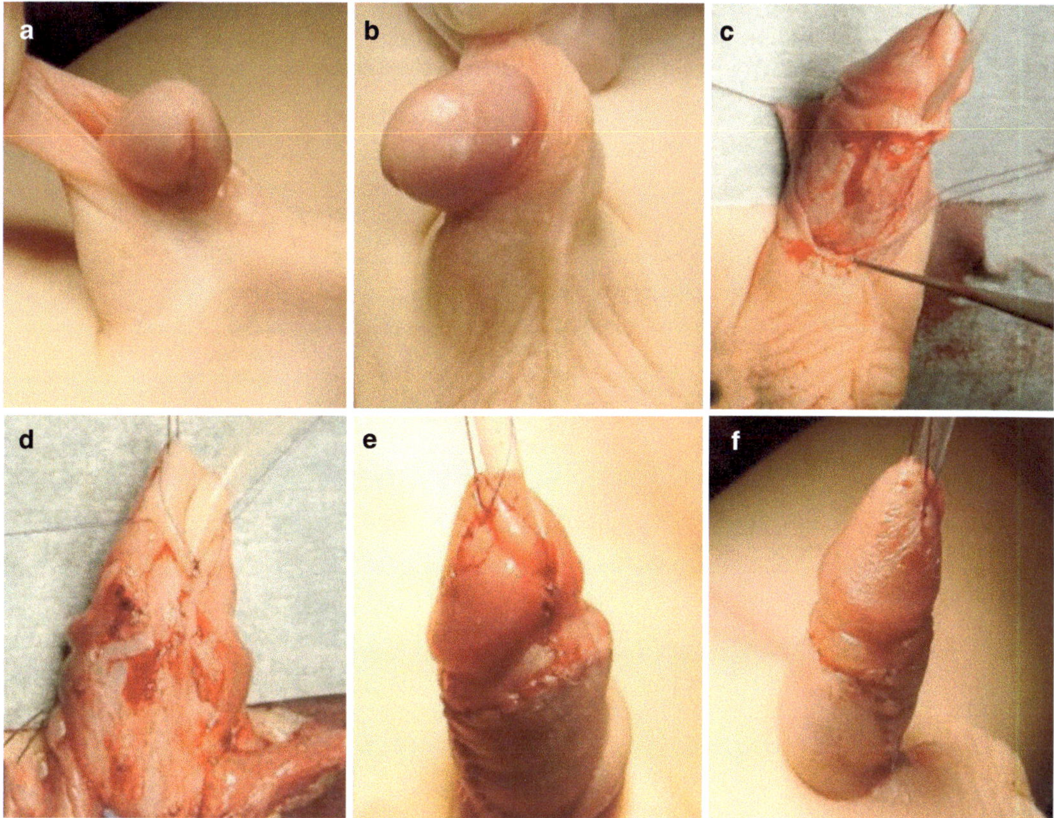

Fig. 22.2 (**a**, **b**) Distal hypospadias with significant penile torsion and abnormal penile skin distribution (**c**) skin degloving (**d**) TIP repair (**e**, **f**) final aspect

where there is an obvious impairment of urinary or sexual functions. Although most parents prefer to have surgical correction for a meatus that is proximal to the glans, most coronal repairs are performed more for cosmetic than functional reasons. The definition of a "distal hypospadias" is often quite generic and lack of precise anatomical definition may generate confusion and unjustified psychological pressure for the parents of an affected child. It is therefore mandatory to distinguish all "minimal" hypospadias, which represent the very mild end of the spectrum, where the true anatomical involvement is very limited to a preputial or a meatal variant (Fig. 22.4). These children do not represent the classic hypospadias population, where an early surgical correction is indicated. An honest and conservative attitude seems more appropriate and should always be discussed with the family. The worse and most devastating scenario is represented by a sequence of interventions initiated by a failed and inappropriate initial repair for "minimal hypospadias" which could have been avoided or postponed to an older age.

The increase in surgical indications for distal hypospadias in the pediatric patients has been highly discussed by adult urologists. They report studies where adult patients, with uncorrected distal variants, showed no psychological or functional impairment [31, 32].

22.4.3 Urethroplasty

Despite the multiple reconstructive techniques available, the authors feel that a very simple and reliable protocol can be applied, which is based on the quality and development of the urethral plate, rather than the preoperative location of the meatus [33]. The choice of the technique is therefore determined intraoperatively by the anatomical characteristics previously described.

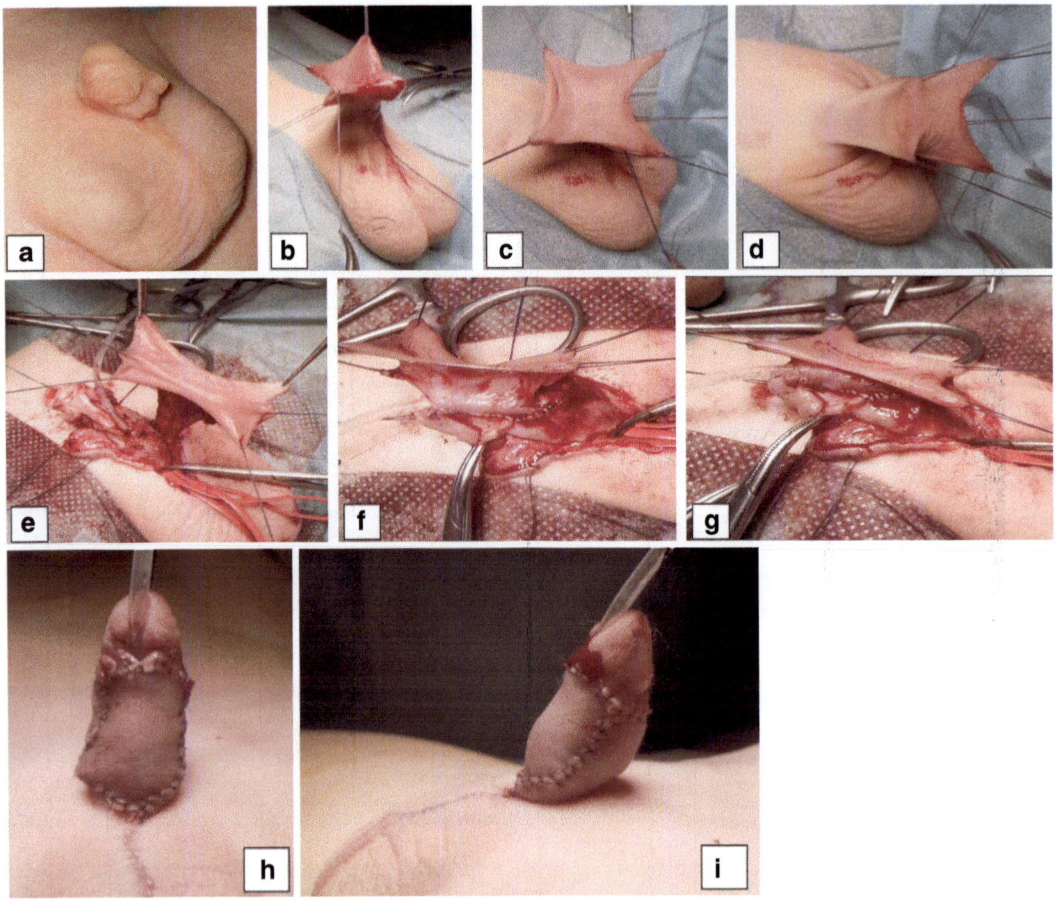

Fig. 22.3 (**a**) Penoscrotal hypospadias with abnormal skin distribution and hypoplastic urethra. (**b–d**) Skin design for repair (three portions: (**b**) inner prepuce, (**c**) outer prepuce, (**d**) penile shaft skin). (**e–g**) The two preputial portions are developed with a single vascular pedicle for OIF and ventral shaft covering (double faced). (**h**, **i**) Final aspect

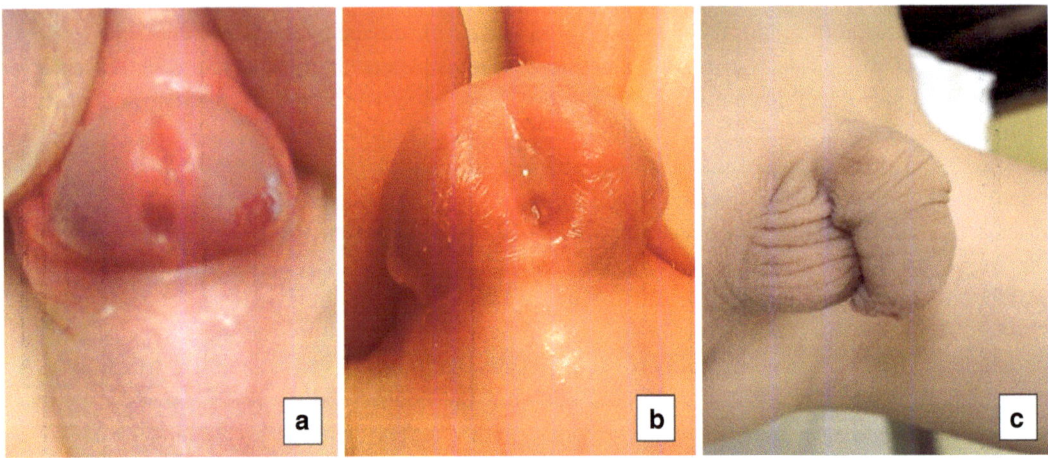

Fig. 22.4 (**a**) Meatal variant. (**b**) Navicular form (substenotic meatus). (**c**) Preputial variant (normal meatus)

Table 22.1 Primary hypospadias: surgical options

Advancement
• MAGPI [34] and modifications [35]
UP tubularization
• TIP [30]/GAP [36]
1-stage UP augmentation
• Dorsal (inlay TIP) [37]
• Ventral (OIF and modifications) [38, 39]
1-stage UP substitution
• TPIF and modifications [40, 41]
2-stage UP substitution
• Bracka [42]

In our institution, the following surgical procedures are applied when dealing with primary hypospadias (Table 22.1).

Meatal advancement with glanuloplasty is indicated for cosmetic purposes and with no risks of fistulas or stricture formation. The correct indication will not result in a retrusive meatus.

TIP repair represents the most common solution for almost all distal forms and Snodgrass's opinion is that the urethral plate width does not represent a limiting factor. His data suggest that a pre-incision plate width less than 8 mm is not a risk factor for complications [43] although this is a very controversial issue [44, 45]. There is still an open debate as to whether an "augmentation" (i.e. inlay) is required in TIP repairs because of the potential risk of neo-urethral functional obstruction. The functional obstruction is thought to be due to a noncompliant urethra that may not become clinically evident until the young boys become continent and off nappies (see Sect. 22.5.1).

Even more controversial (but not the purpose of this chapter) is the debate between performing a two-stage reconstruction or a more demanding and technically challenging single-stage repair. Anatomical abnormalities, progressively revealed during the dissection, may sometime require a different surgical strategy than originally anticipated. This situation may particularly apply to the most severe end of the spectrum, such as the perineal forms, associated with variable degrees of penoscrotal transposition (Fig. 22.5).

22.4.4 Ventral Curvature Correction

The optimal approach to correct ventral curvature is one of the most debated and controversial issues in hypospadias surgery [46].

The incidence of significant ventral curvature associated with distal hypospadias is quite limited. In an extensive review of a very large series, Snodgrass reported only an 11 % incidence and always <30° [43] indicating that a dorsal correction is sufficient to solve the problem. Conversely, in proximal forms, following a sequential approach (degloving and ventral dartos dissection), nearly 50 % will demonstrate a >30° persistent ventral curvature.

In a recent paper, Snodgrass reported the questionable utility of an extensive urethral plate dissection. He feels that this led to areas of ischemia and stricture formation in some patients, and therefore he has abandoned this dissection, concluding that it is safer to transect the plate and provide a staged urethral reconstruction [47].

The option whether a ventral lengthening or a dorsal plication is more appropriate is still open to endless debate. Different options are available with regard to the degree of corporeal disproportion correction. Ventral corporotomies without [48] or with grafting (dermal, SIS, or tunica albuginea) [49–51] versus dorsal plication are performed according to the surgeon's preference. Unfortunately, no long-term data are presently available to corroborate one choice versus the other both in terms of erection outcome or effective shortening of the shaft in the postpubertal age.

22.5 Postoperative Management and Assessment

22.5.1 TIP "Functional Obstruction"

After its introduction in 1994, the tubularized incised plate urethroplasty has gain popularity among hypospadias surgeons. Its capacity to create a wide neo-urethra by increasing the width of the urethral plate, thanks to a reepithelization of its dorsal portion, has been welcomed as a major advance. Since its first publication by Snodgrass

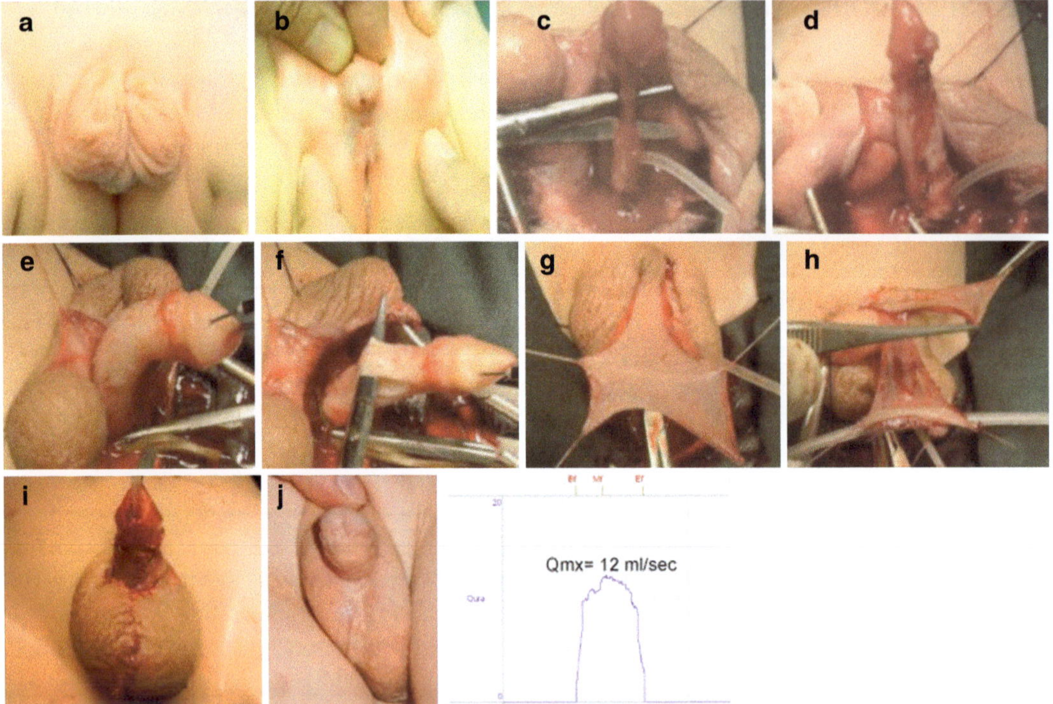

Fig. 22.5 Perineal hypospadias with complete penoscrotal transposition: staged repair originally planned (**a**, **b**). After intraoperative assessment (**c**, **d**) and curvature correction, (**e**, **f**) the available skin allowed to perform a single-stage urethra repair (**g**, **h**), penile shaft resurfacing, and complete correction of penoscrotal transposition (**i**). Four-year follow-up aspect and adequate voiding pattern (**j**)

in 1994, 243 papers can be retrieved in PubMed® accounting for more than 20 publications per year and from every geographical area worldwide.

Despite the popularity of the TIP repair, an increased awareness regarding the fluid dynamics across this tract of neo-urethra carrying a scar has grown since some studies showed changes in uroflow patterns in operated patients [52]. Both clinical and experimental studies revealed that this neo-urethra has a different urodynamic property than the normal urethra showing a tendency for an obstructive pattern despite its adequate caliber.

There are opposing reports on this issue of functional obstruction of the TIP repair. While some authors observed that this impaired flow is present only for a limited period of time [53], other experimental studies revealed that changes in structural and mechanical properties are permanent [54]. In our center, there were three symptomatic cases that resolved only after augmentation of the neo-urethra by incorporating additional tissue as either grafts or flaps [55] (Fig. 22.6).

Future studies and longer follow-up will determine how frequently this complication occurs and if it is related to a variation in technique or to improper patient selection.

22.5.2 Outcome

Little is known about the real prevalence of uncomplicated repairs that fail because of patient dissatisfaction, perhaps owing to an unsatisfactory cosmetic outcome. Certain aspects of the outcome are highly subjective and, therefore, difficult to assess.

Instead, most studies report the prevalence of failed hypospadias by number of complications that require an additional operation [56].

Some attempts were also performed to identify factors that may increase the incidence [57,

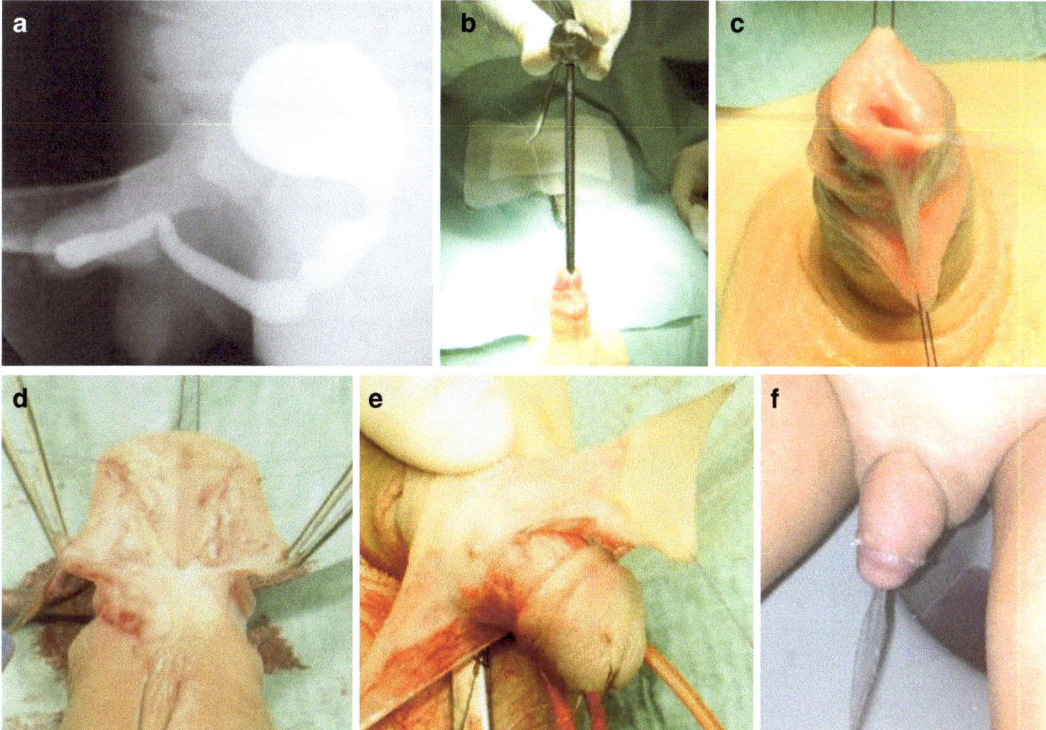

Fig. 22.6 TIP functional obstruction (symptomatic patient): preoperative VCUG showed obstruction of distal urethra (**a**), but EUA demonstrated calibration up to 12 Fr (**b**) and adequate meatal aspect (**c**). Neo-urethra was opened (**d**) and urethral plate augmented by OIF (**e**). Six-month follow-up with normalized micturition (**f**)

58] or to calculate the improvement process of a single institution [59]. Reportedly, overall complication rates after hypospadias repair range from about 5 % in cases of distal hypospadias without associated curvature to 70 % in the most severe cases [60, 61]. A detailed recent review of complications in hypospadias failures is reported in Table 22.2 [62].

A key consideration in the evaluation of complication rates is the duration of follow-up assessment. In the 1980s, many urologists thought that long-term outcomes of hypospadias repair could be predicted after just 2 years of follow-up assessment [63]. However, it is now evident that this is not the case, indicating the need for long-term follow-up when reporting outcomes of a hypospadias repair [64]. In one study to assess the timing of presentation of urethrocutaneous fistulas after hypospadias repair in 26 patients, one-quarter of fistulas were detected more than 2 years after the initial surgery [65]. Another study of 126 patients who had undergone a one-stage hypospadias repair at a mean age of 7 years (ranging from 1 to 14 years) reported that 17 % of the complications were detected after the first 5 years of follow-up assessment [66].

Very few studies have reported outcomes of hypospadias repairs after puberty, which seems to be the most critical period for the development of some complications, such as recurrent curvature [67]. Several surveys have reported an increasing number of patients with failed hypospadias as they pass into adult care [68–70].

All these papers, however, rely on the fact that every complication that does not need further surgery is not to be considered as a true complication. There is a lack of consensus about assessment of results in hypospadias-operated patients.

Some specific tools have been proposed considering only an objective evaluation by the surgeon [71, 72], but the patient's and surgeon's points of view are often not the same [73]. Thus,

Table 22.2 Type of complication after hypospadias repair and proposed correction in literature

Complication	% Incidence	Treatment	% Success
Glans dehiscence	5	TIP redo	74
		GTIP	95.5
		Flaps	70
Fistula	4–28	Fistula closure	75–100
		Redo urethroplasty	n.d.
Urethral dehiscence	Not reported	Redo urethroplasty	n.d.
Meatal stenosis	0–14	Meatotomy	100
Urethral stricture	6–12	DVIU (stricture <1–1.5 cm)	21–40
		Overlap anastomosis	n.d.
		Augmentation urethroplasty	n.d.
		Substitution urethroplasty	n.d.
BXO	15–16 (when prepuce in urethroplasty)	Augmentation urethroplasty	n.d.
		Substitution urethroplasty	n.d.
Symptomatic functional obstruction (non compliant urethra)	Symptomatic not reported (low Q values in 32 %)	Augmentation urethroplasty	n.d.
Hairy urethra	8 % after skin tube flaps	Endoscopic grasping	n.d.
		Laser	100
		Electrolysis	n.d.
		Depilatory cream	100
		Tricholysis	100
		Substitution urethroplasty	n.d.
Urethral ballooning (not associated to stenosis)	4–12	Urethral tapering	100
Penile skin complications	55.2	Penile resurfacing	n.d.
	5 % relevant skin loss	Free grafts	n.d.
		Staged reconstruction with tissue expanders	n.d.
Residual curvature	9.3–31.6	Dorsal plication	n.d.
		Ventral lengthening	n.d.
		Skin de-tethering	n.d.

Reproduced with permission from: Cimador et al. [62]

a subjective evaluation by the patient himself was proposed utilizing validated [70, 74, 75] or unvalidated questionnaires [76, 77]. According to these papers, it seems that patients surgically treated for hypospadias (principally the more proximal forms) are less satisfied than their peers in terms of urinary function. In the same way, there is a higher dissatisfaction with genital appearance and avoidance of sexual relationships. A very recent systematic literature review demonstrated that there is lack of evidence regarding psychosocial adjustment, psychosexual development and HRQoL of children and adolescents with hypospadias [78].

So far, it is almost impossible to effectively measure the exact impact of every factor that influences sexual behavior and experience because these cannot be examined separately [79]. The sexual quality of life (QoL) is affected by many factors (psychological, biological, genetic, social) in an interactive and dynamic bio-psychosocial model. This may affect the future of the patients' development of autonomy and self-confidence. Any attempt to consider a linear model in which psychosexual and social outcomes are hypothesized to be directly determined by the genital deformity and reconstructive surgery seems therefore an oversimplification.

References

1. Paulozzi LJ, Erickson JD, Jackson RJ (1997) Hypospadias trends in two US surveillance systems. Pediatrics 100(5):831–834
2. Lund L, Engebjerg MC, Pedersen L, Ehrenstein V, Nørgaard M, Sørensen HT (2009) Prevalence of hypospadias in Danish boys: a longitudinal study, 1977–2005. Eur Urol 55(5):1022–1026
3. Dolk H, Vrijheid M, Scott JE, Addor MC, Botting B, de Vigan C, de Walle H, Garne E, Loane M, Pierini A, Garcia-Minaur S, Physick N, Tenconi R, Wiesel A, Calzolari E, Stone D (2004) Toward the effective surveillance of hypospadias. Environ Health Perspect 112(3):398–402
4. Elliott CS, Halpern MS, Paik J, Maldonado Y, Shortliffe LD (2011) Epidemiologic trends in penile anomalies and hypospadias in the state of California, 1985–2006. J Pediatr Urol 7(3):294–298
5. Fisch H, Lambert SM, Hensle TW, Hyun G (2009) Hypospadias rates in New York State are not increasing. J Urol 181(5):2291–2294
6. Yang Q, Qu WY, Yang L, Wang K, Tu HY, Wang J (2013) Literature on the aetiology of hypospadias in the last 5 years: molecular mechanism and environmental factors. Andrologia. doi:10.1111/and.12125
7. Kojima Y, Kohri K, Hayashi Y (2010) Genetic pathway of external genitalia formation and molecular etiology of hypospadias. J Pediatr Urol 6(4):346–354
8. Kalfa N, Sultan C, Baskin LS (2010) Hypospadias: etiology and current research. Urol Clin North Am 37(2):159–166
9. Kaya C, Bektic J, Radmayr C, Schwentner C, Bartsch G, Oswald J (2008) The efficacy of dihydrotestosterone transdermal gel before primary hypospadias surgery: a prospective, controlled, randomized study. J Urol 179(2):684–688
10. Gorduza DB, Gay CL, de Mattos E, Silva E, Demède D, Hameury F, Berthiller J, Mure PY, Mouriquand PD (2011) Does androgen stimulation prior to hypospadias surgery increase the rate of healing complications? – A preliminary report. J Pediatr Urol 7(2):158–161
11. Snodgrass WT, Villanueva C, Granberg C, Bush NC (2014) Objective use of testosterone reveals androgen insensitivity in patients with proximal hypospadias. J Pediatr Urol 10(1):118–122
12. Wright I, Cole E, Farrokhyar F, Pemberton J, Lorenzo AJ, Braga LH (2013) Effect of preoperative hormonal stimulation on postoperative complication rates after proximal hypospadias repair: a systematic review. J Urol 190(2):652–659
13. Berrettini A, Tringali V, Vallasciani S, Minoli DG, Manzoni G (2013) Pre-operative androgen stimulation and hypospadias complications: further informations. In: 24th Congress of the ESPU, Genoa
14. van der Griend BF, Lister NA, McKenzie IM, Martin N, Ragg PG, Sheppard SJ, Davidson AJ (2011) Postoperative mortality in children after 101,885 anesthetics at a tertiary pediatric hospital. Anesth Analg 112(6):1440–1447
15. Bush NC, DaJusta D, Snodgrass WT (2013) Glans penis width in patients with hypospadias compared to healthy controls. J Pediatr Urol 9:1188–1191
16. Bermudez DM, Canning DA, Liechty KW (2011) Age and pro-inflammatory cytokine production: wound-healing implications for scar-formation and the timing of genital surgery in boys. J Pediatr Urol 7(3):324–331
17. Schultz JR, Klykylo WM, Wacksman J (1983) Timing of elective hypospadias repair in children. Pediatrics 71(3):342–351
18. American Academy of Pediatrics (1996) Timing of elective surgery on the genitalia of male children with particular reference to the risks, benefits, and psychological effects of surgery and anesthesia. Pediatrics 97(4):590–594
19. Schönbucher VB, Landolt MA, Gobet R, Weber DM (2008) Psychosexual development of children and adolescents with hypospadias. J Sex Med 5(6):1365–1373
20. Weber DM, Schonbucher VB, Gobet R, Gerber A, Landolt MA (2009) Is there an ideal age for hypospadias repair? A pilot study. J Pediatr Urol 5(5):345–350
21. Aaronson IA (1994) Micropenis: medical and surgical implications. J Urol 152(1):4–14
22. Bush NC, Holzer M, Zhang S, Snodgrass W (2013) Age does not impact risk for urethroplasty complications after tubularized incised plate repair of hypospadias in prepubertal boys. J Pediatr Urol 9(3):252–256
23. Perlmutter AE, Morabito R, Tarry WF (2006) Impact of patient age on distal hypospadias repair: a surgical perspective. Urology 68(3):648–651
24. Korvald C, Stubberud K (2008) High odds for freedom from early complications after tubularized incised-plate urethroplasty in 1-year-old versus 5-year-old boys. J Pediatr Urol 4(6):452–456
25. Eassa W, Jednak R, Capolicchio JP, Brzezinski A, El-Sherbiny M (2011) Risk factors for re-operation following tubularized incised plate urethroplasty: a comprehensive analysis. Urology 77(3):716–720
26. Kaplan GW, Lamm DL (1975) Embryogenesis of chordee. J Urol 114:769
27. Kizilcan F, Tanyel FC, Cakar N, Bujukpamukcu N, Hicsonmez A (1994) The effect of intrauterine vascular compromise on further development of corpus spongiosum and urethra. Eur J Pediatr Surg 4:26–29
28. Hollowell JG, Keating MA, Snyder HM 3rd, Duckett JW (1990) Preservation of the urethral plate in hypospadias repair: extended applications and further experience with the Onlay island flap urethroplasty. J Urol 143(1):98–100
29. Orkiszewski M, Madej J, Kilian T (2006) How wide a urethra should we produce? J Pediatr Urol 2(5):473–476
30. Snodgrass W (1994) Tubularized, incised plate urethroplasty for distal hypospadias. J Urol 151(2):464–465

31. Dodds PR, Batter SJ, Shield DE, Serels SR, Garafalo FA, Maloney PK (2008) Adaptation of adults to uncorrected hypospadias. Urology 71(4):682–685
32. Fichtner J, Filipas D, Mottrie AM, Voges GE, Hohenfellner R (1995) Analysis of meatal location in 500 men: wide variation questions need for meatal advancement in all pediatric anterior hypospadias cases. J Urol 154(2 Pt 2):833–834
33. Manzoni G, Bracka A, Palminteri E, Marrocco G (2004) Hypospadias surgery: when, what and by whom? BJU Int 94(8):1188–1195
34. Duckett JW (1981) MAGPI (meatoplasty and glanuloplasty): a procedure for subcoronal hypospadias. Urol Clin North Am 8(3):513–519
35. Vallasciani S, Spagnoli A, Borsellino A, Martini L, Ferro F (2007) Simplifying the surgical approach to glanular and coronal hypospadias: longitudinal urethral incision and glanuloplasty. J Pediatr Urol 3(6):453–456
36. Zaontz MR (1989) The GAP (glans approximation procedure) for glanular/coronal hypospadias. J Urol 141(2):359–361
37. Hayes MC, Malone PS (1999) The use of a dorsal buccal mucosal graft with urethral plate incision (Snodgrass) for hypospadias salvage. BJU Int 83(4):508–509
38. Elder JS, Duckett JW, Snyder HM (1987) Onlay island flap in the repair of mid and distal penile hypospadias without chordee. J Urol 138(2):376–379
39. Rigamonti W, Castagnetti M (2011) Onlay on albuginea: modified onlay preputial island flap urethroplasty for single-stage repair of primary severe hypospadias requiring urethral plate division. Urology 77(6):1498–1502
40. Duckett JW Jr (1980) Transverse preputial island flap technique for repair of severe hypospadias. Urol Clin North Am 7(2):423–430
41. Perovic S, Vukadinovic V (1994) Onlay island flap urethroplasty for severe hypospadias: a variant of the technique. J Urol 151:711–714
42. Bracka A (1995) Hypospadias repair: the two-stage alternative. Br J Urol 76(Suppl 3):31–41
43. Snodgrass W, Bush N (2011) Tubularized incised plate proximal hypospadias repair: continued evolution and extended applications. J Pediatr Urol 7:2–9
44. Holland AJA, Smith GHH (2000) Effect of the depth and width of the urethral plate on tubularized incised plate urethroplasty. J Urol 164:489
45. Sarhan O, Saad M, Helmy T, Hafez A (2009) Effect of suturing technique and urethral plate characteristics on complication rate following hypospadias repair: a prospective randomized study. J Urol 182(2):682–685
46. Springer A, Krois W, Horcher E (2011) Trends in hypospadias surgery: results of a worldwide survey. Eur Urol 60(6):1184–1189
47. Snodgrass WT, Granberg C, Bush NC (2013) Urethral strictures following urethral plate and proximal urethral elevation during proximal TIP hypospadias repair. J Pediatr Urol 9(6 Pt B):990–994
48. Snodgrass W, Prieto J (2009) Straightening ventral curvature while preserving the urethral plate in proximal hypospadias repair. J Urol 182:1720–1725
49. Braga LH, Pippi Salle JL, Dave S, Bagli DJ, Lorenzo AJ, Khoury AE (2007) Outcome analysis of severe chordee correction using tunica vaginalis as a flap in boys with proximal hypospadias. J Urol 178(4 Pt 2):1693–1697
50. Leslie JA, Cain MP, Kaefer M, Meldrum KK, Misseri R, Rink RC (2008) Corporeal grafting for severe hypospadias: a single institution experience with 3 techniques. J Urol 180(4 Suppl):1749–1752
51. Castellan M, Gosalbez R, Devendra J, Bar-Yosef Y, Labbie A (2011) Ventral corporal body grafting for correcting severe penile curvature associated with single or two-stage hypospadias repair. J Pediatr Urol 7(3):289–293
52. Tuygun C, Bakirtas H, Gucuk A, Cakici H, Imamoglu A (2009) Uroflow findings in older boys with tubularized incised-plate urethroplasty. Urol Int 82(1):71–76
53. Andersson M, Doroszkiewicz M, Arfwidsson C, Abrahamsson K, Holmdahl G (2011) Hypospadias repair with tubularized incised plate: does the obstructive flow pattern resolve spontaneously? J Pediatr Urol 7(4):441–445
54. Lalla M, Riis C, Jørgensen CS, Danielsen CC, Jørgensen TM (2011) A biomechanical, histological and biochemical study in an experimental rabbit hypospadias repair model using scanning acoustic microscopy. J Pediatr Urol 7(4):404–411
55. Vallasciani S, Berrettini A, Manzoni G (2012) Urethral obstruction without stenosis: a cautionary tale following TIP repair. In: 23rd ESPU Meeting, Zurich
56. Prasad MM, Marks A, Vasquez E, Yerkes EB, Cheng EY (2012) Published surgical success rates in pediatric urology–fact or fiction? J Urol 188(4 Suppl):1643–1647
57. Lee OT, Durbin-Johnson B, Kurzrock EA (2013) Predictors of secondary surgery after hypospadias repair: a population based analysis of 5,000 patients. J Urol 190(1):251–255
58. Marrocco G, Calisti A, Materia E, Baglio G, Tancioni V (2002) The efficacy of surgical treatment of hypospadias: analysis of hospital data from Lazio region during the three year period (1996–8). Pediatr Med Chir 24(3):223–227
59. Parikh AM, Park AM, Sumfest J (2014) Cumulative summation (CUSUM) charts in the monitoring of hypospadias outcomes: a tool for quality improvement initiative. J Pediatr Urol 10:306–311
60. Snodgrass WT, Bush N, Cost N (2010) Tubularized incised plate hypospadias repair for distal hypospadias. J Pediatr Urol 6(4):408–413
61. Shukla AR, Patel RP, Canning DA (2004) The 2-stage hypospadias repair. Is it a misnomer? J Urol 172(4 Pt 2):1714–1716
62. Cimador M, Vallasciani S, Manzoni G, Rigamonti W, De Grazia E, Castagnetti M (2013) Failed hypospadias in paediatric patients. Nat Rev Urol 10(11):657–666

63. Hinder UT, Duran FR, Caravaca MP (1980) In: Goldwyn RM (ed) Long term results in plastic and reconstructive surgery, 1st edn, 1. Boston Little Brown & Co, USA
64. Spinoit AF, Poelaert F, Groen LA, Van Laecke E, Hoebeke P (2013) Hypospadias repair at a tertiary care center: long-term follow-up is mandatory to determine the real complication rate. J Urol 189(6):2276–2281
65. Wood HM, Kay R, Angermeier KW, Ross JH (2008) Timing of the presentation of urethrocutaneous fistulas after hypospadias repair in pediatric patients. J Urol 180(4 Suppl):1753–1756
66. Nuininga JE, De Gier RP, Verschuren R, Feitz WF (2005) Long-term outcome of different types of 1-stage hypospadias repair. J Urol 174(4 Pt 2):1544–1548
67. Vandersteen DR, Husmann DA (1998) Late onset recurrent penile chordee after successful correction at hypospadias repair. J Urol 160(3 Pt 2):1131–1133
68. Rynja SP, de Jong TP, Bosch JL, de Kort LM (2011) Functional, cosmetic and psychosexual results in adult men who underwent hypospadias correction in childhood. J Pediatr Urol 7(5):504–515
69. Barbagli G, Perovic S, Djinovic R, Sansalone S, Lazzeri M (2010) Retrospective descriptive analysis of 1,176 patients with failed hypospadias repair. J Urol 183(1):207–211
70. Fraumann SA, Stephany HA, Clayton DB, Thomas JC, Pope JC 4th, Adams MC, Brock JW 3rd, Tanaka ST (2014) Long-term follow-up of children who underwent severe hypospadias repair using an online survey with validated questionnaires. J Pediatr Urol 10(3):446–450
71. Holland AJ, Smith GH, Ross FI, Cass DT (2011) HOSE: an objective scoring system for evaluating the results of hypospadias surgery. BJU Int 88(3):255–258
72. Baskin L (2001) Hypospadias: a critical analysis of cosmetic outcomes using photography. BJU Int 87(6):534–539
73. Mureau MA, Slijper FM, Slob AK, Verhulst FC, Nijman RJ (1996) Satisfaction with penile appearance after hypospadias surgery: the patient and surgeon view. J Urol 155(2):703–706
74. Weber DM, Landolt MA, Gobet R, Kalisch M, Greeff NK (2013) The Penile perception score: an instrument enabling evaluation by surgeons and patient self-assessment after hypospadias repair. J Urol 189(1):189–193
75. Ruppen-Greeff NK, Weber DM, Gobet R, Landolt MA (2013) Health-related quality of life in men with corrected hypospadias: an explorative study. J Pediatr Urol 9(5):551–558
76. Chertin B, Natsheh A, Ben-Zion I, Prat D, Kocherov S, Farkas A, Shenfeld OZ (2013) Objective and subjective sexual outcomes in adult patients after hypospadias repair performed in childhood. J Urol 190(4 Suppl):1556–1560
77. Wei Y, Li XD, Xu N, Xue XY, Zheng QS, Jiang T, Huang JB, Sun XL (2014) Penile appearance, sexual function and sexual satisfaction of hypospadias patients after surgery: a long-term follow-up study. Zhonghua Nan Ke Xue 20(1):48–53
78. Schonbucher VB, Weber DM, Landolt MA (2008) Psychosocial adjustment, health-related quality of life, and psychosexual development of boys with hypospadias: a systematic review. J Pediatr Psychol 33(5):520–535
79. Schonbucher V, Schweizer K, Richter-Appelt H (2010) Sexual quality of life of individuals with disorders of sex development and a 46, XY karyotype: a review of international research. J Sex Marital Ther 36(3):193–215

Cryptorchidism

23

Francesca Destro and Mario Lima

23.1 Introduction

The term cryptorchidism refers to the condition of abnormal testicular descent (TD). In this situation the testis is "hidden" and it cannot be identified in its normal position that is inside the scrotum. In fact the term "cryptorchidism" literally means "hidden testicle" and is often used interchangeably with the term "undescended testicle" [1–3]. A normal testicular function is guaranteed by its full descent into the scrotum. Undescended testes carry the risk of malignant transformation and loss of fertility. It is thus mandatory to recognize this condition in order to plan the surgical correction.

The importance of undescended testes (UDT) has been known since ancient times. Indeed the term testis derives from the Latin "witness" because Romans used to hold the testicles during an oath [4]. The condition was first described by Hunter in 1786, but the first successful surgical orchidopexy was performed only by Annandale in 1877 [5].

F. Destro (✉) • M. Lima
Department of Pediatric Surgery,
S. Orsola-Malpighi University Hospital,
Via Massarenti 11, Bologna 40138, Italy
e-mail: francesca_destro@hotmail.com;
mario.lima@unibo.it

23.2 Classification

The lack of a unitary classification and the variability of nomenclature have always caused difficulties in comparing treatment results. The first distinction is between the non-palpable and the palpable testes that could be obtained after a physical examination. Palpable testis represents 92 % of cases. The term refers to the testes that arrest along its normal descending path. It is further divided into palpable UDT, ectopic, and retractile. Non-palpable testes represent 8 % of cases: in 53 % of cases the testes are absent (agenesis – blinding ending) or vanishing (atrophy), and in 47 % of cases although impalpable it is present (intra-abdominal or near the inguinal canal) [1, 2, 5, 6, 7].

23.2.1 Palpable Testes

23.2.1.1 Retractile Testes

A retractile testis is a normal testis that is not in the scrotum but it can be tractioned in it without difficulties or tension. It will remain in place at the end of the maneuver. It is the result of a cremasteric massive contraction.

23.2.1.2 Palpable Undescended Testes (UDT)

It is the most frequent condition. There are three semeiologic varieties:

M. Lima, G. Manzoni (eds.), *Pediatric Urology: Contemporary Strategies from Fetal Life to Adolescence*, DOI 10.1007/978-88-470-5693-0_23, © Springer-Verlag Italia 2015

1. Falling (high inguinal position): the gonad stays at the internal inguinal ring and it can be manipulated in an elusive way at the beginning of the inguinal canal.
2. Medial inguinal position: the gonad is in the center of the inguinal region and it can be pushed toward the external inguinal ring.
3. Emergent: the gonad is near the external ring, and it can be squeezed out of the inguinal canal but it does not remain in the scrotum.

23.2.1.3 Ectopic Testes

The ectopic UDT has deviated the normal path of descent. It is not very frequent. There are five different localizations:

1. Inguinal region: it is the most common variety. The testes are palpable in the inguinal region, over the inguinal canal and between the external oblique muscle aponeurosis and the subcutaneous fascia.
2. Perineum: the gonad appears in the perineal region laterally to the ano-scrotal raphe.
3. Peno-pubic area: the gonad is at the bottom of the penis or near the pubic symphysis.
4. Femoral region: the gonad has made its way through the femoral canal and it is palpable in Scarpa's femoral triangle.
5. Controlateral scrotum (transverse ectopia): it is a rarity. The ectopic gonad migrates contralaterally during the abdominal descent. Both gonads are in the same scrotum in the complete forms (exceptional). More frequently (incomplete forms) one testis is found retained in the inguinal canal while the other is in the scrotum.

23.2.2 Non-palpable Undescended Testes

23.2.2.1 Agenesis or Atrophy

The term anorchia refers to testicular absence and it can be caused by lack of formation (congenital cause – agenesis) or by an acquired damage (atrophy). The reasons of anorchia are embryological alterations that lead to *blind ending vessels and vas* and intrauterine or perinatal vascular accidents that lead to *vanishing testes*.

23.2.2.2 Intra-abdominal Testes (True Cryptorchidism)

It is a normal testis laparoscopically found in the abdomen. It is further classified as *close ring* or *open ring* depending on the status of the internal inguinal ring.

There is also another entity known as *acquired UDT*. A previous palpable testis cannot longer be brought down into the scrotum. It can be due to iatrogenic causes (inguinal surgery).

23.3 Epidemiology

Cryptorchidism is the most frequent abnormality of the urogenital tract and it represents the most common congenital malformation. In prospective studies using similar defined criteria of cryptorchidism, the birth rate varies between 1.6 % and 9 % [8]. Preterm infants have a higher rate of cryptorchidism (up to ten times higher). However, gestational age is not an independent risk factor and low birth weight seems to be the principal determinant. Cryptorchidism represents 3.4 % of term infants weighing more than 2,500 g, 30.3 % of premature infants weighing less than 2,500 g, and 100 % of babies weighing less than 900 g (Table 23.1) [2]. Other factors that predispose to cryptorchidism include genetic predisposition, small size for gestational age, twinning, and maternal exposure to estrogen during the first trimester. The bilateral cryptorchidism has an incidence of 5 %. The left size is affected more than the right one. [2].

Studies have suggested that there are geographical and ethnic differences along with an increasing trend in the incidence of congenital cryptorchidism. This increment is related to unknown reasons and it is of concern given the long-term adverse health effects of UDT. In fact

Table 23.1 Associated anomalies

Patent vaginal duct
Hypospadia
Abdominal wall defects
Müllerian remnants
Mental retardation
Wilms' tumor

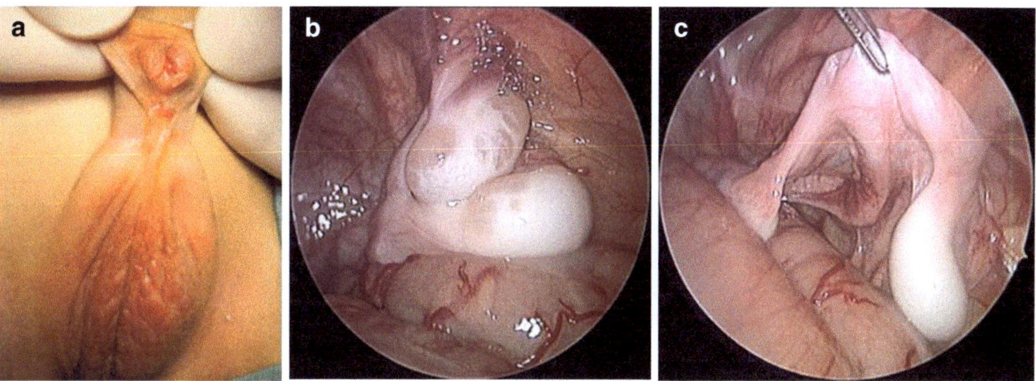

Fig. 23.1 Anomalies that may be associated with cryptorchidism. (**a**) hypospadias and bilateral cryptorchidism (**b**) laparoscopic identification of a crossed testicular ectopia with UDT (**c**) laparoscopic identification of UDT with Müllerian remnant

cryptorchidism has been proposed to be part of a "testicular dysgenesis syndrome" which includes hypospadias, reduced semen quality, and testicular cancer [9]. These conditions seem to have a common origin in prenatal testicular maldevelopment. Familiarity has been demonstrated in 14 % of cases of UDT. The congenital cryptorchidism is usually followed by spontaneous testicular descent that occurs during the first few months of life (approximately 70–77 % of testes will descend by 3 months). Spontaneous descent is more likely in infants with low birth weight, preterm birth, or bilateral cryptorchidism. The incidence of cryptorchidism declines to 0.7–1 % at the end of infancy. Furthermore, although cryptorchidism has been described among school-aged boys, approximately 75 % of these cases show spontaneous descent during puberty. Bilateral presentation is found in 10–20 % of cases. The left side is more common in unilateral cases.

23.4 Associated Anomalies

Cryptorchidism can appear isolated or in a context of syndromes (Table 23.1) and nonchromosomal or chromosomal disorders. In many of these syndromes, there are ambiguous genitalia, hypospadias, or abnormalities of the internal genitalia, such as the persistence of Müllerian remnants that characterize intersexual states (Fig. 23.1) [1–3, 10].

Therefore, a complete screening is indicated in case of cryptorchidism, including: clinical and instrumental evaluation of the urinary tract, ultrasound, and/or abdominal and pelvic MRI to study the gonads.

The prune belly syndrome (absence or severe deficiency of the anterior abdominal wall musculature, urinary tract anomalies, bilateral cryptorchidism) deserves a special mention as it is associated with intra-abdominal testicles in almost all cases [1–3, 11].

UDTs are normal in 70 % of cases (forms, volume, trophism, didymus-epididymis connection). Ipotrophy is more frequent in high retention. Surgical anomalies are described but they are difficult to quantify. Inguinal hernia is often present and when symptomatic requires early surgical correction.

23.5 Embryogenesis

The testis originates early in fetal life. The testis formation is included in a process called sex determination during which the testis produces hormones that initiate and sustain normal male sexual differentiation with simultaneous regression of Müllerian duct structures [12–15]. The SRY gene on the Y chromosome seems to be responsible for male differentiation, and it initiates testicular development.

At 4–6 weeks' gestation, primordial germ cells migrate from the caudal wall of the embryonic yolk sac to the genital ridges. At 7 weeks germ cells differentiate into gonocytes upon entering the testicular cords. In the same period the gubernaculum appears on mesenchymal tissue condensation. It connects the lower pole of the testes to the inguinal canal. Just before testicular descent, the gubernaculum grows in length and mass. The role of the gubernaculum in descent of the testes is still unclear, but it is important for testis fixation to the inguinal canal. There is another mesenchymal structure that anchors the testis cranially. It is called the cranial suspensory ligament (CSL) and it regresses during fetal life. It has no significant role in testicular descent. The testis is initially located between the CSL and the gubernaculum, near the kidney. Androgens seem to mediate regression of the CSL and testis descent. In particular testosterone is produced by Leydig cells that originate at 9 weeks' gestation. At 8 weeks the inguinal canal develops as a caudal evagination of the abdominal wall that is occupied by a herniation of the peritoneum (processus vaginalis).

Testicular descent occurs in 10 % at 24 weeks' gestation, in 50 % at 27 weeks', in 75 % at 28 weeks, and in 80 % at 34 weeks to birth. The descent can be illustrated in three different phases: transabdominal (that seems to be under AMH regulation), transinguinal (under androgen regulation), and extracanalicular (that includes the descent from the external ring to the scrotum).

23.6 Etiopathogenesis

The etiopathogenesis of undescended testis is still unknown and it involves many factors [16].

- *Endocrine*: the integrity of the hypothalamic-pituitary-gonadal axis is fundamental for testis descent. Alterations include gonadotropin production, androgen biosynthesis, or androgen action. Androgens appear to be important for the inguinal scrotal phase of testicular descent (phase 2). Other endocrine factors are MIF (that is more a mediator), estrogens, and an androgen-independent factor that stimulates the growth of gubernaculum.
- *Gubernaculum*: it has been associated with different roles such as the dilator of the inguinal canal to obtain testicular passage, a structure that tractions the testis pulling it into the scrotum, the guide for testes, etc.
- *Epididymis*: this factor was proposed on the base of the evidence that epididymal abnormalities in patients with undescended testes approach 90 %.
- *Intra-abdominal pressure*: it probably affects phase 2 in association with androgen secretion.

23.7 Diagnosis

Cryptorchidism has specific features that make history and clinical examination sufficient to diagnose the condition [17–19]. Imaging and laboratory evaluation are rarely indicated and they are generally used for surgical planning.

23.7.1 History, Physical Examination, and Laboratory Tests

The evaluation of a patient with cryptorchidism starts with a complete history (medical, surgical, and familiar) and a physical examination. Parents should be questioned regarding previous history of normal descended testes during the first year of life or during different moments of the day (e.g., when the patient is relaxed in the bathtub that may suggest excessive cremasteric reflex or retractile testes) and previous inguinal surgery (iatrogenic cryptorchidism). A family history may be present too.

Cryptorchidism is usually an asymptomatic condition, and only rarely it gives the feeling of mild pain or discomfort at the level of the inguinal region. The onset of symptoms may indicate the onset of complications.

The clinical examination (Fig. 23.2) is the most accurate test to diagnose this situation, and it is reliable and less invasive. The aim of the clinical examination is the identification of a palpable gonad and of the lowest position that can be reached and where the testicle can be placed

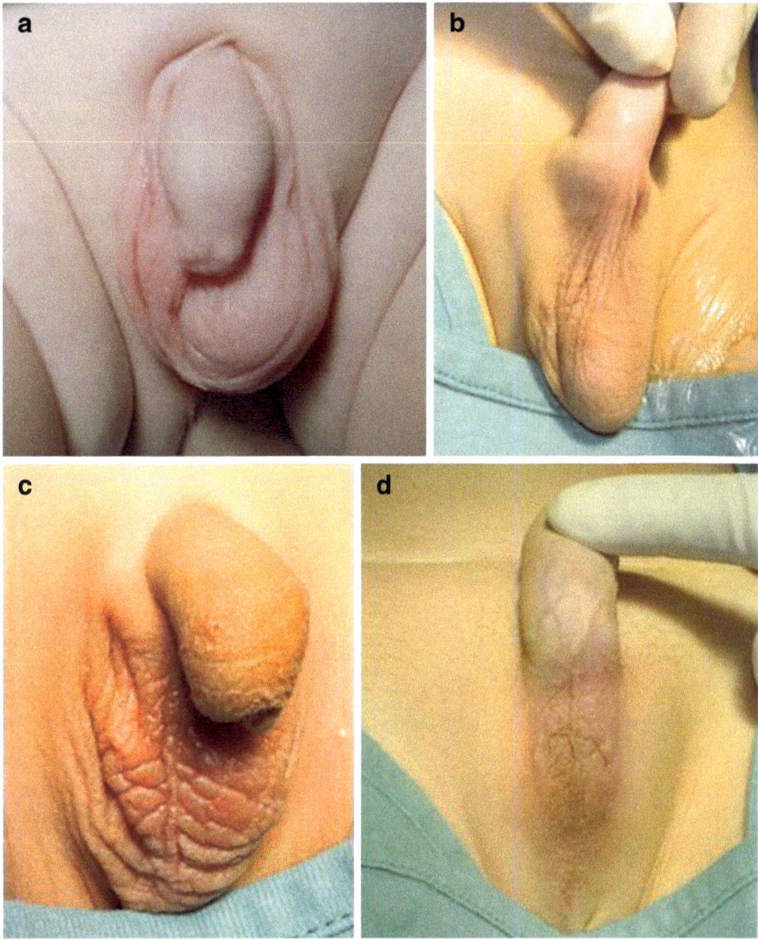

Fig. 23.2 Clinical pictures: (**a**, **b**) inhabited right scrotum; (**c**, **d**) bilateral cryptorchidism (Note scrotal hypotrophy and abnormal folds)

without tension. The evaluation should be performed in a warm environment with the child relaxed over the table. Relaxation is fundamental as evidenced by the fact that 20 % of nonpalpable testes become palpable when the patient is under anesthesia. Children are first examined supine with legs in the frog-like position and then straight or curled in orthostatism. External genitalia are inspected for the appearance of the scrotum and to identify inguinal swellings (high testis or associated hernia). The presence or absence position and size of each testis are evaluated as well as the aspect of the scrotum (asymmetry, hypoplasia) and the presence of surgical scars.

The aspect of the scrotum varies with age: neonates have a thin and pendulous scrotum while children have a small and puckered one. An empty scrotum after a previously normal exam correlates with testicular ascent or a vascular event (atrophy). It may also be iatrogenic or primary (retraction of the processus vaginalis or muscular spasticity). A hypoplastic scrotum has probably never held testicles.

Testes may be visible in an empty scrotum by gentle cranial retraction of the suprapubic skin. The palpation of the inguinal region with a flat hand is effective in detecting a testis. A palpable testis is usually squeezed out of the inguinal canal by pressing on the abdominal wall laterally near the anterosuperior iliac spine and downward toward the scrotum (fingertips are slide through the inguinal canal to appreciate the testis). Once the gonad appears at the external inguinal ring, one hand attempts to push it while the other attempts to grasp it through the scrotum. This

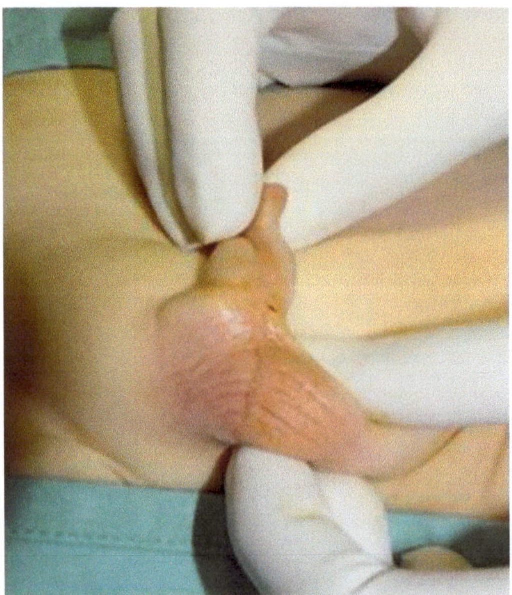

Fig. 23.3 Clinical examination

maneuver permits to determine the lowest level reached by the testis (Fig. 23.3).

The evaluation of the contralateral gonad is important in case of unilateral undescended testis. A hypertrophied gonad (volume >2 mL) may be present when the other testis is absent (atrophy).

The cremasteric reflex is not present in newborns but it later helps identifying the testicle (it is more active between 3 and 9 years).

If the testis is above the scrotum in newborns, the child should be re-evaluated at 3 months of age. If the situation is the same by that age, a diagnosis of UDT can be made; otherwise, close observation should be planned as re-ascent is frequent in these cases.

Clinical examination is important to differentiate normally retractile testes from UDT (Table 23.2).

Common sites of ectopic testis should be examined if the gonad is not found (most commonly the testis lies superficial to the inguinal canal but might be in front of the pubis, in the perineum, or in the upper thigh).

Clinical examination should include observation of the penis to search for hypospadia or ambiguous genitalia and inspection for syndromic features and pubertal signs.

Table 23.2 Normally retracted testes

Easily brought to the bottom of the scrotum
They remain in the scrotum
They are normal in size
They are spontaneously in the scrotum (history)

The follow-up laboratory tests should be performed in case of unilateral cryptorchidism associated with hypospadia and in case of bilateral cryptorchidism (suspected anorchia) [20, 21]:

- LH
- FSH
- 17-OH progesterone
- Testosterone with or without hCG (human chorionic gonadotropin) stimulation
- Inhibin B
- Karyotype

Positive response after hCG stimulation, low levels of FSH, and normal levels of inhibin B mean a functioning testicular tissue is present.

23.7.2 Radiological Evaluation

There are various imaging techniques that have been proposed to identify the position of the testis including: ultrasonography (US), computerized tomography (CT) scanning, routine magnetic resonance (MR) imaging and MR angiography, and venography [22, 23]. Some of these techniques require sedation or anesthesia and they are not free from risks. In addition their overall accuracy is 44 % [23]. Radiological evaluation is not superior to a physical examination in detecting the gonad and thus planning surgery. The rate of false negatives and false positives of ultrasound, computed tomography, and magnetic resonance is significant. Accuracy varies by location of the testicles, with less invasive methods demonstrating poor accuracy for abdominally located testicles and those that are atrophied.

Laparoscopy has now become the most common way to identify the position of an intra-abdominal testis, and it permits a direct observation of the spermatic cord. Surgical exploration is mandatory and it is a key element in differentiating agenesis – atrophy and intra-abdominal testes. No specific imaging technique is able to completely identify anorchia or descent of the testicles and thus eliminate the need for further surgical evaluation. Therefore, imaging is an unnecessary expense, and it should be limited to cases of ambiguous genitalia to evaluate the presence of Müllerian remnants and renal alterations (frequently associated with testicular agenesis or vassal agenesis).

23.8 Therapy

The goal of any intervention for cryptorchidism is to move the undescended testicle to a normal position in the scrotum, in as safe and least invasive way possible [24–40]. Clinical decision making about treatment is influenced by many factors such as bilateralism, palpability, age at presentation, and associated anomalies of medical conditions. In boys under 1 year of age, it may be difficult to distinguish between "true" cryptorchidism and a retractile testicle as the testicle is close to but not quite inside the scrotum. It may be useful to observe the patient until he is 1 year old.

There are different kinds of therapeutic strategies once cryptorchidism is diagnosed: conservative treatment (wait and see), hormonal treatment, or surgery. The type of clinical pathway should be selected through results of hormonal stimulation testing, imaging, and above all clinical evaluation, particularly when the testicle is non-palpable. Hormonal stimulation helps determining the presence of testicular tissue in case of bilateral nonpalpable cryptorchidism. In particular, hormones (such as hCG) stimulate the testes to secrete testosterone. Increased levels of testosterone after administration of hCG suggest that there is at least one viable testicle, while no hormone response suggests anorchia.

23.8.1 Complications of Cryptorchidism

Undescended testes represent an important cause of *infertility*. Unfortunately assessment for fertility is inexact because most studies are retrospective and the ability to have children does not correlate with semen quality. Patients with bilateral cryptorchidism have less sperm cells than the general population (percentage of men with normal semen analysis 25–30 %) and paternity rates at 45–65 %. Germ cell hypoplasia seems to happen early during gestation in patients with undescended testes, and it is related to low cell proliferation and cell destruction. In fact two important prepubertal steps (the transformation of the gonocytes into the adult stem cell pool at 2–3 months and the transformation of spermatogonia into spermatocytes at 4–5 years) are defective in patients with undescended testes. Bilateral cryptorchidism damages fertility more than unilateral cryptorchidism. The long-term prognosis for fertility is better when judged by paternity. Paternity has found to be significantly compromised in men with previous bilateral but not unilateral cryptorchidism (unilateral: paternity rates 80–90 % with normal semen in 55–95 %). Recently biopsy studies have shown an improvement in fertility that is probably related to early orchiopexy (under 2 years of age).

Cryptorchidism has an important association with *testicular malignancies* (the relative risk seems to be 3.8 times greater than normal when orchiopexy had been performed after 9 years of age). The most common tumor developed in undescended testes is seminoma. It is yet inconclusive whether early orchiopexy will protect against the development of malignancies.

Sometimes the undescended testis develops multiple small echogenic foci of calcification in adult age (*microcalcification*). It has been suggested that microcalcification might be a tumor marker when associated with cryptorchidism, infertility, and testicular atrophy. Isolate asymptomatic microcalcification is an incidental finding that requires only ultrasound surveillance.

The undescended testis has an increased susceptibility to rotate around the spermatic cord (*testicular torsion*) because there is a development abnormality between the testis and its mesentery.

23.8.2 Medical Therapy

Human chorionic gonadotropin (hCG) with LH-like action and gonadorelin (GnRH) are the main hormones used in the medical treatment of cryptorchidism. These hormones have been used alone or in combination with other drugs.

Hormonal therapy is associated with some temporary harms of treatment. The hCG may cause scrotal hyperemia, swelling of the genitals, frequent erections (as a result of the increase in testosterone circulating levels), and restlessness which usually subside a few weeks after discontinuation of therapy. The GnRH usually has a virilizing side effect and it is rarely responsible for restlessness.

With regard to the effectiveness of hormone therapy in inducing permanent descent of the testis into the scrotum, it seems that:

- Different regimens offer similar results with a reported success rate between 6 and 75 %.
- The gonad location is the main factor that influences the positive response to hormonal therapy. In particular, the higher the position of the testicle, the lower the rate of response.
- Effectiveness of hormonal therapy is not influenced by patients' age.

Unfortunately there are not definitive conclusions regarding the expected effect rate for any hormonal or combined medical therapy as most scientific studies are of poor quality.

23.8.3 Surgical Therapy

The optimal therapeutic option is still a matter of debate. Considering the efficacy and the side effects of the various options, surgery is considered the primary choice. The success rate of surgery, defined as scrotal testis position without atrophy, depends on three elements: the type of UDT, the type of procedure chosen, and the age at time of surgery. It is estimated to be between 74 % (abdominal testes) and 92 %. In the past decade percentages have increased up to >85–90 % for abdominal testes and >95 % for inguinal testes. Surgery seems also to improve sperm cell count in uni- and bilateral cases and Leydig cell function, especially if it is performed in early childhood.

There are different surgical strategies (Fig. 23.4). In particular primary orchiopexy with creation of a subdartos pouch is used in lower testes (closer to the scrotum). The Bianchi single high scrotal incision technique may be an option in case of testes distal to the external inguinal ring. The retroperitoneal dissection is crucial for the success of both techniques. Bilateral cases can be done during the same procedure. Fowler-Stephens orchiopexy (whether 1 or 2 stage) is reserved for higher testes which are more difficult to treat and have higher rates of after surgery retraction. In the context of minimally invasive surgery, laparoscopy has been recently widely used in children because of technological advances and postoperative advantages in terms of toleration and cosmesis. If both testes are nonpalpable, the patient should be immediately referred to endocrinologic evaluation. In these cases laparoscopy is used to determine surgical therapy (Fig. 23.3). Two or more stage procedures are performed in order to do one side at a time and to evaluate the result before proceeding to the other side. Testicular biopsy is usually not performed, and it is reserved in case of ambiguous genitalia or chromosomal disorders.

The optimal age for treatment should be established on the base of its influence on future spermatogenesis, hormonal production, and risk for tumors. Actually there are not certain data but many studies report that early intervention is the most beneficial (<1 years of age). Orchiopexy in patients born with UDT should not be performed before 6 months in order to give the possibility to the testes to descent. In addition it is generally accepted that truly retractile testes require no therapy as fertility potential is normal. Unfortunately some retractile testes are outside the scrotum for most of the time during childhood, and they descend only during puberty. This situation may lead to impaired function that can be prevented by early intervention.

23.8.3.1 Orchiopexy: Palpable UDT

Multiple operative techniques have been described and they are associated with various success rates. The surgical procedure has four key steps: complete mobilization of the testes and spermatic cord, repair of the processus vaginalis, tension-free placement of the testis in the scrotum, and creation of a superficial pouch to

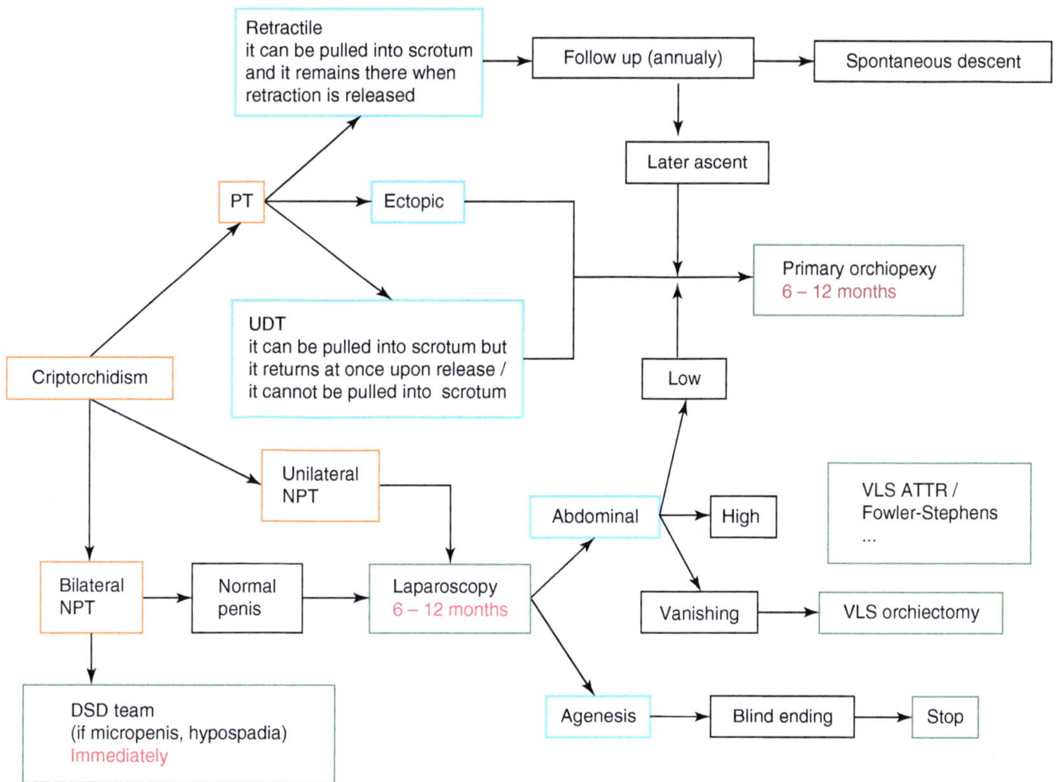

Fig. 23.4 Surgical management of children with cryptorchidism

place and fix the gonad. Inguinal orchiopexy is the most common surgical approach.

A transverse skin incision is performed in the midway between the pubis and the anterior-superior iliac spine (Fig. 23.5).

The dermis and subcutaneous tissues are opened with electrocautery; Scarpa's fascia is cut with cold scissors that are used for blunt dissection. Retractors are used to improve the view over the external oblique muscle fascia. Care should be taken to avoid damages of the gonad in case of superficial ectopies. The inguinal canal is entered by opening the external oblique fascia in case of intracanalicular testes (be careful to avoid the ilio-inguinal nerve). The testicular tunics are grasped and the gubernaculum is dissected distally (be careful not to damage the vas deferens and remember that the vas can have unconventional pathways). Fibers and the cremasteric muscle are dissected to mobilize the spermatic cord to

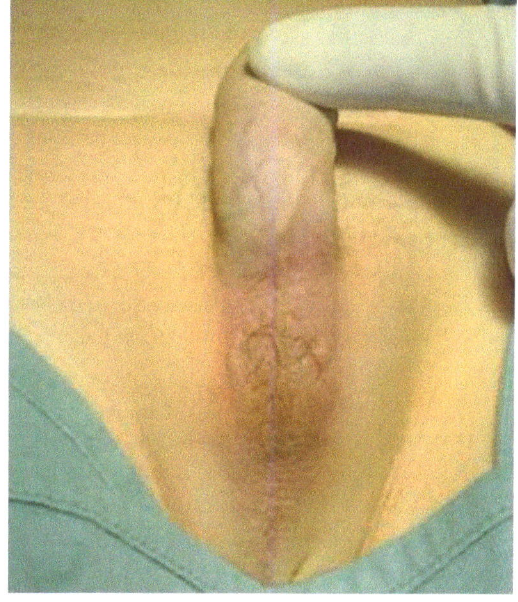

Fig. 23.5 Skin incision

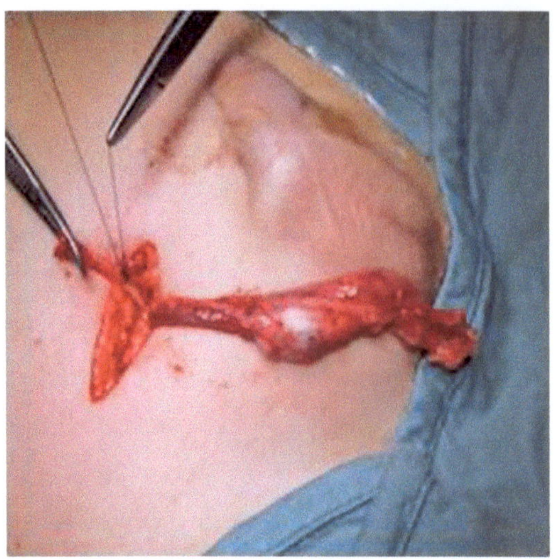

Fig. 23.6 The patent vaginal duct is isolated, ligated, and dissected at the internal inguinal ring

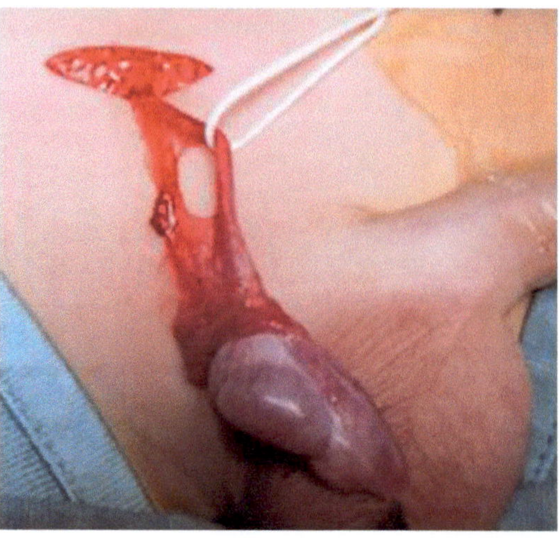

Fig. 23.7 At the end of the dissection, the testis can be brought down without tension

the internal inguinal ring. The tunica vaginalis is then opened over the testis that is exposed and evaluated (shape, dimensions, integrity, presence of embryological remnants).

The tension-free placement is obtained by complete mobilization f the spermatic cord that should not damage paratesticular structures or devitalize the vascular supply. During this part of the operation, the patent processus vaginalis is divided from the elements of the spermatic cord.

Once the hernia sac is completely isolated, it is twisted, suture ligated at the level of the internal inguinal ring, and amputated (Fig. 23.6).

The division of the processus vaginalis and cremasteric muscle attachments (with cotton tipped applicators, sponge, etc.) usually provides adequate length (Fig. 23.7). In all other cases dissection continues in the retroperitoneal space and the Prentiss maneuver may be necessary (the testis and spermatic cord are moved medial to the inguinal canal).

Once the desired length is obtained, the surgeon uses its finger or a large surgical clamp to create a tunnel for the gonad that extends from the inguinal canal to the scrotum. A transverse scrotal incision is then performed. A clamp is anchored to the surgeon's glove and its tip is guided into the inguinal canal by withdrawing the finger. The clamp is then used to grasp the

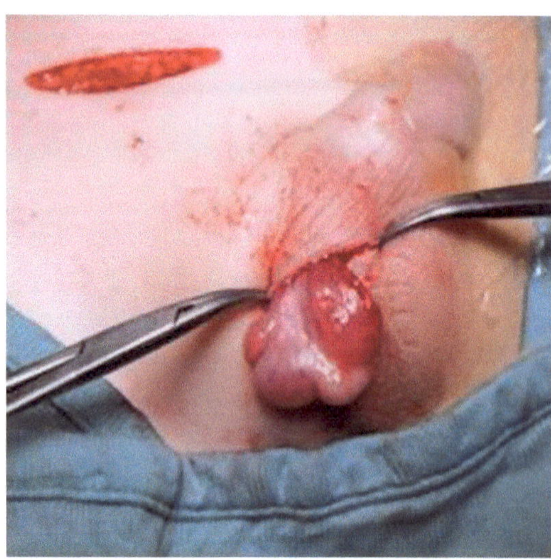

Fig. 23.8 A scrotal incision allows the testes to descend

tunica vaginalis and to locate the testis into the scrotum (Fig. 23.8). The position of the spermatic cord should be tested to avoid torsions. There are two distinct surgical techniques to fix the testis. The classical one (transfixation orchiopexy) provides for a suture to be passed through the tunica albuginea to fix it to the scrotum (with or without external pledget). The other one (dartos pouch) consists in the creation of a pouch under the scrotal skin that extends inferiorly from the scrotal incision. The testes are placed within the dartos pouch avoiding the

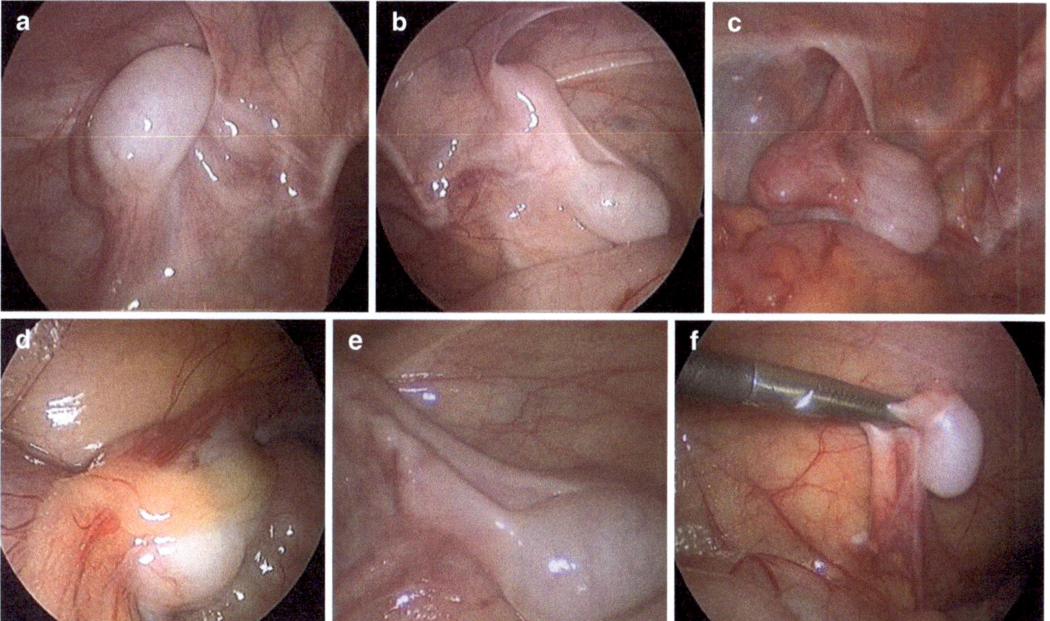

Fig. 23.9 Laparoscopic view of intra-abdominal testes: low iuxta-canalicular testes (**a–c**); high iliac and pelvic testes (**d–f**)

suture of the tunica albuginea (it causes significant testicular inflammation although it prevents later testicular torsion).

Scrotal skin is closed with 4/0 interrupted absorbable suture. The external oblique fascia is closed with running absorbable suture and the inguinal canal is re-created. Above tissues are closed with intradermal absorbable suture for the skin.

Another common operation is the prescrotal (Bianchi) orchiopexy that involves making an incision along the edge of the scrotum, mobilizing the testis and spermatic cord, repairing the inguinal hernia, and placing the testis in the scrotum. It is ideal for the ascending or retractile testis.

23.8.3.2 Laparoscopy: Unilateral Nonpalpable UDT

Laparoscopy is useful to determine which surgical approach should be taken. The patient is placed in supine decubitus with distended legs and arms. The sterile field extends between the xiphoid region to the perineum (external genitalia are included) and laterally below the anterior-superior iliac spine. The Trendelenburg position aids in better visualization of the lower abdomen and pelvis and a Foley catheter draining the bladder maximizes the operating space. A 5 mm port is inserted through the umbilicus for the 0° optic and pneumoperitoneum is created with 0.5–1 L/min of flow and 8–10 mmHg of pressure. The abdominal cavity is explored starting from the internal inguinal ring. It is important to have the comparative image of the opposite side. The exploration proceeds to the pelvis and the iliac regions to the origin of the internal spermatic vessels. This is important especially in case of testicular agenesis where a second or third trocar can be inserted to search for rare anatomical anomalies as spleno-gonadic fusion.

Laparoscopic findings can be different:

1. *Low abdominal testis* (<2 cm from the inguinal ring) (Fig. 23.9a–c): the testis is normal and it is near the internal inguinal ring (*iuxta-canalicular*); the ring is usually patent and the testis can enter intermittently the ring (*peeping testis*). In these cases the inguinal pressure pulls the testes in the abdomen while the scrotal traction takes it down in the canal. Inguinal orchiopexy is performed at the same time.

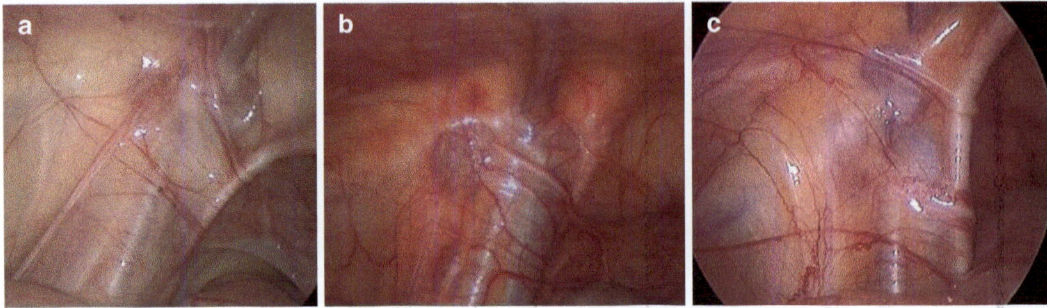

Fig. 23.10 Laparoscopic view of intraperitoneal vanishing testes: the spermatic vessels appear slender, tortuous, and almost vanishing at the internal inguinal ring that is closed (**a–c**)

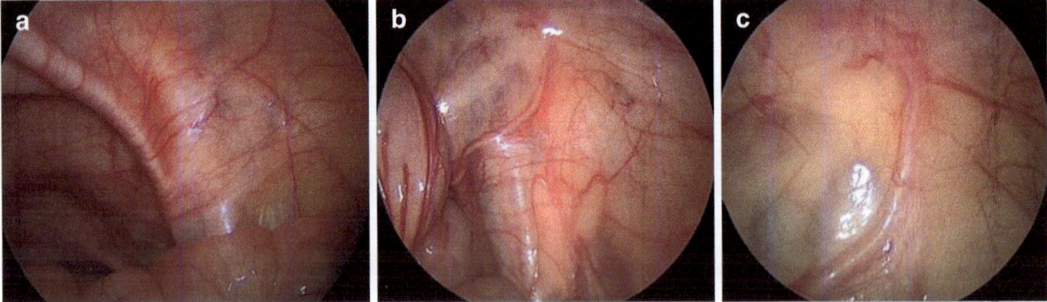

Fig. 23.11 Laparoscopic view of testicular agenesis: spermatic vessels are absent and the vas is hypotrophic (**a–c**)

2. *High abdominal testis* (>2 cm from the internal inguinal ring) (Fig. 23.9d, e): the testis usually lies on the posterior abdominal wall (retroperitoneal-iliac); rarely it is behind the bladder (pelvic). The internal inguinal ring is usually closed.
3. *Abdominal atrophy* of the testes (Fig. 23.10): hypoplastic vas and vessels are seen to end in a small unformed testis (abdominal *vanishing testis*). If the testis is hypotrophic or atrophic, an orchiectomy should be performed.
4. *Abdominal agenesis* of the testes (Fig. 23.11): the internal spermatic vessels are absent or hypotrophic and they end blindly in the abdomen (abdominal *blind ending*). The terminal part of the deferential artery is serpiginous and the vas is narrow. Pathological evaluation of the tip of the vessels may show remnants of testicular tissue or hemosiderin that are indicative of testicular resorption.
5. *Intracanalicular atrophy/agenesis* of the testes: there are hypoplastic vas and vessels going into the internal inguinal ring (intracanalicular "vanishing testis"). In these cases the need of an inguinal exploration may be useful to remove the atrophic testes and to reduce the risk of cancer even if the need of this operation is still debated. The complete absence of the vessels is typical of the intracanalicular testis agenesis (intracanalicular "blind ending testis") that does not require an open inguinal exploration.

The inguinal exploration after laparoscopy is recommended in case of obese children, in opened internal inguinal ring (insufflations may have pushed the testis downward), and, as previously said, when the presence of an atrophic-hypotrophic testis is suspected.

The inguinal approach is unsuccessful in case of high abdominal testes. A two stage orchiopexy is preferred when the vessels are too short. This procedure consists of mobilization and fixation of the testes as low as possible (e.g., at the pubic tubercle or inguinal ligament) followed by the second stage after 6–12 months. The advantage is that the testicular artery is

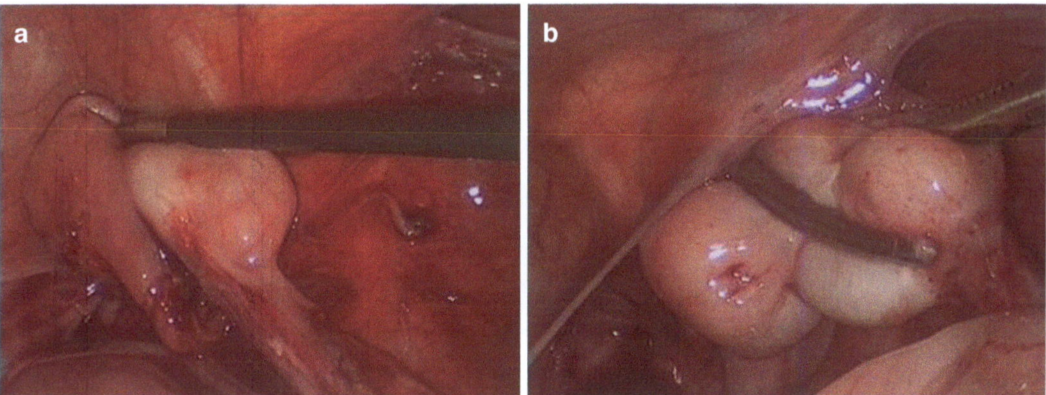

Fig. 23.12 The gonad is brought near the internal inguinal ring once the laparoscopic mobilization is completed (**a**); a clamp through the scrotum is used to catch the gonad and to place it in the scrotal pouch (**b**)

preserved; the disadvantage is that some elements (the vas deferens, the epididymis, and the testicular blood supply) may be injured during the second stage.

23.8.3.3 Fowler-Stephens Orchiopexy: Unilateral Nonpalpable UDT

The Fowler-Stephens orchiopexy is used in case of high nonpalpable testis (testes located more than 3 cm from the ipsilateral internal inguinal ring), and it consists of ligation of the spermatic vessels leaving the testicular vascularization to the vassal, cremasteric, and gubernacular arteries. The technique requires integrity of these collateral vessels, and for this reason, it is not a good option after inguinal exploration that may have led to vascular impairment. The technique is usually performed in two steps: vessels are first ligated laparoscopically or by laparotomy. The second stage involves the section of the vessels and the completion of the orchiopexy. A waiting period of at least 6 months is required between the two steps in order to allow the collateral circulation to develop.

23.8.3.4 Koff-Sethi: Unilateral Nonpalpable UDT

The Koff and Sethi procedure is an alternative to the Fowler-Stephens (also called one-step Fowler-Stephens). The ligation of the spermatic vessels takes place in a lower position (at least 3–4 cm away from the testes) decreasing tension and enhancing viability. This maneuver is allowed thanks to the singular testicular vascular anatomy. Orchiopexy is thus performed in a single-step procedure. Sometimes the testes may be mobilized through a retroperitoneal dissection starting from a high suprainguinal incision. The main disadvantage is the risk of testicular atrophy due to possible vasospasm of small deferential vessels. The surgeon may also decide to leave the testes at the lower position reached and to conclude the procedure after a year, during a second operation.

23.8.3.5 Laparoscopic-Assisted Orchiopexy

This technique has been developed to preserve the spermatic vessels. Patient and trocar position is the same as for a standard laparoscopy. The testicular vessels and the vas are mobilized from the posterior peritoneum in order to free the testes leaving the tissue between spermatic vessels and vas intact. The testis is brought down to the scrotum through the internal inguinal ring or a neo-ring created between the umbilical artery and the inferior epigastric vessels (Fig. 23.12). The creation of a neo-ring may be useful also in case of short cord (Prentiss maneuver: a 12 mm expandable port or a blunt clamp is introduced through the base of the scrotum and it is used to create a neoring medial to the epigastric vessels) because it shortens the path to the scrotum.

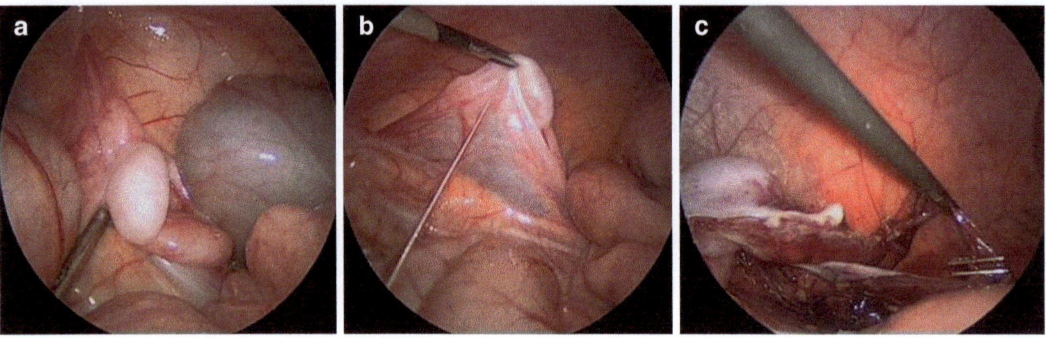

Fig. 23.13 Laparoscopic step: identification of the gonad (**a**) and its isolation (**b**) followed by vascular section after clip ligation (**c**)

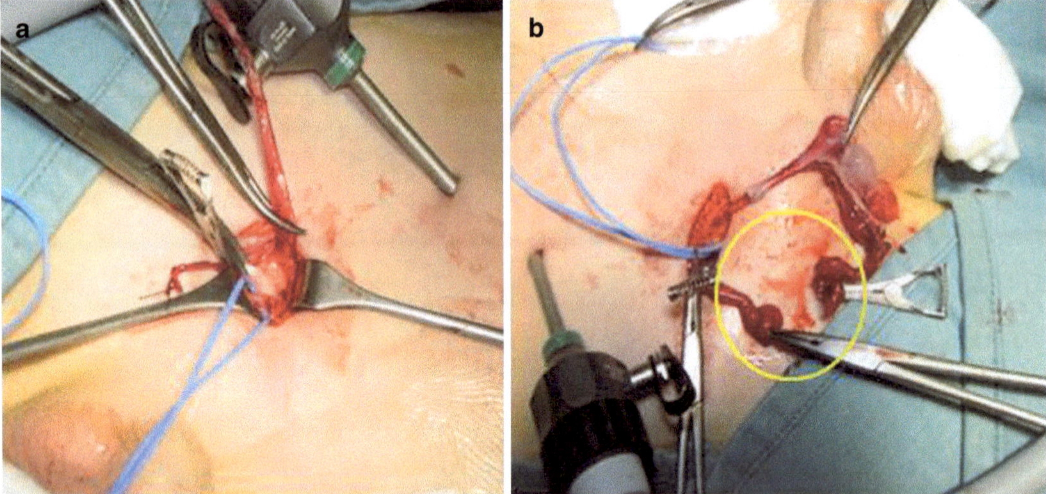

Fig. 23.14 Inguinal step: vessels are isolated (**a**) and prepared for microvascular anastomosis (**b**). The yellow circle in b shows the extremities that will be anastomosed.

23.8.3.6 Microvascular Orchiopexy (Silber-Kelly): Unilateral Nonpalpable UDT

This technique was developed in order to preserve a better vascular testicular supply. It requires long operative times, special skills, and dedicated instrumentation. This procedure should be performed around 3 years of age. Testicular vessels are divided and a microvascular anastomosis between the testicular artery and vein and the inferior epigastric vessels is performed. It has a success rate of 80 %.

An alternative procedure is the "ATTR" (literally "testicular wastewater autotransplantation") proposed by Lima and colleagues. It provides for the section of the vascular spermatic pedicle and the microsurgical venous anastomosis between the spermatic vein and the inferior epigastric vein. The gonad is then freed and brought down to the scrotum. The effectiveness of this technique is related to the fact that the deferential circle is able to offer a good supply of arterial blood but not an adequate venous drainage when the spermatic circle is excluded. The venous anastomosis permits to overcome this problem, and it is safer than the Fowler-Stephens and simpler than the Silber-Kelly.

ATTR procedure:

Figures 23.13, 23.14, 23.15, and 23.16

23.8.3.7 Complications of Surgery

Wound infection and hematoma are rare but are described as immediate complications after orchiopexy. Recurrent cryptorchidism is possible, and

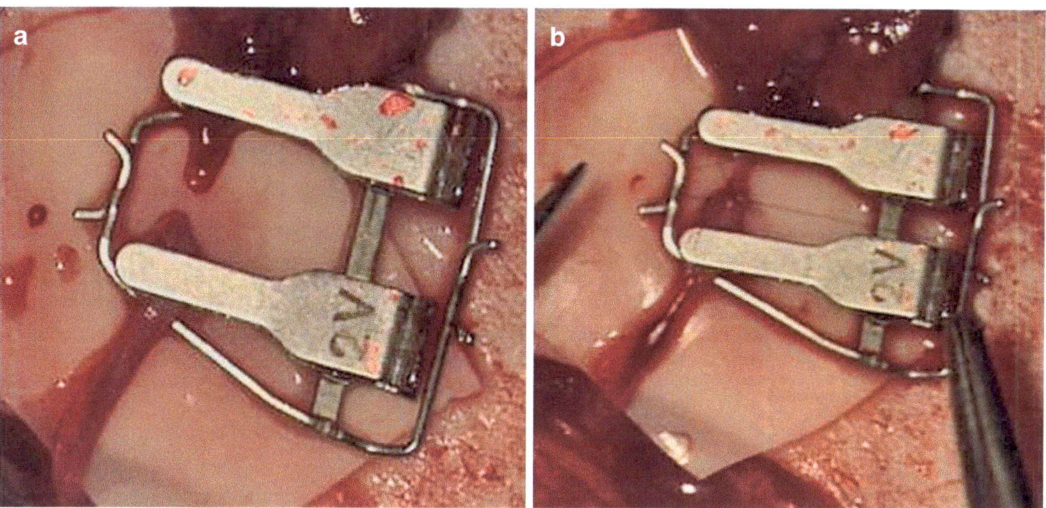

Fig. 23.15 Appearance of vessels before (**a**) and after (**b**) microvascular anastomosis. The anastomosis is performed with operative microscope (8-12x) in nylon 10/0 and long needle.

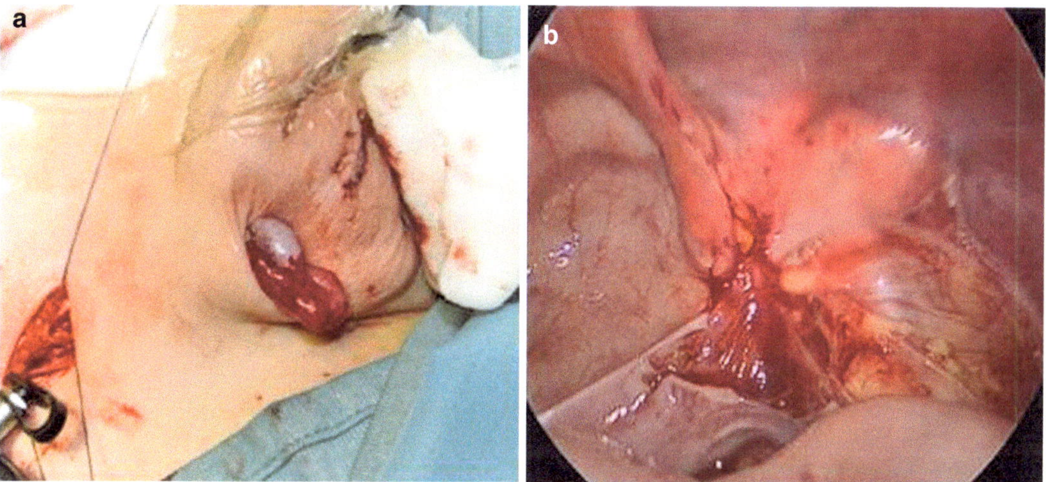

Fig. 23.16 The procedure ends with a standard orchiopexy (**a**) and the final laparoscopic control (**b**)

it is often related to inadequate inguinal hernia repair, to insufficient retroperitoneal dissection, or to patent processus vaginalis. Testicular atrophy and hypotrophy are the most important complications. They are related to ischemic injuries. Clinical follow-up should be done 12 months after surgery with ultrasound evaluation to define testicular volume. Re-evaluation at early puberty is necessary in bilateral cases. Patients with retractile testis require evaluation at 3, 5, 7, and 10 years old to detect later ascent. A close follow-up is required also in patients with spontaneous descent. Success of surgery is assessed by testicular position, presence of testicular atrophy, and, later in life, by fertility and risk of cancer.

References

1. Dòmini R, Lima M (1998) Criptorchidismo. In: Chirurgia delle malformazioni urinarie e genitali, vol 26. Piccin, Padova, pp 505–521
2. Spinelli C, Lima M, Signoretti P, Bertelloni S, Franchi G (2001) Il Criptorchidismo. Fisiopatologia, Clinica, Terapia Medica e Chirurgica. Piccin, Padova
3. Dòmini R, Belbusti F, Lima M, Signoretti P, Jasonni V (1991) Criptorchidia. In: Argomenti di andrologia

chirurgica pediatrica. Applicazioni di tecniche microchirurgiche. Piccin, Padova, pp 7–59
4. Hudson JM (2006) Undescended testes. In: Stringer MD, Oldhans K, Mouriquand PDE (eds) Pediatric surgery and urology. Cambridge University Press, New York, pp 652–663
5. Turek PJ, Ewalt DH, Snyder H (1994) The absent cryptorchid testis: surgical findings and their implications for diagnosis and etiology. J Urol 151:718–721
6. Hudson JM (2006) Undescended testes, torsion and varicocele. In: Grosfeld JL (ed) Pediatric surgery. Elsevier, Philadelphia, pp 1193–1214
7. Tennenbaum SY, Lerner SE, McAleer I (1994) Preoperative laparoscopic localization of the nonpalpable testis: a critical analysis of a 10-year experience. J Urol 151:732–734
8. Gapany C, Frey P, Cachat F et al (2008) Management of cryptorchidism in children: guidelines. Swiss Med Wkly 138(33–34):492–498
9. Thorup J, Haugen S, Kollin C et al (2001) Surgical treatment of undescended testes. Acta Paediatr 96(5):631–637
10. Lima M, Dòmini M, Gargano T, Ruggeri G, Gentili A, Manuele R (2010) Transverse testicular ectopia and persistent mullerian duct syndrome: video-assisted treatment. Eur J Pediatr Surg 20(1):53–4
11. Schneck FX, Bellinger MF (2007) Abnormalities of the testes and scrotum and their surgical management: chapter 127. In: Wein AJ et al (eds) Campbell-Walsh urology, 9th edn. Saunders Elsevier, Philadelphia
12. Kubota Y, Temelcos C, Bathgate RAD et al (2002) The role of insulin 3 testosterone, MIS and relaxin in rat gubernaculum growth. Hum Mol Reprod 8:900–905
13. Abacı A, Çatlı G, Anık A, Böber E (2013) Epidemiology, classification and management of undescended testes: does medication have value in its treatment? J Clin Res Pediatr Endocrinol 5(2):65–72
14. Hrabovszky Z, Farmer PJ, Hutson JM (2000) Does the sensory nucleus of the genitofemoral nerve have a role in testicular descent? J Pediatr Surg 35:96–100
15. Ritzen EM (2008) Undescended testes: a consensus on management. Eur J Endocrinol 159:S87–S90
16. Ritzen EM, Bergh A, Bjerknes R et al (2007) Nordic consensus on treatment of undescended testes. Acta Pediatr 96(5):638–643
17. Esposito C, Caldamone AA, Settimi A, El-Ghoneimi A (2008) Management of boys with nonpalpable undescended testis. Nat Clin Pract Urol 5:252–260
18. Hutson JM, Balic A, Nation T, Southwell B (2010) Cryptorchidism. Semin Pediatr Surg 19(3):215–224
19. Lao OB, Fitzgibbons RJ Jr, Cusick RA (2012) Pediatric inguinal hernias, hydroceles, and undescended testicles. Surg Clin N Am 92(3):487–504
20. Lee PA, Houk CP (2013) Cryptorchidism. Curr Opin Endocrinol Diabetes Obes 20(3):210–216
21. Penson D, Krishnaswami S, Jules A et al (2013) Effectiveness of hormonal and surgical therapies for cryptorchidism: a systematic review. Pediatrics 131(6):e1897–e1907
22. Ashley RA, Barthold JS, Kolon TF (2010) Cryptorchidism: pathogenesis, diagnosis, treatment and prognosis. Urol Clin N Am 37:183–193
23. Huston JM, Clarke MC (2007) Current management of undescended testicle. Semin Pediatr Surg 16:64–70
24. Bruijnen CJ, Vogels HD, Beasley SW (2012) Age at orchidopexy as an indicator of the quality of regional child health services. J Paediatr Child Health 48(7):556–559
25. Casanova NC, Johnson EK, Bowen DK et al (2013) Two-step Fowler-Stephens orchiopexy for intra-abdominal testes: a 28-year single institution experience. J Urol 190(4):1371–1376
26. Docimo SG, Moore RG, Adams J (1995) Laparoscopic orchiopexy for the high impalpable testis: preliminary experience. J Urol 154:1513–1515
27. Dòmini R, Lima M, Dòmini M (1997) Microvascular autotransplantation of the testis: the "Refluo" technique. Eur J Pediatr Surg 7:288–291
28. Esposito C (2008) Laparoscopic treatment of nonpalpable testis: chap 101. In: Bax K, Georgeson K, Rothemberg S, Valla JS, Yeung CK (eds) Endoscopic surgery in infants and children. Springer, Berlin, pp 753–758
29. Holcomb GW (2003) Laparoscopy for the nonpalpable testis: chap 8. In: Lobe TE (ed) Pediatric laparoscopy. Landes Bioscience, Georgetown, pp 83–89
30. Hutsocn JM (2006) Orchidopexy: chap 53. In: Puri P, Höllwarth M (eds) Pediatric surgery. Springer, Berlin/New York, pp 555–568
31. Kollin C, Stukenborg JB, Nurmio M et al (2012) Boys with undescended testes: endocrine, volumetric and morphometric studies on testicular function before and after orchidopexy at nine months or three years of age. J Clin Endocrinol Metab 97:4588–4595
32. Lima M, Esposito C, Papparella A, Mattioli G (2004) Criptorchidismo: chap 8. In: Laparoscopia, Toracoscopia e Retroperitoneoscopia pediatrica, vol 4. CLUEB, Bologna, pp 185–195
33. Loughlin KR (2012) Changes in male fertility in the last two decades. Urol Clin N Am 39(1):33–36
34. Papparella A, Zamparelli M, Cobellis G (1999) Laparoscopy for non palpable testis: is inguinal exploration always necessary when the cord structures enter the inguinal ring? J Laparoendosc Adv Surg Technol B 1:29–33
35. Powell C, McIntosh J, Murphy JP et al (2013) Laparoscopic orchiopexy for intra-abdominal testes-a single institution review. J Laparoendosc Adv Surg Technol A 23(5):481–483
36. Rozanski TA, Wojno KI, Bloom DA (1996) The remnant orchiectomy. J Urol 155:712–714

37. Schleef J, Von Bismarck S (2002) Groin exploration for non-palpable testes: laparoscopic approach. J Pediatr Surg 37:1552–1555
38. Shnorhavorian M, Jacobs MA, Stearns G et al (2012) Practice variation and clinical confusion regarding undescended testes and retractile testes among primary care respondents: a multiregional survey study in the United States. Pediatr Surg Int 28:635–639
39. Tasian GE, Yiee JH, Copp HL (2011) Imaging use and cryptorchidism: determinants of practice patterns. J Urol 185(5):1882–1887
40. Thorup J, McLachlan R, Cortes D et al (2010) What is new in cryptorchidism and hypospadias – a critical review on the testicular dysgenesis hypothesis. J Pediatr Surg 45(10):2074–2086

Part VI

Uro-genitals Tumors

Adrenal Tumors

24

Andrea Pession, Federico Baronio, Marco Togni, and Arcangelo Prete

24.1 Introduction

The adrenals are small retroperitoneal glands, located on the upper pole of kidneys within the fascia of Gerota. Each gland is composed of two functional endocrine sections, the adrenal *cortex* and *medulla*, essential to normal physiologic functioning.

The adrenal cortex is divided into three zones with distinct endocrine function: zona glomerulosa, zona fasciculata, and zona reticularis that produce mineralocorticoids, glucocorticoids, and androgens, respectively.

The cortex is derived from mesothelial cells of the primitive coelom adjacent to the mesonephric tubules and gonadal ridges [1]. By the second week of life, the inner part, called "the fetal cortex," that is hormonally active during pregnancy involutes [2]. At birth zonae glomerulosa and fasciculata are already formed, while zona reticularis is completed during the first 3 years of life [3]. The normal adrenal cortex is 80–90 % of the volume of the normal gland. The adrenal medulla synthesizes and secretes catecholamines; it derives from *neural crest* and develops with sympathetic nervous system.

Adrenal tumors are rare in childhood and the classification could be made by their origin (medulla or cortex) and function (hyperfunctioning or nonfunctioning tumors). Cancers arising from the medulla originate from the neural crest, and for this reason they may be found also along the sympathetic neural chain. This group of tumors, defined as peripheral neuroblastic tumors (PNTs), includes neuroblastoma (NBL), ganglioneuroma (GN), ganglioneuroblastoma (GNB), and pheochromocytoma. The adrenocortical tumors (ACTs) include both adrenocortical carcinoma and adenoma.

24.2 Epidemiology

In children, NBL is the second most common abdominal neoplasm, after Wilms' tumor, represents 90 % of adrenal cancers, and, after leukemia and central nervous system tumors, is the third most common cancer, accounting for 10 % of all pediatric malignancies.

The large part of patients is diagnosed between 1 and 5 years of age, but NBL is the most frequent malignancy diagnosed in the first month of life (30–50 %), and it is the most common cancer among infants of less than

A. Pession (✉) • F. Baronio
Department of Pediatrics,
S. Orsola-Malpighi University Hospital,
Via Massarenti 11, Bologna 40138, Italy
e-mail: andrea.pession@unibo.it;
federico.baronio@aosp.bo.it

M. Togni • A. Prete
Department of Pediatrics – Pediatric Hematology and Oncology "Lalla Seràgnoli",
S. Orsola-Malpighi University Hospital,
Via Massarenti 11, Bologna 40138, Italy
e-mail: marco.togni4@unibo.it;
arcangelo.prete@aosp.bo.it

M. Lima, G. Manzoni (eds.), *Pediatric Urology: Contemporary Strategies from Fetal Life to Adolescence*,
DOI 10.1007/978-88-470-5693-0_24, © Springer-Verlag Italia 2015

12 months of age [4]. In Italy, 130 new cases per year are reported (AIEOP http://www.aieop.org/index.php?q=node/370).

GNs are rare tumors and in children <15 years of age the incidence in the USA is one case per million/year. The median age at diagnosis is 7 years. Approximately only 20 % of GNs occur in the adrenal gland [5].

Pheochromocytomas are rare (less than 5 % of incidence) in childhood, often occurring in the adrenal gland (80 %) [6], and in 25 % of cases both glands are involved; these tumors are often familial and inherited as autosomal dominant trait. Pheochromocytomas could be associated in a minor number of cases with multiple endocrine neoplasia syndromes (type II), neurofibromatosis, hemihypertrophy, and Von Hippel-Lindau syndrome. The tumors are usually diagnosed in older children (mean age 11 years) and, from 10 % up to 30 % of cases (in the inherited cancer syndromes), could be multiple [7].

According to the National Registry of Childhood Tumors, the incidence of benign and unspecified pheochromocytomas is 0.11 per million children, whereas the incidence of the malignant form is 0.02 per million children [8].

Adrenocortical neoplasms that include both carcinomas and adenomas are very rare in children (0.2 % of pediatric cancers) [9], with a worldwide incidence of 0.3/1 million/year below 15 years of age. These tumors are less frequent than NBL but more common than pheochromocytoma. In the pediatric population these cancers are typically diagnosed below 5 years of age, with a small predominance of female sex; a second peak of incidence is reported during adolescence [10].

In Southern Brazil the incidence of ACTs is 15 times higher than worldwide and most cases show a p53 germline mutation [11].

24.3 Etiology and Pathogenesis

24.3.1 Medullary Tumors

The etiology of neuroblastic tumors is poorly understood. Preconceptual or gestational environment events as exposure to drugs or viruses, maternal factors as gestational diabetes mellitus [12], folate deficiency [13], or opiate consumption [14] have been considered as possible etiologic factors, since the early age of onset of these cancers. NBLs are in the large part of cases of sporadic tumors; however, they could be found in patients with neurofibromatosis type 1, Turner's syndrome [15], suggesting some genetic etiology. Familial NBL accounts for <2 % of all cases and is associated with a younger age at diagnosis [16]. Activating mutations in the tyrosine kinase domain of the anaplastic lymphoma kinase (*ALK*) oncogene and loss-of-function mutations in the homeobox gene *PHOX2B* have been reported as the two major predisposition mutations in familial NBL [17, 18]. About 6–10 % of sporadic NBLs show somatic *ALK* oncogene activating mutations, and an additional 3–4 % have a high frequency of *ALK* oncogene amplification [18], indicating that ALK is an oncogenic driver gene in both familial and sporadic NBLs [19]. Despite the clear involvement of *ALK* oncogene in the development of NBL, the most common focal genetic lesion in sporadic NBL is the amplification of *MYCN* oncogene. Located on 2p24, *MYCN* amplification occurs in 25 % of newly diagnosed NBLs and represents a powerful biomarker for an aggressive phenotype and poor outcome [20].

Recently GN and GNB have been found in children with rapid-onset obesity with hypothalamic dysfunction, hypoventilation, and autonomic dysregulation as a manifestation of a global disorder of neural crest-derived cells [21].

Adrenal pheochromocytoma arises from catecholamine-producing cells in the adrenal medulla. It is an uncommon hormon producing neoplasm, which is potentially curable, shows an identifiable germline mutation in 60–70 % of cases. These mutations predispose to pheochromocytoma interfering with normal cell life cycle of sympathetic neuronal cell precursor [22].

24.3.2 Adrenocortical Tumors

In more than 50 % of cases in USA and Europe, and in 95 % of Brazilian cases, predisposing genetic factors are implicated in the etiology and pathogenesis of ACTs in children. The molecular mechanism of tumor genesis of these cancers is not completely understood; however, *TP53* germline mutations seem to be always involved in ACTs etiology. The high incidence of adrenocortical tumor in Beckwith-Wiedemann syndrome (imprinting defects in the 11p15 genomic region) and hemihypertrophy syndromes [23] suggests the importance of a deregulation of the insulin growth factor system (IGF 2 and IGF receptor) in the development of these tumors. Overexpression of the steroidogenic factor-1 transcription factor seems to be another pathogenic factor of ACTs [24].

24.4 Classification and Clinical Features

24.4.1 PNTs

Peripheral neuroblastic tumors, originating from the primordial neural crest cells of the sympathetic nervous system, are histologically related and are classified according to the prevalence of neural-type cells and Schwann-type cells. These tumors show different degrees of *differentiation* and a broad spectrum of *clinical phenotype*, from benign to extremely aggressive. They are classified as NBL, which is the most common and malignant type; GNB, which is subclassified in two distinct forms (nodular and intermixed) both with malignant potential behavior; and GN, essentially the most differentiated and benign form that could arise de novo or follow a spontaneous or treatment-induced differentiation of NBL or GNB [25].

The degree of differentiation and stromal component of PNTs can be predictive of outcome and is used in the determination of Children's Oncology Group (COG) risk category for treatment.

24.4.1.1 Neuroblastoma

NBL staging is necessary in order to define prognosis and to design the best treatment for the patient. The International NBL Staging System (INSS) is used to stage patients with NBL after initial surgical resection. However, because surgical approaches differ from one institution to another, INSS stage for patients can vary substantially. Therefore, a new International Neuroblastoma Risk Group Staging System (*INRGSS*) was developed [26]. Currently, the risk assessment of NBL according to INRG classification schema includes the criteria INRGSS stage, age, histologic category, grade of tumor differentiation, MYCN status, presence/absence of 11q aberrations, and tumor cell ploidy. However, despite the advances made by the INRG committee, further insight in NBL biology will improve the classification of patients into classes of risk and directing them toward more efficient treatment.

About 70 % of primary NBLs occur within the abdomen, with half of these arising in the adrenal glands. Most of the remainder originates in the paraspinal sympathetic ganglia. The clinical presentation is highly variable, ranging from a mass that causes no symptoms to a primary tumor that causes critical illness as a result of local invasion, widely disseminated disease, or both [27]. About 50 % of children with NBL show a disseminated disease at diagnosis. Metastatic spread, which is more common in children younger than 1 year at diagnosis, occurs via local invasion or distant hematogenous or through the lymphatic system. The most frequent sites of metastasis are the regional or distant lymph nodes, bone marrow, long bones and skull, liver, and skin. Metastases in the lung and brain are rare (<3 %) [28]. Metastatic disease is usually associated with aspecific symptoms, including fever, pallor, irritability, anorexia, and bone pain [29]. Hallmarks of disseminated NBL include periorbital ecchymoses, proptosis, or both.

24.4.1.2 Ganglioneuroma

GN is the most differentiated PNT and is predominantly composed of Schwannian cells studded with maturing or fully mature ganglion cells. This tumor is generally diagnosed in children 5–7 years of age and shows benign characteristic although it can disseminate [30].

De novo GN is often asymptomatic and affects older children more than malignant PNTs, and the production of catecholamines is normal or slightly elevated. Symptoms can result from the compressive effect of the tumor on neighboring tissues [30].

Significant clinical differences between GN and the other malignant PNTs are the predominance of female sex (62 vs 45 %), older age at diagnosis (79 vs 21 months), tumor localization (thorax, 42 vs 17 %), and dissemination (50 vs 100 %) [25].

24.4.1.3 Ganglioneuroblastoma

GNB has mixed histological features and borderline malignant behavior and is classified into two forms, "intermixed stroma rich" and "nodular stroma rich" according to the grade of neuroblastic differentiation and Schwannian stromal development. The neuroblasts are clustered together and have a more mature appearance than in NBL [31]. As suggested by the International NBL Pathology Classification (INPC), the GNB intermixed stroma rich has a favorable histology, whereas the prognosis of the nodular form depends on the characteristics of the neuroblastic component [32]. There is no difference in sex distribution. The localization of tumor is predominantly in the adrenal medulla (1/3 of cases), retroperitoneum (1/3), and posterior mediastinum (1/3), while other extra-adrenal sites as neck and pelvis are less frequent. GNB is most commonly diagnosed in young children <10 years of age [5]. Clinical features at diagnosis of patients with adrenal GNB are related to the presence of a growing abdominal mass, with abdominal distension and pain caused by either the primary tumor or metastatic disease (mainly in bones, liver, and skin).

24.4.2 Pheochromocytoma

The clinical features of pheochromocytoma are determined by tumor mass and production of hormones that usually are epinephrine and norepinephrine or in rare case vasoactive intestinal peptide (VIP). Symptoms are hypertension, tachycardia, hypertensive encephalopathy, sweating, headaches, visual blurring, papilla edema, flushing, diarrhea, weight loss, and chronic diarrhea.

In a study by Pham et al., 30 % of children with pheochromocytoma showed abdominal pain and distension or back pain caused by the mass effect of the tumor, while 64 % had hypertension [33]. In the majority of cases, hypertension is sustained rather than paroxysmal [34]; malignant hypertension can occur [35].

Malignant form of pheochromocytoma in children and adolescents (up to 47 % of cases) is more frequent than in adults (10 %) [33]. Unfortunately benign and malign forms show the same histological and biochemical features, and the only difference is regional invasion or distant metastases that could occur later (up to 20 years) after surgery [36].

24.4.3 Adrenocortical Tumors

In children the distinction between adrenocortical adenoma (10–20 % of cases) [37] and carcinoma is difficult. Macroscopically, adenomas tend to be smaller and not invasive, whereas carcinomas are >200 cm^3 of volume with lobulation, hemorrhage, and areas of necrosis. Morphological criteria and histopathological features are not sufficient to discriminate benign and malignant behavior, and other variables have been proposed, as mitotic rate, IGF2 expression, venous, capsular, or adjacent organ invasion. In the large part of cases, pediatric adrenocortical tumors are hormonally active, and the clinical features are determined by endocrine abnormalities. In these patients diagnosis is made early after the onset of the first signs [38–40]: most children (50–80 % of cases) with ACTs show virilization and pseudo-precocious puberty, hirsutism, and clitoridomegaly or penis enlargement; in 20–40 % of cases patients may develop Cushing's syndrome, secondary to glucocorticoid overproduction often associated with hyperandrogenism. In less than 10 % of pediatric cases, these tumors are hormonally inactive [41].

24.5 Diagnosis

24.5.1 Introduction

Physical examination and history of children with clinical signs of functioning tumors (virilization, hirsutism, acne, hypertension, headache, and sweating) or abdominal pain and distension should be carefully performed. In smaller children

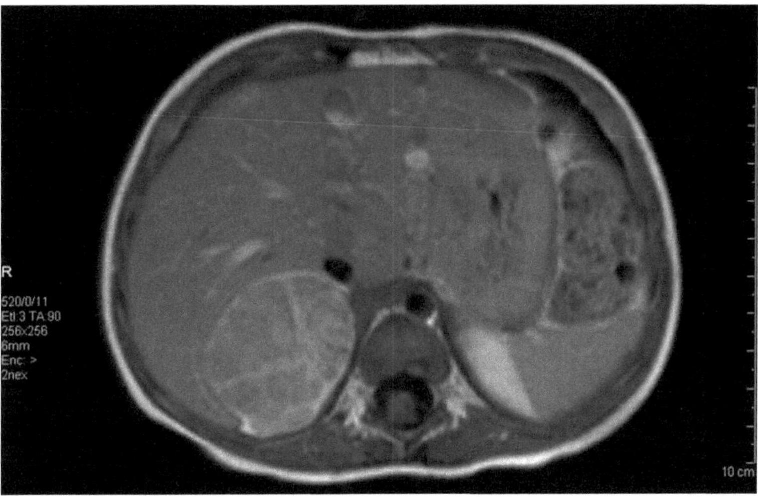

Fig. 24.1 MRI of a right adrenal neuroblastoma

adrenal masses could be palpated, but biochemical (adrenal steroids, vanillylmandelic acid, homovanillic acid, and urinary or serum catecholamines) and imaging studies as abdominal computerized axial tomography scans, ultrasounds, magnetic resonance imaging studies, and metaiodobenzylguanidine (*MIBG*) scintiscans are necessary to characterize the mass and evaluate tumor size, organ of origin, tissue invasion, vascular encasement, adenopathy, and calcifications [42]. Imaging has fundamental importance in the diagnosis and follow-up of NPTs, and ultrasonography (US) is the first-line method in children. Computed tomography and magnetic resonance imaging are needed when more accurate descriptions are required on location, tumor relation to neighboring organs and vessels, and eventual spinal invasion and obviously to accurately plan surgery.

Age at *diagnosis*, related symptoms, and biochemical and imaging results should be integrated for a correct interpretation of the adrenal mass. Furthermore, positron emission tomography (PET), single-photon emission CT (SPECT), and 1–4 PET-CT can be used for diagnosis and follow-up of recurrences or metastasis [43].

24.5.2 NBL

The diagnosis of NBL is based on the presence of characteristic histopathological features of tumor tissue or the presence of tumor cells in a bone marrow aspirate or *biopsy*, accompanied by raised concentrations of urinary catecholamines (HVA and VMA). Presence of tumor-specific genetic markers and histopathological assessment are crucial factors of treatment planning. Therefore, tumor biopsies are highly recommended at the time of diagnosis. Computed tomography (CT), magnetic resonance imaging (MRI) (Fig. 24.1), and 99mTc-diphosphonate scintigraphy (bone scan) (Fig. 24.2) are usual methods for assessment of NBL. Enhanced sensitivity and specificity for detecting possible multiple sites of disease, including bone and soft tissue, are provided by MIBG scintigraphy [44].

24.5.3 Adrenal Ganglioneuromas

Adrenal GNs are generally diagnosed in older asymptomatic children, often as incidental findings. However, in a minor number of cases, they could be symptomatic, as palpable masses, with diarrhea, hypertension, or back pain if they invade the vertebral spine. Urinary catecholamine levels are usually in normal range. The mass shows on US a homogeneous solid structure. On CT, GNs are well-defined masses with mild enhancement after contrast injection. In 50 % of cases calcifications are seen [45]. On MR imaging, GNs show low signal intensity on T1 and often heterogeneous high signal intensity on

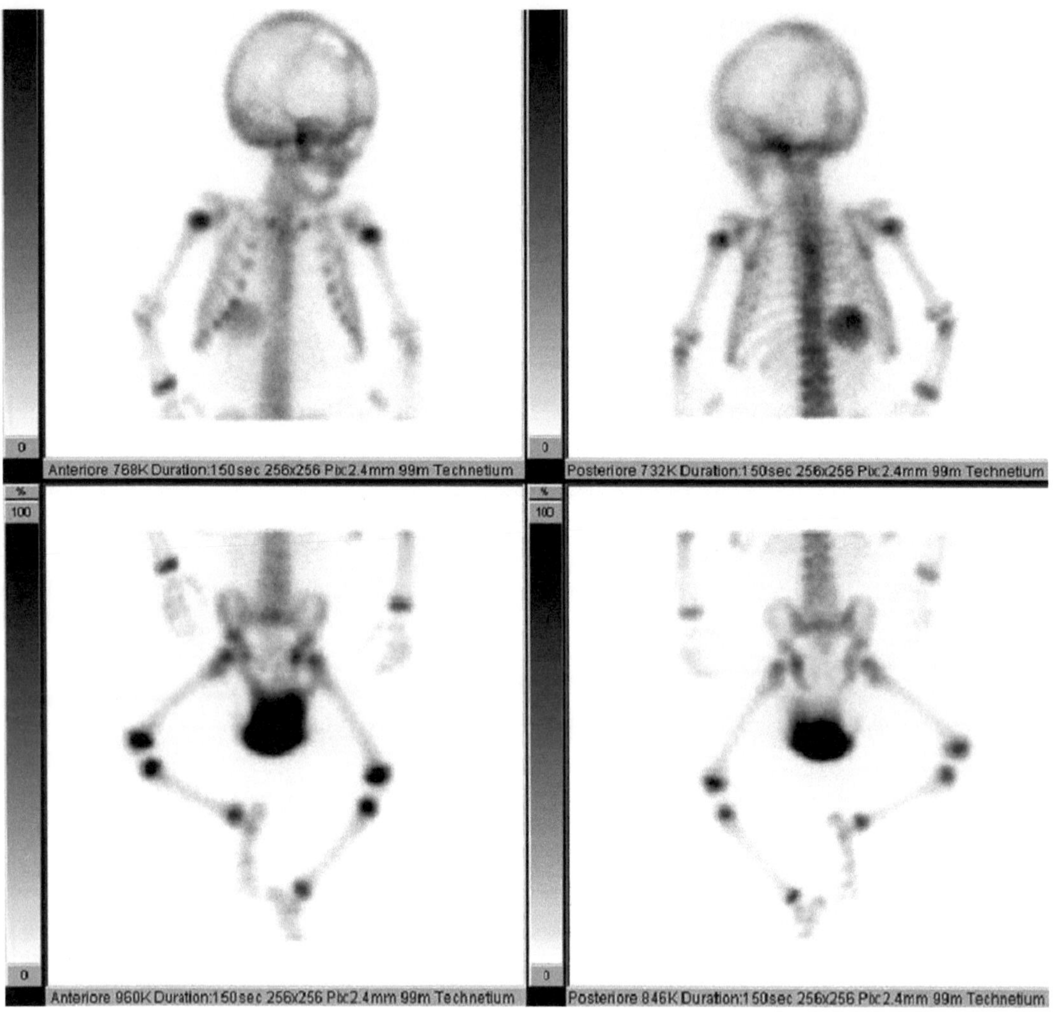

Fig. 24.2 99mTc-diphosphonate scintigraphy in a patient with right adrenal neuroblastoma

T2-weighted images [46]. However, despite these radiological features, they cannot be securely differentiated from NBL, and histology should be evaluated for definitive diagnosis.

24.5.4 Adrenal Ganglioneuroblastomas

Adrenal GNBs are diagnosed in symptomatic younger children (mean age of onset 2 years) that may show abdominal pain, distension, hypertension, and *cushingoid* features or incidentally during abdominal US performed for other reasons. CT and MRI are required to characterize these masses that appear mainly solid, predominantly cystic, or heterogeneous with in some cases irregular margins. These tumors tend to produce catecholamines (vanillylmandelic acid and homovanillic acids) that are important diagnostic markers.

GNs and GNBs appear radiologically identical, as well-circumscribed, smooth, or lobulated masses with or without calcifications. The presence of distant metastases could help differentiate malignant GNBs from GNs [5, 46]. At histological evaluation the presence of mature ganglion cell is the most striking feature of GN; on the contrary immature ganglion cells, necrosis, mitosis, neuropil, and *calcifications* are present in ganglioneuroblastoma and NBL. In differential diagnosis of PNTs, fine-needle aspiration biopsy or core biopsy may fail to detect immature components of GNB. Obviously a complete resection of the mass is mandatory, completed by immunohistochemistry and electron microscopy studies [47].

24.5.5 Pheochromocytoma

The diagnosis of adrenal pheochromocytoma relies on detection of overproduction of catecholamines or vasoactive intestinal peptide (rare) in combination with imaging. The *catecholamines* collection in a 24-h urine or plasma fractionated metanephrines determination are the most appropriate first-line biochemical assays [48]. On US, the pheochromocytomas appear as a soft tissue mass, with possible areas of hemorrhage or necrosis and calcifications. MIBG scanning is recommended for its diagnostic sensitivity and for detecting multifocal disease, while CT and MR image studies should precede surgery. Typically pheochromocytomas have reduced low signal intensity on T1-weighted MRI images and markedly high signal intensity on T2 [49].

24.5.6 Adrenocortical Tumors

In children the majority of adrenocortical tumors are symptomatic, and the diagnosis of these masses should be made on the basis of biochemical/endocrine assessment and adrenal imaging. In children with virilization, urinary 17 ketosteroids and serum levels of adrenal steroids (DHEA, DHEA-S, androstenedione) are elevated. Patients with Cushing's syndrome lose serum cortisol circadian rhythm and show blunted adrenocortical hormone levels along with elevated 24-h urinary free cortisol. In suspicious cases of adrenocortical tumor, US evaluation of adrenal glands should be firstly performed, followed by CT and MRI, to study focal tumor invasion or spread. US is recommended to evaluate tumor invasion of vena cava. Lung CT should be always performed at diagnosis of ACTs because lungs are the most common site for distant metastasis. Imaging and even histologic characterization do not always clearly define the malignity or benignity of the ACTs. Size greater than 5–10 cm, weight more than 200 g, aggressive growth features, and the presence of local and distant *metastases* (lung, liver, bone) suggest the malignity of the tumor [49].

24.6 Therapeutic Management and Outcome

As reported by the consensus statement of National Institute of Health (2002), *adrenalectomy* should be considered both in patients with clinically unapparent functional adrenal tumors and in those with nonfunctional adrenal incidentalomas >6 cm. Adrenalectomy should be strongly recommended if imaging findings suggest that the lesion is not an adenoma with rapid growth rate and decreased lipid content [50].

In children, a higher proportion of adrenal tumors are malignant. Since the size of masses or the imaging cannot safely discriminate malignant from benign forms, it is recommended to remove all adrenal masses discovered in children older than 3 months [51].

24.6.1 Medullary Masses

24.6.1.1 Neuroblastoma

Different therapeutic approaches (surgery, radiotherapy, and chemotherapy) can be applied on children with NBL, according to the risk group assigned to the tumor. The treatment for low-risk NBL is surgery with cure rates over 90 % without further therapies [52]. In low-risk stage 4S/MS cases, the NBL usually undergoes spontaneous regression without any therapy. However, chemotherapy and low-dose radiotherapy could be required for patients with large tumors or massive hepatomegaly causing mechanical obstructions, respiratory insufficiency, or liver dysfunction [53].

The intermediate-risk group encompasses a wide spectrum of conditions with an overall survival probability of about 90 %. The challenge is to identify patients for whom the intensity of treatment could be safely reduced. Moderate-dose multi-agent chemotherapy, followed by surgical resection of the tumor, is the typical treatment for this group of patients, although for invasive locoregional tumors with unfavorable biological features, intensive *multimodal therapy* is often needed to achieve a cure [54].

Despite recent advances, the outcomes for high-risk NBL remain poor, with a long-term survival around 40 % [55] and 50–60 % of patients who have a relapse [27]. These children are generally treated with dose-intensive multi-agent chemotherapy [56], and, whether the conditions allow it, chemotherapy is followed by surgical resection of the primary tumor plus consolidation phase with myeloablative cytotoxic agents followed by stem cell rescue. However, despite that most high-risk NBLs initially respond to therapy, relapse is a frequent occurrence. To date, relapsed NBLs still remain a clinical challenge, and in the last years several novel agents and therapeutic approach, such as targeted radiotherapy, immunotherapy, retinoids, and angiogenesis, MYCN and tyrosine kinase inhibitors [57] have been developed in order to improve the prognosis of this group of NBLs.

24.6.1.2 Ganglioneuroma

Total resection of adrenal ganglioneuroma in children is mandatory since preoperative diagnosis of benignity is difficult. Careful image monitoring alone is advisable in asymptomatic patients in which complete resection of large tumor is impossible. Biopsy should be promptly performed when any change in size or appearance would suggest malignant transformation [46].

24.6.1.3 Ganglioneuroblastoma

The prognosis of these cancers has been recently well described, and it is strictly related to histology (criteria of the INPC). Tumors with favorable histology are often localized and could be completely resected with excellent prognosis. However, patients with unfavorable histology have often distant metastases at diagnosis and poor prognosis [32].

24.6.1.4 Pheochromocytomas

Surgery is the treatment of choice for patients with *pheochromocytoma*. However, medical treatment is mandatory before surgery. This should include alpha-adrenergic blockade with the nonselective irreversible medication phenoxybenzamine (2 weeks before surgery), followed by beta-adrenergic blockade (to blunt reflex tachycardia) and fluid volume correction. Laparoscopy is often used for tumors <10 cm of maximum diameter, although total adrenalectomy is performed for unilateral tumors or cortex-sparing bilateral adrenalectomy for bilateral adrenal pheochromocytomas. Intraoperative careful monitoring and meticulous anesthesia are needed to early detect and treat unpredictable *hypertensive* crisis, stroke, and arrhythmias due to tumor manipulation [58]. High-dose ^{131}I-MIBG may be used in patients who develop metastatic disease.

Histological evaluation unfortunately cannot help discriminate malignant forms of these cancers that can be diagnosed with documented metastases [59]. The resolution of symptoms generally follows the removal of a benign pheochromocytoma; persistent hypertension (beyond 24 h after surgery) suggests retained tumor [60].

Follow-up (blood pressure and catecholamine assay every 6 months and later every year) of these cases is lifelong to detect the possible development of metachronous tumors and tumors at other sites. Pediatric endocrinologist and clinical geneticist should be early involved in the management of these children, since the endocrine implications (i.e., adrenal insufficiency after bilateral adrenalectomy) and the genetic syndromes may affect the patient as a predisposing condition to develop further tumors [8].

24.6.1.5 Adrenocortical Tumors

The therapeutic approach to the ACTs is multidisciplinary. Surgery in combination with systemic therapy is the treatment of choice [61]. In children with localized disease (2/3 of cases at diagnosis), surgery is curative in 70–75 % of cases, while chemotherapy with *mitotane* and cisplatin-based regimens, usually incorporating doxorubicin and etoposide, should be reserved to patients with advanced disease [62, 63].

An aggressive approach (that may involve neighboring organs to reach radical curative results) is recommended, bearing in mind tumor *friability* and the chance of capsule rupture and spillage (20 % of initial resections, 43 % of subsequent resections) [38].

Thus, open adrenalectomy is the gold standard surgical approach, whereas fine-needle aspiration biopsy and laparoscopic approach are not recommended to avoid tumor rupture and peritoneal carcinomatosis [64]. Radiotherapy is not generally utilized in these tumors since they are considered *radioresistant*. Moreover, ionizing radiations could increase the risk of secondary tumors in those patients who carry germline TP53 mutations.

After surgery these patients should be carefully monitored with regular biochemical and imaging (US/MRI/radiography) follow-up. Metastases usually involve liver, lungs, bones, and locoregional lymph nodes. Adrenal insufficiency after surgery should be prevented with regular administration of *corticosteroids* from the day of surgery for 3–4 days with adequate dose tapering.

References

1. Moore KL, Dalley AF (1999) Clinically oriented anatomy. Lippincott, Baltimore, p 279
2. Perrier ND, Boger MS (2005) Adrenal glands: diagnostic aspects and surgical therapy. In: Linos D, van Heerden JA (eds) Surgical anatomy. Springer, New York, p 7
3. Brunt LM, Halverson JD (2002) The endocrine system. In: O'Leary JP (ed) The physiologic basis of surgery. Lippincott, Philadelphia, p 351
4. Brodeur GM, Hogarty MD, Mosse YP et al (2011) Neuroblastoma. In: Pizzo PA, Poplack DG (eds) Principles and practice of pediatric oncology. Lippincott Williams & Wilkins, Philadelphia, p 886
5. Lonergan GJ, Schwab CM, Suarez ES et al (2002) Neuroblastoma, ganglioneuroblastoma, and ganglioneuroma: radiologic-pathologic correlation. Radiographics 22:911–934
6. Lenders JW, Eisenhofer G, Mannelli M et al (2005) Phaeochromocytoma. Lancet 366:665–675
7. Bhansali A, Rajput R, Behra A et al (2006) Childhood sporadic pheochromocytoma: clinical profile and outcome in 19 patients. J Pediatr Endocrinol Metab 19:749–756
8. British Society of Paediatric Endocrinology & Diabetes (2005) Paediatric endocrine tumours. A multidisciplinary consensus statement of best practice from a Working Group Convened Under the Auspices of the BSPED and UKCCSG. http://www.bsped.org.uk/clinical/docs/RareEndocrineTumour_final.pdf. Accessed 14 Sept 2013
9. Agrons GA, Lonergan GJ, Dickey GE et al (1999) Adrenocortical neoplasms in children: radiologic-pathologic correlation. Radiographics 19:989–1008
10. Bonfig W, Bittmann I, Bechtold S et al (2003) Virilising adrenocortical tumours in children. Eur J Pediatr 162:623–628
11. Figueiredo BC, Sandrini R, Zambetti GP et al (2006) Penetrance of adrenocortical tumours associated with the germline TP53 R337H mutation. J Med Genet 43:91–96
12. Chow EJ, Friedman DL, Mueller BA (2007) Maternal and perinatal characteristics in relation to neuroblastoma. Cancer 109:983–992
13. French AE, Grant R, Weitzman S et al (2003) Folic acid food fortification is associated with a decline in neuroblastoma. Clin Pharmacol Ther 74:288–294
14. Cook MN, Olshan AF, Guess HA et al (2004) Maternal medication use and neuroblastoma in offspring. Am J Epidemiol 15:721–731
15. Blatt J1, Olshan AF, Lee PA, Ross JL (1997) Neuroblastoma and related tumors in Turner's syndrome. J Pediatr 131(5):666–70
16. Maris JM, Weiss MJ, Mosse Y et al (2002) Evidence for a hereditary neuroblastoma predisposition locus at chromosome 16p12-13. Cancer Res 22:6651–6658
17. Mossé YP, Laudenslager M, Longo L et al (2008) Identification of ALK as a major familial neuroblastoma predisposition gene. Nature 455:930–935
18. Trochet D, Bourdeaut F, Janoueix-Lerosey I et al (2004) Germline mutations of the paired-like homeobox 2B (PHOX2B) gene in neuroblastoma. Am J Hum Genet 74:761–764
19. Berry T, Luther W, Bhatnagar N et al (2012) The ALK(F1174L) mutation potentiates the oncogenic activity of MYCN in neuroblastoma. Cancer Cell 22:117–130
20. Cohn SL, Tweddle DA (2004) MYCN amplification remains prognostically strong 20 years after its "clinical debut". Eur J Cancer 40:2639–2642
21. Ize-Ludlow D, Gray JA, Sperling MA et al (2007) Rapid-onset obesity with hypothalamic dysfunction, hypoventilation, and autonomic dysregulation presenting in childhood. Pediatrics 120:179–188
22. Waguespack SG, Rich T, Grubbs E et al (2010) A current review of the etiology, diagnosis, and treatment of pediatric pheochromocytoma and paraganglioma. J Clin Endocrinol Metab 95:2023–2037

23. Hoyme HE, Seaver LH, Jones KL et al (1998) Isolated hemihyperplasia (hemihypertrophy): report of a prospective multicenter study of the incidence of neoplasia and review. Am J Med Genet 79:274–278
24. El Wakil A, Doghman M, Latre De Late P et al (2011) Genetics and genomics of childhood adrenocortical tumors. Mol Cell Endocrinol 336:169–173
25. De Bernardi B, Gambini C, Haupt R et al (2008) Retrospective study of childhood ganglioneuroma. J Clin Oncol 1:1710–1716
26. Cohn SL, Pearson AD, London WB et al (2009) The International Neuroblastoma Risk Group (INRG) classification system: an INRG Task Force report. J Clin Oncol 27:289–297
27. Maris JM (2010) Recent advances in neuroblastoma. N Engl J Med 362:2202–2211
28. Zage PE, Ater JL (2012) Neuroblastoma. In: Stanton B, St.Geme J, Schor N, Behrman RE, Kliegman RM (eds) Nelson textbook of pediatrics, 19th edn. Elsevier, Philadelphia, p 492
29. Quinn JJ, Altman AJ (1979) The multiple hematologic manifestations of neuroblastoma. Am J Pediatr Hematol Oncol 1:201–205
30. Geoerger B, Hero B, Harms D et al (2001) Metabolic activity and clinical features of primary ganglioneuromas. Cancer 15:1905–1913
31. Schwab M, Shimada H, Joshi V et al (2000) Neuroblastic tumours of adrenal gland and sympathetic nervous system. In: Kleihues P, Cavenee WK (eds) World Health Organization classifications of tumors. Pathology and genetics of tumours of the nervous system. IARC Press, Lyon, France, p 153
32. Okamatsu C, London WB, Naranjo A et al (2009) Clinicopathological characteristics of ganglioneuroma and ganglioneuroblastoma: a report from the CCG and COG. Pediatr Blood Cancer 53:563–569
33. Pham TH, Moir C, Thompson GB et al (2006) Pheochromocytoma and paraganglioma in children: a review of medical and surgical management at a tertiary care center. Pediatrics 118:1109–1117
34. Caty MG, Coran AG, Geagen M et al (1990) Current diagnosis and treatment of pheochromocytoma in children. Experience with 22 consecutive tumors in 14 patients. Arch Surg 125:978–981
35. Januszewicz P, Wieteska-Klimczak A, Wyszyńska T (1990) Pheochromocytoma in children: difficulties in diagnosis and localization. Clin Exp Hypertens A 12:571–579
36. Pattarino F, Bouloux PM (1996) The diagnosis of malignancy in phaeochromocytoma. Clin Endocrinol (Oxf) 44:239–241
37. Wooten MD, King DK (1993) Adrenal cortical carcinoma. Epidemiology and treatment with mitotane and a review of the literature. Cancer 72:3145–3155
38. Michalkiewicz E, Sandrini R, Figueiredo B et al (2004) Clinical and outcome characteristics of children with adrenocortical tumors: a report from the International Pediatric Adrenocortical Tumor Registry. J Clin Oncol 22:838–845
39. Weiss LM (1984) Comparative histologic study of 43 metastasizing and nonmetastasizing adrenocortical tumors. Am J Surg Pathol 8:163–169
40. van Slooten H, Schaberg A, Smeenk D et al (1985) Morphologic characteristics of benign and malignant adrenocortical tumors. Cancer 55:766–773
41. Ribeiro RC, Sandrini Neto RS, Schell MJ et al (1990) Adrenocortical carcinoma in children: a study of 40 cases. J Clin Oncol 8:67–74
42. Ciftici AO, Senocak ME, Tanyel FC et al (2001) Adrenocortical tumors in children. J Pediatr Surg 36:549–554
43. Kleis M, Daldrup-Link H, Matthay K et al (2009) Diagnostic value of PET/CT for the staging and restaging of pediatric tumors. Eur J Nucl Med Mol Imaging 36:23–36
44. Voute PA, Hoefnagel CA, Marcuse HR et al (1985) Detection of neuroblastoma with 131I-metaiodobenzylguanidine. Prog Clin Biol Res 175:389–398
45. Ichikawa T, Ohtomo K, Araki T et al (1996) Ganglioneuroma: computed tomography and magnetic resonance features. Br J Radiol 69:114–121
46. Guo YK, Yang ZG, Li Y et al (2007) Uncommon adrenal masses: CT and MRI features with histopathologic correlation. Eur J Radiol 62:359–370
47. Domanski H (2005) Fine-needle aspiration of ganglioneuroma. Diagn Cytopathol 32:363–366
48. Gardet V, Gatta B, Simonnet G et al (2001) Lessons from an unpleasant surprise: a biochemical strategy for the diagnosis of pheochromocytoma. J Hypertens 19:1029–1035
49. McHugh K (2007) Renal and adrenal tumours in children. Cancer Imaging 7:41–51
50. Grumbach MM, Biller BM, Braunstein GD et al (2003) Management of the clinically inapparent adrenal mass ("incidentaloma"). Ann Intern Med 138:424–429
51. Masiakos PT, Gerstle JT, Cheang T et al (2004) Is surgery necessary for incidentally discovered adrenal masses in children? J Pediatr Surg 39:754–758
52. Perez CA, Matthay KK, Atkinson JB et al (2000) Biologic variables in the outcome of stages I and II neuroblastoma treated with surgery as primary therapy: a children's cancer group study. J Clin Oncol 18:18–26
53. Nickerson HJ, Matthay KK, Seeger RC et al (2000) Favorable biology and outcome of stage IV-S neuroblastoma with supportive care or minimal therapy: a Children's Cancer Group study. J Clin Oncol 18:477–486
54. Maris JM, Hogarty MD, Bagatell R et al (2007) Neuroblastoma. Lancet 369:2106–2120
55. De Bernardi B, Nicolas B, Boni L et al (2003) Disseminated neuroblastoma in children older than one year at diagnosis: comparable results with three consecutive high-dose protocols adopted by the Italian Co-Operative Group for Neuroblastoma. J Clin Oncol 21:1592–1601
56. Cheung NK, Kushner BH, LaQuaglia M et al (2001) N7: a novel multi-modality therapy of high risk

neuroblastoma (NB) in children diagnosed over 1 year of age. Med Pediatr Oncol 36:227–230
57. Matthay KK, George RE, Yu AL (2012) Promising therapeutic targets in neuroblastoma. Clin Cancer Res 18:2740–2753
58. Bravo EL, Tarazi RC, Gifford RW et al (1979) Circulating and urinary catecholamines in pheochromocytoma. Diagnostic and pathophysiologic implications. N Engl J Med 301:682–686
59. DeLellis RA, Lloyd RV, Heitz PU et al (2004) World health organization classification of tumours, pathology and genetics of tumours of endocrine organs. IARC Press, Lyon
60. Edmonds S, Fein DM, Gurtman A (2011) Pheochromocytoma. Pediatr Rev 32:308–310
61. Allolio B, Fassnacht M (2006) Adrenocortical carcinoma: clinical update. J Clin Endocrinol Metab 91:2027–2037
62. Rodriguez-Galindo C, Figueiredo BC, Zambetti GP et al (2005) Biology, clinical characteristics, and management of adrenocortical tumors in children. Pediatr Blood Cancer 45:265–273
63. Zancanella P, Pianovski MA, Oliveira BH et al (2006) Mitotane associated with cisplatin, etoposide, and doxorubicin in advanced childhood adrenocortical carcinoma: mitotane monitoring and tumor regression. J Pediatr Hematol Oncol 28:513–524
64. Gonzalez RJ1, Shapiro S, Sarlis N et al (2005) Laparoscopic resection of adrenal cortical carcinoma: a cautionary note. Surgery 2005;138(6):1078–85

25 Renal Tumors

Fraia Melchionda, Francesco Corazza, Claudio Antonellini, and Andrea Pession

25.1 Introduction

Renal tumors represent more than 6 % of total cancer diagnoses among children younger than 15 years of age and comprise a spectrum of several histologic subtypes that in recent years have been recognized as distinct pathologic entities. Wilms tumor, also called nephroblastoma, is the most frequently occurring (87 %); the other rare histologic types are classified as non-Wilms tumor category and encompass clear cell sarcoma of the Kidney, rhabdoid tumor of the kidney, congenital mesoblastic nephroma, multilocular cystic renal tumor, renal cell carcinoma, angiomyolipoma, renal medullary carcinoma, and leukemia/lymphomas (Table 25.1) [1, 2]. Due to their histological heterogeneity and variable grade of malignancy, renal neoplasms in children may have a different response to therapies and mortality. Multimodality therapies have resulted in a significant improvement in outcome from approximately 30 % in the 1930s to more than 85 % in the modern era, representing a successful example of tumor treatment.

F. Melchionda • F. Corazza • A. Pession (✉)
Department of Pediatrics,
S. Orsola-Malpighi University Hospital,
Via Massarenti 11, Bologna 40138, Italy
e-mail: andrea.pession@unibo.it

C. Antonellini
Department of Pediatric Surgery,
S. Orsola-Malpighi University Hospital,
Via Massarenti 11, Bologna 40138, Italy

25.2 Epidemiology

Renal tumor epidemiology in childhood is notably age dependent (Table 25.2), being more frequent in younger children and representing 9.7 % of malignancies diagnosed among children younger than 5 years of age, 5.4 % in children 5–9 years of age, 1.1 % in children 10–14 years of age, and only 0.6 % in adolescents 15–19 years of age. Incidence rate is slightly higher for black population and substantially lower in Asians. Male-to-female ratio is 0.92:1.00 and 0.6:1.00 for unilateral and bilateral disease, respectively. The average age at diagnosis of unilateral renal tumor is 3 ½ years, whereas bilateral forms are generally diagnosed in younger children [3, 4].

25.3 Histology and Pathogenesis

Histologic characteristics are the most powerful prognostic indicators for renal tumors. The National Wilms Tumor Study Group (NWTSG) and the International Society of Pediatric Oncology (SIOP) studies have shown a strong relationship between response, recurrence rate, and the histology of tumor [5, 6]. It is possible to identify

M. Lima, G. Manzoni (eds.), *Pediatric Urology: Contemporary Strategies from Fetal Life to Adolescence*,
DOI 10.1007/978-88-470-5693-0_25, © Springer-Verlag Italia 2015

patients with different risk distribution (Tables 25.3 and 25.4) according to the presence of anaplasia and histologic variants as clear cell sarcoma of the kidney or rhabdoid tumor of the kidney. Identification of patient histology risk, together with tumor stage, may guide to select children having a greater survival rate to receive a less intense chemotherapy regimes, while those at higher risk to benefit from more intensive chemotherapy and, in selected cases, radiotherapy (Table 25.5).

25.3.1 Wilms Tumor

Wilms tumor (WT) is the most frequent renal tumor in children accounting for 87 % of renal neoplasms. The vast majority of patients with WT have a good prognosis with current treatment, but approximately 10 % have histopathologic features that are associated with a poorer prognosis. WT can be separated into prognostic groups on the basis of histopathology: favorable histology, anaplastic histology, and nephrogenic rests.

- *Favorable histology*: WT cell mimics development of a normal kidney with three cell types: blastemal, epithelial (tubules), and stromal. Nevertheless not all tumors are triphasic, and monophasic patterns may present diagnostic difficulties. Even if associations between histological features and prognosis or responsiveness to therapy have been suggested, with the exception of anaplasia, none of these features have reached statistical significance and therefore they do not direct the initial therapy [7].
- *Anaplastic histology*: Anaplastic histology accounts for about 5–10 % of WT, usually

Table 25.1 Renal tumors histologic distribution in children

Histology	Percentage (%)
Wilms tumor	87
Congenital mesoblastic nephroma	3
Clear cell sarcoma of the kidney	3
Rhabdoid tumor of kidney	2
Miscellaneous	5
Metanephric stromal tumor	
Papillary renal carcinoma	
Angiomyolipoma	
Renal medullary carcinoma	
Lymphoma	
PNET	
Other rare tumors	

Table 25.3 Risk distribution according to histology of untreated tumor

Low risk	Congenital mesoblastic nephroma
	Cystic partially differentiated nephroblastoma and variants
Intermediate risk	Wilms tumor without anaplasia
	Wilms tumor with focal anaplasia
High risk	Wilms tumor with diffuse anaplasia
	Clear cell sarcoma of the kidney
	Rhabdoid tumor of the kidney

Table 25.2 Age distribution renal neoplasms

Renal neoplasm	Age range	Peak age
Wilms tumor		
Unilateral	1–11 years	3½ years
Bilateral	2 months–2 years	15 months
Nephroblastomatosis	Any age	6–18 months
Renal cell carcinoma	6 months –60 years	10–20 years[a]
Congenital mesoblastic nephroma	0–1 year	1–3 months
Clear cell sarcoma of the kidney	1–4 years	2 years
Rhabdoid tumor of kidney	6 months–9 years	6–12 months
Multilocular cystic renal tumor	3 months–4 years	1–2 years
Angiomyolipoma	6–41 years	10 years[b]
Lymphoma		
Hodgkin	>10 years	Late teen
Non-Hodgkin	Any age	<10 years

[a]von Hippel–Lindau syndrome
[b]von Hippel–Lindau syndrome; neurofibromatosis; tuberous sclerosis

with a higher incidence in older children (aged 10–16 years) [8]. Diffuse anaplasia is the single most important histologic predictor of response and survival in patients with WT; it is an indicator of chemotherapy resistance and correlates with a marked increase of recurrent disease. The impact of anaplasia is more remarkable when it is diffusely distributed, but less important when anaplasia is only focal [9].

- *Nephrogenic rests*: Nephrogenic rests are embryonic kidney precursor cells that abnormally persist in postnatal life. They are found in almost 35 % of kidneys with unilateral Wilms tumors and in nearly 100 % of kidneys with bilateral Wilms tumors. When nephrogenic rests are diffused configure a condition called nephroblastomatosis. Patients with any type of nephrogenic rest in a kidney removed for WT may have an increased risk for tumor formation in the remaining kidney tissue [10].

WT arise from the same tissue of normal kidney, the primitive metanephric blastema; particularly, WT may contain tissues not usually present in the developing normal kidney, as skeletal muscle, cartilage, and squamous epithelium. WT is usually monolateral, even if in more than 10 % of cases it has a multicentric origin. Almost 7 % of children indeed have a bilateral WT at diagnosis.

Table 25.4 Risk distribution according to histology of pretreated tumor

Low risk	Congenital mesoblastic nephroma
	Cystic partially differentiated nephroblastoma
	Completely necrotic Wilms tumor
Intermediate risk	Wilms tumor epithelial type
	Wilms tumor stromal type
	Wilms tumor mixed type
	Wilms tumor regressive type
	Wilms tumor with focal anaplasia
High risk	Wilms tumor blastemal type
	Wilms tumor with diffuse anaplasia
	Clear cell sarcoma of the kidney
	Rhabdoid tumor of the kidney

Table 25.5 Staging systems

	NWTSG staging (pre-chemotherapy)	SIOP staging (post-chemotherapy)
Stage I	The tumor confined within one kidney and completely resected	Tumor limited to the kidney, complete resection
	No penetration of the renal capsule or involvement of renal sinus vessels	No previous biopsy
		Vessels of sinus clear
		Hilar lymph nodes examined and negative
Stage II	Tumor extends beyond the kidney but fully resected (negative margins and lymph nodes)	Tumor extending outside the kidney, complete excision
	At least one of the following has occurred	Invasion beyond the capsule, perirenal/perihilar
	Penetration of renal capsule	Invasion of regional lymph nodes. Invasion of extrarenal vessels or ureter
	Invasion of renal sinus vessels	
	Tumor biopsy	
	Tumor thrombus in vessels outside the kidney is stage II if the thrombus is removed en bloc with the tumor	
Stage III	Gross or microscopic residual tumor remains postoperatively, including	Incomplete excision, without hematogenous perioperative or preoperative tumor rupture
	Inoperable tumor	Invasion of extra-regional nodes
	Positive surgical margins	
	Diffuse tumor spillage	
	Regional lymph node metastases	
	Transected tumor thrombus	
Stage IV	Distant metastases	Distant metastases
Stage V	Bilateral renal tumor at diagnosis	Bilateral renal tumor at diagnosis

A germline mutation is thought to be the cause of about 10–15 % of Wilms tumor. The Wilms tumor suppressor gene (*WT1*) on chromosome 11p13 was identified in 1990, and it encodes a transcriptional factor containing a domain of four zinc finger motifs; it was among the first tumor suppressor genes cloned, and it is involved in kidney and gonadal development. The specific role of *WT1* in early urogenital development and in kidney differentiation can be deduced from its expression pattern in fetal kidneys and various cells of the genital system. It has been reported that a germline mutation in *WT1* predisposes to the development of tumors with stromal predominant histology [11]. *WT1* irregularities are estimated to account for less than 20 % of sporadic tumors. Indeed it is known that up to 10 % of newly diagnosed WT occurs in children with congenital anomalies, as urinary tract anomalies, cryptorchidism, hypospadias, and hemihypertrophy; moreover, *WT1*-associated syndromes, such as WAGR and Denys–Drash syndrome, have been strongly associated with Wilms tumor. There are several definite syndromes where it is known that a genetic abnormality correlates with tumor development; these syndromes may be with or without phenotypic prenatal and postnatal overgrowth [12, 13].

Overgrowth Syndromes

- Beckwith–Wiedemann syndrome (macroglossia, gigantism, midline abdominal wall defects as omphalocele/exomphalos, umbilical hernia, diastasis recti, ear creases or ear pits, and neonatal hypoglycemia)
- Sotos syndrome (characterized by cerebral gigantism)
- Simpson–Golabi–Behmel syndrome (characterized by macroglossia, macrosomia, renal and skeletal abnormalities, and increased risk of embryonal cancers)
- Perlman syndrome (characterized by fetal gigantism, renal dysplasia, Wilms tumor, islet cell hypertrophy, multiple congenital anomalies, and mental retardation)
- Isolated hemihypertrophy (asymmetric regional body overgrowth due to differences in the growth of bone, soft tissue, or both)

Syndromes Without Overgrowth

- Genitourinary anomalies including hypospadias, undescended testis, and others are associated with *WT1* gene mutations (prevalence is over 6 % of children with Wilms tumor) [14]. Children with pseudo-hermaphroditism and/or renal disease (glomerulonephritis or nephrotic syndrome) who develop Wilms tumor may have the Denys–Drash or Frasier syndrome (characterized by male hermaphroditism, primary amenorrhea, chronic renal failure, and other abnormalities), both of which are associated with mutations in the WT1 gene. Specifically, germline missense mutations in the WT1 gene are responsible for most Wilms tumors that occur as part of the Denys–Drash syndrome [15, 16].
- WAGR syndrome (aniridia, genitourinary anomaly, and mental retardation). Prevalence is about 0.4 % of children with Wilms tumor, and incidence of bilateral Wilms tumor in children with WAGR syndrome is about 15 % [17, 18].
- Isolated aniridia.
- Bloom syndrome.
- Alagille syndrome.
- Trisomy 18.
- Li–Fraumeni syndrome

25.3.2 Clear Cell Sarcoma of the Kidney (CCSK)

CCSK is not a WT variant, but it is an important primary renal tumor (3 % of renal neoplasms in children) associated with a significantly higher rate of relapse and death than favorable histology WT [19]. The mean age of patients at onset of CCSK is 36 months; however, CCSK is rare in children below 6 months. In several studies CCSK has been reported a male predominance ratio of about 2:1 [20].

Unfortunately clinical presentation of CCSK does not differ from WT symptoms of patients and includes abdominal distension, abdominal pain, constipation, hypertension, fever, and gross hematuria. When bone pain or masses are present, they may be due to bone metastases. CCSK may present metastases also to the lungs, lymph nodes, liver, and brain [7, 20].

Even if historically CCSK had an inferior survival compared to WT, in the recent years the use of more intensive chemotherapy regimens, including multiagent chemotherapy and radiotherapy, combined with nephrectomy dramatically improved outcomes on CCSK patients [20].

Relapses occur in about 20–40 % of children, with a large variability across studies [20]. With current therapies, relapse of CCSK after 3 years is uncommon even if in the past it has been reported up to 10 years after frontline chemotherapy; moreover, the pattern of relapse has changed from the historical data where bone, followed by lungs, represented the most frequent site recurrence, but more recently cooperative studies identified brain as the more frequent site of recurrence [20].

To date, as CCSK lacked a specific diagnostic immunohistochemical pattern or reproducible genetic aberrations able to reliably distinguish it from other renal tumors, diagnosis has been only based on histological features [21].

Only little is known about the biology of CCSK, and recently t(10;17)(q22;p13) has been identified in near 12 % of cases. t(10;17)(q22;p13) results in rearrangement of *YWHAE* on chromosome 17 and a member of the *FAM22* gene family on chromosome 10. Elucidation of molecular mechanisms for development of specific tumor may lead to identify potential therapeutic targets and open chance to design targeted therapy-based protocols. Furthermore identifying genetic mutations, characteristic of rare kidney tumors as CCSK, will improve their diagnosis otherwise more difficult solely on histology [21].

25.3.3 Rhabdoid Tumor of the Kidney (RTK)

Rhabdoid tumor of kidney is rare in children accounting for 2 % of kidney neoplasms; even if it does not demonstrate muscle differentiation, it took this denomination because of the resemblance to rhabdomyoblasts of its tumor cells. RTK occurs in young children, median age is 11 months, and up to 80 % of tumors are diagnosed within the first 2 years of life. Unlike other renal tumors with predilection of infant as congenital mesoblastic nephroma, RTK is highly lethal. Typical clinical presentation includes fever, hematuria, and high tumor stage at diagnosis; RTK tends to metastasize to brain and lungs; indeed more than 10 % of patients with RTK have also CNS lesions [22]. Relapses occur early (median time from diagnosis is 8 months) [23]. Some characteristic molecular abnormality, as well as morphologic delineation, has helped to better differentiate RTK from CMN; indeed rhabdoid tumors, in all anatomical locations, show a common genetic abnormality with the mutation and/or deletion of the SMARCB1 (also called hSNF5 or INI1) gene located at chromosome 22q11 [24, 21].

25.3.4 Congenital Mesoblastic Nephroma (CMN)

CMN is a low-grade fibroblastic sarcoma of kidney. CMN represents 5 % of childhood kidney tumors, it is the most frequent kidney tumor diagnosed in infant between 1 and 3 months of age, 90 % of CMN are diagnosed within 1 year, and it is extremely rare after the 2 years. CMN carries an excellent prognosis, when diagnosed in the first 7 months of life, the 5-year event-free survival (EFS) rate is 94 % and the overall survival (OS) rate is 96 %; indeed relapse and hematogenous metastases are very rare. The risk of relapse may be due the difficulties experienced in obtaining radical margin. Moreover this tumor can generally be cured by complete surgical excision with no need of chemotherapy. The recent recognition of distinctive tumors that mimic CMN in older children and adults (such as metanephric stromal tumor, mixed epithelial stromal tumor, and renal synovial sarcoma) has reaffirmed that CMN essentially never occurs after the age of 3 years [25].

At imaging CMN appears as unilateral masses, indistinguishable from nephroblastoma.

25.3.5 Renal Cell Carcinoma (RCC)

While RCC represents the most common primary malignancy of the kidney in adults, it occurs rarely in children younger than 15 years (2–5 % of renal tumor). In the oldest age group of adolescents (aged 15–19 years), approximately two-thirds of renal malignancies are RCC [26]. Pediatric patients with RCC typically present as the adult cases of frank hematuria, palpable abdominal mass, and abdominal pain; however, up to one-fourth of cases are totally asymptomatic. Metastatic disease may involve the lungs, liver, bone, and brain. RCC may be associated with other conditions, including the following: von Hippel–Lindau (VHL) disease and tuberous sclerosis [27]. RCCs have been described as second malignant neoplasm in patients previously treated for pediatric malignancies such as neuroblastoma, rhabdomyosarcoma, and leiomyosarcoma. RCC in young patients has a different histological, genetic, and morphologic spectrum than that seen in older adults. Childhood RCCs are more frequently of the papillary subtype (20–50 % of pediatric RCCs), and they can sometimes occur in the setting of Wilms tumor, metanephric adenoma, and metanephric adenofibroma. Although the two main morphological subgroups of papillary and clear cell can be identified, about 25 % of RCCs show heterogeneous features that do not fit into either one of these categories [26].

25.3.6 Multilocular Cystic Nephroma

Multilocular cystic nephroma is benign lesions consisting of cysts lined by renal epithelium. It arises from an error in embryogenesis, but its pathogenesis is still debated. These lesions can occur bilaterally and a familial pattern has been rarely reported. Multilocular cystic nephroma has been associated with pleuropulmonary blastomas, so radiographic imaging studies of the chest should be followed in patients with multilocular cystic nephroma.

Although only benign lesions have been described, it is difficult to differentiate MCN from more aggressive neoplasms by imaging studies alone. For this reason, radical nephrectomy has been the standard of care. Recurrence has been reported following tumor spillage at surgery [28].

25.3.7 Cystic Partially Differentiated Nephroblastoma (CPDN)

CPDN is a rare cystic variant of Wilms tumor (1 %) with unique pathologic characteristics; indeed the tumor mass is surrounded by a pseudocapsule, and it is composed of cysts with thin septa as the solid portion of the tumor. The septa contain blastemal cells in any amount with or without embryonal, stromal, or epithelial cell types also resembling mature renal tubules.

These histopathologic features distinguish CPDN from other cystic neoplasms as cystic nephroma (multilocular cystic nephroma), multilocular cystic renal cell carcinoma, cystic hamartoma, and cystic atypical mesoblastic nephroma. The clinical presentation of CPDN is similar to WT and represented by large, palpable abdominal mass, usually reported before the age of 2 years. Patients with stage I disease have a 100 % survival rate with surgery alone. Patients with stage II have an excellent outcome with tumor resection followed by postoperative vincristine and dactinomycin [29].

25.4 Clinical Aspects

Frequently renal neoplasms are asymptomatic and the majority of children with renal neoplasms are brought to medical attention because of abdominal swelling or the presence of an abdominal mass, often noted by parents occasionally while bathing or dressing the child. However, in up to a third of all newly diagnosed children, the abdominal mass can lead to abdominal pain, gross hematuria, fever, anorexia, and hypertension probably due to increased renin activity. At physical exam it appears as a large flank mass not moving with respiration. It is important to specifically note the presence of congenital abnormalities typical of renal tumor-associated syndromes as aniridia, BWS-associated facial dysmorphism, partial or complete hemihypertrophy, genitourinary abnormalities including hypospadia, cryptorchidism, and pseudohermaphroditism reported in almost 30 % of cases [5, 30].

25.5 Diagnosis

The workup of a child with suspected renal tumor begins with appropriate diagnostic imaging studies to define the extent of disease and to help plan the surgical intervention, but even if imaging studies are fundamental to define the anatomy of the renal mass and the involvement of contiguous organs and vessels, they do not substitute histological diagnosis. Indeed imaging cannot reliably distinguish non-WTs such as RTK, CCSK, primitive neuroectodermal tumor (PNET), and RCC from WT [31].

Ultrasonography represents the first test for children suspected of having renal tumor because it provides a panoramic view of the abdomen, including the patency of the inferior vena cava. Moreover, it carries no risk for radiation exposure.

Computed tomography (CT) produces a higher-resolution image of the pelvic and abdominal structures as well as lymph nodes.

Magnetic resonance imaging (MRI) is not a routine component of the evaluation of renal tumor, although MRI is being used with increasing frequency because it does not involve radiation exposure. MRI may facilitate the distinction between Wilms tumor and nephrogenic rests.

Positron emission tomography (PET) is not a routine component of the initial evaluation of renal tumor, though most Wilms tumors take up the radiotracer fluorodeoxyglucose. PET may play a role in the detection of occult metastatic sites at recurrence [32].

25.5.1 Staging

Two major staging systems are currently used, the first is developed by the National Wilms Tumor Study Group (NWTSG staging system) and consists in a pre-chemotherapy, surgery-based system; the second developed by the International Society of Pediatric Oncology (SIOP staging system) is a post-chemotherapy-based system (Table 25.4). Both staging systems have proven valuable in predicting outcomes and designated five tumor stages, where higher stages are associated with greater recurrence risk [4, 33, 34].

25.6 Therapeutic Management

Remarkable progress has been made in the treatment and understanding of children with renal tumors. Particularly for WT patients, multidisciplinary cooperative groups, conducting large clinical trials, have developed multiagent chemotherapy regimens that improved survival dramatically. Treatment for patients with renal tumor includes surgery, chemotherapy, and radiotherapy.

Management of renal tumor differs substantially between protocols developed by the two major international study groups, NWTSG and SIOP. The US protocols developed by the NWTSG recommend primary surgery with nephrectomy, followed by chemotherapy basing on pathologic tumor stage. There are some exceptions as bilateral tumors, extension of tumor thrombus in the suprahepatic cava or heart, and extensive metastatic disease causing respiratory distress, where up-front surgery should be avoided. Major advantages of this approach consist in the accurate and complete staging of untreated tumor, collection of tumor specimen adequate for histology, and biological studies for prognostic evaluation. NWTSG protocols thus may provide appropriate chemoradiotherapy program according to stage from the beginning of treatment. However, there is a higher incidence of tumor rupture and intraoperative spillage and higher rate of surgical complications [31].

Instead the International Society of Pediatric Oncology protocols suggest up-front chemotherapy followed only later by nephrectomy. The rationale behind presurgical chemotherapy is to reduce the incidence of intraperitoneal tumor spillage thus obtaining a more favorable stage distribution and reducing the treatment burden as confirmed by reduced tumor rupture frequency in SIOP-5 study [35]. The other advantage of preoperative chemotherapy is to evaluate tumor responsiveness to the standard chemotherapy. On the other side the main disadvantages of this management are the possibility to administer an incorrect chemotherapy for the little group of non-Wilms renal neoplasm and to overtreat benign tumors or to undertreat high-risk tumors as CCSK or RTK [31].

Thus the NWTSG approach provides a better pathological view of the untreated tumor, while the SIOP approach elicits information on the tumor's response to chemotherapy [36].

Despite the different approaches, overall survival is similar in patients managed according to European and US protocols. Modern treatment regimens yield OS rates of 90 for patients with Wilms tumor. Therefore, current goals aim to reduce the morbidity associated with therapy. Chemotherapy includes for both approaches the use of vincristine and dactinomycin for stage I and II favorable histology Wilms tumor and vincristine, dactinomycin, and doxorubicin for stage III and IV favorable histology disease. Treatment for anaplastic Wilms tumor or high-risk patients includes vincristine, dactinomycin, doxorubicin, cyclophosphamide or ifosfamide, etoposide, and carboplatin [31].

Despite these good results, there are still a group of patients where treatment is not satisfactory as anaplastic or bilateral WT or patient at relapse. Nevertheless, substantial progress has been made in the cure of relapsed patients, where intensive-dose chemotherapy regimens may lead to 60 % of survival [34, 37].

The goals of surgery include complete removal of the tumor with avoidance of tumor rupture or injury to contiguous organs. The standard procedure for unilateral Wilms tumor is the radical nephrectomy with a transverse abdominal transperitoneal approach to properly assess extrarenal tumor extension, whereas flank incision should be avoided. Inspection of abdominal cavity is suggested to identify possible peritoneal implants, intravascular invasion, and metastasis as well as the exploration of the contralateral kidney with the aim of excluding bilateral disease before nephrectomy. A sampling of regional lymph nodes should be included (hilar and ipsilateral para-aortic or caval nodes) to consent an accurate staging of disease. No intraoperative biopsies of the primary tumor are performed unless the tumor is deemed unresectable. Some possible postoperative complications are represented by bowel obstruction (5.1 %), extensive hemorrhage (1.9 %), wound infection (1.9 %), extensive vascular injuries (1.4 %), and injuries to other visceral organs (1 %). These occur less in patients treated with chemotherapy front line (SIOP protocols) than in those where surgery is done up front (NWTSG studies); this is probably due to the decreased tumor size after chemotherapy [31].

The advanced minimally invasive techniques have been applied for nephron-sparing surgery (NSS) [38], which represents the treatment of choice for selected cases of renal tumor as children with bilateral WT, WT occurring in patient with a single kidney, or in case of benign tumors. Moreover, laparoscopic approach for NSS is an interesting alternative for patients at risk of metachronous WT, as child with predisposing genetic syndrome [39]. However, to date, the indication of laparoscopic nephroureterectomy (Fig. 25.1) is debated, even if it may be advocated to decrease postoperative complications [40]. Also NSS remains a controversial approach for children with WT and a normal contralateral kidney; also knowing it may reduce the risk of hyperfiltration injury and late renal failure [41]. Further controlled trials are needed to better identify patients who may take advantage of these less invasive techniques.

Although flank or whole-abdomen radiotherapy (RT) represents an important therapeutic tool in the multimodality therapy of renal tumors, the improved response to modern chemotherapy regimens led to the identification of subgroup of children, basing on age, stage, and histology, where RT gives a therapeutic advantage. This enables us to decrease the number of patients treated with RT and thus to minimize treatment-related morbidity and mortality. Indeed radiotherapy may cause both acute and late toxic effects. Most important acute side effects involve gastrointestinal tract with nausea, vomiting, diarrhea, and abdominal pain; hemopoietic system with leucopenia, anemia, and thrombocytopenia, also worsened by concomitant use of chemotherapy; and liver with ascites, hypertransaminasemia, and radiation hepatitis. Late effects include renal toxicity, gastrointestinal complications, gonadal damage, musculoskeletal abnormalities, respiratory disease, and second malignancies [42, 43].

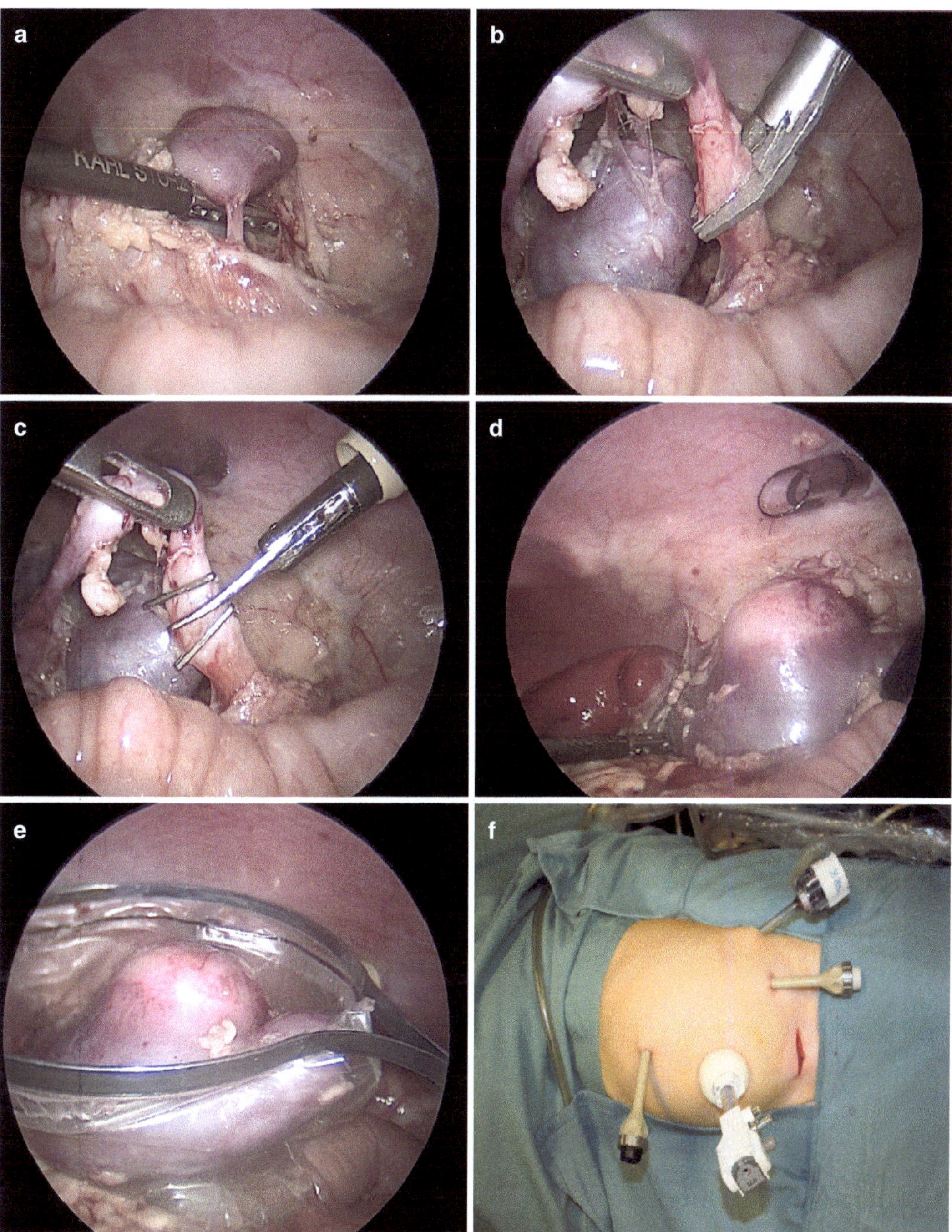

Fig. 25.1 Transperitoneal laparoscopic-assisted nephroureterectomy. (**a**) Laparoscopic view of the kidney. (**b**) Ureter identification and dissection after clip ligation. (**c**) Tumor mass detail. (**d**) Placement into endobag of affected kidney. (**e**) Port placement for transperitoneal laparoscopic-assisted nephroureterectomy and Pfannenstiel incision needed for endobag extraction

References

1. Pastore G, Znaor A, Spreafico F et al (2006) Malignant renal tumours incidence and survival in European children (1978–1997): report from the Automated Childhood Cancer Information System project. Eur J Cancer 42(13):2103–2114
2. Argani P, Ladanyi M (2003) Recent advances in pediatric renal neoplasia. Adv Anat Pathol 10(5):243–260
3. Bernstein L, Linet M, Smith MA et al (1999) Cancer incidence and survival among children and adolescents: United States SEER Program 1975–1995, SEER Program, vol 99. National Cancer Institute NIH Pub, Bethesda, p 4649
4. Lowe LH, Isuani BH, Heller RM et al (2000) Pediatric renal masses: Wilms tumor and beyond. RadioGraphics 20:1585–1603
5. Fernandez C, Geller JI, Ehrlich PF, et al. Renal tumors (2011). In: Pizzo P, Poplack D (eds) Principles and practice of pediatric oncology, 6th edn. Lippincott, Williams & Wilkins, Philadelphia Pa, pp 861–885
6. Vujanić GM, Sandstedt B, Harms D et al (2002) Revised International Society of Paediatric Oncology (SIOP) working classification of renal tumors of childhood. Med Pediatr Oncol 38(2):79–82
7. Perlman EJ (2005) Pediatric renal tumors: practical updates for the pathologist. Pediatr Dev Pathol 8(3):320–338
8. Popov SD, Sebire NJ, Pritchard-Jones K et al (2011) Renal tumors in children aged 10–16 years: a report from the United Kingdom Children's Cancer and Leukaemia Group. Pediatr Dev Pathol 14(3): 189–193
9. Vujanić GM, Harms D, Sandstedt B et al (1999) New definitions of focal and diffuse anaplasia in Wilms tumor: the International Society of Paediatric Oncology (SIOP) experience. Med Pediatr Oncol 32(5):317–323
10. Beckwith JB (1993) Precursor lesions of Wilms tumor: clinical and biological implications. Med Pediatr Oncol 21(3):158–168
11. Schumacher V, Schneider S, Figge A et al (1997) Correlation of germ-line mutations and two-hit inactivation of the WT1 gene with Wilms tumors of stromal-predominant histology. Proc Natl Acad Sci U S A 94:3972–3977
12. Lapunzina P (2007) Risk of tumorigenesis in overgrowth syndromes: a comprehensive review. Am J Med Genet C: Semin Med Genet 137(1):53–71
13. Chu A, Heck JE, Ribeiro KB (2010) Wilms' tumour: a systematic review of risk factors and meta-analysis. Paediatr Perinat Epidemiol 24:449–469
14. Barbosa AS, Hadjiathanasiou CG, Theodoridis C et al (1999) The same mutation affecting the splicing of WT1 gene is present on Frasier syndrome patients with or without Wilms' tumor. Hum Mutat 13(2): 146–153
15. Koziell AB, Grundy R, Barratt TM et al (1999) Evidence for the genetic heterogeneity of nephropathic phenotypes associated with Denys-Drash and Frasier syndromes. Am J Hum Genet 64(6):1778–1781
16. Royer-Pokora B, Beier M, Henzler M et al (2004) Twenty-four new cases of WT1 germline mutations and review of the literature: genotype/phenotype correlations for Wilms tumor development. Am J Med Genet A 127(3):249–257
17. Fischbach BV, Trout KL, Lewis J et al (2005) WAGR syndrome: a clinical review of 54 cases. Pediatrics 116(4):984–988
18. Breslow NE, Norris R, Norkool PA et al (2003) Characteristics and outcomes of children with the Wilms tumor-Aniridia syndrome: a report from the National Wilms Tumor Study Group. J Clin Oncol 21(24):4579–4585
19. Argani P, Perlman EJ, Breslow NE et al (2000) Clear cell sarcoma of the kidney: a review of 351 cases from the National Wilms Tumor Study Group Pathology Center. Am J Surg Pathol 24(1):4–18
20. Gooskens SLM, Furtwangler R, Vujanić GM et al (2012) Clear cell sarcoma of the kidney: a review European. J Cancer Educ 28:2219–2226
21. O'Meara E, Stack D, Lee CH et al (2012) Characterization of the chromosomal translocation t(10;17)(q22;p13) in clear cell sarcoma of kidney. J Pathol 227(1):72–80
22. Tomlinson GE, Breslow NE, Dome J et al (2005) Rhabdoid tumor of the kidney in the National Wilms' Tumor study: age at diagnosis as a prognostic factor. J Clin Oncol 23(30):7641–7645
23. Amar AM, Tomlinson G, Green DM et al (2001) Clinical presentation of rhabdoid tumors of the kidney. J Pediatr Hematol Oncol 23(2):105–108
24. Eaton KW, Tooke LS, Wainwright LM et al (2011) Spectrum of SMARCB1/INI1 mutations in familial and sporadic rhabdoid tumors. Pediatr Blood Cancer 56(1):7–15
25. Van den Heuvel-Eibrink MM, Grundy P, Graf N et al (2008) Characteristics and survival of 750 children diagnosed with a renal tumor in the first seven months of life: a collaborative study by the SIOP/GPOH/SFOP, NWTSG, and UKCCSG Wilms tumor study groups. Pediatr Blood Cancer 50(6): 1130–1134
26. Ahmed HU, Arya M, Levitt G et al (2007) Part I: primary malignant non-Wilms' renal tumours in children. Lancet Oncol 8(9):842–848
27. Linehan WM, Pinto PA, Bratslavsky G et al (2009) Hereditary kidney cancer: unique opportunity for disease-based therapy. Cancer 115(10):2252–2261
28. Ashley RA, Reinberg YE (2007) Familial multilocular cystic nephroma: a variant of a unique renal neoplasm. Urology 70(1):179.e9—10
29. Blakely ML, Shamberger RC, Norkool P et al (2003) Outcome of children with cystic partially differentiated nephroblastoma treated with or without chemotherapy. J Pediatr Surg 38(6):897–900
30. Ahmed HU, Arya M, Tsiouris A et al (2007) An update on the management of Wilms' tumour. Eur J Surg Oncol 33(7):824–831

31. Kembhavi SA, Qureshi S, Vora T et al (2013) Understanding the principles in management of Wilms' tumour: can imaging assist in patient selection? Clin Radiol 68(7):646–653
32. Moinul Hossain AK, Shulkin BL, Gelfand MJ et al (2010) FDG positron emission tomography/computed tomography studies of Wilms' tumor. Eur J Nucl Med Mol Imaging 37:1300–1308
33. D'Angio GJ, Breslow N, Beckwith JB et al (1989) Treatment of Wilms' tumor. Results of the Third National Wilms' Tumor Study. Cancer 64:349–360
34. Metzger ML, Dome JS (2005) Current therapy for Wilms' tumor. Oncologist 10(10):815–826
35. Green DM, Breslow NE, D'Angio GJ et al (2014) Outcome of patients with stage II/favorable histology Wilms tumor with and without local tumor spill: a report from the National Wilms Tumor Study Group. Pediatr Blood Cancer 61(1):134–139
36. Sonn G, Shortliffe LM (2008) Management of Wilms tumor: current standard of care. Nat Clin Pract Urol 5(10):551–560
37. Spreafico F, Bisogno G, Collini P et al (2008) Treatment of high-risk relapsed Wilms tumor with dose-intensive chemotherapy, marrow-ablative chemotherapy, and autologous hematopoietic stem cell support: experience by the Italian Association of Pediatric Hematology and Oncology. Pediatr Blood Cancer 51(1):23–28
38. Pichè N, Barrieras D (2012) Minimally invasive nephron-sparing surgery for unilateral Wilms tumor. J Pediatr Surg 47(7):E 1–E 4
39. Romão RL, Pippi Salle JL, Shuman C et al (2012) Nephron sparing surgery for unilateral Wilms tumor in children with predisposing syndromes: single center experience over 10 years. J Urol 188(4): 1493–1498
40. Javid PJ, Lendvay TS, Acierno S et al (2011) Laparoscopic nephroureterectomy for Wilms' tumor: oncologic consideration. J Pediatr Surg 46(5): 978–982
41. McLorie GA (2001) Wilms' tumor (nephroblastoma). Curr Opin Urol 11(6):567–570
42. Jairam V, Roberts KB, Yu JB (2013) Historical trends in the use of radiation therapy for pediatric cancers: 1973–2008. Int J Radiat Oncol Biol Phys 85(3): e151–e155
43. Levitt G (2012) Renal tumours: long-term outcome. Pediatr Nephrol 27:911–916

Gonadal Tumors

26

Riccardo Masetti, Daniele Zama,
Francesca Vendemini, and Andrea Pession

26.1 Introduction

Gonadal tumors raise the challenge to pediatric surgeons and pediatric oncologists to cure the tumor while preserving fertility. The first issue is to discriminate between benign and malignant tumor, considering that risk of malignancy is estimated as 50 % in males and about 10–25 % in females, including both solid and cystic lesions.

A conservative surgical procedure, such as tumorectomy with gonadal preservation, should be attempted when possible in benign tumors. With the introduction of recent international protocols patients diagnosed with malignant tumors have good prognosis after adequate surgical treatment and, possibly, chemotherapy [1]. Current chemotherapy protocols, based on platinum and bleomycin, have demonstrated to be very effective, even for advanced-stage tumors [2, 3]. Thus, with the improvement of chemotherapy and the recognition that many of these tumors respond in a similar manner, the management of gonadal tumors is being clarified.

The main consequences of the treatment of gonadal tumors are the sterility due to the failure of gamete production and the lack of sex hormone production which prevents the progression of natural puberty and the development of secondary sexual characteristics. This latter effect can be managed by lifelong hormonal substitution, while sterility may result important psychological consequents [4].

Improvements in discovery, diagnosis, minimally invasive surgery management and chemotherapy have required changes in clinical practice, which is aimed at reducing morbidity without compromising cure rates. However, because of the low incidence of these tumors, cooperative group studies will be necessary to extend future therapeutic advances.

26.2 Epidemiology

Gonadal tumors are rare in childhood, with a rate of 0.5–2.0 cases per 100,000 children and representing approximately 2–3 % of tumors diagnosed in persons younger than 15 years [5], with an incidence slightly higher in male.

The peak of incidence of ovarian tumors is at 8–9 years and at 19–20 years [6]. As for testicular tumors, the frequency of ovarian germ cell tumors increases with the gonadotropin release, implicating hormonal factors in their etiology [7].

R. Masetti • D. Zama • F. Vendemini
Department of Pediatrics – Pediatric Hematology and Oncology "Lalla Seràgnoli",
S. Orsola-Malpighi University Hospital,
Via Albertoni 5, Bologna 40138, Italy
e-mail: riccardo.masetti@gmail.com

A. Pession (✉)
Department of Pediatrics,
S. Orsola-Malpighi University Hospital,
Via Albertoni 5, Bologna 40138, Italy
e-mail: andrea.pession@unibo.it

M. Lima, G. Manzoni (eds.), *Pediatric Urology: Contemporary Strategies from Fetal Life to Adolescence*,
DOI 10.1007/978-88-470-5693-0_26, © Springer-Verlag Italia 2015

Table 26.1 Classification of pediatric gonadal tumors

Ovarian	Testicular
Germ cell	
Teratoma	Endodermal sinus tumor (yolk sac tumor)
Mature (solid, cystic)	Embryonal carcinoma
Immature (Grade 0–3)	Teratoma
Associated with malignant germ cell tumor component	Teratocarcinoma
Associated with malignant somatic component	Gonadoblastoma
Dysgerminoma	Others (seminoma, choriocarcinoma, mixed germ cell)
Endodermal sinus tumor (yolk sac tumor)	
Mixed malignant germ cell tumor	
Choriocarcinoma	
Gonadoblastoma	
Non-germ cell	
Epithelial (serous, mucinous)	Sex cord stromal (Leydig cell, Sertoli cell)
Sex cord-stromal cell (granulosa, Leydig cell, Sertoli cell)	

Differently from adult ovarian tumors, about 60 % of pediatric ovarian tumors are of germ cell origin, while tumors of epithelial and stromal origin are less frequent [8]. In order of decreasing frequency, the categories are dysgerminoma, endodermal sinus tumor (yolk sac carcinoma), immature teratoma, mixed germ cell tumor, and embryonal carcinoma (Table 26.1).

Pediatric testicular tumors resemble those seen in adults, but they differ with respect to incidence, clinical manifestations, histopathology, and prognosis [8]. Approximately three-quarter of childhood testicular tumors are of germ cell origin, as compared with more than 90 % of those found in the adult population [9]. More than half of the germ cell tumors are endodermal sinus tumors and a smaller portion are teratomas. Rarely, a mixture of germ cell and stromal components (gonadoblastoma) is noted in a phenotypic female patient with dysgenetic gonads and male karyotype.

26.3 Ethiology and Pathogenesis

The gonads contain three cell types that have neoplastic potential. Germ cells give rise to germ cell tumors, the cells of the sex cords that rarely may develop into stromal tumors (testicular Sertoli or Leydig cell tumors, ovarian granulosa cell tumors, or mixtures of these components) and last, coelomic epithelium covering the ovary may evolve into epithelial neoplasms, found most often in adults.

26.3.1 Germ Cell Tumors

Germ cell tumors result from arrested or aberrant migration of common progenitor cells. These primitive cells originate near the allantois of the embryonic yolk sac endoderm and migrate to the genital ridge at 4–5 weeks gestational age.

The localization of the tumor in extragonadal locations is due to the abnormal deposition of these cells and includes the central nervous system, neck, mediastinum, retroperitoneum, and sacrococcygeal region. Most childhood germ cell tumors are benign, and include mature and immature teratomas. Teratomas contain elements from one or more of the embryonic germ layers and contain tissue foreign to the site of origin [10]. Immature teratomas contain primitive neuroepithelium and are graded between I and III [11].

In infancy and childhood, Yolk sac tumors, also called endodermal sinus tumor, are the most common malignant histologic variants. For this subtype of tumor, the main sites of metastases are lymph nodes or lungs. Other malignant histologic types include choriocarcinoma and embryonal carcinoma.

Germinoma (seminoma and dysgerminoma) are not usual in infancy and childhood. In the adolescent age germinoma are typically localized in the central nervous system and mediastinum as well as at the gonadal sites. Malignant elements coexist in approximately a quarter of pediatric germ cell tumors [12] and benign elements (teratoma) are often present with malignant tumors particularly in the mediastinum [13] and ovary [14].

26.3.2 Gonadal Stromal Tumors

Gonadal stromal tumors (sex cord tumors) are rare in children (5–10 % of cases). They arise from stromal components and frequently produce hormones, such as estrogen or androgen. The hormone production can cause clinical apparent changes in the patient. Two types are distinguished according to the initial cell: granulosa–theca cell tumors and the Sertoli–Leydig cell tumors (arrhenoblastoma). Both of them are frequently benign. In these tumors hormonal production and potential malignancy are not correlated.

26.3.3 Epithelial Tumors

Epithelial tumors are specific for the ovary and account for 15 % of gonadal tumors. They are typically benign (serous and mucinous cystadenoma), bilateral and tend to spread locally within the pelvis. Few cases are malignant (serous or mucinous adenocarcinoma). An elevation of serum levels of CA-125 tumor antigen is typically found in these tumors.

26.3.4 Gonadoblastoma

In gonadoblastoma tumors both germ cells and stroma cells can be found. They are considered a pseudotumoral dysgenetic gonad rather that a true tumor, usually associated with an intersex disorder with a Y-chromosome or evidence of some Y-chromatin. Mixed gonadal digenesis, pure gonadal digenesis, WAGR syndrome, true hermaphroditism, DRASH syndrome, Turner and Turner-like syndromes, and FRASER syndrome are associated to gonadoblastoma. The typical age of onset is in post puberty, but sometimes they may be seen also in childhood. They are well encapsulated, slow-growing tumors; bilateral in the 40 % of cases. Usually they are asymptomatic, but should be removed prophylactically in infancy or early childhood for the high risk of malignant transformation, that is estimated from 10 to 50 %.

26.3.5 Genetic and Risk Factors

26.3.5.1 Testicular Tumors

Children with intersex disorders, such as undescended testes and Klinefelter's syndrome are associated with thoracic teratoma. These children have also an increased risk of germ cell tumors. Gonadoblastoma, in situ lesion with the capability of transforming into dysgerminoma, yolk sac tumor, immature teratoma, or choriocarcinoma [15], has an increased frequency in children with intersex disorders. The presence of a Y chromosome is thought to be the risk factor and thus includes male pseudohermaphrodites (under-androgenized males) with lack of testosterone, androgen insensitivity syndrome, or 5α reductase deficiency as well as mixed gonadal dysgenesis [16]. The risk of malignancy in complete androgen insensitivity varies around 3 % at age of 20–22 % at 30 [17]. In these children is recommended a gonadectomy.

Undescended testes are also a universally recognized risk factor for the occurrence of testicular cancer in boys. The incidence of undescended testes in general population is approximately 0.4 %; however, the incidence among males with testicular cancer is 3.5–12 % [18]. The seminal study of Campbell and coworkers [19] demonstrated the risk appears even higher with intra-abdominal testes, so they firstly notes that this site accounts for only 14.3 % of undescended testes, but 48.5 % of the tumors in undescended testes. In these patients also the contralateral testes are at increased risk of developing a tumor, as 20 % of tumors in patients with undescended testes occur in the controlateral scrotal testes [20]. Seminomas occur with an increased frequency in the undescended testes compared with descended testes [21], and though some authors have reported a decreased rate of seminoma after orchiopexy [22], the exact effect of orchiopexy on the frequency of testicular cancer is not known.

26.3.5.2 Ovarian Tumors

The genetic biology of ovarian germ cell tumors is more complex than that of testicular germ cell tumors.

The cytogenetic assessment of ovarian mature teratomas demonstrates that 95 % have a normal karyotype. In only 5 % of mature teratomas gains of single whole chromosomes have been found, the identity of which differs from case to case [23]. Studies of molecular loci have revealed that most of mature ovarian teratomas have entered but not completed meiosis [23, 24]. Thus, these tumors are diploid, genetically unique, due to the fact the majority of their genome is isodisomic.

Ovarian immature teratomas are heterogeneous: some have a meiotic stem-cell origin, while others show a mitotic origins, suggesting failure of early meiotic arrest [25]. The frequency of chromosomal abnormalities in immature teratoma is higher than in mature teratoma, but no recurrent abnormalities, have been found. Apparently a correlation exists between the histologic grade of immature teratoma and DNA content: grades 1 and 2 are diploid, and grade 3 tumors are aneuploidy [26].

Most malignant ovarian germ cell tumors are aneuploid. The main frequent genetic lesions are i(12p), gains of chromosomes 21 and 1q and loss of chromosomes 13 and 8. The same lesions can be detected in malignant testicular germ cells tumors with a lower rate. In conclusion, though malignant ovarian germ cell tumors appear to have the same origin of their adolescent testicular counterparts, immature and mature ovarian teratoma remain unique subcategories of germ cell tumors likely to have a different mechanism of origin.

26.4 Clinical Aspects

26.4.1 Ovarian Tumors

The possibility of an ovarian tumor should be always carefully considered in a girl presenting with pelvic pain, an abdominal mass, precocious puberty or virilization, [12, 13, 14, 27, 28].

The benign nature of the tumor is highly probable as in pure cystic lesions and also in neonatal tumors that represent the most part of cases. Benign or functional cysts (follicular cyst, corpus luteum cyst, simple cyst) may be often discovered occasionally in the fetus during the last trimester of pregnancy or postnatally or around puberty. Their finding is much more frequent now that ultrasound scanning is readily available and, so they currently represent more than half of all ovarian cysts in children and adolescents. These benign cysts may regress spontaneously or may cause complications such as intracystic bleeding and adnexal torsion. Benign mature teratomas, including dermoid cysts, which represent a monophasic teratoma, generally are easily identified with instrumental evaluation and tumor markers are within normal limits. They can occur at any age.

Large (>10 cm) and rapidly growing solid tumor associated with signs of local invasion, ascites or metastases are highly suspicious for malignancy since the presentation. One third of ovarian masses are discovered because of torsion and nearly three-quarters of twisted ovaries contain an underlying cystic or solid mass [29]. Preoperative ultrasonography is a poor discriminant of simple ovarian torsion and torsion of an ovarian mass.

26.4.2 Testicular Tumors

A testicular mass is the typical presentation finding of a testicular tumor (Fig. 26.1). It may be noted by the patient himself or detected during a routine examination. Occasionally, a hydrocele is found and may delay the diagnosis. Otherwise, the patient may present with an acute scrotum due to a bleeding or a torsion or, more rarely, with precocious puberty or gynecomastia. Benign tumors are more likely in these situations: the neonatal period, when they are associated to an endocrine disorder, or in patients with a micro/multicystic lesion associated with homolateral renal agenesis. This last situation is highly suggestive of cystic dysplasia of the rete testis [15, 30].

An emergency presentation is quite rare in boys, but relatively frequent in girls, and include

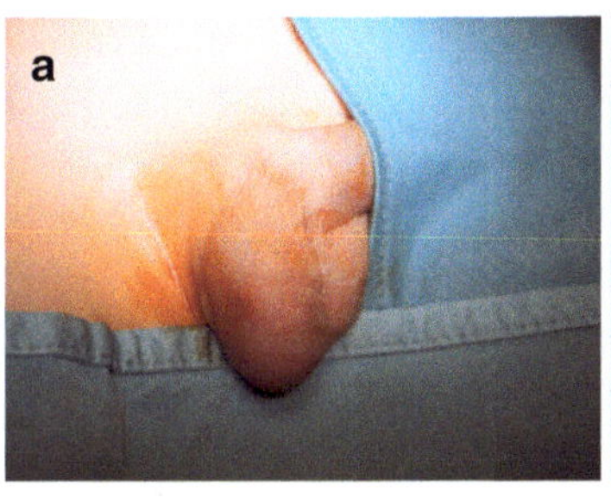

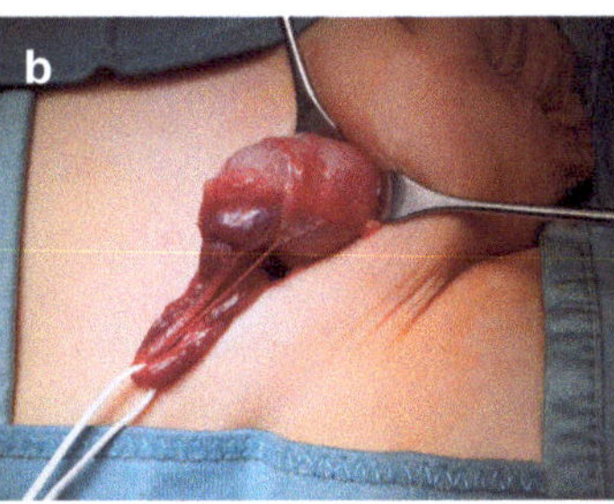

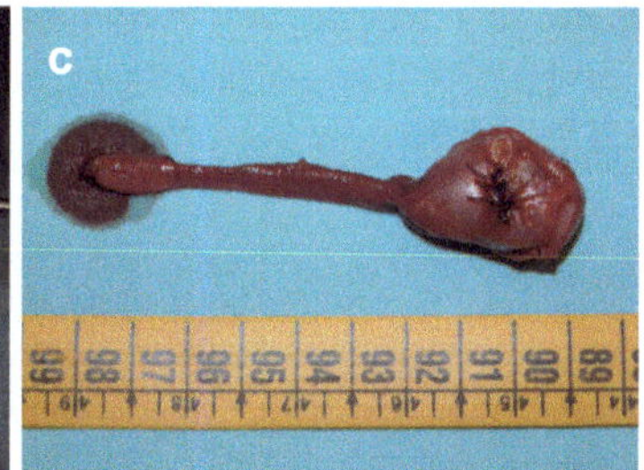

Fig. 26.1 (**a**) A right testicular mass noted by the parents of a 5-years old boy. (**b**) The patients underwent radical inguinal orchiectomy with en bloc excision of spermatic cord structures and testis. (**c**) The surgical specimen. The histological examination showed endodermal sinus tumor (yolk sac tumor)

cases of acute torsion or bleeding of a gonadal tumor. These presentations should be carefully evaluated, because they can be quite misleading and the diagnostic delay may compromise the long-term outcome.

26.5 Diagnosis

26.5.1 Tumor Markers

Most germ cell tumors secrete either serum alfa-Fetoprotein (AFP) and beta subunit of Human Chorionic Gonadotropine (hCG) and levels of both substances should be obtained prior to surgical exploration. AFP is normally elevated during the fetal life, decrease gradually after birth and should reduce to normal after 9 months of age: the AFP plasmatic half-life is 5 days [31]. Serum AFP levels are increased in patients with yolk sac tumors and correlate with the clinical course of patients. Indeed, after surgical excision of the tumor, serum AFP levels decrease progressively: failure to return to normal levels or subsequent elevation of this marker may indicate the presence of residual, recurrent or progressive disease, respectively [32]. Serum AFP levels may be increased when there are foci of yolk sac tumors in teratomas.

Serum beta hCG levels are always increased in infant or neonate with choriocarcinoma: the syncytiotrophoblastic component of the tumor produced the protein whose [33] half-life is of 16 h.

Lactate dehydrogenase isoenzyme-1 (LDH-1) is a non-specific marker which increases in patients with germ cell tumors including yolk sac tumor, dysgerminoma, and choriocarcinoma [34]: high serum levels correlate with tumor mass (i.e. metastasis) and response to treatment lead to a gradual reduction of the protein levels.

26.5.2 Pre-operative Staging

Ultrasonography is the technique of choice for the initial evaluation of patients with abdominal, pelvic or scrotal masses and will differentiate cystic from solid lesions. In the suspect of testicular tumor, ultrasonography is useful for distinguishing a simple hydrocele from a reactive hydrocele associated with the tumor. In case of teratoma ultrasound evaluation showed a sonolucent cystic area with intermixed solid portions.

Computed tomography (CT) of the abdomen and pelvis is helpful in identifying the site of origin, the extent of tumor and metastatic disease. Because patients with ovarian or testicular tumors can develop metastatic disease to the thoracic lymph nodes, lung and bone, staging evaluation should include chest CT and scintigraphy with 99mTC-pertechnetate.

26.5.3 Surgical Staging

The goal of initial surgery in patients with gonadal tumors is to evaluate the extent of disease (staging) and to resect all tumor if feasible, while sparing uninvolved reproductive organs. The exploration consist of a thorough examination of the omentum, peritoneal surfaces and liver, with removal of any suspicious lesions or

Table 26.2 Pediatric Oncology Group/Children Cancer Group (POG/CCG) staging system for pediatric ovarian germ cell tumors

Stage	
I	Limited to the ovary (ovaries) Peritoneal washing negative. No clinical, radiographic, or histologic evidence of disease beyond the ovaries
II	Microscopic residual or positive lymph nodes (<2 cm); peritoneal evaluation negative. Tumor markers positive or negative
III	Lymph node involvement (>2 cm); gross residual or biopsy only; contiguous visceral involvement (omentum, intestine, bladder); peritoneal evaluation positive for malignancy. Tumor markers positive or negative
IV	Distant metastases, including liver

Table 26.3 Pediatric Oncology Group/Children Cancer Group (POG/CCG) staging system for pediatric testicular germ cell tumors

Stage	
I	Limited to testis (testes). Completely resected by high inguinal orchiectomy. Tumor markers normal after appropriate half-life decline (AFP, 5 days; hGC 16 h). Patients with normal or unknown tumor markers at diagnosis must have a negative ipsilateral retroperitoneal node sampling to confirm Stage I disease if radiographic studies demonstrate lymph nodes >2 cm
II	Transcrotal orchiectomy: microscopic disease in scrotum or high spermatic cord (< 5 cm from proximal end); retroperitoneal lymph node involvement (<2 cm) and/or increased tumor markers after appropriate half-life decline
III	Retroperitoneal lymph node involvement, but no visceral or extra-abdominal involvement. (Involvement means lymph nodes >4 cm by CT or >2 and <4 cm with biopsy proof)
IV	Distant metastases, including liver

any enlarged retroperitoneal or pelvic lymph nodes. Additionally, if malignant germ cell tumor is suspected, bilateral retroperitoneal lymph node sampling are required. Ascitic fluid, if present, or peritoneal washings are to be sent for cytologic examination.

If the initial surgical procedure did not include an exploration of the omentum, peritoneal surfaces or liver and there is evidence of residual tumor, it should be considered to perform a re-exploration with resection of any visible residual disease. In Tables 26.2 and 26.3 the Pediatric Oncology Group/Children Cancer Group (POG/CCG) Staging System for ovarian germ cell and testicular tumors are reported.

26.6 Therapeutic Management

26.6.1 Surgery

Surgical resection alone is the therapy of choice in benign tumors, such as mature teratomas. In the presence of malignant tumors, removal is indicated if possible, but resection should not be undertaken up to sacrificing vital structure. In this situation, only biopsy or debulking followed by adjuvant chemotherapy are recommended.

26.6.1.1 Ovarian Tumors

Teratomas are benign lesion that are treated by surgical excision alone. Rarely, mature or immature teratomas may have peritoneal and omental implantation of mature glial tissue, also called "gliomatosis peritonei" [35]. In this case, sampling of the lesions should be performed in order to confirm the diagnosis.

For malignant ovarian tumors the Children Oncology Group guidelines recommend to collect ascitic fluid or peritoneal washings for cytology, to examine entire peritoneal surface and liver and excise suspicious lesions. The tumoral resection consists of unilateral oophorectomy and, only if suspected, wedge biopsy of contralateral ovary is indicated. Omental inspection is recommended and omentectomy is indicated if adherence or nodules are observed; biopsy of suspicious or enlarged retroperitoneal or pelvic lymph nodes is suggested. In case of bilateral tumors, in the attempt to preserve residual ovarian function it is possible to consider the resection of the least involved ovary, particularly if a clear demarcation is evident between the tumor and normal ovarian tissue.

Laparoscopy has been widely utilized in the management of ovarian lesions in childhood (Fig. 26.2). The main controversy surrounds the possibility to perform an adequate oncologic surgical procedure in cases where the benign

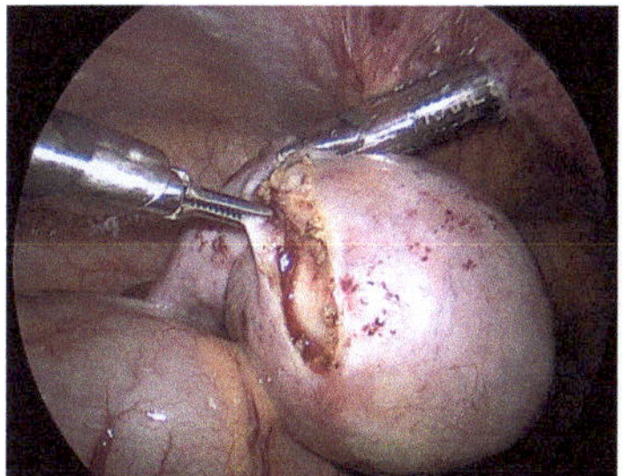
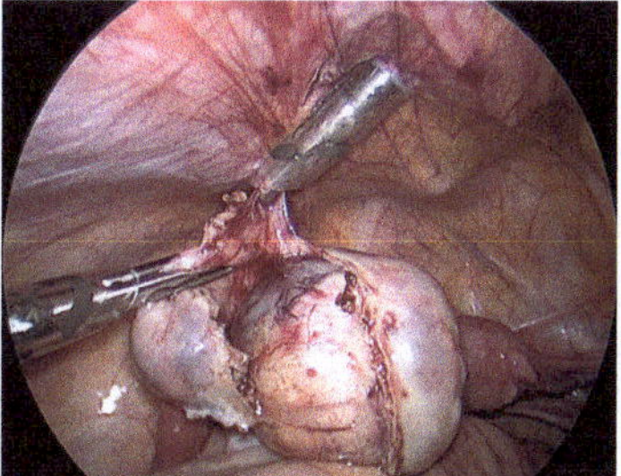
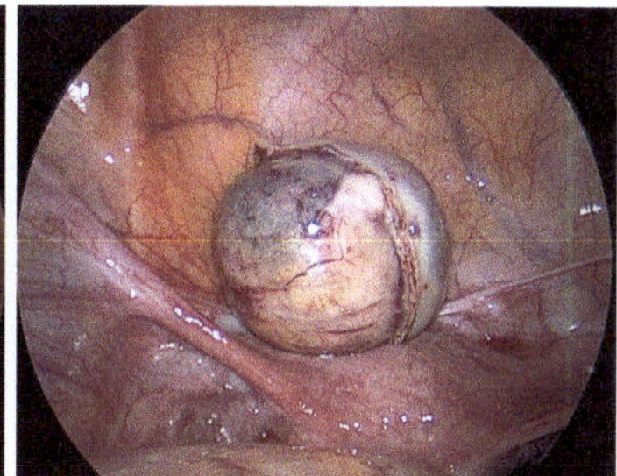

Fig. 26.2 Laparoscopic resection of ovarian teratoma. The sequence showed the gonadal sparing surgery that allow to remove the tumor while preserving ovarian tissue

or malignant nature of the lesion cannot be determined pre-operatively. If the lesion is primarily solid or if the serum markers are elevated, an open procedure is indicated whereas if the serum markers are normal and the lesion is primarily cystic a less invasive technique may be considered; however, avoidance of tumor spill must be assured.

26.6.1.2 Testicular Tumors

The surgical approach for both diagnosis and treatment of a solid testicular mass is radical inguinal orchiectomy with en bloc excision of spermatic cord structures and testis. If the mass appears to involve a portion of the testis or has cystic feature consistent with a teratoma, it can be treated with enucleation. An extemporaneous histological examination should be performed in this case in order to confirm the diagnosis.

26.6.2 Chemotherapy

Before the advent of multimodal therapy, children with malignant germ cell tumors could expect poor outcomes [36, 37]. On the basis of a paucity of clinical trials in pediatric patients, subsequent therapy was based on the larger adult experience with gonadal cancer. Cyclophosphamide-based therapy improved the outcome for patients with localized malignant germ cell tumors [38], but for patients with advanced disease, outcome remained poor. The subsequent introduction of cisplatin-based therapy, dramatically improved the survival for all-stage disease [39].

26.6.2.1 Ovarian Tumors

Malignant germ cell tumors are treated using different protocols in Europe and the USA. In Europe (SIOP protocol TGM55 and TGM90), in patients with localized non-seminomatous tumors (stage I and II) that has been completely removed no further therapy is needed. The Associazione Italiana Ematologia Oncologia Pediatrica (AIEOP) recommends treating stage I malignant ovarian germ cell tumor with surgery followed by a close observation, considering the relatively low risk of recurrence [40]. However, the use of chemotherapy in localized tumors is still controversial since in the prospective study POG9048/CCG 8891 the POG/CCG proposed to treat patients with stage I ovarian tumor with four cycles of cisplatin-etoposide-bleomycin (PEB) [41]. Both in european and in POG/CCG protocols the therapeutic approach for stage III - IV tumors consist of four PEB cycles followed by the surgical excision of the residual mass and metastasis in stage IV disease [40, 42].

Considering ovarian sex cord stromal tumor, among which the Sertoli-Leydig cell tumor was the most aggressive variety, a cisplatin-based chemotherapy was useful in patients with residual disease after surgery or metastatic spread; however, the optimal role of chemotherapy is still to be defined [43].

For non-secreting malignant tumors such as immature teratoma with some foci of yolk sac tumor surgical resection is the primary treatment. The prognostic significance of gliomatosis peritonei in patients with teratomas remain unclear. Although having peritoneal implants does not up-stage the patient's disease, some author have reported malignant transformation of these elements and adverse outcome [35]. However, the experience in the intergroup study from the POG/CCG [44] supports to treat patients affected by teratoma with complete resection only, followed by close observation of serum tumor markers and diagnostic imaging. Chemotherapy with its potential side effects can be reserved for patients who develop recurrent disease.

26.6.2.2 Testicular Tumors

In case of complete excision of germ cell tumor and no evidence of disease outside the scrotum (Stage I) the tumoral markers can be followed to assure a normal decline. If a normal decline occurs, the child can be treated with observation alone. Some case of relapse in patients with stage I disease were reported but the salvage rate with chemotherapy was extremely high [44, 45]. For stage II-III disease POG/CCG recommend to proceed with four PEB cycles after surgery. Stage IV disease is treated with four neoadiuvant PEB cycles followed by surgical removal of residual disease [40, 42].

Considering testis sex cord stromal tumor, platinum-based chemotherapy is suggested when residuals are left after surgical excision and in those rare cases with metastatic spread [46].

26.7 Results and Aftercare

26.7.1 Prognosis

The introduction of cisplatinum chemotherapy and current advances in the surgical treatment have resulted in a dramatic improvement of the prognosis of children with gonadal tumors.

The survival for stage I germ cell gonadal tumors and all immature teratomas at any site is excellent and these are mainly managed by surgical excision alone and subsequent observation. The results of POG 9048/CCG 8891 protocol are testimony to the excellent outcome of gonadal tumor, especially in the localized form: for stages I and II ovarian and stage II testicular malignant germ cell tumors the 6-year EFS was 94.5 % and the OS was 95.7 % [41].

For high risk patients, such as stage III - IV malignant gonadal germ cell tumors, the results of the last POG/CCG Intergroup trial showed good prognosis after treatment with PEB cycles and surgery: the 6-years EFS and OS for stage III tumors were 94–96 and 98–100 %, whereas for stage IV tumors the EFS and OS were 86–88 and 90–93 %, respectively [42].

26.7.1.1 Malignant Tumors

In case of secreting tumors, follow-up includes measurement of serum markers every 2 weeks for 3 months, then strictly for 2 years. Marker levels must return to normal within 3 months of surgery. As mentioned above, failure to return to normal levels or subsequent elevation of serum markers may indicate the presence residual, recurrent or progressive disease and impose to perform further diagnostic evaluations.

Abdominal CT scan or ultrasound evaluation is required every 3 months during the 1st and the 2nd year since therapy interruption. During the 3rd year is recommended to evaluate the patients twice or three times a year and subsequently once a year until the 5th year since therapy suspension.

26.7.1.2 Benign Tumors

After removal of a benign tumor, an appropriate follow up comprises testes evaluation by palpation and regular ultrasound scans and ultrasound scan of ovaries in order to find possible ipsilateral recurrence or development of controlateral tumor. There is no consensus on follow up but an annual check up can be proposed at least in the early years after the enucleation.

26.7.2 Gonadal Function

The improvement of the prognosis in patients diagnosed with ovarian or testicular tumors raises the problem of preservation of gonadal function. After tumor enucleation without gonadectomy, gonadal function is usually normal wheres after unilateral gonadectomy without chemotherapy, gonadal function is slightly impaired in both sexes. Moreover, in synchronous or metachronous bilateral tumors, or in advanced disease treated with gonadectomy followed by chemotherapy, gonadal function can be markedly impaired. The pubertal age is considered to be at high risk of chemotherapy-induced damage in gonadal function due to the high vulnerability of ovarian and testicular germ cell which, during this period, cease to be on quiescent state. Gonadotropin releasing hormone analogs suppress the hypothalamic-pituitary-gonadal axis and render the gonad quiescent, decreasing the germ cell vulnerability to therapy. Therefore, although the effectiveness of this intervention is still controversial, it can be considered in pubertal adolescent that undergo chemotherapy for gonadal tumors [47]. Another option to be considered to preserve the fertility can be sperm cryopreservation in pubertal patients and ovarian tissue cryopreservation that could be realize also in pre-pubertal children [48].

Surgery continues to play a crucial role in the treatment of gonadal tumors. Benign tumors are treated only with conservative surgery and, when possible, the laparoscopic approach is the treatment of choice.

For malignant tumors, the aim of current treatments is to improve survival rates on the one hand and reduce treatment-induced adverse effects on the other. Future progress can be achieved by improving the understanding of tumor biology, the risk-stratification of patients, the modulation of chemotherapy and the use of laparoscopic techniques.

References

1. Mertens AC, Yasui Y, Neglia JP et al (2001) Late mortality experience in five-year survivors of childhood and adolescent cancer: the Childhood Cancer Survivor Study. J Clin Oncol 19:3163–3172
2. Bosl GJ, Geller NL, Bajorin D et al (1988) A randomized trial of etoposide and cisplatin versus vinblastine + bleomycin + cisplatin + cyclophosphamide + dactinomycin in patients with good prognosis germ cell tumors. J Clin Oncol 6:1231
3. Williams S, Birch R, Einhorn L (1987) Treatment of disseminated germ cell tumors with cisplatin, bleomycin, and either vinblastine or etoposide. N Engl J Med 316:1435
4. Landier W, Wallace WH, Hudson MM. Long-term follow-up of pediatric cancer survivors: education, surveillance, and screening. Pediatr Blood Cancer. 2006;46(2):149–58
5. AIRTUM Workin Group. Italian Cancer Figures – Report 2012 (2012) Childhood cancer: incidence, survival, trends. Epidemiol Prev 37(1):164–169
6. Ries LA, Gurney JG, Linet M et al (1999) Cancer incidence and survival among children and adolescents: United States SEER Program 1975–1995, National Cancer Institute, SEER Program. NIH Pub, Bethesda
7. Cronen PW, Nagaraj HS (1988) Ovarian tumors in children. South Med J 81:464
8. Brosman SA (1979) Testicular tumors in prepubertal children. Urology 13:581
9. Weissbach L, Altwein JE, Stiens R (1984) Germinal testicular tumors in childhood. Eur Urol 10:73
10. Malogolowkin MH, Ortega JA, Krailo M et al (1989) Immature teratomas: identification of patients at risk for malignant recurrence. J Natl Cancer Inst 81:870–874
11. Norris HJ, Zirkin HJ, Benson WL (1976) Immature (malignant) teratoma of the ovary: a clinical and pathological study of 58 cases. Cancer 37:2359–2372
12. Gobel U, Schneider DT, Calaminus G et al (2000) Germ cell tumors in childhood and adolescence. Ann Oncol 11:263–271
13. Billmire D, Vinocur C, Rescorla F et al (2001) Malignant mediastinal germ cell tumors: an intergroup study. J Pediatr Surg 36:18–24
14. Billmire D, Vinocur C, Rescorla F et al (2004) Outcome and staging evaluation in malignant germ cell tumors of the ovary in children and adolescents: an intergroup study. J Pediatr Surg 39:424–429
15. Ross JH, Rybicki L, Kay R (2002) Clinical behavior and contemporary management algorithm for prepubertal testis tumors: a summary of the prepubertal testis tumor registry. J Urol 168:1675–1679
16. Rutgers JL, Scully RE (1992) Pathology of the testes in intersex syndromes. Semin Diagn Pathol 4:275–291
17. Manuel M, Katayama PK, Jones HW Jr (1976) The age of occurrence of gonadal tumors in intersex patients with a Y chromosome. Am J Obstet Gynecol 124:293–300
18. Fonkalsrud EW (1978) The undescended testis. Curr Probl Surg 15:1–56
19. Campbell HE (1942) Incidence of malignant growth of the undescended testicle. Arch Surg 44:353–369
20. Johnson DE, Woodhead DM, Pohl DR et al (1968) Cryptorchidism and testicular tumorigenesis. Surgery 63:919–922
21. Sohval AR (1954) Testicular dysgenesis as an etiologic factor in cryptorchidism. J Urol 72:693–702
22. Jones BJ, Thornhill JA, O'Donnell B et al (1991) Influence of prior orchiopexy on stage and prognosis of testicular cancer. Eur Urol 19:201–203
23. Surti U, Hoffner L, Chakravarti A et al (1990) Genetics and biology of human ovarian teratomas: I. Cytogenetic analysis and mechanism of origin. Am J Hum Genet 47:635
24. Inoue M, Fujita M, Azuma C et al (1992) Histogenetic analysis of ovarian germ cell tumors by DNA fingerprinting. Cancer Res 52:6823

25. Ohama K, Nomura K, Okamoto E et al (1985) Origin of immature teratoma of the ovary. Am J Obstet Gynecol 152:896
26. Silver SA, Wiley JM, Perlman EJ (1994) DNA ploidy analysis of pediatric germ cell tumors. Mod Pathol 7:951
27. Brennan BM, Rahim A, Mackie EM et al (1998) Growth hormone status in adults treated for acute lymphoblastic leukaemia in childhood. Clin Endocrinol 48:777–783
28. Littley MD, Shalet SM, Beardwell CG et al (1999) Hypopituitarism following external radiotherapy for pituitary tumours in adults. Q J Med 70:145–160
29. Didcock E, Davies HA, Didi M et al (1995) Pubertal growth in young adult survivors of childhood leukaemia. J Clin Oncol 13:2503–2507
30. Valla JS for the Group d'Etude en Urologie Pediatrique (2001) Testis sparing surgery for benign testicular tumor in children. J Urol 165:2280–2283
31. Wu JT, Book L, Sudar K (1981) Serum alpha fetoprotein (AFP) levels in normal infants. Pediatr Res 15(1):50–52
32. Harms D, Janig U (1986) Germ cell tumors of childhood. Virchows Arch 409:223–229
33. Belchis DA, Mowry J, Davis JH (1993) Infantile choriocarcinoma. Cancer 72:2028–2032
34. Lahdenne P, Pitkänen S, Rajantie J et al (1997) International Germ Cell Cancer Collaborative Group: International Germ Cell Classification: a prognostic factor-based staging system for metastatic germ cell cancer. J Clin Oncol 15:594–603
35. Müller AM, Söndgen D, Strunz R, Müller KM (2002) Gliomatosis peritonei: a report of two cases and review of the literature. Eur J Obstet Gynecol Reprod Biol 100(2):213–222
36. Mulligan RM (1975) Pathogenesis of teratoid tumors of the ovary and testis. Pathol Annu 10:271–298
37. Kurman RJ, Norris H (1976) Endodermal sinus tumor of the ovary: a clinical and pathologic analysis of 71 cases. Cancer 38:2404–2419
38. Cangir A, Smith J, van Eys J (1978) Improved prognosis in children with ovarian cancers following modified VAC (vincristine sulfate, dactinomycin, and cyclophosphamide) chemotherapy. Cancer 42:1234–1238
39. Pinkerton CR, Pritchard J, Spitz L (1986) High complete response rate in children with advanced germ cell tumors using cisplatin- containing combination chemotherapy. J Clin Oncol 4:194–199
40. Protocollo TCMG AIEOP (2004) https://www.aieop.org/index.php
41. Rogers PC, Olson TA, Cullen JW, Pediatric Oncology Group 9048; Children's Cancer Group 8891 et al (2004) Treatment of children and adolescents with stage II testicular and stages I and II ovarian malignant germ cell tumors: a Pediatric Intergroup Study – Pediatric Oncology Group 9048 and Children's Cancer Group 8891. J Clin Oncol 22(17):3563–3569
42. Cushing B, Giller R, Cullen JW et al (2004) Pediatric Oncology Group Randomized comparison of combination chemotherapy with etoposide, bleomycin, and either high-dose or standard-dose cisplatin in children and adolescents with high-risk malignant germ cell tumors: a pediatric intergroup study – Pediatric Oncology Group 9049 and Children's Cancer Group 8882.9049; Children's Cancer Group 8882. J Clin Oncol 22(13):2691–2700
43. Cecchetto G, Ferrari A, Bernini G et al (2010) Sex cord stromal tumors of the ovary in children: a clinicopathological report from the Italian TREP project. Pediatr Blood Cancer 56(7):1062–1067
44. Marina N, Cushing B, Giller R et al (1999) Complete surgical excision is effective treatment for children with immature teratomas with or without malignant elements: a Pediatric Oncology Group/Children's Cancer Group Intergroup Study. J Clin Oncol 17: 2137–2214
45. Giguere JK, Stablein DM, Spaulding JT, McLeod DG, Paulson DF, Weiss RB (1988) The clinical significance of unconventional orchiectomy approaches in testicular cancer: a report from the Testicular Cancer Intergroup Study. J Urol 139(6):1225–1228
46. Cecchetto G, Alaggio R, Bisogno G et al (2010) Sex cord-stromal tumors of the testis in children. A clinicopathologic report from the Italian TREP project. J Pediatr Surg 45(9):1868–1873
47. Fallat ME, Hutter J, American Academy of Pediatrics Committee on Bioethics; American Academy of Pediatrics Section on Hematology/Oncology; American Academy of Pediatrics Section on Surgery (2008) Preservation of fertility in pediatric and adolescent patients with cancer. Pediatrics 121(5): e1461–e1469
48. Aubard Y, Piver P, Pech JC, Galinat S, Teissier MP (2001) Ovarian tissue cryopreservation and gynecologic oncology: a review. Eur J Obstet Gynecol Reprod Biol 97(1):5–14

Part VII

Nephro-urology

Renal Function from Fetus to Adulthood

27

Gaetano La Manna, Irene Capelli, and Giorgio Feliciangeli

27.1 The Kidney During the Fetal Period

27.1.1 Introduction

The embryological development of the urogenital system, which includes two embryologically and anatomically interconnected units, the urinary tract and genital tract, has been well understood from decades. Only in the last few years, a significant amount of data on the genetic regulation of these developmental processes has been produced, largely through studies of mutant mouse models and a growing number of human studies [1]. Among the most recent concepts, the nephron endowment is of particular interest for its significance in the relationship between the effects of changes in fetal microenvironment on renal development on one hand and the risk of renal and cardiovascular disease in the adult kidney on the other hand [2]. In fact, adverse events during fetal development may predispose an individual to increased cardiovascular risk in adulthood, establishing what is referred to by many researchers as "fetal programming" of adult cardiovascular disease. Indeed current literature reflects a growing interest on the relationship between the reduced number of nephrons at birth and the consequences it entails in terms of cardiovascular risk [3]. In the human species, the number of nephrons at birth is extremely variable, mirroring the extreme variability of the development of the kidney and urinary tract and different effectiveness in responding to the challenges of postnatal life.

G. La Manna • I. Capelli • G. Feliciangeli (✉)
Dialysis, Nephrology and Transplantation Unit, Department of Experimental, Diagnostic and Specialty Medicine, S. Orsola-Malpighi University Hospital, via Massarenti 9, Bologna 40138, Italy
e-mail: gaetano.lamanna@unibo.it; irene.capelli@gmail.com; giorgio.feliciangeli@aosp.bo.it

27.1.2 Kidney Development Stages

The normal development of the urinary tract consists of three different stages, all derived predominantly from intermediate mesoderm but also with some contribution from paraxial mesoderm. They develop in a temporal and craniocaudal sequence:

- *Pronephros* or "primitive kidneys," a transient not functioning structure that develops from the cervical region of the intermediate mesoderm and regresses at the embryonic age of 4 weeks.
- *Mesonephros* or "middle kidneys," a structure that replaces the pronephros from the fifth gestational week and that develops from the paravertebral mesoderm.

  At the beginning of the 4th week of intrauterine life, during the regression of the pronephric kidney, the primitive mesonephric tubules appear. They quickly lengthen, forming an S-shaped body, and acquire a tuft of capillaries that constitute a glomerulus at the medial end. Around the glomerular tuft tubules forms the

M. Lima, G. Manzoni (eds.), *Pediatric Urology: Contemporary Strategies from Fetal Life to Adolescence*,
DOI 10.1007/978-88-470-5693-0_27, © Springer-Verlag Italia 2015

Bowman's capsule, resulting in the formation of the renal corpuscle. The side of the tubule is connected to a longitudinal collecting tubule, the mesonephric duct or Wolffian duct. The mesonephros as a whole produces urine from the 6th through the 10th week of development. Between the 6th and 8th weeks, cranial tubules and glomeruli undergo degenerative processes, while the caudal ones are still in the phase of differentiation and in the male persist to form together with the mesonephric duct the genital system. In the female, instead, these structures disappear at the end of the 8th week.

- *Metanephros* or "permanent kidneys," the ureteric bud, an outgrowth of the mesonephric duct, invades the metanephric blastema leading to the formation of the metanephros or definitive kidney. Growing within the metanephric blastema, the ureteric bud gives rise to the pelvis and calyceal system. The advance of the bud also induces mesenchymal cells of the blastema to differentiate into epithelial cells to form glomeruli and renal tubules. Metanephric development is the result of the expression of numerous genes in the ureteric bud cells and metanephric blastema: they both send signals that induce organogenesis. From about the 10th week of gestation throughout intrauterine life, the kidney produces urine that becomes part of the amniotic fluid. However, at the intrauterine level, the kidneys do not play a fundamental role in maintaining fetal homeostasis. Around the 36th week, the formation of nephrons ends, even if "nephrogenesis" seems to continue for a few weeks of extrauterine life in preterm infants. It is not clear if extrauterine preterm nephrogenesis is able to lead to full nephron completion. The development of metanephric kidney instead continues beyond the end of nephrogenesis with significant growth, differentiation, and remodeling of the renal tissue [4].

27.1.3 The Kidney Ontogeny

The process of renal ontogeny is given mainly to the complex interaction between two key factors: the ureteric bud and the metanephric blastema. A primary defect of one of the two elements inevitably leads to an altered development of the other.

The molecular basis of renal embryogenesis is largely still to be identified. It is well known, however, that this process requires an interaction between molecules such as transcription factors, growth factors, cell adhesion molecules, and extracellular matrix proteins that are essential for the control of the cell cycle, proliferation, differentiation, and morphogenesis during embryonic development.

There are a large number of genes involved in this process, including those coding for proteins that control differentiation and cellular transcription (signaling molecules), apoptosis (survival cells), growth factors, and structural genes regulating the extracellular matrix [5].

27.1.3.1 Ureteric Branching Morphogenesis

The final collecting tubules of the kidney develop from the ureteric bud, a protrusion that originates from the mesonephric duct (Wolffian duct). Its localization is regulated by BMP4 (bone morphogenetic protein 4), expressed by a subpopulation of mesenchymal cells adjacent to the mesonephric duct. This factor inhibits ureteric branching, a process controlled by the expression of GREM1 (gremlin 1). It is by the action of these two factors that the normal development of the kidney and urinary tract is determinated [1]. The epithelium of the ureteric bud invades the metanephric blastema that is shaped like a cap on its distal end. The mesenchyme can respond to induction by the expression of several transcription factors such as EYA1, PAX2, ODD1, and WT1. WT1, expressed by the same mesenchyme, regulates the production of GDNF (glial cell line-derived neurotrophic factor) as well as other factors. These factors stimulate ureteral branching, forming several generations of tubules through the interaction with the receptors c-RET and GFRα1, expressed from the ureteric bud, establishing a signaling pathway between the two tissues to prevent the risk of ectopic ramifications [1, 6].

Subsequently, the ureteric bud widens, forming the primitive renal pelvis, and divides into a cranial and a caudal portion, constituting the future major calyces. The peripheral development of more tubules, which continues until the 20th week, will lead to the formation of minor chalices with the establishment of the renal pyramid through the elongation and convergence in the minor chalices of collecting tubules of the fifth and the following generations. The ureteric bud thus creates the ureter, the renal pelvis, the major and minor chalices, and the collecting tubules, by means of successive branches that are realized only at the periphery of the kidney, in the so-called nephrogenic zone. This area, in the course of kidney development, becomes more and more distant from the medullary portion of the kidney and renal pelvis [1].

27.1.3.2 Nephrogenesis and Nephron Endowment

Nephrogenesis is the process of generating new nephrons, which is realized in the nephrogenic zone, at the end of the precursor structure of the system of collecting ducts. Nephron endowment represents the number of nephrons at the end of the nephrogenesis process. During the late stages of ureteral branching, about four nephrons are induced by each ureteral end, thus increasing exponentially renal endowment [3].

The cells of the metanephric mesenchyme condense at the ureteral ends to form the mesenchymal cap structures responsible for the formation of all the epithelial components of the nephron. The mesenchymal cap differs following the sequence: pretubular aggregates→epithelial renal vesicles→S-shaped bodies→ renal corpuscles and tubules. The mesenchymal cap cells that express the factors GDNF, PAX2, and WT1 to promote ureteral branching ramifications can be classified into distinct subpopulations based on the expression of specific genetic markers. All mesenchymal cells express SIX2 factor, markers of renal stem cells; CITED1, EYA1, FLK-1, and WNT4 are additional genetic markers of mesenchymal cap subpopulations. The loss of expression of SIX2 determined by exposure of the mesenchymal cap to the action of the epithelial-derived factors WNT9B, TGFβ2, FGF-2, and LIF initiates the phase of epithelialization of the pretubular aggregates, which begins the formation of all cell types of the kidney epithelium [1].

The first sign of the process of epithelialization is represented by the conversion from a mesenchymal cell phenotype into a columnar phenotype, in order to form the kidney vesicles, which in turn give rise to small S-shaped tubules. These tubules, together with their glomeruli, which arise from a pocket at one end of the tubule, originate the nephrons or excretory units. The proximal portion of each nephron forms the Bowman's capsule. The distal portion is opened in one of the collecting tubules, thereby establishing a passage between the Bowman's capsule and the connection unit [6].

The continuous extension of the excretory tubule leads to the formation of the proximal convoluted tubule, the loop of Henle, and the distal convoluted tubule. This process is called segmentation and its molecular regulation is poorly understood. Recent studies have highlighted the role of gamma secretase, and other factors are currently under investigation, including the expression of PAX2 in the distal portion of the renal vesicle, the expression of WT1 and NOTCH2 for the differentiation of podocytes and of the epithelium of the proximal tubule, and the function of genes BRN1 and IRX3 in the loop of Henle.

The modifications of the extracellular matrix are also complex. Fibronectin and collagens I/III are replaced by laminin and collagen IV; the cell adhesion molecules, the syndecans and E-cadherins, that are essential for the condensation of mesenchymal cells in the peripheral epithelium are synthesized. If in the past the renal stroma was considered an inert support structure for the development of nephrons, now it is considered as an essential part of the process of ureteric branching. The kidney stroma in addition to expressing the retinoic acid receptors α and β2, essential for the expression of c-RET, also secretes cytokines with stimulatory and inhibitory action on glomerulogenesis and tubulogenesis. Furthermore, the cells of the renal stroma are necessary for the formation of the renal capsule and the definition of the sites in which the development of the kidney takes place [6].

There is still a lack of knowledge about renal vascularization. In contrast to the previous extra-renal vascular cell hypothesis, at present there is increasing evidence to indicate that a population of progenitor cells endogenously expressing FLK-1, localized at the level of the metanephric mesenchyme, are responsible for all the renal vasculature and the development of glomerular capillaries [1, 6].

Nephron endowment can be considered a measure of the success of kidney development. The studies of the last 25 years have highlighted the role of genetic and environmental regulation in the establishment of nephron endowment and consequences in adult life of its depletion at birth. Among the first studies, an important contribution was given by Brenner et al. who pointed out that the reduction in the number of nephrons at birth represents a major risk factor for the development of hypertension in adult life [2, 7]. Furthermore, the results of a study by Barker et al. have demonstrated an inverse relationship between birth weight and systolic blood pressure in adulthood, thus supporting the important role of intrauterine development on cardiovascular risk in adulthood. This correlation is known as the Barker hypothesis of fetal programming of adult hypertension. The inverse relationship is applicable to infants with an unfavorable intrauterine environment to normal fetal development and therefore is small for their gestational age, as happens, for example, in cases of restriction of dietary protein or exposure to high levels of glucocorticoids and alteration of the renin–angiotensin system. A suboptimal intrauterine environment is likely to reduce the ability of human adaptation to the challenges of extrauterine life, thus increasing the risk for diseases in adult life. This setting has been recently referred to as "developmental origins of adult health and disease" hypothesis [7].

27.2 The Kidney During Neonatal Period and Adulthood

At birth, each human kidney contains about one million nephrons that cannot be regenerated. Each nephron consists of:

1. A glomerulus
2. A renal tubule

The glomerulus arises from specialized capillaries adherent to the mesangium, wrapped by an invagination of the tubule, the Bowman's capsule, in turn formed by two layers that are reflected at the level of the vascular pole: the visceral layer is adherent to the glomerulus and consists of the podocytes and the parietal one that continues with the proximal convoluted tubule [8].

The basal membrane develops at the interface between the capillaries and the glomerular mesangium from one side and the layer of podocytes from the other side. The space between the two epithelial cell layers of Bowman's capsule is the urinary space that at the level of the urinary pole is in continuity with the tubular lumen.

The capillaries together with the mesangium are covered by epithelial cells (podocytes) forming the visceral epithelium of Bowman's capsule. At the level of the vascular pole, the visceral epithelium is reflected to become the parietal epithelium of the capsule. The basal membrane develops at the interface between the capillaries and the mesangium at one side and the layer of podocytes on the other side (glomerular basement membranes, GBM). The space between the two layers of epithelial cells of Bowman's capsule constitutes the urinary space and, at the level of the urinary pole, is in continuity with the tubular lumen [8]. The wall of the glomerular capillaries is formed by three layers.

27.2.1 The Endothelium

The endothelial cells of the glomerular capillaries contain numerous pores or fenestrations. They occupy about 20 % of the endothelial surface. The glomerular filtration rate depends on the area of the section (fractional area) of the fenestrations, and the restriction of protein passage is enabled through the glycocalyx contained in them. Another feature of glomerular endothelium is the presence, at the luminal surface, of a coating of negative electric charges, thanks to a glycoprotein called podocalixina. Any dysfunction of glomerular endothelial fenestrations can trigger renal failure or proteinuria; the pathophysiological importance of fenestration is well characterized in conditions such as preeclampsia or diabetic nephropathy [9].

27.2.2 Glomerular Basement Membrane

The glomerular basement membrane is much thicker than the other basement membranes and seems to be drawn from both capillary endothelial cells and podocytes. The principal components of the GBM are type IV collagen, laminin, and proteoglycans. The main feature of the GBM is the specific spectrum of isoforms of type IV collagen and laminin [8]. The mature form of GBM is made of type IV collagen that consists of chains α3, α4, and α5 (those found in other types of basal membrane composed of chains α1 and α2) and laminin 11, formed by chains α5, β2, and γ1. Congenital or acquired abnormalities of members of the GBM determine glomerular nephropathies such as Goodpasture's disease (an autoimmune disease in which the target antigen is type IV collagen) or Alport syndrome (mutations in the genes that encode the chains α3, α4, and α5 of type IV collagen).

Electron microscopy reveals that the glomerular basement membrane consists of three layers:

- The lamina rara interna, adjacent to the endothelium
- The lamina densa, placed centrally
- The lamina rara externa, in contact with the outer layer of podocytes
- Both lamina rara interna and externa are charged negatively and together constitute the primary filter for plasma proteins larger than 7–10 nm.

27.2.3 The Podocytes

These monostratified epithelial cells wrap the glomerular capillaries and have long cytoplasmic extensions called primary processes, which in turn give rise to short secondary processes (pedicels) that intersect the primary processes. The secondary processes rely directly on the lamina rara externa [10]. The spaces between the interdigitations are called filtration slit and present uniform dimensions (30–40 nm). They are closed by a thin diaphragm (slit diaphragm) 4 nm thick, highly permeable to water and small solutes, limiting the passage of larger proteins owing to their small openings (5–15 nm) at the level of the diaphragm. The latter is formed as the main component of nephrin, linked to actin cytoskeleton by CD2AP (CD2-associated protein), podocin, and several other structural proteins [8]. For each glomerulus, there are approximately 500–600 glomerular podocytes. Thanks to an extended actin cytoskeleton, the podocytes have contractile properties to oppose the hydrostatic pressure of the glomerular capillary (~60 mmHg), of greater intensity than other capillary beds. The main functions performed by the podocytes are not limited to a structural role or to the composition of the glomerular filtration barrier. The podocytes are also able to synthesize and repair the GBM, as well as to secrete growth factors that contribute to endothelium integrity or the differentiation and chemotaxis of mesangial cells within the mesangium. Furthermore, the podocyte plays another important role in terms of immunological function, as a component of the innate immune system due to its possible involvement in the surveillance against pathogens or abnormal proteins at the level of urinary space [8].

By the process of selective filtration, the free hemoglobin (65 kDa) and smaller molecules pass freely through the glomerular filter, while albumin (68 kDa) and larger molecules are retained [11].

There are three factors that determine the permeability to macromolecules:

- The electric charge
- The size
- The three-dimensional configuration

The mesangium forms the central portion of the renal glomerulus with a support function of the renal corpuscle. It consists of a cellular component, the mesangial cell, wrapped in the mesangial extracellular matrix. The mesangium contained in the renal corpuscle, intraglomerular mesangium, is related to the extraglomerular mesangium and to the juxtaglomerular apparatus [8, 10, 11].

The mesangial cells constitute 30–40 % of the cell population of the renal glomerulus. They contain actin and myosin, presenting contractile properties, which allow them to reduce the capillary lumen and to alter the blood flow within the renal glomerulus, thus influencing the filtration process. One of the most noteworthy features of mesangial cells is their ability to remove circulating immune complexes and to produce inflammatory mediators and growth factors and to regulate the synthesis of mesangial matrix [12].

The extraglomerular cells constitute a conical mass, whose apex is in continuity with the intraglomerular mesangium. From a functional point of view, they are part of the juxtaglomerular apparatus, consisting of a vascular component, the juxtaglomerular cells, and of a tubular component, the cells of the macula densa. The mesangial extraglomerular cells participate to a complex feedback mechanism between the tubule and the glomerulus, through which changes of the concentration of sodium, at the level of the macula densa, evoke regulatory signals of glomerular blood flow. The cells of the macula densa and endothelial cells act, respectively, as chemoreceptors and mechanoreceptors, detecting the first variations of the sodium concentrations and second variations of blood glomerular pressure [11]. The juxtaglomerular cells, containing granules of renin, and the cells of the tunica muscularis of the afferent arterioles, under both paracrine and endocrine stimulation, behave as effector cells in the regulation of vascular tone and renin secretion. This physiological response is indicated by the term renal autoregulation.

The renal tubule is divided into several segments: the proximal convoluted tubule, the loop of Henle, the distal convoluted tubule, the collecting tubule, and the collecting duct (although the latter segment for embryological reasons cannot be fully considered as a part of the nephron) [13]. The loop of Henle includes the straight portion of the proximal tubule (thick descending branch), the descending and ascending thin branch, and the thick ascending branch [8]. The distal convoluted tubule is sited in continuity with the thick ascending branch, which together with the collecting tubule, histologically similar to it, constitutes the distal portion of the nephron. The collecting duct begins in the renal cortex and penetrates deep into the medullary, gathering several collecting tubules of most nephron units. At the level of the renal pyramids, the collecting ducts converge at an acute angle between them to form larger ducts, papillary ducts (of Bellini) which, in number of 15–30, open at the apex of each renal papilla [13].

The renal tubules are lined by a monolayer epithelium resting on its basement membrane. At the apical (luminal) side, tubular epithelial cells are connected by junction systems represented most frequently by tight junctions (tight junction, zonula occludens), adherens junctions, and desmosomes, less commonly [8]. The result of such an organization is the formation of two different ways of transport through the epithelium: transcellular transport which occurs through the cell membrane and the cytoplasm and the paracellular pathway which occurs through the occluding junctions (tight junctions) of the lateral intercellular spaces. This transport modality has functional characteristics determined by the type of tight junctions expressed at various levels of the renal tubule. Conversely, transcellular transport is achieved through the expression of specific channels, carriers, and transporters localized to the apical and basolateral cell membranes. The various segments of the renal tubule differ markedly for the type of function and distribution of transport proteins [14].

27.3 Renal Function Development

27.3.1 Glomerular Filtration Rate

Renal function is measured or estimated by determining or calculating the glomerular filtration rate (GFR) or the total rate at which fluid is filtered into all the nephrons [8].

Because the homeostasis in the fetus is almost entirely maintained by maternal–fetal exchanges that take place through the placenta,

Table 27.1 Kidney function in different intra- and extrauterine life period

Intrauterine life		Extrauterine life	
Fetal period (weeks)	GFR (mL/min)	Life period	GFR (mL/min)
4–5 (pronephros)	Not functioning	At birth	20
6–10 (mesonephros)	Not functioning	2–4 weeks	40–60
From 10 (metanephros)	0–20	1–2 years	120

GFR glomerular filtration rate

fetal GFR is low, but it increases progressively. Within the last months of gestation, there is a progressive rise in GFR with gestational age until the 36th week, which is due to an expansion in the number and size of nephrons. Thereafter, GFR develops more slowly up to the time of birth. At birth, GFR is still relatively low: measured by inulin clearance, it is almost 20 mL/min/1.73 m^2 in term neonates [15, 16]. In term infants, there is a large increase in GFR during the first 2 weeks of life. There are many factors that contribute to the important increase of GFR in the first weeks of life: increases in systemic blood pressure and consequently hydrostatic pressure of glomeruli, pore size of glomerular capillary wall (as well as glomerular capillary surface area) and ultrafiltration coefficient, and plasma flow rate secondary to increase in caliber of afferent and efferent arterioles and the decrease in these arterioles' resistance. All these factors play some role in maturational increase in early postnatal GFR [15].

Although the weight of each factor on the increase in postnatal GFR is still to be determined [17, 18], it is known that GFR doubles during the first 2 weeks of life and reaches 50 ± 10 mL/min/1.73 m^2 between the second and fourth postnatal week. After the 1st month of life, GFR increases progressively and reaches adult levels between 1 and 2 years of life [15, 19]. This occurs in conjunction with changes in the tubular function (see Table 27.1). The most accurate technique for measuring GFR is the direct methods, which involve injection of a tracer, characterized by being filtered freely in the glomeruli, without renal reabsorption, secretion, or metabolization in the kidneys as inulin. They are also relatively invasive and expensive.

Therefore, much simpler methods are applied when estimating renal function: among them, creatinine clearance is a widely used test to estimate the glomerular filtration rate (GFR) [20]. Due to the small size and lack of protein binding, creatinine passes the glomerulus freely. However, it is also actively secreted by the proximal tubules at an unpredictable rate related to the level of renal function and/or type of renal disease [21, 22]. With decreasing GFR, the fraction of tubular creatinine secretion increases, which leads to a GFR overestimation of 10–40 % compared to inulin clearance [21]. In patients with glomerulopathies, the overestimation may be even higher [22]. A decrease in GFR is reflected by an increase in plasma creatinine. Moreover, plasma creatinine levels may change independently of glomerular function in case of dietary intake of meat, malnutrition, muscle atrophy, hepatic disease, or increased tubular creatinine secretion [23].

In order to find a more accurate and precise method for GFR estimation function, cystatin C was investigated. CysC is a low-molecular-weight protein with a function of a potent inhibitor of cysteine proteinases. Because of its low molecular weight and positive charge, at physiological pH, CysC is practically freely filtered in the glomeruli. A study of radiolabeled human CysC performed in rats showed a 94 % renal plasma clearance of 51Cr-EDTA and a subsequent tubular reabsorption and complete catabolization without any tubular secretion [24, 25]. Serum CysC has proved to give a better estimation of GFR in comparison with plasma creatinine [26].

In children the estimation of GFR from plasma creatinine can be particularly difficult. One reason is the constant and muscle-mass related increase in plasma creatinine levels in children above 2 years, with a constant GFR of 104 mL/min/1.73 m^2 (measured by 51Cr-EDTA) [23, 27–30]. The direct creatinine clearance method involves precise urine collection for 24 h, which is hard to obtain in children, time-consuming, and impractical for routine use. This imprecision is exemplified by a high day-to-day variation in children of 13.8 %, compared to only 4.8 and 6.9 %, respectively, for venous and capillary blood samples for determination of 51Cr-EDTA plasma clearance [31, 44, 45].

As for the adults, also for the pediatric population, alternative formulas have been proposed to achieve a more reliable estimation of glomerular filtration rate.

The most widely used formula for estimating glomerular filtration rate (eGFR) in children is the Schwartz formula, published in 1976 [32]. As the endogenous 24-h creatinine clearance is less precise than the Schwartz estimate [33], creatinine clearance is better estimated from the plasma level of creatinine using the Schwartz formula taking the mentioned limitations into account.

As several studies in children have shown, differently from creatinine, the levels of CysC remain stable after the first year of life [27–29]. Furthermore, CysC has been proven to be independent of gender, height, and weight in both pediatric and adult population [27–29, 34] indicating that CysC is a robust biomarker, especially applicable not only in children but also in elderly patients and other populations with low muscle mass, where serum creatinine measurements do not perform well. So CysC has been largely used to measure children's GFR, and accordingly, Schwartz formula has been recently revised using a combination of creatinine and CysC [35].

Moreover, many other formulas have been proposed: they intended to be more reliable in the estimation of glomerular filtration rate. None of these, however, have been introduced in the current routine clinical practice [35, 36].

27.3.2 Tubular Function

The renal tubule is classically divided into proximal tubule, loop of Henle, distal tubule, and collecting duct.

The *proximal tubule* as a whole is responsible for the bulk of Na+, K+, Cl−, and HCO3− reabsorption and almost complete reabsorption of glucose, amino acids, and low-molecular-weight proteins (e.g., retinol-binding protein, α- and β-microglobulins) that have penetrated the filtration barrier. Most other filtered solutes are also reabsorbed to some extent in the proximal tubule (e.g., ~60 % of calcium, ~80 % of phosphate, ~50 % of urea). The proximal tubule is highly permeable to water, so no quantitatively significant osmotic gradient can be established; thus, most filtered water (~65 %) is also reabsorbed at this site. In the final section of the proximal tubule, there is some secretion of weak organic acids and bases [8].

Animal studies have been very useful for the assessment of the maturation of tubular function, which is the focus of a recent comprehensive review on this topic [37]. Initials studies indicated that the overall transport rate of volume reabsorption in the neonatal rabbit was about one-fourth of the adult transport rate [38]. In addition, bicarbonate and glucose transport rates were also found to be one-fourth to one-third of the adult rate. Further investigations, using in vitro perfusion techniques that allowed measurement of the Na–H exchange rate, have shown that the activity of this transporter in the neonatal tubule was about one-third of the adult rate [39]. The paracellular permeability for bicarbonate in the neonatal tubule was also found to be extremely low; thus, the low reabsorption rate in the neonate was due to a decrease in the active transport of bicarbonate and not to passive backleak [40]. Molecular studies then revealed that the expression of NHE3 in the neonatal proximal tubule had a maturational increase mirroring the functional data. On closer examination, the sodium–proton exchange activity in the neonatal proximal tubule was always higher than expected in comparison with the NHE3 expression data. This raised the question of whether or not there could be a different NHE isoform in the neonatal tubule. Molecular studies of NHE8 expression indicated that this might be the isoform in the luminal membrane of the neonatal proximal tubule [41]. Although NHE8 is also found in the adult tubule, it is primarily located in the intracellular compartment, whereas in the neonate, it is found primarily on the luminal membrane, where it can function in bicarbonate reabsorption. The tubular reabsorption of glucose is also lower in the neonate as compared with the adult [38]. This is reflected clinically by the fact that infants born before 30 weeks of gestation can show a renal glucosuria [42, 43]. The tubular control of phosphate is different from that of other solutes because the neonatal renal tubules seem to have an increase in reabsorption of phosphate. Thus, the fractional reabsorption of phosphate is much higher in the neonate than in the adult [44]. The paracellular pathway for passive transport was also proven to undergo extensive changes during development. The permeability of the neonatal proximal tubule to bicarbonate is very low and the chloride permeability is almost zero [40, 45].

The *loop of Henle* is defined anatomically as comprising the pars recta of the proximal tubule (thick descending limb), the thin descending and ascending limbs, the thick ascending limb, and the macula densa. Besides its role in the continuing reabsorption of solutes (Na^+, Cl^-, K^+, Ca^{2+}, Mg^{2+}), this part of the nephron is responsible for the kidney's ability to generate a concentrated or diluted urine [8].

The *distal tubule* and the collecting duct system are made up of the straight part or thick ascending limb of the loop of Henle and distal convoluted tubule, where thiazide-sensitive NaCl reabsorption occurs; the connecting tubule, whose function is essentially intermediate between that of the distal connecting tubule and that of the next segment; and the collecting duct. Two cell types compose the cortical collecting duct. The predominant type is the principal cell, responsible for Na^+ reabsorption and K^+ secretion (as well as for water reabsorption); the other cell type, the intercalated cell, is responsible for secretion of H^+ (by α-intercalated cell) or HCO_3^- (by β-intercalated cell) into the final urine [8].

The serum potassium concentration in the preterm infant can be very high [42]. The excretion of potassium tends to be much lower in the neonate than in the adult because the infant needs to remain in positive potassium balance for growth. Studies have shown that this is because of a decrease in the expression of potassium channels in the collecting duct principal cells. In particular, the maxi-K channel has little or no expression in the neonate and then increases to the adult level. This channel is activated by a rise in flow through the tubule to produce a "flow-mediated" response. Perfusion of collecting ducts from neonatal rabbits showed no flow-mediated increase in potassium secretion [37]. As a result, it is critical to limit the amount of potassium given to these neonates [42].

27.3.3 Water Balance

The kidney regulates water homeostasis either by excreting excess free water or by conserving free water through urine concentration. The generation of free water is dependent upon the delivery of tubular fluid to the diluting segment, which comprises the thick ascending limb and the distal convoluted tubule. In the neonate, free water excretion is generally limited by the low GFR and the subsequent limited delivery of fluid distally. The diluting segment is capable of reabsorbing solute to dilute the urine so that the neonate can excrete urine with an osmolality of 50 mOsm/kg water [45]. The ability of the neonate to concentrate the urine is limited, and it does not reach the adult level until about 2 years of life [46–48]. The implicated factors include the medullary osmotic gradient and the tubular response to antidiuretic hormone (ADH). The fetal and neonatal pituitary gland can respond to osmotic changes and secrete adequate amounts of ADH [49]; however, the collecting duct principal cells have a blunted response to ADH. Initial studies indicated that the reduced response might be due to the effects of prostaglandins. When neonatal tubules were incubated with indomethacin, the production of cAMP in response to ADH was enhanced [50]. However, the osmotic water permeability response in the neonatal tubules was not augmented by indomethacin, suggesting a defect that was distal to cAMP production [51]. A more recent study showed that overexpression of phosphodiesterase in the neonatal tubule was the major contributing factor to the declined ADH response. When the neonatal tubules were incubated with isobutylmethylxanthine or rolipram (a specific type 4 phosphodiesterase inhibitor), the water permeability response to ADH was corrected to the same level as the adult tubules [52]. The limitation in the ability to excrete free water is due to the low GFR of the neonate, preventing the delivery of fluid to the diluting segment. Infants drink milk that is naturally low in sodium, but typically have no problems in excreting free water. When the milk or formula is watered down, the infant will drink a far greater amount as the caloric density is much lower. The increased intake exceeds the ability of the neonatal kidney to excrete free water and leads to hyponatremia.

27.3.4 Kidney Function in Preterm Neonates

The condition of the preterm infant (gestational age <37 weeks) is characteristic. In these infants, an increase in creatinine blood values has been described in the first 24–48 h of life. This increase was also inversely related to infant's gestational age. Only after this period, the creatinine values tend to decrease and reach values comparable to term infant (0.4–0.5 mg/dl). This reduction, however, is slow and progressive and can take up to 4 weeks for complete normalization [53, 54].

The rise in serum creatinine that occurs in the first hours of life reflects the balance between the release of creatinine from muscle deposits and renal clearance of the molecule. Infants are known to have a small muscle mass, and then it is feasible that the increase in serum creatinine in the first days of life is due to a reduced clearance, attributable to a delay in reaching the normal filtration process secondary to a still incomplete nephrogenesis or to a resorption process characteristic of immature tubule, as found in animal models [55].

In the preterm neonates, the changes in tubular transport explain also some of the findings. For example, the serum bicarbonate in term neonates averages 22 mEq/L and can be much lower in preterm infants (14–18 mEq/L) [56, 57]. The low bicarbonate is due to the low reabsorption rate by the proximal tubule that can make it difficult to correct [26]. Due to the immaturity of the proximal tubule, the glucose reabsorption rate can be less than the filtered load. This will result in renal glycosuria, which is common in preterm infants born before 34 weeks of gestation [28, 29]. Moreover, sodium entry into the collecting duct principal cell is via the epithelial sodium channel (ENaC). The preterm infant has been shown to have a high fractional excretion of sodium [42, 43]. Part of the reason for the excess excretion of sodium seems to be resistance to the effect of aldosterone on sodium transport in the tubule [58]. Transport of sodium has been shown to be low in the neonatal collecting duct and to increase with maturation [59, 60]. This is reflected by an increase in the expression of EnaC as the infant matures [61].

Bibliography

1. Walker KA, Bertram JF (2011) Kidney development: core curriculum 2011. Am J Kidney Dis 57(6): 948–958
2. Luyckx VA, Bertram JF, Brenner BM et al (2013) Effect of fetal and child health on kidney development and long-term risk of hypertension and kidney disease. Lancet 382(9888):273–283
3. Bertram JF, Cullen-McEwen LA, Egan GF et al (2013) Why and how we determine nephron number. Pediatr Nephrol. doi:10.1007/s00467-013-2600-y
4. Nelson (2002) XVI Trattato di Pediatria. Minerva Medica, Torino
5. 3°Convegno Pediatrico. Anomalie Congenite Renali; http://www.msditalia.it/altre/manuale/sez19/2612385d.html
6. Sadler TW (2013) Embriologia medica di Langman, edizione italiana a cura di Raffaele De Caro, Sergio Galli. V ed Elsevier, Italia, p 392
7. Madsen K, Tinning AR, Marcussen N, Jensen BL (2013) Postnatal development of the renal medulla; role of the renin-angiotensin system. Acta Physiol (Oxf) 208:41–49
8. Floege J, Johnson JR, Feehally J (2010) Renal anatomy in comprehensive clinical nephrology, 4th edn. Elsevier
9. Satchell SC, Braet F (2009) Glomerular endothelial cell fenestrations: an integral component of the glomerular filtration barrier. Am J Physiol Renal Physiol 296(5):F947–F956
10. Jefferson JA, Nelson PJ, Najafian B, Shankland SJ (2011) Podocyte disorders: core curriculum 2011. Am J Kidney Dis 58(4):666–677

11. Young B, Heath JW (2001) Il sistema urinario in Atlante di istologia e anatomia microscopica del Wheater, IIIth edn. Casa Editrice Ambrosiana, Milano, pp 286–309
12. Schlöndorff D, Banas B (2009) The mesangial cell revisited: no cell is an island. J Am Soc Nephrol 20(6):1179–1187
13. Balboni GC et al (2000) Apparato Urinario. Anatomia Umana, vol 2. Ed. Ermes, Italia, pp 355–390
14. Christov M, Alper SL (2010) Tubular transport: core curriculum. Am J Kidney Dis 56:1202–1217
15. Hunley TE, Kon V, Ichikawa J (2009) Glomerular circulation and function. In: Avner ED, Harmon WE, Niaudet P, Yoshikawa N (eds) Pediatric nephrology, 6th edn. Springer, Berlin, pp 31–64
16. Vogt BA, Dell KM (2008) The kidney and urinary tract. In: Martin R, Fanaroff A, Walsh M, (eds) Fanaroff and Martin's neonatal perinatal medicine, 9th edn. Elsevier, pp 1681–704
17. Guignard JP, Gouyon JB (2008) Glomerular filtration rate in neonates. In: Polin RA (ed) Nephrology and fluid electrolyte physiology. Saunders, Philadelphia, pp 79–96
18. Turner AJ, Brown RD, Carlstrom M et al (2008) Mechanisms of neonatal increase in glomerular filtration rate. Am J Physiol Regul Integr Comp Physiol 295:916–921
19. Otukesh H, Hoseini R, Rahimzadeh N, Hosseini S (2012) Glomerular function in neonates. Iran J Kidney Dis 6:166–172
20. Rose BD and Post T (2001). Clinical Physiology of Acid-Base and Electrolyte Disorders. McGraw Hill Professional, Boston
21. Perrone RD, Madias NE, Levey AS (1992) Serum creatinine as an index of renal function: new insights into old concepts. Clin Chem 38(10):1933–1953
22. Hood B, Attman PO, Ahlmen J, Jagenburg R (1971) Renal hemodynamics and limitations of creatinine clearance in determining filtration rate in glomerular disease. Scand J Urol Nephrol 5(2):154–161
23. Schwartz GJ, Brion LP, Spitzer A (1987) The use of plasma creatinine concentration for estimating glomerular filtration rate in infants, children, and adolescents. Pediatr Clin N Am 34(3):571–590
24. Andersen TB (2012) Estimating renal function in children: a new GFR-model based on serum cystatin C and body cell mass. Dan Med J 59(7):B4486
25. Tenstad O, Roald AB, Grubb A, Aukland K (1996) Renal handling of radiolabelled human cystatin C in the rat. Scand J Clin Lab Invest 56(5):409–414
26. Andersen TB, Eskild-Jensen A, Frøkiaer J, Brøchner-Mortensen J (2009) Measuring glomerular filtration rate in children; can cystatin C replace established methods? A review. Pediatr Nephrol 24(5):929–941
27. Bökenkamp A, Domanetzki M, Zinck R et al (1998) Reference values for cystatin C serum concentrations in children. Pediatr Nephrol 12(2):125–129
28. Finney H, Newman DJ, Thakkar H et al (2000) Reference ranges for plasma cystatin C and creatinine measurements in premature infants, neonates, and older children. Arch Dis Child 82(1):71–75
29. Helin I, Axenram M, Grubb A (1998) Serum cystatin C as a determinant of glomerular filtration rate in children. Clin Nephrol 49(4):221–225
30. Piepsz A, Tondeur M, Ham H (2006) Revisiting normal (51)Cr-ethylenediaminetetraacetic acid clearance values in children. Eur J Nucl Med Mol Imaging 33(12):1477–1482
31. Brøchner-Mortensen J, Rohbrandt K, Lauritzen RB (1977) Precision of single injection [51Cr]EDTA plasma clearance and endogenous creatinine clearance determinations in children. Scand J Clin Lab Invest 37(7):625–629
32. Schwartz GJ, Haycock GB, Edelmann CM, Spitzer A (1976) A simple estimate of glomerular filtration rate in children derived from body length and plasma creatinine. Pediatrics 58(2):259–263
33. Aufricht C, Balbisi A, Gerdov C et al (1995) Formula creatinine clearance as a substitute for 24-hour creatine clearance in children with kidney transplantation. Klin Padiatr 207(2):59–62
34. Bökenkamp A, Domanetzki M, Zinck R et al (1998) Cystatin C- a new marker of glomerular filtration rate in children independent of age and height. Pediatrics 101(5):875–881
35. Chehade H, Cachat F, Jannot AS et al (2013) Combined serum creatinine and cystatin C Schwartz formula predicts kidney function better than the combined CKD-EPI formula in children. Am J Nephrol 38(4):300–306
36. Chehade H, Cachat F, Jannot AS et al (2014) New combined serum creatinine and cystatin C quadratic formula for GFR assessment in children. Clin J Am Soc Nephrol 9(1):54–63
37. Quigley R (2012) Developmental changes in renal function. Curr Opin Pediatr 24(2):184–190
38. Schwartz GJ, Evan AP (1983) Development of solute transport in rabbit proximal tubule. I. HCO-3 and glucose absorption. Am J Physiol 245:F382–F390
39. Baum M (1992) Developmental changes in rabbit juxtamedullary proximal convoluted tubule acidification. Pediatr Res 31:411–414
40. Quigley R, Baum M (1990) Developmental changes in rabbit juxtamedullary proximal convoluted tubule bicarbonate permeability. Pediatr Res 28:663–666
41. Becker AM, Zhang J, Goyal S et al (2007) Ontogeny of NHE8 in the rat proximal tubule. Am J Physiol Renal Physiol 293:F255–F261
42. Wilkins BH (1992) Renal function in sick very low birth weight infants. Arch Dis Child 67:1162–1165
43. Arant BS Jr (1978) Developmental patterns of renal functional maturation compared in the human neonate. J Pediatr 92:705–712
44. Johnson V, Spitzer A (1986) Renal reabsorption of phosphate during development: whole-kidney events. Am J Physiol 251:251–256
45. Baum M, Quigley R (2005) Maturation of rat proximal tubule chloride permeability. Am J Physiol Regul Integr Comp Physiol 289:1659–1664

46. Heller H (1944) The renal function of newborn infants. J Physiol 102:429–440
47. Edelmann CM Jr, Barnett HL (1960) Role of the kidney in water metabolism in young infants: physiologic and clinical considerations. J Pediatr 56:154–179
48. Polacek E, Vocel J, Neugebauerova L et al (1965) The osmotic concentrating ability in healthy infants and children. Arch Dis Child 40:291–295
49. Leake RD, Weitzman RE, Weinberg JA, Fisher DA (1979) Control of vasopressin secretion in the newborn lamb. Pediatr Res 13:257–260
50. Bonilla-Felix M, John-Phillip C (1994) Prostaglandins mediate the defect in AVP stimulated cAMP generation in immature collecting duct. Am J Physiol 267:F44–F48
51. Bonilla-Felix M, Vehaskari VM, Hamm LL (1999) Water transport in the immature rabbit collecting duct. Pediatr Nephrol 13:103–107
52. Quigley R, Chakravarty S, Baum M (2004) Antidiuretic hormone resistance in the neonatal cortical collecting tubule is mediated in part by elevated phosphodiesterase activity. Am J Physiol Renal Physiol 286:F317–F322
53. Gallini F, Maggio L, Romagnoli C et al (2000) Progression of renal function in preterm neonates with gestational age <32 weeks. Pediatr Nephrol 15:119–124
54. Miall LS, Henderson MJ, Turner AJ et al (1999) Plasma creatinine rise dramatically in the first 48 hours of life in preterm infants. Pediatrics 104(6): e76
55. Matos P, Duarte-Silva M, Drukker A et al (1998) Creatinine reabsorption by the newborn rabbit kidney. Pediatr Res 44:639–641
56. Baum M, Quigley R (1995) Ontogeny of proximal tubule acidification. Kidney Int 48:1697–1704
57. Drukker A, Guignard GP (2002) Renal aspects of term and preterm infants: a selective update. Curr Opin Pediatr 14:175–182
58. Aperia A, Broberger O, Herin P, Zetterstrom R (1979) Sodium excretion in relation to sodium intake and aldosterone excretion in newborn preterm and full-term infants. Acta Paediatr Scand 68:813–817
59. Vehaskari VM (1994) Ontogeny of cortical collecting duct sodium transport. Am J Physiol 267:F49–F54
60. Satlin LM, Palmer LG (1996) Apical Na conductance in maturing rabbit principal cell. Am J Physiol 270:F391–F397
61. Vehaskari VM, Hempe JM, Manning J et al (1998) Developmental regulation of ENaC subunit mRNA levels in rat kidney. Am J Physiol 274:C1661–C1666

28 Urinary Tract Infections: An Overview of Urine Collection, Imaging, and Prevention

Claudio La Scola, Claudia Guiducci, and Giovanni Montini

28.1 Definitions

1. Febrile urinary tract infection (fUTI) or pyelonephritis or upper UTI: infection of the renal parenchyma associated with systemic symptoms of inflammation, mainly fever
2. Nonfebrile UTI or cystitis or lower UTI (lUTI): infection limited to the urethra and the bladder in association with localized symptoms (dysuria, frequency, malodorous urine, daytime and night time urinary incontinence)
3. Asymptomatic or covert bacteriuria (AB): any growth of bacteria in the urine in the absence of symptoms or specific abnormalities on urine screening tests (presence of leucocituria and nitrites)

28.2 Introduction

Diagnosis of UTI is common in every day pediatric clinical practice. During the first 6 years of life, the annual incidence is around 1.7/1,000 for boys and 3.1/1,000 for girls, while approximately 6–7 % of girls and 2.5 % of boys will develop a UTI during this period [1]. In the first 2 years of life, fUTIs prevail in both sexes, and then the rate of non febrile UTI increases, particularly in girls [1, 2]. The rate of bacteriuria is more difficult to ascertain. Screening studies have demonstrated a prevalence of 1.9 % in schoolgirls and 0.2 % in schoolboys aged 5–18 years [3, 4]. During thc follow-up period of the Italian Renal Infection Study 2 [5], a randomized controlled study (RCT) carried out in order to determine the effectiveness of 12-month antimicrobial prophylaxis in preventing UTI recurrences, 2,052 urinalyses and urine cultures were performed in children of both sexes, aged between 2 and 36 months. In this cohort of children, considered to be at risk because of a previous fUTIs, with or without associated vesicoureteral reflux, a 1.5 % rate of asymptomatic bacteriuria was detected (personal series).

The management of children with a UTI has always been a matter of debate as far as diagnosis, imaging, and antibiotic prophylaxis are concerned. While some recent trials have succeeded in leading to agreement on certain issues, other important points of contention remain. Here we focus on several of the most controversial.

28.3 Urine Collection

When a UTI is suspected, a sterile urine specimen should be collected for urinalysis and urine culture before antibiotic therapy is initiated.

C. La Scola • C. Guiducci • G. Montini (✉)
Pediatric Nephrology and Dialysis Unit,
Department of Pediatrics,
S. Orsola-Malpighi University Hospital,
Via Massarenti 11, Bologna 40138, Italy
e-mail: clasc1976@gmail.com;
giovanni.montini@aosp.bo.it

M. Lima, G. Manzoni (eds.), *Pediatric Urology: Contemporary Strategies from Fetal Life to Adolescence*,
DOI 10.1007/978-88-470-5693-0_28, © Springer-Verlag Italia 2015

Table 28.1 Methods of urine collection, their relative advantages and disadvantages and cutoff points for bacterial growth

Urine collection method	Pros	Cons	Cutoff growth
SPA	Low risk of contamination	Invasive, painful, variable rate of success	$\geq 10^3$ CFU/ml
U-CATH	Low risk of contamination	Invasive and painful (but less than SPA), risk of infection	$\geq 10^4$ CFU/ml
Clean voided	Comfortable for child, cheap	Time consuming	$\geq 10^5$ CFU/ml
Sterile bag	Easy and cheap	High risk of contamination, discomfort, time consuming	$\geq 10^5$ CFU/ml

Table 28.2 Urine collection methods in non-toilet-trained children: a comparison of recent guidelines

Guidelines	SPA	U-CATH	Clean catch	Sterile bag
NICE [20]		Second option[a]	First choice	Not recommended[b]
AAP [12]		First choice	Not considered	Under no circumstances
ISPN [21]	Not considered	In severely ill children	First choice	Second option[c]

[a]If other noninvasive methods (pads) are not possible
[b]If clean catch is not possible, other noninvasive methods (pads) are recommended
[c]If febrile children are in good clinical condition

Methods of urine sample collection can be either invasive or noninvasive. Invasive techniques include suprapubic bladder aspiration (SPA) and urethral catheterization (U-CATH), while noninvasive methods include the clean-voided method (midstream and clean catch) and the sterile bag (Table 28.1). The cutoff point for the growth of a single pathogen necessary for a positive urine culture test varies according to the collection method used; it is lower for invasive methods due to the lower risk of contamination. Considering that urine is sterile when it leaves the bladder, some authors suggest that any growth should be evaluated as positive when a specimen is collected using SPA [6], whereas others prefer to account for a hypothetical risk of skin contamination and suggest a cutoff growth of more than 10^3 colony forming unit/ml (CFU) [7]. The threshold reported for U-CATH is, instead, higher than 10^4 CFU/ml [8]. As regards the noninvasive methods, which are considered to carry a higher risk of contamination from organisms not present in the bladder, a growth of more than 10^5 CFU/ml is generally considered acceptable [9, 10].

Essentially, the choice of method depends on whether or not the child is able to control his/her bladder. For toilet-trained children, it is generally agreed that clean-voided midstream collection, obtained after thorough perineal/genital cleaning, is the best method. Washing the perineum and genitalia with soap significantly reduces the rate of contamination, which is described as around 20 % [11]. In children who are not toilet trained, collecting a clean sample is more difficult and this is why the use of invasive methods is considered (Table 28.2). The authors of the American Academy of Pediatrics (AAP) guidelines [12] recommend collecting urine samples by invasive methods only. They suggest SPA as the standard method and U-CATH as an alternative, except in boys with phimosis or girls with tight labial adhesions. Both methods are reliable with a low contamination rate (2 % for SPA and 12.5 % for U-CATH) [13, 14], but their execution requires expert personnel and, as well as having variable success rates, the experience is painful for the child. In addition, some authors warn that during catheterization, bacteria can be introduced into the urinary tract and cause local or systemic infection and therefore suggest an antibiotic therapy following the procedure [15].

The success rate for obtaining a sample using SPA ranges widely from 20 to 90 % and is lower than that reported for U-CATH, which is between 72 and 100 % [12, 16, 17]. Two RCTs involving infants younger than 2 months of age were carried out in order to understand which of the invasive methods caused more discomfort [18, 19]. Results confirmed that SPA was more painful than U-CATH. In particular, Kozer et al., using the Douleur Aigue du Nouveaune Score (DAN), a neonatal acute pain scale that scores pain from 0 (no pain) to 10 (maximum pain), demonstrated a mean score of 7 (±1.9) in children randomly assigned to SPA vs 4.5 (±2.1) in those who were assigned to U-CATH (difference between means, 2.5; 95 % confidence interval, 1.4–3.7) [18].

The National Institute for Clinical Excellence (NICE) [20] and Italian Society of Pediatric Nephrology (ISPN) guidelines [21], unlike those recommended by the AAP, suggest clean catch as the method of choice, while invasive techniques are recommended only in specific clinical situations (e.g., a febrile child in poor general health or severely ill in appearance). The clean-catch method is associated with acceptable diagnostic accuracy when compared to SPA, with a sensitivity range between 75 and 100 % and specificity ranging from 57 to 100 % [22–27]. The contamination rate for this technique is about 15 % [13, 14] and is mainly due to errors in collection (contamination of the container by commensal bacteria) and in catching (initial stream). The major drawback of this technique is that trying to obtain a sample from a child can be time consuming [28]. Recently, Fernández et al. reported a safe procedure that permitted the collection of a midstream clean-catch urine sample in newborns in a mean time of about 1 min [29]. The described technique consisted in three steps: (1) feed the baby and clean the genitals 25 min after feeding; (2) stimulate the bladder by tapping the suprapubic area at a frequency of 100 taps per minute for 30 s, while someone holds the baby under their armpits with their legs dangling; and (3) massage the paravertebral lumbar area with light circular movements for 30 s.

The other noninvasive collection method, the sterile bag, has been repeatedly criticized for various reasons including discomfort, the length of time it takes to obtain a sample and, mainly, for the associated high risk of contamination, which varies between 37 and 63 % compared to SPA, especially in children at low risk for UTI [13, 14, 22, 30–34]. Shroeder et al. reported that despite ambiguous cultures being more common in bag specimens compared to U-CATH (7.4 % vs 2.7 %), 21 catheterized specimens are needed to avoid each ambiguous bag result. In general, the use of bag-collected specimens is not recommended [15]. Only the ISPN guidelines recommend bag-collected specimens for dipstick tests or microscopy, and consider it for urine culture, as a second option, when clean-catch collection is unsuccessful and the child is in good general health. The authors consider this procedure to be reliable as a second option, when correctly performed: (1) wash hands and wear disposable polyethylene gloves, (2) disinfect external genitalia, (3) place a sterile bag over the external genitalia (changing it every 30 min), and (4) remove the bag after urine is voided. In this case, a count $>10^5$ of the same single organism in two consecutive bag specimens would indicate the likelihood of a real infection.

In a "real-life" setting, the choice of method varies although noninvasive methods are generally preferred to invasive ones, the latter being used mainly in the neonatal period [13, 14]. Two recent studies, carried out in a hospital setting, evaluated the preferred methods of urine collection for UTI diagnosis in children in two different pediatric departments, one in Turkey [13], which reported a population aged 0–16 years, and the other in Australia [14], which looked at a population younger than 2 years of age. In the Turkish study, considering only the subjects aged 2 years and under (532), the sterile bag was the most frequently used method and was used in 90 % of cases, followed by clean catch in 7 %. Invasive methods were utilized less in this setting (SPA 2 %, U-CATH 1 %) and were mostly restricted to the newborn age group [13]. In the Australian study (599 children), the preferred methods were clean catch with a rate of 34 %, followed by U-CATH 16 %, SPA 14 %, while sterile bag collection was used in only 2 % of cases (no data was available for the remaining 34 %) [14]. As far as primary care is concerned, in a recent survey of general practitioners in the West of Ireland, the implementation of the NICE UTI guidelines in children was evaluated [35]. When asked how they would collect a urine sample from a child older than 1 year of age, 80 % of respondents preferred the use of bag, while 20 % opted for the clean-catch method.

In conclusion, all urine collection methods carry a risk of contamination by bacteria not present in the bladder. The mean contamination rate, which is not influenced by age or sex, is approximately 25 % [13, 14, 36]. In our opinion, clean-voided (midstream and clean catch) methods should be the first choice as they are relatively easy to perform, reliable, cost-effective, and acceptable to children, parents, and caregivers. We suggest using invasive methods only when a child is in poor general health. Finally, the sterile bag remains one of the most widely used methods, especially in primary care, and is often preferred by parents for home collection over clean catch. We believe that this method could be reliable when the correct procedure is followed and we suggest using this method as a second choice, when the child is in good general health. However, in order to obtain a reliable result, two consecutive specimens must be collected [37].

28.4 Imaging After Urinary Tract Infection

The need for imaging after UTI has long been debated, especially after a first fUTI in young children. Over the last four decades, the consensus regarding imaging has moved from the widespread diagnostic approach [38, 39], characterized mainly by the use of ultrasound (US), voiding cystourethrography (VCUG), and technetium-99-dimercapto-succinic acid (DMSA) scanning, to a less aggressive approach [12, 20, 21, 40].

The more intensive procedures were justified by the spectrum of "reflux nephropathy" and its long-term sequelae (hypertension and renal failure) [41]. This pathologic entity has been directly related to the relationship between UTI, vesicoureteral reflux (VUR), and acquired pyelonephritic scarring. Therefore, a complete imaging workup was considered essential in order to enable, primarily, the detection of children who would develop scars and ensure their long-term clinical follow-up and, secondly, the identification of children with VUR of any grade. All this was done with the aim of starting antibiotic prophylaxis and/or performing surgical correction of the reflux, with the expectation of reducing the recurrence of infections and the appearance of renal scarring [42].

The improvement and wider diffusion of antenatal ultrasonography and pediatric registries for chronic renal failure have highlighted the fact that much of the renal damage, previously related to acquired pyelonephritic scarring, is in fact congenital in nature, due to alterations in kidney development, particularly hypodysplasia [43–47] (Fig. 28.1). In some cases, it is associated with urinary tract anomalies, such as obstruction or high-grade VUR. Moreover, a recent systematic review concerning the long-term consequences of UTI in children reported a low incidence of unfavorable sequelae. In this systematic review, Toffolo et al. stated that, of the 1,029 children evaluated in prospective studies and with normal renal function at the time of the UTI, only 0.4 % showed a deterioration in function during the follow-up period [48]. Salo et al. reported that in the absence of structural kidney abnormalities evident in imaging studies after the first childhood UTI, the etiologic fraction of recurrent childhood UTIs as a main cause of CKD was, at most, 0.3 % [49]. Moreover, no study has been able to prove the clinical effectiveness of routine imaging in children with confirmed UTI, while only one study has demonstrated that it has no bearing on recurrence of infection or renal scarring [40]. At the same time, the role of surgery [42, 50] and of antibiotic prophylaxis [5, 51–55] in children with VUR has been revaluated in recent times (see below).

These new insights led the authors of the current guidelines for the management of a first fUTI to consider less aggressive imaging strategies. However, consensus on the nature of malformations, degree of reflux and damage that merits detection remains controversial, so the approaches recommended in recent guidelines

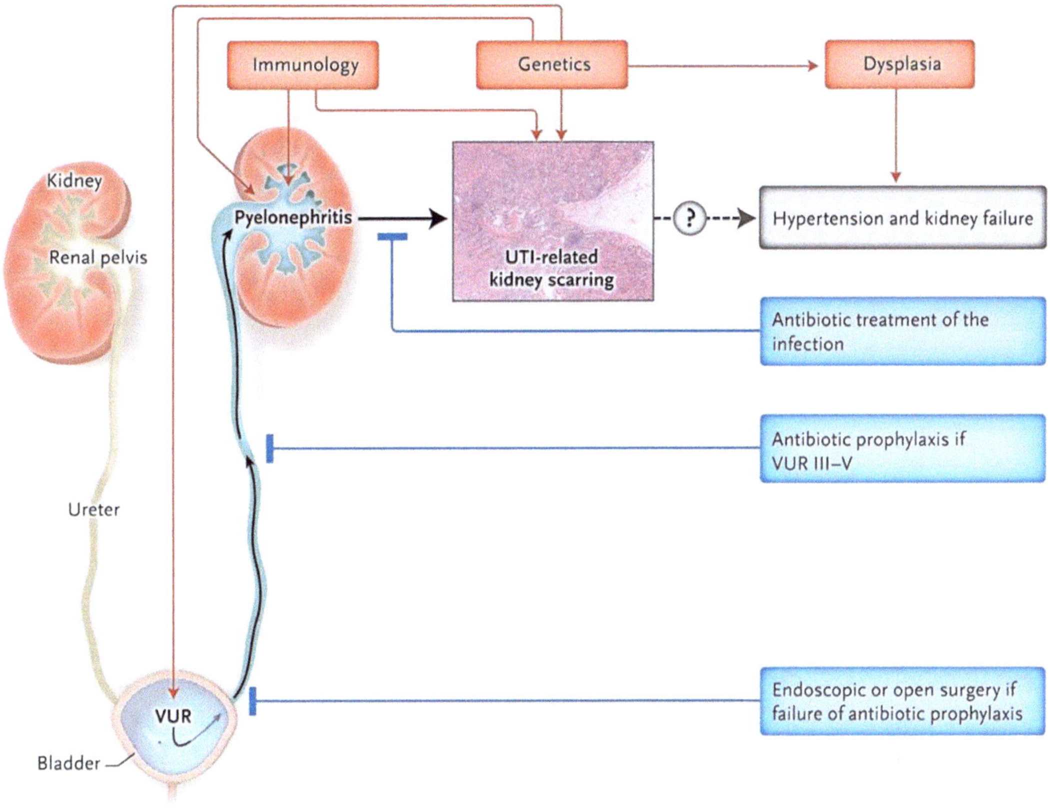

Fig. 28.1 Current understanding of febrile urinary tract infections and renal scarring (Reproduced with permission from Montini et al. [56])

are not uniform, especially as far as the execution of DMSA scintigraphy is concerned [56].

AAP guidelines suggest performing a routine renal and bladder US and recommend VCUG execution only if hydronephrosis, scarring, or other anomalies are detected at the US [12]. Moreover, they indicate VCUG in the presence of "other atypical or complex clinical circumstances," but these situations are not specified in detail. In any case, a DMSA scan is not recommended. NICE [20] and ISPN [21] consider the presence of risk factors together with the results of ultrasonography as the first step in the selection of children for further imaging (VCUG and/or DMSA scan) and, like AAP, discourage routine imaging. However, in clinical practice what is known as the top-down approach (TDA) is often used even though it is not a formal guideline [57]. TDA involves performing an initial DMSA scan in all children during the acute phase of the infection and a subsequent VCUG only in those children whose scan shows the presence of localized infection in the renal parenchyma. Details of the imaging algorithms are summarized in Table 28.3. So these new algorithms were proposed in order to identify a high-risk population, for which a full imaging workup is necessary. Identifying this high-risk population allows for a reduction in the number of unnecessary imaging tests, in psychological stress, and in economic and radiation costs.

In a recent study [58], we retrospectively simulated the application of AAP, NICE, ISPN, and TDA algorithms to a cohort of children aged 2–24 months from the Italian Renal Infection Study 1 [2], an RCT comparing the efficacy of oral antibiotic treatment alone with initial parenteral treatment, in children with a first fUTI. All

Table 28.3 Imaging strategies following the first febrile urinary tract infection: comparison between different guidelines

Guidelines	Ultrasound	Voiding cystogram	Late DMSA scan
NICE [20]	Yes	If positive US and/or atypical UTI[a]	If atypical UTI[a]
<6 months ≥6 months	If atypical UTI[a]	If children with risk factors[b]	If atypical UTI[a]
AAP [12]	Yes	If positive US	No
ISPN [21]	Yes	If positive US and/or children with risk factors[c]	If positive US and/or VUR
TDA [57]	No	If positive acute DMSA	If positive acute DMSA

[a]Seriously ill, poor urine flow, abdominal or bladder mass, raised creatinine, septicemia, failure to respond to correct antibiotic treatment within 48 h, infection with non *E. coli* organisms

[b]Dilatation on US, poor urine flow, non *E. coli* infection, family history of VUR

[c]Abnormal prenatal US of the urinary tract, family history of VUR, septicemia, renal failure, age <6 months in a male infant, likely noncompliance of the family, abnormal bladder emptying, no clinical response to correct antibiotic treatment within 72 h, non *E. coli* infection

recruited children underwent a complete imaging workup (US, VCUG, and acute and late DMSA scan). The missed rate of reflux grades III–V was 27 % for ISPN (LR+2.1, LR- 0.4), 50 % for NICE (LR+5.1, LR- 0.5), 61 % for AAP (LR+3.3, LR- 0.7), and 15 % for the TDA (LR+1.7, LR- 0.3), while the rate of missed scars was 53 % for ISPN (LR+3.2, LR- 0.6), 62 % for NICE (LR+2.4, LR- 0.7), and 100 % for AAP (LR not available). Obviously, the TDA detected the presence of all scars (LR+2.2, LR- 0) [58]. So, these diagnostic approaches, as expected, have a low sensitivity, failing to identify a good proportion of VUR and scars, except for the TDA.

Data on missed anomalies together with the poor related likelihood ratio suggest that all three diagnostic algorithms from the formal guidelines are not highly reliable, either for ruling in or ruling out children with high-grade VUR or scarring. Today, the role that these results play in the management of fUTIs is still unclear because of the following: (1) As far as the long-term consequences are concerned, the clinical significance of missing some of the refluxes remains undefined; (2) The majority of recommendations require that children undergo full imaging workup after a second infection, meaning that those children who slipped through the net the first time round would be correctly diagnosed at this point. These children would constitute the high-risk group open to recurrent infection; (3) The TDA, which identifies the vast majority of VUR and renal scars, carries the greatest burden in terms of financial and radiation costs. However, the new approaches significantly reduce the number of investigations performed [58–61], avoiding what are now deemed as unnecessary imaging tests in children after an uncomplicated first febrile UTI, who are at low risk of significant anomalies.

The rate of infants with any grade of VUR after a first febrile UTI is 20–30 % but, when considering high-grade refluxes, the rate drops to 1–4 % for grade IV–V [2, 12, 62, 63]. The rate of infants with high-grade VUR is higher for children with recurrent infections. The prevalence of VUR decreases with age of the child at the first febrile UTI. The prevalence of renal scarring after a first febrile UTI at late DMSA scan is 15 %, while less than 1 % had preexisting renal scarring and/or dysplasia [63]. High-grade refluxes (III to V) are reported as being at increased relative risk for developing renal scarring compared to those with lower grade (RR: 2.1 [95 % CI: 1.4–3.2]) [63].

Finally, a less aggressive imaging follow-up leads to a substantial reduction in economic costs and radiation exposure [64, 65]. The latter is between 4 and 15 times lower compared to a full imaging workup. The radiation risks connected to radiographic and scintigraphic imaging should not be underestimated. A recent article on pediatric cancer associated with exposure to diagnostic radiation in infancy demonstrated an increased risk of lymphoma (odds ratio, 5.14; 95 % CI, 1.27–20.78) [65]. Therefore, such procedures have to be adequately justified.

In conclusion, we believe that, in light of current knowledge, a less aggressive diagnostic approach should be adopted after a first fUTI. Further diagnostic procedures should be limited to those children who have recurrent febrile infections or documented renal developmental anomalies (e.g., hypo-dysplasia) that represent an independent risk factor for the development of chronic kidney disease. However, we suggest performing an US even though, as reported by a systematic review [22], it is considered a poor test both for ruling in and for ruling out the localization of UTI (pooled likelihood ratio was 3.11 [95 % CI 2.3–3.4] and pooled negative likelihood ratio was 0.62 [95 % CI 0.53–0.73]) and VUR (pooled likelihood ratio was 1.9 [95 % CI 1.2–2.9] and pooled negative likelihood ratio was 0.76 [95 % CI 0.63–0.93]). Conversely, US is a reasonably good test for the prediction of scarring (pooled positive likelihood ratio, 10.7 [95 % CI 4.5–25.7]), while it is less useful for ruling it out (pooled negative likelihood ratio, 0.40 [95 % CI 0.19–0.86].

However, considering the high rate of spontaneous resolution of VUR with age and the good renal outcome for patients with scarring but without major congenital renal abnormalities, we discourage the routine execution of VCUG and DMSA scans.

28.5 Antibiotic Prophylaxis and Complementary Strategies for UTI Prevention

Recurrent febrile UTIs are significantly associated with DMSA abnormalities at 1 year [66], as well as causing discomfort and psychological stress for children and apprehension for parents. This has led to an effort to identify risk factors for UTI recurrence and strategies that may help prevent this phenomenon.

There is a lack of solid evidence and some controversy regarding the risk factors predisposing to recurrence (Table 28.4). Panaretto et al. evaluated risk factors that predispose for recurrent UTIs in a cohort of 290 children (aged up to 5 years) following a first symptomatic UTI, who developed 46 relapses. The authors identified age of less than 6 months (OR 2.9) and grade 3–5 reflux (OR: 3.5) as independent risk factors for recurrence [66]. Conway et al. identified risk factors for recurrent

Table 28.4 Summary of risk factors relating to recurrence of urinary tract infections

	Study					
Risk factors	Panaretto et al. [66]	Shaikh et al. [69]	Stauffer et al. [70]	Bratslavsky et al. [71]	Bakker et al. [72]	Conway et al. [67]
Gender	NS	NE	NE	NS	NE	NS
Age	++[a]	NE	NE	NE	NE	++[b]
Family history	NE	NE	++	NS	NE	NE
Constipation/ functional stool retention/ encopresis	NE	++	++	NS	NE	NE
Circumcision	NE	NE	NE	NS	NE	NE
Dysfunctional voiding/inadequate toilet habits	NE	++	++	NE	++	NE
Poor fluid intake	NE	NE	++	NE	NE	NE
All grades of VUR	NS	++	NE	NE	NE	NS
High grades of VUR	++[c]	NE	NE	NE	NE	++[d]

NE not evaluated, *NS* not significant
[a]<6 months
[b]3–5 years
[c]Grade 3–5 VUR
[d]Grade 4–5 VUR

UTIs during the study of a cohort of 611 children under 6 years of age, recruited from a network of 27 pediatric primary care centers, 83 of whom developed recurrent UTI [67]. Multivariate analysis showed that factors associated with an increased risk of recurrence of UTI were white race (0.17 per person-year; hazard ratio [HR], 1.97; 95 CI, 1.22–3.16), age between 3 and 4 years (0.22 per person-year; HR, 2.75; 95 % CI, 1.37–5.51), age between 4 and 5 years (0.19 per person-year; HR, 2.47; 95 % CI, 1.19–5.12), and grade 4–5 vesicoureteral reflux (0.60 per person-year; HR, 4.38; 95 % CI, 1.26–15.29). Sex, grade 1–3 vesicoureteral reflux, and no circumcision were not associated with risk of recurrence. A recent meta-analysis reports lack of circumcision as an important risk factor of UTIs [68]. Other described risk factors relating to recurrence were family history of UTI, dysfunctional voiding syndrome, poor fluid intake, and functional stool retention [20, 69–72].

While some of the described risk factors are not modifiable (age, white race, familiarity), others (presence of reflux, voiding habits, phimosis, bladder function, constipation, and fluid intake) can be modified through behavioral changes and/or medical interventions. Historically, antibiotic prophylaxis represented the corner stone for the prevention of recurrent UTI, especially if VUR was detected, so much so that the three most recent guidelines almost exclusively consider antibiotic prophylaxis as a preventative measure [12, 20, 21], but none of them actually advocate a routine use (Table 28.5). However, ISPN recommends prophylaxis in children with reflux grades III to V and in children with recurrent (≥3 febrile UTIs within 12 month) febrile UTIs [21].

Several RCTs have been conducted in pediatric settings with the aim of assessing whether or not long-term antibiotic prophylaxis is effective in reducing recurrence of UTI. Two systematic reviews have been published summarizing evidence up to 2010 [73, 74]. Most of the included studies had limitations in methodological design, particularly inadequate sample size, allocation concealment and no blinding, and questionable primary outcome (such as repeated positive urine culture). Both reviews showed that the benefit of long-term prophylaxis is small, with a modest and not statistically significant decrease in the amount of recurrence of symptomatic UTI. Moreover, long-term antibiotics increased the development of resistant bacteria to the treatment drug. A significant reduction (RR 0.68, 95 % CI 0.48–0.95) with no heterogeneity was found only when data of the two of the later and larger studies with an adequate allocation concealment [5, 54] were analyzed [74]. These studies were reported as "the least biased and therefore likely to reflect the true effect of prophylactic antibiotic treatment" [74].

Table 28.5 Antibiotic prophylaxis and complementary strategies for UTI prevention: comparison between different guidelines

Guidelines	Antibiotic prophylaxis	Others interventions
NICE [20]	Not for routine use	Treat dysfunctional elimination syndromes and constipation Drink an adequate amount of fluid Do not delay voiding
AAP [12]	Not for routine use	Not considered
ISPN [21]	For reflux III–V Recurrent febrile UTI[a]	Not considered

[a]≥3 febrile UTIs within 12 months

Neither of the reviews analyzed data from the Swedish Reflux Study which showed that antibiotic prophylaxis is capable of reducing the recurrence of pyelonephritis and scarring in the few infants and young children with high-grade (III–IV) dilating reflux, particularly in girls [55].

Another medical option which helps to prevent urinary tract recurrence, mainly cystitis in girls, is drinking cranberry juice or taking products containing cranberry. Cranberries contain a substance able to inhibit bacterial adhesion to the uroepithelium of the bladder. Recently, a Cochrane review of 24 studies demonstrated that cranberry products did not significantly reduce the occurrence of symptomatic UTI overall (RR 0.86, 95 % CI 0.71–1.04) or for any of the subgroups such as women with recurrent UTIs (RR 0.74, 95 % CI 0.42–1.31), children with recurrent UTI (RR 0.48, 95 % CI 0.19–1.22), and people with neuropathic bladder or spinal injury (RR 0.95, 95 % CI: 0.75–1.20) [75].

The role of circumcision was evaluated by two systematic reviews with contradictory results [68, 76]. The first, published in 2005, demonstrated that circumcision reduces the risk of UTI but that 111 circumcisions are required to prevent one UTI when this intervention is applied to non predisposed infant boys. In boys with recurrent UTI or high-grade VUR, the numbers needed to treat are 11 and 4, respectively [76]. A more recent review regarding circumcision, published in 2013, demonstrated that lack of circumcision confers a 23 % chance of UTI during lifetime, with a lower number needed to treat of 4 [68]. The authors therefore favor circumcision.

Only NICE guidelines suggest addressing dysfunctional elimination syndromes and constipation in infants and children who have had a UTI, encouraging children to drink an adequate amount of fluid, and have ready access to clean toilets when required and not delay voiding [20]. These interventions have never been tested in randomized controlled trials.

In conclusion, we suggest, based on current evidence, that antibiotic prophylaxis should be proposed in children with reflux of grade III and above and in the case of recurrent febrile UTIs; co-amoxiclav, cotrimoxazole, cephalosporins, and nitrofurantoin are the preferred antibiotics. The latter, although more effective, is burdened by adverse side effects and the risk of poor compliance [73, 74]. We think that a reasonable duration for antibiotic prophylaxis is 2 years in young girls and 1 year in young boys. Circumcision should not be routine practice but reserved for males with recurrent UTI if associated with a high-grade reflux. We recommend assessing whether constipation is present or not and evaluating voiding habits to see whether any irregularities are present, which should then be corrected. Moreover, children should drink an adequate amount of fluid every day.

References

1. Mårild S, Jodal U (1998) Incidence rate of first-time symptomatic urinary tract infection in children under 6 years of age. Acta Paediatr 87:549–552
2. Montini G, Toffolo A, Zucchetta P et al (2007) Antibiotic treatment for pyelonephritis in children: multicentre randomised controlled non-inferiority trial. BMJ 335:386
3. Savage DC, Wilson MI, McHardy M et al (1973) Covert bacteriuria of childhood. A clinical and epidemiological study. Arch Dis Child 48(1):8–20
4. Fitzgerald A, Mori R, Lakhanpaul M (2012) Interventions for covert bacteriuria in children. Cochrane Database Syst Rev 15(2):CD006943
5. Montini G, Rigon L, Zucchetta P, Fregonese F, Toffolo A, Gobber D et al (2008) Prophylaxis after first febrile urinary tract infection in children? A multicenter, randomized, controlled, noninferiority trial. Pediatrics 122(5):1064–1071
6. Hansson S, Brandstrom P, Jodal U et al (1998) Low bacterial counts in infants with urinary tract infection. J Pediatr 132:180–182
7. Goldraich NP, Manfroi A (2002) Febrile urinary tract infection: escherichia coli susceptibility to oral antimicrobials. Pediatr Nephrol 17:173–176
8. Cheng Y-W, Wong S-N (2005) Diagnosing symptomatic urinary tract infections in infants by catheter urine culture. J Paediatr Child Health 41:437–440
9. Pryles CV, Luders D, Alkan MK (1961) A comparative study of bacterial cultures and colony counts in paired specimens of urine obtained by catheter versus voiding from normal infants and infants with urinary tract infection. Pediatrics 27:17–28
10. Guidoni EB, Berezin EN, Nigro S et al (2008) Antimicrobial agent resistance patterns of pediatric community-acquired urinary infections. Braz J Infect Dis 12:321–323
11. Vaillancourt S, McGillivray D, Zhang X et al (2007) To clean or not to clean: effect on contamination rates in midstream urine collections in toilet-trained children. Pediatrics 119(6):e1288–e1293
12. Roberts KB (2011) Subcommittee on Urinary Tract Infection, Steering Committee on Quality Improvement and Management. Urinary tract infection: clinical practice guideline for the diagnosis and management of the initial UTI in febrile infants and children 2 to 24 months. Pediatrics 128(3):595–610
13. Karacan C, Erkek N, Senel S et al (2010) Evaluation of urine collection methods for the diagnosis of urinary tract infection in children. Med Princ Pract 19(3):188–191
14. Tosif S, Baker A, Oakley E et al (2012) Contamination rates of different urine collection methods for the diagnosis of urinary tract infections in young children: an observational cohort study. J Paediatr Child Health 48(8):659–664
15. Schroeder AR, Newman TB, Wasserman RC et al (2005) Choice of urine collection methods for the diagnosis of urinary tract infection in young, febrile infants. Arch Pediatr Adolesc Med 159:915–922
16. Pollack CV Jr, Pollack ES, Andrew ME (1994) Suprapubic bladder aspiration versus urethral catheterization in ill infants: success, efficiency and complication rates. Ann Emerg Med 23:225–230
17. Chen L, Hsiao AL, Moore CL et al (2005) Utility of bedside bladder ultrasound before urethral catheterization in young children. Pediatrics 115:108–111

18. Kozer E, Rosenbloom E, Goldman D et al (2006) Pain in infants who are younger than 2 months during suprapubic aspiration and transurethral bladder catheterization: a randomized, controlled study. Pediatrics 118:e51–e56
19. El-Naggar W, Yiu A, Mohamed A et al (2010) Comparison of pain during two methods of urine collection in preterm infants. Pediatrics 125(6):1224–1229
20. National Institute for Health and Clinical Excellence (2012) Urinary tract infection in children: diagnosis, treatment and long term management. www.nice.org.uk/nicemedia/pdf/CG54fullguideline.pdf. Accessed Aug 2013
21. Ammenti A, Cataldi L, Chimenz R et al (2012) Febrile urinary tract infections in young children: recommendations for the diagnosis, treatment and follow-up. Acta Paediatr 101(5):451–457
22. Whiting P, Westwood M, Bojke L, et al (2006) Clinical and cost-effectiveness of tests for the diagnosis and evaluation of urinary tract infection (UTI) in children: a systematic review and economic model. Health Technol Assess 10(36):iii–iv, xi–xiii, 1–154
23. Aronson AS, Gustafson B, Svenningsen NW (1973) Combined suprapubic aspiration and clean-voided urine examination in infants and children. Acta Paediatr Scand 62:396–400
24. Hardy JD, Furnell PM, Brumfitt W (1976) Comparison of sterile bag, clean catch and suprapubic aspiration in the diagnosis of urinary infection in early childhood. Br J Urol 48:279–283
25. Morton RE, Lawande RI (1982) The diagnosis of urinary tract infection: comparison of urine culture from suprapubic aspiration and midstream collection in a children's out-patient department in Nigeria. Ann Trop Paediatr 2:109–112
26. Pylkkanen J, Vilska J, Koskimies O (1979) Diagnostic value of symptoms and clean-voided urine specimen in childhood urinary tract infection. Acta Paediatr Scand 68:341–344
27. Ramage IJ, Chapman JP, Hollman AS et al (1999) Accuracy of clean-catch urine collection in infancy. J Pediatr 135:765–767
28. Liaw LC, Nayar DM, Pedler SJ et al (2000) Home collection of urine for culture from infants by three methods: survey of parents' preferences and bacterial contamination rates. BMJ 320(7245):1312–1313
29. Herreros Fernández ML, González Merino N, Tagarro García A et al (2013) A new technique for fast and safe collection of urine in newborns. Arch Dis Child 98(1):27–29
30. Downs SM (1999) Technical report: urinary tract infections in febrile infants and young children. The Urinary Tract Subcommittee of the American Academy of Pediatrics Committee on Quality Improvement. Pediatrics 103(4):e54
31. Li PS, Ma LC, Wong SN (2002) Is bag urine culture useful in monitoring urinary tract infection in infants? J Paediatr Child Health 38:377–381
32. Al-Orifi F et al (2000) Urine culture from bag specimens in young children: are the risks too high? J Pediatr 137(2):221–226
33. PID note (2004) Bag urine specimens still not appropriate in diagnosing urinary tract infections in infants. Paediatr Child Health 9:377–378
34. McGillivray D, Mok E, Mulrooney E et al (2005) A head-to-head comparison: "clean-void" bag versus catheter urinalysis in the diagnosis of urinary tract infection in young children. J Pediatr 147(4): 451–456
35. Kennedy KM, Glynn LG, Dineen B (2010) A survey of the management of urinary tract infection in children in primary care and comparison with the NICE guidelines. BMC Fam Pract 26:11–16
36. Verrier-Jones K, Hockley B, Scrivener R et al (2001) Diagnosis and management of urinary tract infections in children under two years: assessment of practice against published guidelines. Royal College of Paediatrics and Child Health, London
37. Whiting P, Westwood M, Watt I et al (2005) Rapid tests and urine sampling techniques for the diagnosis of urinary tract infection (UTI) in children under five years: a systematic review. BMC Pediatr 5:4
38. Kass EJ, Kernen KM, Carey JM (2000) Paediatric urinary tract infection and the necessity of complete urological imaging. BJU Int 86(1):94–96
39. Cincinnati Children's Hospital Medical Center (2006) Evidence-based care guideline for medical management of first urinary tract infection in children 12 years of age or less. Cincinnati Children's Hospital Medical Center, Cincinnati
40. Westwood ME, Whiting PF, Cooper J (2005) Further investigation of confirmed urinary tract infection (UTI) in children under five years: a systematic review. BMC Pediatr 5(1):2
41. Bailey RR (1973) The relationship of vesico-ureteric reflux to urinary tract infection and chronic pyelonephritis-reflux nephropathy. Clin Nephrol 1(3):132–141
42. Smellie JM, Barratt TM, Chantler C et al (2001) Medical versus surgical treatment in children with severe bilateral vesicoureteric reflux and bilateral nephropathy: a randomised trial. Lancet 357(9265): 1329–1333
43. Adissino G, Daccò V, Testa S et al (2003) ItalKid project. Epidemiology of chronic renal failure in children: data from the ItalKid project. Pediatrics 111(4 Pt 1): e382–e387
44. North American Pediatric Renal Trials and Collaborative Studies. Annual report, 2008. Available at: https://web.emmes.com/study/ped. Accessed 30 Jan 2012
45. Wennerström M, Hansson S, Jodal U, Stokland E (2000) Primary and acquired renal scarring in boys and girls with urinary tract infection. J Pediatr 136(1):30–34
46. Broyer M, Chantler C, Donckerwolcke R, Ehrich JH, Rizzoni G, Schärer K (1993) The paediatric registry of the European Dialysis and Transplant Association: 20 years' experience. Pediatr Nephrol 7(6):758–768
47. Esbjörner E, Berg U, Hansson S (1997) Epidemiology of chronic renal failure in children: a report from Sweden 1986–1994. Pediatr Nephrol 11(4):438–442

48. Toffolo A, Ammenti A, Montini G (2012) Long-term clinical consequences of urinary tract infections during childhood: a review. Acta Paediatr 101(10): 1018–1031
49. Salo J, Ikäheimo R, Tapiainen T et al (2011) Childhood urinary tract infections as a cause of chronic kidney disease. Pediatrics 128(5):840–847
50. American Urological Association. Clinical guidelines 2010 http://www.auanet.org/content/guidelines-and-quality-care/clinical guidelines.cfm?sub=vur
51. Garin EH, Olavarria F, Garcia Nieto V, Valenciano B, Campos A, Young L (2006) Clinical significance of primary vesicoureteral reflux and urinary antibiotic prophylaxis after acute pyelonephritis: a multicenter, randomized, controlled study. Pediatrics 117(3):626–632
52. Pennesi M, Travan L, Peratoner L, Bordugo A, Cattaneo A, Ronfani L et al (2008) Is antibiotic prophylaxis in children with vesicoureteral reflux effective in preventing pyelonephritis and renal scars? A randomized, controlled trial. Pediatrics 121(6):e1489–e1494
53. Roussey-Kesler G, Gadjos V, Idres N, Horen B, Ichay L, Leclair MD et al (2008) Antibiotic prophylaxis for the prevention of recurrent urinary tract infection in children with low grade vesicoureteral reflux: results from a prospective randomized study. J Urol 179(2):674–679
54. Craig JC, Simpson JM, Williams GJ, Lowe A, Reynolds GJ, McTaggart SJ et al (2009) Antibiotic prophylaxis and recurrent urinary tract infection in children. N Engl J Med 361(18):1748–1759
55. Brandstrom P, Esbjorner E, Herthelius M, Swerkersson S, Jodal U, Hansson S (2010) The Swedish reflux trial in children: III. Urinary tract infection pattern. J Urol 184(1):286–291
56. Montini G, Tullus K, Hewitt I (2011) Febrile urinary tract infections in children. N Engl J Med 365(3): 239–250
57. Preda I, Jodal U, Sixt R (2007) Normal dimercaptosuccinic acid scintigraphy makes voiding cystourethrography unnecessary after urinary tract infection. J Pediatr 151(6):581–584
58. La Scola C, De Mutiis C, Hewitt IK et al (2013) Different guidelines for imaging after first UTI in febrile infants: yield, cost, and radiation. Pediatrics 131(3):e665–e671
59. Schroeder AR, Abidari JM, Kirpekar R et al (2011) Impact of a more restrictive approach to urinary tract imaging after febrile urinary tract infection. Arch Pediatr Adolesc Med 165(11):1027–1032
60. Deader R, Tiboni SG, Malone PS et al (2012) Will the implementation of the 2007 National Institute for Health and Clinical Excellence (NICE) guidelines on childhood urinary tract infection (UTI) in the UK miss significant urinary tract pathology? BJU Int 110(3):454–458
61. Jerardi KE, Elkeeb D, Weiser J et al (2013) Rapid implementation of evidence-based guidelines for imaging after first urinary tract infection. Pediatrics 132(3):e749–e755
62. Finnell SM, Carroll AE, Downs SM Subcommittee on Urinary Tract Infection (2011) Technical report diagnosis and management of an initial UTI in febrile infants and young children. Pediatrics 128(3):e749–e770
63. Shaikh N, Ewing AL, Bhatnagar S, Hoberman A (2010) Risk of renal scarring in children with a first urinary tract infection: a systematic review. Pediatrics 126(6):1084–1091
64. Perisinakis K, Raissaki M, Damilakis J et al (2006) Fluoroscopy-controlled voiding cystourethrography in infants and children: are the radiation risks trivial? Eur Radiol 16(4):846–851
65. Rajaraman P, Simpson J, Neta G et al (2011) Early life exposure to diagnostic radiation and ultrasound scans and risk of childhood cancer: case-control study. BMJ 342:d472
66. Panaretto KS, Craig JC, Knight JF et al (1999) Risk factors for recurrent urinary tract infection in preschool children. J Paediatr Child Health 35(5): 454–459
67. Conway PH, Cnaan A, Zaoutis T et al (2007) Recurrent urinary tract infections in children: risk factors and association with prophylactic antimicrobials. JAMA 298:179–186
68. Morris BJ, Wiswell TE (2013) Circumcision and lifetime risk of urinary tract infection: a systematic review and meta-analysis. J Urol 189(6):2118–2124
69. Shaikh N, Hoberman A, Wise B et al (2003) Dysfunctional elimination syndrome: is it related to urinary tract infection or vesicoureteral reflux diagnosed early in life? Pediatrics 112(5):1134–1137
70. Stauffer CM, van der Weg B, Donadini R et al (2004) Family history and behavioral abnormalities in girls with recurrent urinary tract infections: a controlled study. J Urol 171(4):1663–1665
71. Bratslavsky G, Feustel PJ, Aslan AR et al (2004) Recurrence risk in infants with urinary tract infections and a negative radiographic evaluation. J Urol 172 (4 Pt 2):1610–1613
72. Bakker E, Van Gool J, Van Sprundel M et al (2004) Risk factors for recurrent urinary tract infection in 4,332 Belgian schoolchildren aged between 10 and 14 years. Eur J Pediatr 163(4–5):234–238
73. Dai B, Liu Y, Jia J, Mei C (2010) Long-term antibiotics for the prevention of recurrent urinary tract infection in children: a systematic review and meta-analysis. Arch Dis Child 95(7):499–508
74. Williams G, Craig JC (2011) Long-term antibiotics for preventing recurrent urinary tract infection in children. Cochrane Database Syst Rev 16(3):CD001534
75. Jepson RG, Williams G, Craig JC (2012) Cranberries for preventing urinary tract infections. Cochrane Database Syst Rev 10:CD001321
76. Singh-Grewal D, Macdessi J, Craig JC (2005) Circumcision for the prevention of urinary tract infection in boys: a systematic review of randomised trials and observational studies. Arch Dis Child 90: 853–858

Chronic Kidney Disease 29

Francesca Mencarelli, Marco Busutti, and Giovanni Montini

29.1 Introduction

Chronic kidney disease (CKD) is a clinical condition characterized by an irreversible deterioration of renal function that gradually progresses to end-stage renal disease (ESRD), the terminal stage of CKD, when treatment with renal replacement therapy (RRT) becomes necessary to sustain life. The Kidney Disease Outcomes Quality Initiative (KDOQI) working group of the National Kidney Foundation (NKF) defined CKD as "evidence of structural or functional kidney abnormalities (abnormal urinalysis, imaging studies, or histology) that persist for at least 3 months, with or without a decreased glomerular filtration rate (GFR), as defined by a GFR of less than 60 ml/min per 1.73 m^2" [1].

The above definition is not applicable to children younger than 2 years, because they normally have a low GFR, even when corrected for body surface area. In these patients, calculated GFR based on serum creatinine can be compared with normative age-appropriate values (Table 29.1) to detect renal impairment.

F. Mencarelli • M. Busutti • G. Montini (✉)
Pediatric Nephrology and Dialysis Unit,
Department of Pediatrics,
S. Orsola-Malpighi University Hospital,
Via Massarenti 11, Bologna 40138, Italy
e-mail: francesca.mencarelli@aosp.bo.it; marco.busutti@live.com; giovanni.montini@aosp.bo.it

According to the KDOQI scheme, CKD is characterized by stage 1 through stage 5 (ESRD), as depicted in Table 29.2.

Table 29.1 Normal GFR values for age

Age	Medium GFR ± SD (mL/min/1.73 m^2)
1 week (male e female)	41 ± 15
2–8 weeks (male e female)	66 ± 25
8 weeks–2 years (male e female)	96 ± 22

Clinical practice guidelines for chronic kidney disease: evaluation, classification, and stratification
KDOQI clinical practice guidelines

Table 29.2 NKF-KDOQI stages of chronic kidney disease

Stage	Description	GFR (mL/min/1.73 m^2)
1	Kidney damage with normal or increased GFR	>90
2	Kidney damage with mild decrease in GFR	89–60
3	Moderate decrease in GFR, biochemical abnormalities, poor growth and appetite	59–30
4	Severe decrease in GFR, more severe symptoms	29–15
5	Kidney failure, renal replacement therapy required	<15 or dialysis

Clinical practice guidelines for chronic kidney disease: evaluation, classification, and stratification (Reprinted from National Kidney Foundation [1] with permission from Elsevier)

M. Lima, G. Manzoni (eds.), *Pediatric Urology: Contemporary Strategies from Fetal Life to Adolescence*, DOI 10.1007/978-88-470-5693-0_29, © Springer-Verlag Italia 2015

29.2 Epidemiology and Causes of CKD

The earlier stages of CKD are both underdiagnosed and underreported, as patients are often asymptomatic. Most of the information on CKD in children originates from data available on ESRD. Epidemiological studies that have been performed provide evidence that ESRD only represents the "tip of the iceberg" of CKD, suggesting that patients in the earlier stages of the disease are likely to exceed those reaching ESRD by as many as 50 times [2]. Incidence and prevalence are 20 times lower in children than in adults [3]. The incidence of ESRD in Europe, according to the ESPN/ERA-EDTA Registry, is 6.5 children per year per million of age-related population (pmarp), ranging from 2.3 in Hungary to 12.3 in Finland [3]. The highest incidence of ESRD is in adolescence (8 pmarp/year), the lowest in late childhood (4.6 pmarp/year), and the intermediate (6.7 pmarp/year) in children younger than 5 years of age. The prevalence of ESRD children is around 65 pmarp in Australia, Canada, and Europe, with the exception of Finland, where a higher prevalence of ESRD in infants is due to congenital nephrotic syndrome of the Finnish type. In the United States, prevalence is higher (85 pmarp), while in Japan it is much lower (34 pmarp). ItalKid is an Italian registry of children affected by chronic renal failure which collected data from 1990 to 2000. ItalKid reported a mean incidence of 12.1 cases per year per million in the age-related population and a prevalence of 74.7 per million [4], which are values that are significantly lower than those mentioned above. This discrepancy is probably due both to the fact that ItalKid selected patients using a different definition of CKD (GFR <75 mL/min/1.73 m^2) and patients in the early stages are often asymptomatic and therefore the condition is underdiagnosed.

Causes of CKD are very different in children compared to adults; differences exist also as far as the age of onset within the pediatric range is concerned, as depicted in Table 29.3.

Table 29.3 Principle CKD diseases according to most frequent age onset

0–5 years	5–18 years
CAKUT	IgA nephropathy
Autosomal recessive polycystic kidney disease	Henoch-Schonlein nephritis
Congenital nephrotic syndrome	Lupus nephritis
Genetic syndromes	Nephronophthisis and medullary cystic kidney disease
Hemolytic uremic syndrome	Focal segmental glomerulosclerosis
	Alport syndrome
	Membranoproliferative glomerulonephritis
	Fanconi syndrome (cystinosis, Dent's disease, Lowe syndrome, mitochondrial cytopathies)
	Primary hyperoxaluria

The primary causes of CKD in adults are diabetic nephropathy and hypertension, which do not exist in pediatric patients. In children, the most common causes are congenital anomalies of the kidney and urinary tract, also known as CAKUT, accounting for 57.5 % of CKD children [4]. CAKUT include mainly renal agenesis and hypodysplasia from the nephrological viewpoint and vesicoureteral reflux, hydrouretero-nephrosis, and posterior urethral valves from the urological point of view. CAKUT predominates in younger patients and nowadays these anomalies are often detected at prenatal ultrasound. These conditions are usually associated with other comorbidities and are included in the framework of many genetic syndromes that also have kidney involvement, as depicted in Table 29.4. A multidisciplinary approach is always recommended in order to provide adequate counseling and prognosis.

Other causes of CKD manifesting in the first 2 years of life are ciliopathies (Joubert syndrome, autosomal recessive polycystic kidney disease) and congenital nephrotic syndrome [4]. Glomerulopathies, such as IgA nephropathy and Alport syndrome, are the leading cause in children older than 12 years of age, together with nephronophthisis and medullary cystic kidney disease.

The aforementioned diseases are well-established pediatric nephropathies; however, new conditions are emerging as causes of or predisposing factors for CKD in children: low birth

Table 29.4 Genetic syndromes with renal involvement

Disease	Kidney abnormalities
William's syndrome	Renal ipo-agenesis, nephrocalcinosis, renal artery stenosis
Down syndrome	Renal hypodysplasia associated to uropathies
Turner, Noonan, DiGeorge	Various structural abnormalities
Brachio-oto-renal syndrome	Renal agenesis, hypodysplasia associated to uropathies
Tuberous sclerosis	Renal angiomyolipomas and cysts
Bardet-Biedl syndrome	Cystic dysplasia
Meckel-Gruber syndrome	Cystic dysplasia
Vacter-vacterl	Renal agenesis, hypodysplasia associated to uropathies
Denys-Drash syndrome	Congenital nephrotic syndrome, Wilms tumor
Frasier syndrome	Congenital nephrotic syndrome, Wilms tumor

weight and prematurity, chemotherapy-induced nephropathies, solid organ transplantation, and obesity. Low birth weight and prematurity are a relatively frequent condition in the current population, considering that 13 million infants are born prematurely each year [5]. People with low birth weight and prematurity show an increased risk of developing primary renal diseases and progressing to CKD; the loss of nephron mass associated with premature birth seems to be the main explanation for this. Both prenatal and postnatal factors are implicated: nephrogenesis reaches completion between 34 and 36 weeks of gestation, so the strong connection between the week of birth and kidney development is evident. Postnatal factors include the high prevalence in preterm infants of acute kidney injury during the perinatal period and the effects of perinatal drugs on kidney growth [6]. Raised blood pressure and decreased renal function, usually manifesting in early childhood, often progress to overt disease in adulthood [5]. Confirming this hypothesis are data from a meta-analysis of 32 studies [7], which reported the odds ratio for CKD (including ESRD) associated with low birth weight as 1.73 (95 % CI 1.44–2.08).

Obesity also seems to play a role, both directly and indirectly, in the development of CKD in pediatric patients [8]: glomerular hyperfiltration, hypertension, and renin-angiotensin-aldosterone system activation induce glomerular damage and progressive kidney failure, especially in patients with an initial renal "hit." Furthermore, obesity-associated dyslipidemia contributes to progressive CKD promoting blood vessel inflammation and endothelial dysfunction [9]. Evidence for a link between dyslipidemia and reduced renal function in children was recently noted in a population-based study from Turkey (CREDIT-C study), where higher BMI, hypertriglyceridemia, and hypercholesterolemia were associated with a lower GFR [10].

Table 29.5 Patients who need to be followed by a pediatric nephrologist

Family history of chronic renal disease
Prematurity and low birth weight
Solitary kidney or major nephro-urologic malformations
Obesity
High blood pressure
Past history of acute kidney injury
Growth retardation and polyuria

The causes of CKD vary across races; for example, focal segmental glomerulosclerosis, the main cause of glomerular disease, is three times more common in blacks than in whites and especially among black adolescents [11]; primary hyperoxaluria type 1 is seen with higher frequency in Tunisia and the Canary Islands [12]; congenital nephrotic syndrome with NPHS1 mutation is predominant in Finland [13].

Diagnosis of CKD in its early stages is crucial for achieving an adequate control of metabolic parameters and blood pressure in order to slow down the progression of the disease and avoid the appearance of complications and comorbidities. In Table 29.5, the categories of patients who need to be followed (annual urine analysis and blood pressure measurement) as they are potentially at risk of developing CKD are listed. For example, children with solitary kidney need to be followed as they are at risk of developing CKD even when they have a normal renal function. Two important studies pointed out that in these patients hypertension, proteinuria, and renal failure are more frequent than in healthy children [14, 15].

29.3 Progression of the Disease: Modifiable and Non-modifiable Risk Factors

Our aim as pediatric nephrologists is to slow down the progression of CKD. At present, our knowledge regarding the pathogenesis of chronic renal damage has been able to provide some important targets for drug therapies and diagnostic tools. Two models have been suggested for the progression of kidney injury to CKD, focusing principally on both the involvement of the glomeruli and the tubulointerstitium. The "fibrosis hypothesis" suggests that a variety of initial insults to the kidney cause tubulointerstitial damage, leading to inflammation and injury that proceeds to CKD. The "overload hypothesis," on the other hand, states that a decrease in the number of functioning nephrons leads to kidney injury. In response, the remaining nephrons compensate for this loss by increasing their functional capacity. This, in turn, causes ulterior nephron damage and loss, generating a feedforward circuit that ultimately leads to ESRD. These pathways,

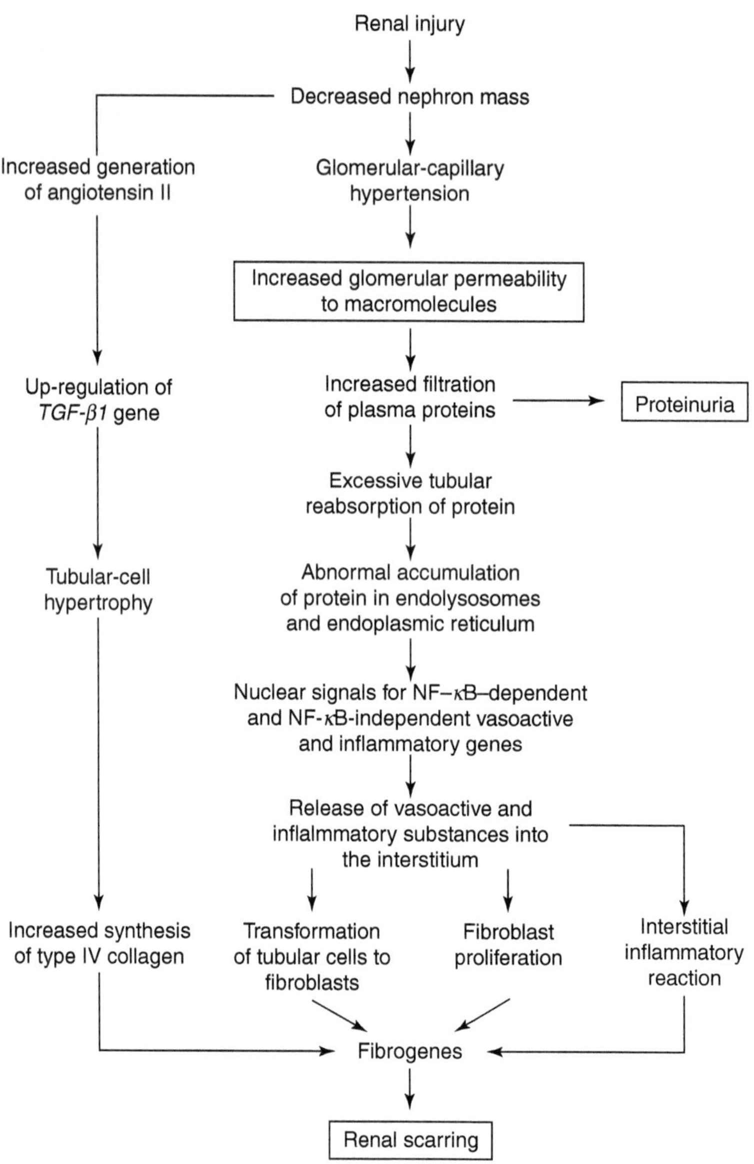

Fig. 29.1 Pathophysiology of the kidney injury (From Remuzzi and Bertani [51]. Copyright © 1998 Massachusetts Medical Society. Reprinted with permission from Massachusetts Medical Society)

depicted in Fig. 29.1, give us two distinct ideas about the mechanism by which CKD progresses, yet they can be simultaneous [16].

The natural evolution of the early stages is variable and often unpredictable, especially because of the limited epidemiological data available for these children. Conversely, patients in the advanced stages of CKD will develop ESRD, either in the short or long term, as shown in Fig. 29.1. Patients with earlier stages of CKD often have a normal or near-normal serum creatinine concentration. When a critical amount of nephron mass has been lost, renal function will decline more or less progressively, leading to the development of irreversible CKD, which results in ESRD. The abovementioned adaptive hyperfiltration leads to long-term damage to the residual nephrons, which causes pathological proteinuria and a gradual loss of kidney function. The increase in urinary protein is "toxic" for tubular cells and interstitium, while systemic hypertension causes glomerular hypertension, hypertrophy, and injury. It is obvious that kidney diseases progress in different ways depending on their particular pathogenesis. Glomerulopathies progress more rapidly to ESRD than CAKUT, probably because proteinuria and hypertension are always present at onset in the former, while they appear later in CAKUT [17].

29.3.1 Modifiable Risk Factors

The principle modifiable risk factors for renal failure progression are: proteinuria, hypertension, obesity, dyslipidemia, hyperuricemia, metabolic acidosis, oxidative stress, disorders of mineral metabolism, and hyperparathyroidism. In the routine clinical management of CKD children, pediatric nephrologists strive to keep as many of these factors under control as possible.

Proteinuria and hypertension are the two principal risk factors associated with a more rapid decline in kidney function [18–21]. They are both frequent and can appear in the first stages of CKD. In a study of almost 400 children with CKD, the prevalence of hypertension and proteinuria was 70 and 11.5 %, respectively. In children with CKD stages IV and V, the prevalence of proteinuria approached 40 % [22]. The ItalKid Project evaluated the role of proteinuria in the disease progression of children with hypodysplastic kidneys. Patients with a higher protein value at baseline (protU/creatU >0.9) had a faster decline of renal function and poorer kidney survival after 5 years. Inhibition of the renin-angiotensin system (RAS) has been the most extensively studied anti-hypertensive and anti-proteinuric strategy for renoprotection in CKD and represents the mainstay of current preventive strategies for CKD progression. RAS antagonists act through several pathways, reducing filtration by lowering intraglomerular pressure and inhibiting vasoactive and pro-inflammatory signaling [23]. Interestingly, a significant reduction in renal failure progression and proteinuria was obtained through strict blood pressure control with an ACE inhibitor (ramipril) in the ESCAPE trial (Effect of Strict Blood Pressure Control and ACE Inhibition on the Progression of CRF in Pediatric Patients). The ESCAPE study enrolled 468 European children with CKD. They were randomized into two groups: patients subjected to intensified blood pressure control (mean 24 h BP <50th percentile) and patients subjected to conventional blood pressure control (mean 24 h BP: 50–90° percentile). All patients were treated with ramipril. Children with hypodysplasia and glomerulopathies under intensified BP control had a significant reduction in relative risk (35 %) of losing 50 % of kidney function or progressing to ESRD in a long-term follow-up of 5 years. The anti-proteinuric effect of ramipril was observed for the first 6 months, after which an increase in proteinuria was noted, although good blood pressure control persisted. In another trial, 300 CKD children with proteinuria were treated with losartan or enalapril. Here, the reduction in proteinuria was sustained for 3 years [24, 25]. The use of a combined therapy, ACE inhibitor and angiotensin type 1 receptor blockers, can prolong and increase the anti-proteinuric effect when there is a resistance to ACE inhibitors alone.

29.3.2 Non-modifiable Risk Factors

There are various significant non-modifiable risk factors: genetics, ethnicity, age, low birth weight and/or prematurity, and gender.

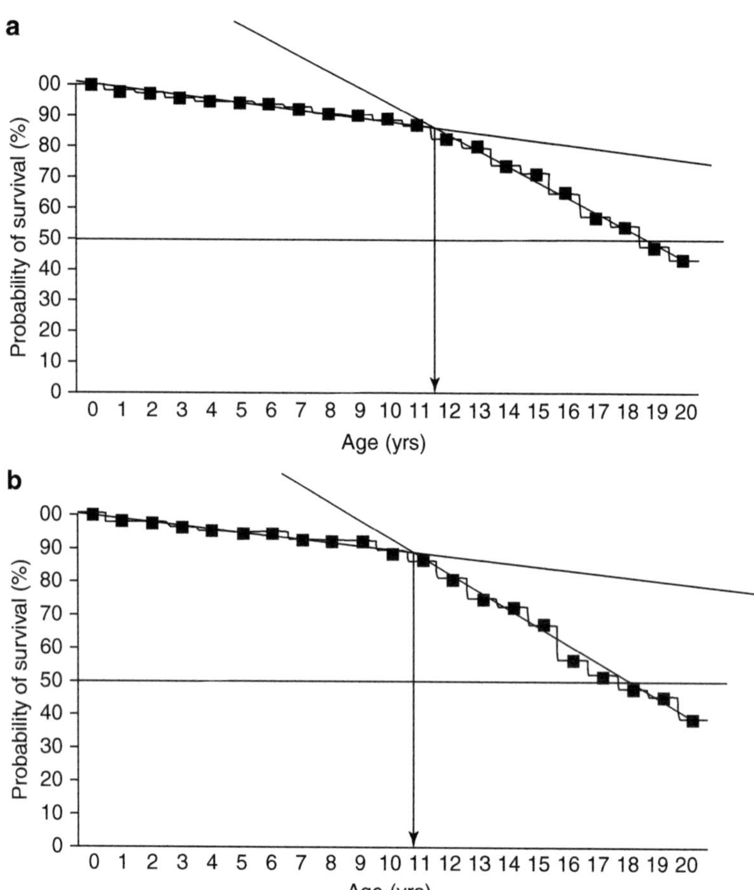

Fig. 29.2 Estimated kidney survival in children with CKD by age (From Ardissino et al. [26] with permission from BMJ Publishing Group Ltd)

Puberty is the period of life during which CKD children are at higher risk of suffering a rapid decline in renal function. This has been well documented by the abovementioned ItalKid Project [26]. Figure 29.2 shows the rapid downward slope of the kidney survival curve at the start of adolescence. This progression, observed also in other chronic human diseases, may be due to rapid growth and sex hormone activity.

Current research is focused on the attempt to clarify the genetic susceptibility to CKD and the role of genetics in CKD progression. It is well known that there is a hereditability in CKD and research is currently being carried out into the involvement of several candidate genes.

Several population-based studies with genome-wide association have recently been published on genotypic variation and kidney function. UMOD, for example, is the gene that encodes for uromodulin, the major protein secreted in the urine. Its expression is linked to hypertension and CKD [27].

29.4 Growth, Development, and Prognosis of Children with CKD

Growth failure has long been recognized in children with CKD. Over the last two decades, the efforts of pediatric nephrologists have focused especially on improving growth and development in CKD children; however, growth retardation is still a common problem, especially in infants [28]. Impairment of growth can begin when there is a 50 % fall in GFR, and it becomes an evident problem once GFR falls below 25 % [29]. The etiology of growth failure is multifactorial, reflecting abnormalities in the growth hormone/insulin-like growth factor axis, decreased nutrition, and metabolic disturbances. In order to grow, these children require aggressive medical treatment that includes maximization of nutrition, prompt correction of metabolic acidosis, prevention of renal osteodystrophy and hyperparathyroidism, correction of anemia, and salt supplementation as needed. In the last decade, several studies have documented that growth hormone therapy (rhGH) promotes catch-up growth in CKD children [30, 31]. Advances in the management of CKD patients, and particularly in the treatment of the factors mentioned above, have produced a significant improvement in the final height of CKD children. A recent publication reported growth data from 1,612 patients enrolled in the European Registry of RRT [32]. All the enrolled children started RRT before the age of 19 years and reached adult height between 1990 and 2011. The data showed that children who reached adulthood between 2006 and 2011 were significantly taller than the children who reached adulthood between 1990 and 1995 (−1.33 vs. −2.06 SDS, respectively). This gain in height led to psychological benefit and an increase in physical and social functioning together with an improvement in quality of life [33].

Currently, the great challenge for pediatric nephrologists is to further increase the long-term survival prospects of CKD children through the early recognition of the known comorbidities. A great number of recent studies have looked at cardiovascular disease as it is the major cause of mortality in children on ESRD [34–38]. A retrospective cohort study from the United States Renal Data System (USRDS) analyzed data from more than 20,000 dialyzed children between 1990 and 2010 and showed that cardiac arrest was the most common cardiovascular cause of death, both in children younger (53 %) and older (49 %) than 5 years of age [37]. In CKD, there are several factors that increase the pre- and post-cardiac load (fluid retention, hypertension, anemia, chronic inflammation). Left ventricular hypertrophy is a precocious sign, it begins as a compensatory mechanism in order to increase the cardiac output, but it can be quickly associated with systolic and/or diastolic dysfunction. High systolic blood pressure, hyperparathyroidism, hypercalcemia, and hyperphosphatemia, as well as long-term dialysis, have been described as important risk factors for cardiovascular disease [36]. In 2009, a consortium of pediatric nephrologists in Europe started a prospective observational study in order to better understand the causes and consequences of cardiovascular comorbidity in children with progressive CKD. The trial is called the "4C" Study – Cardiovascular Comorbidity in Chronic Kidney Disease in Children – and is following 737 children from 12 European countries as they advance through successive stages of CKD [39]. Patients undergo regular noninvasive cardiac and vessels examinations such as pulse-wave velocity, carotid intima-media thickness, echocardiography, and 24-h blood pressure monitoring in order to detect when the early signs of disease appear and which of the possible risk factors are more heavily involved.

Over the last two decades, a reduction in mortality has been observed which is probably due to improved pre-dialysis care and better control of CV risk factors. The USRDS data illustrates a gradual decrease in mortality rate (deaths per 1,000 person-years of observation) in patients who started dialysis in four approximately equal time periods between 1990 and 2010. Patients who started dialysis in the last decade had a significantly lower mortality rate than those who started in the previous decades [37].

29.5 Special Issues in Management of End-Stage Renal Disease: Preemptive Transplantation and Best Renal Replacement Therapy

29.5.1 Preemptive Transplantation

It is known that expected remaining lifetime is much lower in dialysis children compared to those who have undergone renal transplant [40] and we have already talked about cardiovascular comorbidities and the risk of cardiac death in dialyzed children. Therefore, the current strategy is to reduce time on ESRD and, if possible, avoid dialysis by performing preemptive kidney transplantation. Preemptive kidney transplantation is indeed the gold standard treatment for ESRD. Children are in a privileged position as far as transplantation is concerned. The opportunity of preemptive transplantation due to the availability of living donors, particularly parents, and pediatric deceased donor waiting lists makes transplantation a real possibility in a relatively short time. However, there are some situations in which transplantation should be delayed, such as in very small babies or immunologically sensitized children.

Pre-transplant assessment of the recipient takes time, requires a multidisciplinary approach, and has to be performed "not too early and not too late," in order to be ready for preemptive transplantation. In the context of pediatric urology, the evaluation of patients with lower urinary tract dysfunction is of particular interest, especially when we consider that CAKUT are the most frequent causes of CKD. These patients have to be carefully evaluated as they can have urological and infection-related complications of the graft. Before transplantation, an accurate urodynamic assessment is mandatory in order to evaluate cystometric bladder capacity and detrusor pressure. A voiding cystography is also required to detect the presence of vesicoureteric reflux (VUR). VUR is present in many patients as an underlying diagnosis, and urinary tract infections could affect the native and the transplanted kidney. Some authors recommend native nephrectomies with VUR to decrease the risk of native-kidney UTI after transplantation, although no data from controlled studies are available [41], and, in any case, this not our current policy. In effect several studies have shown that pretransplant antireflux surgery does not reduce the risk of febrile UTI after transplantation and VUR does not need to be corrected before transplantation, unless it is causing symptoms or infection [42, 43].

29.5.2 Infants with ESRD

The number of infants in ESRD in the first year of life has increased over the last decades. This is due to advances in prenatal diagnosis and early referral to specialized renal units where clinical care has made significant developments as well. According to international registries, infants constitute 11 % of all children initiating renal replacement therapy (RRT), and their management represents a particular challenge for pediatric nephrologists [44]. They may need to remain on dialysis for a prolonged period, in order to reach a suitable weight for transplantation. The prognosis for all infants has improved over the last decade. Most deaths occur in the first year of life, with a 1-year survival rate of around 85 % as stated in the NAPRTCS (North American Pediatric Renal Trials and Collaborative Studies report) and in the UK series, compared to a 95 % 1-year survival rate in children starting dialysis after infancy [44]. The majority of patients under 1 year of age in CKD stage 5 have either CAKUT or other congenital diseases, which were considered practically incurable, until a couple of decades ago, such as autosomal recessive polycystic kidney disease (ARPKD) or congenital nephrotic syndrome. A close collaboration between surgeons and nephrologists is absolutely necessary in all these conditions, in order to set up the best program for RRT. Infants awaiting transplant can require nephrectomy of one or both of the native kidneys. For example, ARPKD patients may undergo a nephrectomy because their kidneys take up too much space in the abdomen, while children with congenital nephrotic syndrome often undergo a nephrectomy because their native kidneys are responsible for heavy proteinuria, hypoproteinemia, severe edema, and possible thrombosis.

Transplantation in infants still raises a number of concerns regarding their small size. The target weight suitable for transplantation varies from center to center and is based on the experience of each individual unit. Living-related donor renal transplantation obviously requires great expertise, as there are hemodynamic and technical concerns related to adult-sized kidneys grafted into infants and small children, the risk of hypovolemia and graft thrombosis. Recently, interesting data have been published about a successful experience in living-related donor transplantation in infants. In 2010, NAPRTCS reported a very high proportion of living donor transplantations (75 %) in infants less than 1 year of age [45]. In 2012, pediatric nephrologists from the Karolinska Hospital in Sweden reported that 40 % of children from a population younger than 4 years of age received a living donor graft. The median weight at transplantation was 9.5 kg [46].

29.5.3 Recent Advances in Dialysis

Over the last decade, there have been remarkable advances in dialysis techniques, and, as already mentioned, there are several situations in which transplantation has to be delayed and dialysis is the only option. There are obvious signs and symptoms that lead to dialysis initiation, such as no controlled fluid and electrolyte balance, metabolic acidosis, and hypertension. However, in children, dialysis is generally started when adequate growth and nutritional levels become increasingly more difficult to maintain. The choice of dialysis modality, peritoneal or hemodialysis, depends on several factors, including patient and family choice, distance from the renal center, and comorbidities associated with the renal disease that can affect one treatment compared to another. The aim of pediatric nephrologists is to plan dialysis in order to permit, as far as possible, a normal life for children and parents. Chronic peritoneal dialysis (PD) represents a well-established dialysis modality for pediatric patients, and it is the preferred treatment for infants and children with ESRD in developed countries. Peritoneal dialysis has several advantages over hemodialysis. Technically speaking, it is easier to perform, it does not require vascular access or anticoagulation therapy, it is better tolerated in terms of hemodynamic stability during the procedure, and it provides good metabolic control. Peritoneal dialysis can be easily performed at home thanks to an automatic machine, a cycler that delivers and drains the dialysate into and out of the abdomen of the patient through a peritoneal catheter. Automated PD is usually performed during the night and so children and their families are free to go about their usual daily activities. Absolute contraindications to the use of PD are quite rare, such as omphalocele/gastroschisis, bladder exstrophy, diaphragmatic hernia, obliterated peritoneal cavity, and peritoneal membrane failure due to recent major abdominal surgery [47]. However, in some of these situations, such as in bladder exstrophy or abdominal surgery, peritoneal dialysis remains the modality of choice as hemodialysis could cause more complications in small infants. Chronic conventional hemodialysis (three times a week) is usually less well tolerated in ESRD children; they usually have poorly controlled blood pressure, with subsequent left ventricular hypertrophy and left ventricular dysfunction, episodes of hemodynamic instability during the dialysis session, and poor nutrition and growth control. New, intensified hemodialysis procedures, such as hemodiafiltration and even daily hemodialysis, seem to be more successful in promoting growth, obtaining good phosphate control, and reducing cardiovascular morbidity [48, 49]. Home hemodialysis could be a good alternative for children for whom PD is not possible. Like PD, home hemodialysis gives the patient the opportunity to have a better quality of life, as they are able to attend school and have an active social life. Home hemodialysis allows for daily treatments which almost mimic normal renal function with an improvement in metabolic control and fewer complications than conventional hospital hemodialysis sessions. Good organization is obviously necessary in terms of dialysis equipment and parental/caregiver participation, and there are even advantages regarding cost-effectiveness, but unfortunately not many centers are able to provide this modality of dialysis for children [50].

References

1. National Kidney Foundation (2002) K/DOQI clinical practice guidelines for chronic kidney disease: evaluation, classification, and stratification. Am J Kidney Dis 39(2 Suppl 1):S1–S266
2. Coresh J, Astor BC, Greene T, Eknoyan G, Levey AS (2003) Prevalence of chronic kidney disease and decreased kidney function in the adult US population: third National Health and Nutrition Examination Survey. Am J Kidney Dis 41:1–12
3. Karlijn J, van Stralen E, Tizard J, Verrina E, Schaefer F, Kitty J, Jager on behalf of the European Society for Paediatric Nephrology/European Renal Association-European Dialysis and Transplant Association (ESPN/ERA-EDTA) registry study group (2010) Demographics of paediatric renal replacement therapy in Europe: 2007 annual report of the ESPN/ERA-EDTA registry. Pediatr Nephrol 25:1379–1382
4. Ardissino G, Dacco V, Testa S (2003) Epidemiology of chronic renal failure in children: data from the ItalKid project. Pediatrics 111(4 Pt 1):e382–e387
5. Luyckx VA, Bertram JF, Brenner BM, Caroline F, Hoy WE, Ozanne SE, Vikse BE (2013) Effect of fetal and child health on kidney development and long-term risk of hypertension and kidney disease. Lancet 382:273–283
6. Schreuder MF, Bueters RR, Huigen MC, Russel FG, Masereeuw R, van den Heuvel LP (2011) Effect of drugs on renal development. Clin J Am Soc Nephrol 6(1):212–217
7. White SL, Perkovic V, Cass A (2009) Is low birth weight an antecedent of CKD in later life? A systematic review of observational studies. Am J Kidney Dis 54:248–261
8. Doyon A, Schaefer F (2013) The prodromal phase of obesity-related chronic kidney disease: early alterations in cardiovascular and renal function in obese children and adolescents. Nephrol Dial Transplant 28(Suppl 4):iv50–iv57
9. Ruan XZ, Varghese Z, Moorhead JF (2009) An update on the lipid nephrotoxicity hypothesis. Nat Rev Nephrol 5:713–721
10. Soylemezoglu O, Duzova A, Yalcinkaya F et al (2012) Chronic renal disease in children aged 5–18 years: a population-based survey in Turkey, the CREDIT-C study. Nephrol Dial Transplant 27(Suppl 3):146–151
11. Harambat J, van Stralen KJ, Kim JJ, Tizard EJ (2012) Epidemiology of chronic kidney disease in children. Pediatr Nephrol 27(3):363–373
12. Leumann E, Hoppe B (2001) The primary hyperoxalurias. J Am Soc Nephrol 12(9):1986–1993
13. Holmberg C, Laine J, Rönnholm K, Ala-Houhala M, Jalanko H (1996) Congenital nephrotic syndrome. Kidney Int Suppl 53:S51–S56
14. Westland R, Kurvers RA, van Wijk JA, Schreuder MF (2013) Risk factors for renal injury in children with a solitary functioning kidney. Pediatrics 131(2): e478–e485
15. Corbani V, Ghiggeri GM, Sanna-Cherchi S (2011) Congenital solitary functioning kidneys: which ones warrant follow-up into adult life? Nephrol Dial Transplant 26(5):1458–1460
16. Hodgkins KS, Shnaper HW (2012) Tubulointerstitial injury and the progression of chronic kidney disease. Pediatr Nephrol 27(6):901–909
17. Schaefer B, Wühl E (2012) Educational paper: progression in chronic kidney disease and prevention strategies. Eur J Pediatr 171(11):1579
18. Ardissino G, Testa S, Dacco V, Vigano S, Taioli E, Claris-Appiani A, Procaccio M, Avolio L, Ciofani A, Dello Strologo L et al (2004) Proteinuria as a predictor of disease progression in children with hypodysplastic nephropathy. Data Ital Kid Proj Pediatr Nephrol 19:172–177
19. Peterson JC, Adler S, Burkart JM, Greene T, Hebert LA, Hunsicker LG, King AJ, Klahr S, Massry SG, Seifter JL (1995) Blood pressure control, proteinuria, and the progression of renal disease. The modification of diet in renal disease study. Ann Intern Med 123:754–762
20. Wong CS, Pierce CB, Cole SR, Warady BA, Mak RH, Benador NM, Kaskel F, Furth SL, Schwartz GJ (2009) Association of proteinuria with race, cause of chronic kidney disease, and glomerular filtration rate in the chronic kidney disease in children study. Clin J Am Soc Nephrol 4:812–819
21. Mitsnefes M, Ho PL, McEnery PT (2003) Hypertension and progression of chronic renal insufficiency in children: a report of the North American Pediatric Renal Transplant Cooperative Study (NAPRTCS). J Am Soc Nephrol 14:2618–2622
22. Wong H, Mylrea K, Feber J, Drukker A, Filler G (2006) Prevalence of complications in children with chronic kidney disease according to KDOQI. Kidney Int 70:585–590
23. Wühl E, Schaefer F (2010) Can we slow the progression of chronic kidney disease? Curr Opin Pediatr 22(2):170–175
24. Webb NJ, Lam C, Loeys T, Shahinfar S, Strehlau J, Wells TG, Santoro E, Manas D, Gleim GW (2010) Randomized, double- blind, controlled study of losartan in children with proteinuria. Clin J Am Soc Nephrol 5:417–424
25. Webb NJ, Shahinfar S, Wells TG, Massaad R, Gleim GW, Santoro EP, Sisk CM, Lam C (2012) Losartan and enalapril are comparable in reducing proteinuria in children. Kidney Int 82:819–826
26. Ardissino G, Testa S, Daccò V, Paglialonga F, Viganò S, Felice-Civitillo C, Battaglino F, Bettinelli A, Bordugo A, Cecchetti V, De Pascale S, La Manna A, Li Volti S, Maringhini S, Montini G, Pennesi M, Peratoner L (2012) Puberty is associated with increased deterioration of renal function in patients with CKD: data from the ItalKid Project. Arch Dis Child 97(10):885–888
27. Trudu M, Janas S, Lanzani C, Debaix H, Schaeffer C, Ikehata M, Citterio L, Demaretz S, Trevisani F, Ristagno G, Glaudemans B, Laghmani K, Dell'antonio

G, Swiss Kidney Project on Genes in Hypertension (SKIPOGH) team, Bochud M, Burnier M, Devuyst O, Martin PY, Mohaupt M, Paccaud F, Pechère-Bertschi A, Vogt B, Ackermann D, Ehret G, Guessous I, Ponte B, Pruijm M, Loffing J, Rastaldi MP, Manunta P, Devuyst O, Rampoldi L (2013) Common noncoding UMOD gene variants induce salt-sensitive hypertension and kidney damage by increasing uromodulin expression. Nat Med 19(12):1655–1660
28. Mahan JD, Warady BA (2008) Assessment and treatment of short stature in pediatric patients with chronic kidney disease: a consensus statement. Pediatr Nephrol 21:917–930
29. Tonshoff B, Mehls O (1995) Growth retardation in children with chronic renal insufficiency: current aspects of pathophysiology and treatment. J Nephrol 8:133–142
30. Mahesh S, Kaskel F (2008) Growth hormone axis in chronic kidney disease. Pediatr Nephrol 23(1):41–48
31. Haffner D, Schaefer F, Nissel R, Wühl E, Tönshoff B, Mehls O (2000) Effect of growth hormone treatment on the adult height of children with chronic renal failure. German study group for growth hormone treatment in chronic renal failure. N Engl J Med 343(13):923–930, 28
32. Harambat J, Bonthuis M, van Stralen KJ, Ariceta G, Battelino N, Bjerre A, Jahnukainen T, Leroy V, Reusz G, Sandes AR, Sinha MD, Groothoff JW, Combe C, Jager KJ, Verrina E, Schaefer F, for the ESPN/ERA-EDTA Registry (2013) Adult height in patients with advanced CKD requiring renal replacement therapy during childhood. Clin J Am Soc Nephrol 9(1):92–99
33. Al-Uzri A, Matheson M, Gipson DS, Mendley SR, Hooper SR, Yadin O, Rozansky DJ, Moxey-Mims M, Furth SL, Warady BA, Gerson AC (2013) The impact of short stature on health-related quality of life in children with chronic kidney disease, Chronic Kidney Disease in Children Study Group. J Pediatr 163(3): 736–741
34. Parekh RS, Carroll CE, Wolfe RA, Port FK (2002) Cardiovascular mortality in children and young adults with end-stage kidney disease. J Pediatr 141: 191–197
35. Mitsnefes MM, Kimball TR, Witt SA, Glascock BJ, Khoury PR, Daniels SR (2003) Left ventricular mass and systolic performance in pediatric patients with chronic renal failure. Circulation 107:864–868
36. Shroff R, Weaver DJ Jr, Mitsnefes MM (2011) Cardiovascular complications in children with chronic kidney disease. Nat Rev Nephrol 7:642–649
37. Mitsnefes MM, Laskin BL, Dahhou M, Zhang X, Foster BJ (2013) Mortality risk among children initially treated with dialysis for end-stage kidney disease, 1990–2010. JAMA 309:1921–1929
38. Lilien MR, Groothoff JW (2009) Cardiovascular disease in children with CKD or ESRD. Nat Rev Nephrol 5(4):229–235
39. Querfeld U, Anarat A, Bayazit AK, Bakkaloglu AS, Bilginer Y, Caliskan S, Civilibal M, Doyon A, Duzova A, Kracht D, Litwin M, Melk A, Mir S, Sözeri B, Shroff R, Zeller R, Wühl E, Schaefer F, 4C Study Group (2010) The cardiovascular comorbidity in children with chronic kidney disease (4C) study: objectives, design, and methodology. Clin J Am Soc Nephrol 5(9):1642–1648
40. Foley RN, Murray AM, Li S, Herzog CA, McBean AM, Eggers PW, Collins AJ (2005) Chronic kidney disease and the risk for cardiovascular disease, renal replacement, and death in the United States Medicare population, 1998 to 1999. J Am Soc Nephrol 16(2): 489–495
41. Casale P, Grady RW, Mitchell ME, Healey P (2005) Recurrent urinary tract infection in the post-transplant reflux nephropathy patient: is reflux in the native ureter the culprit? Pediatr Transplant 9:324–327
42. Basiri A, Otookesh H, Simforoosh N, Hosseini R, Hosseini-Moghaddam SM, Sharifian M (2006) Does pre-transplantation antireflux surgery eliminate post-renal transplantation pyelonephritis in children? J Urol 175:1490–1492
43. Luke PP, Herz DB, Bellinger MF, Chakrabarti P, Vivas CA, Scantlebury VP, Hakala TR, Jevnikar AM, Jain A, Shapiro R, Jordan ML (2003) Long-term results of pediatric renal transplantation into a dysfunctional lower urinary tract. Transplantation 76:1578–1582
44. Zurowska AM, Fischbach M, Watson AR, Edefonti A, Stefanidis CJ, on behalf of the European Paediatric Dialysis Working Group (2013) Clinical practice recommendations for the care of infants with stage 5 chronic kidney disease (CKD5). Pediatr Nephrol 28:1739–1748
45. NAPRTCS 2010 Annual Transplant Report. https://web.emmes.com/study/ped/annlrept/2010_Report.pdf
46. Herthelius M, Celsi G, Edström Halling S, Krmar RT, Sandberg J, Tydén G, Asling-Monemi K, Berg UB (2012) Renal Transplantation in infants and small children. Pediatr Nephrol 27(1):145–150
47. National Kidney Foundation (2006) KDOQI clinical practice recommendations for 2006 updates: hemodialysis adequacy, peritoneal dialysis adequacy and vascular access. Am J Kidney Dis 48(Suppl 1):S1–S322
48. De Camargo MF, Henriques CL, Vieira S, Komi S, Leão ER, Nogueira PC (2013) Growth of children with end-stage renal disease undergoing daily hemodialysis. Pediatr Nephrol 29(3):439–444
49. Fischbach M, Fothergill H, Zaloszyc A, Menouer S, Terzic J (2011) Intensified daily dialysis: the best chronic dialysis option for children? Semin Dial 24(6):640–644
50. Hothi DK, Stronach L, Harvey E (2013) Home hemodialysis. Pediatr Nephrol 28(5):721–730
51. Remuzzi G, Bertani T (1998) Pathophysiology of progressive nephropathies. N Engl J Med 339: 1448–1456

Urolithiasis

30

Sajid Sultan

30.1 Introduction

Urolithiasis has been known for a very long time, with the first evidence found in Egyptian mummies [1]. Hippocrates was perhaps the first to describe stone disease [2, 3], yet it is still a mysterious pathology involving multiple etiological factors, including genetics, anatomy, diet, environment, and infection, which may work alone or in combination, thus giving stone disease its complex pathogenesis [4]. In simple terms, stones are endemic or idiopathic, genetic (metabolic), or infective. Nevertheless, there is still large gap in our knowledge. For example, with cystine or xanthine stones, a kidney with no obvious or visible anatomical defect forms recurrent stones, while the contralateral kidney remains stone free. Therefore, the focus of the chapter has been on management rather than etiology. There have been tremendous advances in technology for diagnostic imaging. In addition, small-size pediatric endoscopic instruments can be used to manage or remove stones by various minimally invasive surgical procedures. Unfortunately, the same level of progress has not been achieved in understanding the etiology of the disease, such as why stones form and why they recur.

This review provides a perspective from a developing country, with an overview of the present understanding of the disease, as well as the principles and rationale of current management options.

30.2 Epidemiology

There is great variation in the incidence and prevalence of stone disease in different regions of the world. Variation is also found in age, gender, presentation, and stones composition. In Europe, infective stones prevail while in Pakistan, ammonium hydrogen urate (AHU) stones are predominant [5] – upper tract stones in the developed world and lower tract stones in the developing world [5, 6]. However, historically, a comparison of stone types in the McCarrison study in 1931 interestingly showed the same stone types in both the United Kingdom and India, where the main reason is malnutrition and dietary risk factors [7].

Recently there has also been a progressive increase in the incidence of pediatric urolithiasis, especially in the developed world – the so-called "stone wave" – with reports of a fivefold increase in stone disease in North America and Turkey [8].

The Afro-Asian stone belt region, with high incidence and prevalence of stone disease, extends from Sudan and Egypt in Africa to Saudi Arabia, Iran, Turkey, Pakistan, and India in Asia,

S. Sultan
Department of Pediatric Urology,
Sindh Institute of Urology and Transplantation,
Karachi 74200, Pakistan
e-mail: info@siut.org

M. Lima, G. Manzoni (eds.), *Pediatric Urology: Contemporary Strategies from Fetal Life to Adolescence*,
DOI 10.1007/978-88-470-5693-0_30, © Springer-Verlag Italia 2015

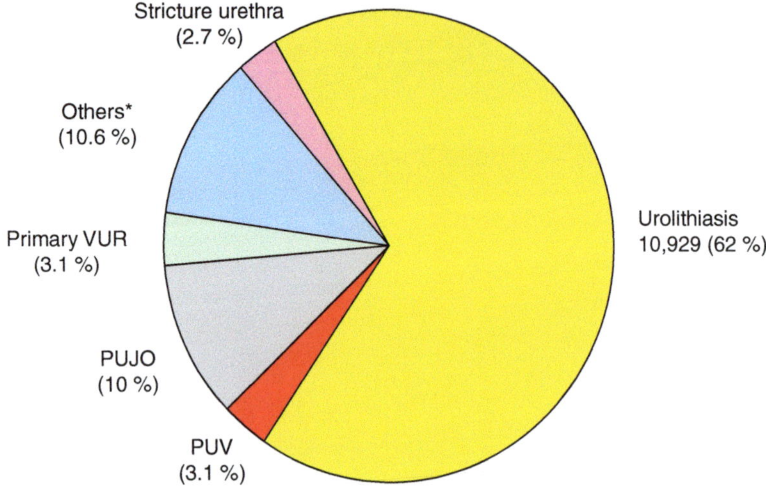

Fig. 30.1 Pediatric urological workload at SIUT from 1998 to 2013 (n = 17,629)

extending as far east as the Philippines in the Far East [7–10]. In our experience, urolithiasis amounts to 60 % of the pediatric urology workload (Fig. 30.1) [11].

Advances in imaging techniques, improved socioeconomic conditions, obesity, and increased consumption of protein-rich diets and dairy products are some of the factors contributing to the increased incidence in the West, where a chronically inadequate dietary intake of proteins (malnutrition), dehydration, and diarrheal disease have long been known and still remain the major contributory factor to the high prevalence of the disease in developing countries [9].

30.3 Demography of Stone Patients

In all, 10,929 patients were seen in the period 1998–2013, with a mean age at the time of presentation of 6.5 ± 3.5 years (range <1–15 years). There was a slight male to female predominance of 2.5:1. Two hundred and nine patients presented in infancy (<1 year), with a male to female ratio of 5:1 (Fig. 30.2). The youngest patient presented to us at the outpatient clinic was 53 days old; however, there are reports of picking up urolithiasis prenatally using ultrasonography [12, 13].

30.4 Clinical Presentation

The commonest presentation is abdominal pain, vague in young children, and more localized flank pain in older children. Other features include hematuria, fever, lower urinary tract symptoms such as frequency, urgency, and dysuria, with or without urinary tract infections [14, 15]. Occasionally stones are identified as an incidental finding on ultrasounds carried out for other pathologies. Some patients present with renal or ureteric colic, and others with strangury because of vesical calculi and even with acute retention of urine, secondary to small stones getting stuck in the urethra.

In our setting, many children present with calculus oligo-anuria with advanced renal failure, fever, tachypnoea, hypotension, severe acidosis, and uraemia, secondary to bilateral obstructing stones or solitary kidney with obstruction [15]. These children develop chronic renal stone disease, caused by neglect and delay in seeking treatment, where they develop a large stone burden with pyeonephrosis, xanthogranulomatous pyelonephritis, renal cortical atrophy, chronic renal failure, advanced uraemia, and even ESRD (end stage renal disease) [15]. Many require resuscitation and urgent renal replacement therapy for stabilization, and further management of the stone disease.

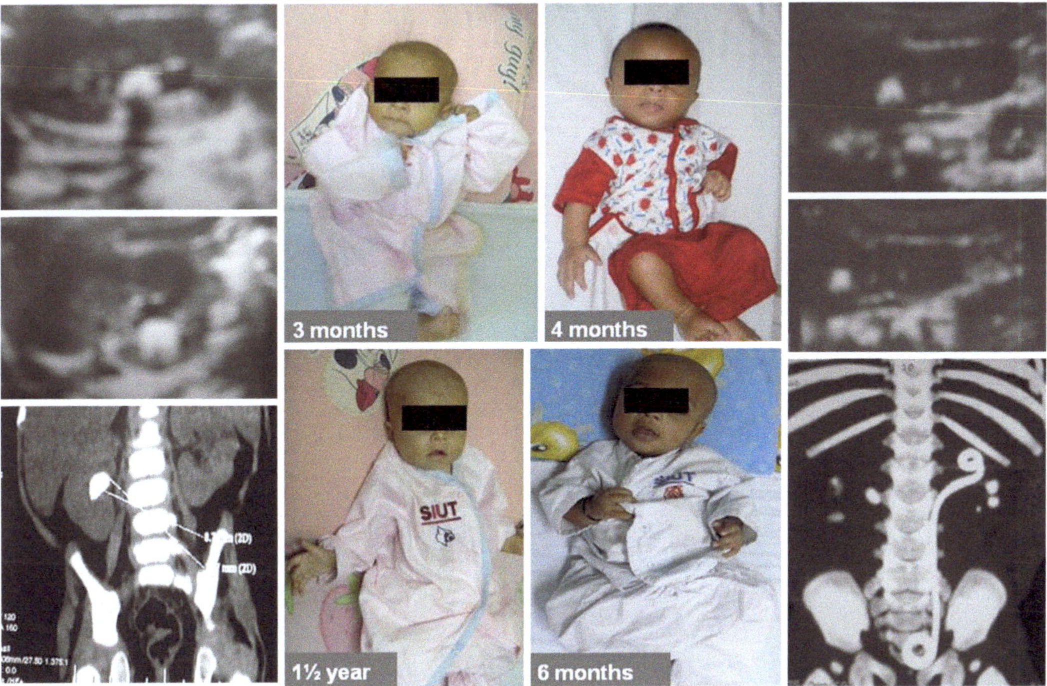

Fig. 30.2 Urolithiasis in infancy

30.5 Diagnostic Investigation

Baseline investigation includes ultrasound and x-ray KUB complete blood picture, urea, creatinine, electrolytes, urine analysis and culture and sensitivity depending on the associated clinical conditions, i.e., renal failure, advanced uraemia, or urosepsis. The following investigations are undertaken on a case–by-case basis: arterial blood gases (ABGs), blood culture, serology of hepatitis B and C, clotting profile, and chest X-ray.

30.6 Evaluation and Management

30.6.1 Evaluation

All the patients presenting to our outpatient department or emergency are evaluated according to protocol (Fig. 30.3).

30.6.1.1 Metabolic Risk Factors

Metabolic analyses identify abnormalities which contribute to the risk of urolithiasis. This analysis is especially important in children because the risk factors identified are corrected to prevent recurrence. Our protocol includes blood tests for urea, creatinine, electrolytes, calcium, phosphate, uric acid, and magnesium. A 24-h urine sample is evaluated in all children to determine volume, pH, protein, electrolytes, magnesium, phosphate, calcium, uric acid, citrate, and oxalate. It is a cumbersome procedure as compliance is poor in children, particularly because of involuntary voiding. In some cases we place an indwelling catheter and in others we collect timed urine or spot urine, and calculate levels by solute to creatinine ratio. Metabolic studies in 2563 children are given in Table 30.1. A separate analysis is also given for the predominant stone types AHU and calcium oxalate (CaOx).

In our population, we were able to identify some predominant factors which contributed to stone formation including hyperoxaluria, hypocitraturia, hypovolemia, and hyperuricosuria.

Calcium levels in our population are not as high as seen in the West because of low dietary intake of dairy products, and this contributes to

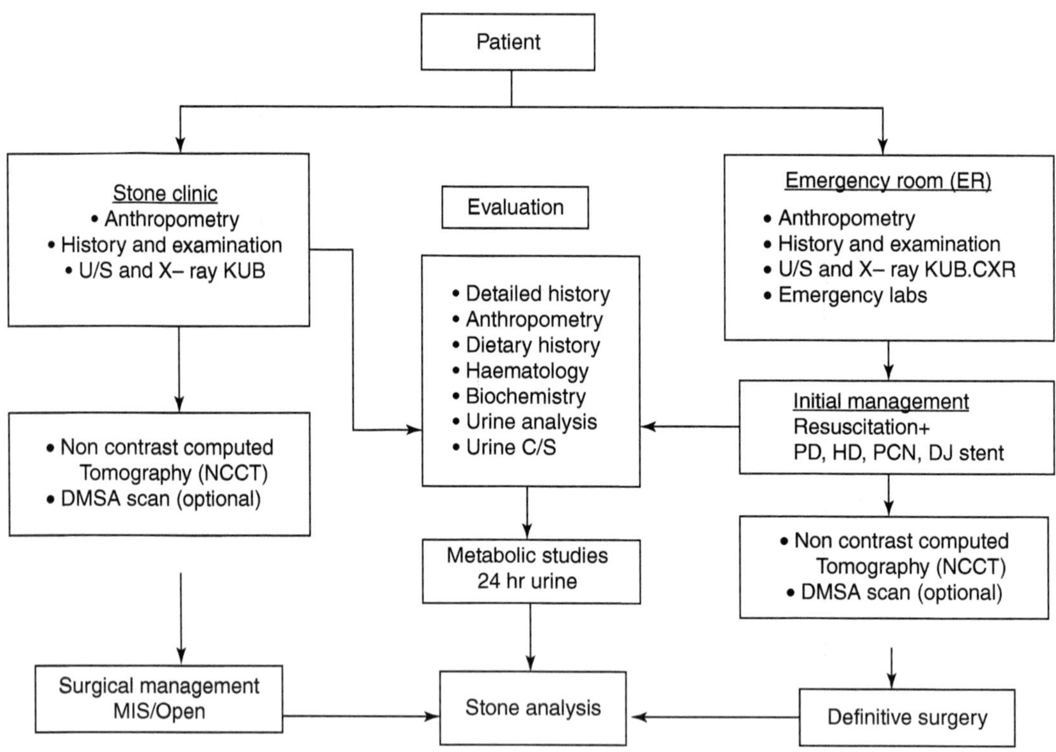

Fig. 30.3 Evaluation protocol for pediatric stone formers

Table 30.1 Metabolic risk factors in 24 h urine of pediatric stone formers

n=2,563				
Parameter	Mean±SD	Overall	AHU stone formers	CaOx stone formers
		n=2,563	n=232	n=312
Urine volume	965.6±810	↓32 %	↓50 %	↓18 %
Uric acid	14.2±19.5	↑27 %	↑47 %	↑19 %
Calcium	4.0±10.2	↑28 %↓21 %	↑15 %↓31 %	↑33 %↓14 %
Phosphorus	15.1±27.2	↑23 %↓19 %	↑29 %↓18 %	↑14 %↓14 %
Sodium	68.1±41.1	↑14 %↓42 %	↑6 %↓58 %	↑22 %↓25 %
Potassium	17.4±10.6	↓48 %	↓42 %	↓41 %
Magnesium	3.8±11.2	↓13 %	↓18 %	↓11 %
Ammonium	21.2±28.5	↑11 %	↑16 %	↑14 %
Protein	220±331	↑41 %	↑44 %	↑36 %
Oxalate	1.84±6.2	↑44 %	↑61 %	↑32 %
Citrate	4.2±14.1	↓87 %	↓84 %	↓92 %
pH	6.01±2.5	↓51 %↑11 %	↑15 %↓44 %	↑9 %↓51 %

the high urinary oxalate levels, as little calcium is available to chelate the dietary oxalate, leading to high levels of oxalate excretion.

Hypocitraturia is found in 87 % of the stone-forming children. In a prospective analysis we compared the urinary citrate levels of our stone-forming children with their non-stone-forming siblings and found that 79 % of these siblings have lower levels of citrate. Hypocitraturia is reported from other developed countries [16], although it remains to be determined whether hypocitraturia has a genetic or dietary origin in our region.

Hypovolumia is a significant contributing factor, as nearly half of the children with AHU stones had low urinary volumes with low sodium levels.

Urinary uric acid levels are the fourth most important contributing factor. Uric acid levels are higher, due to the high intake of legumes and wheat grain. Other than the dietary effect, the role of metabolic derangement cannot be ruled out in uric acid stone formers. In our experience, a properly collected urine specimen can identify the risk factors in more than 90 % of stone-forming children with idiopathic stones. Dietary and medicinal intervention normalizes the risk factors in more than 70 % of these children.

30.6.1.2 Stone Analysis

Chemical composition of stones is the hallmark of studies on etiology, risk factors, and management strategies. Stone analysis is undertaken by Fourier Transformation Infrared Spectroscopy (FTIR), depending on the size of the stone and the fragments available by minimally invasive surgery (MIS) or open surgery. Separate analysis of the core and surface is undertaken whenever possible.

Of 4,648 stone analyzed, 1,794 (38.6 %) were pure stones with single constituent and 2,854 (61.4 %) were mixtures. The frequency of compounds in stones from different sites is given in Table 30.2. Calcium oxalate is the main component in 69–72 % of the stones, followed by ammonium hydrogen urate in 52–55 %. The frequency of compounds in pure stones shows an interesting variation with age (Fig. 30.4).

Children younger than 5 years have predominantly AHU stones, whereas those older than 6 years have mostly CaOx stones. Many of the children younger than 5 years present with malnutrition, diarrheal disease, and dehydration,

Table 30.2 Frequency of compounds in pediatric stone formers

(Pure = 1,794, Mixed = 2,854)	Renal	Bladder	Ureter
	$n=2,798$	$n=1,273$	$n=577$
Calcium oxalate	2,031 (72 %)	873 (69 %)	397 (69 %)
Ammonium hydrogen urate	1,482 (53 %)	703 (55 %)	298 (52 %)
Calcium phosphate apatite	743 (26 %)	272 (21 %)	140 (24 %)
Struvite	278 (10 %)	187 (15 %)	49 (8 %)
Uric acid	207 (7 %)	130 (10 %)	32 (6 %)
Sodium urate	84 (3 %)	7 (0.5 %)	13 (2 %)
Cystine	20 (0.7 %)	7 (0.5 %)	5 (0.8 %)
Xanthine	49 (1.8 %)	20 (16 %)	13 (2 %)
Protein	18 (0.6 %)	–	–
Others	11 (0.4 %)	20 (16 %)	7 (1 %)

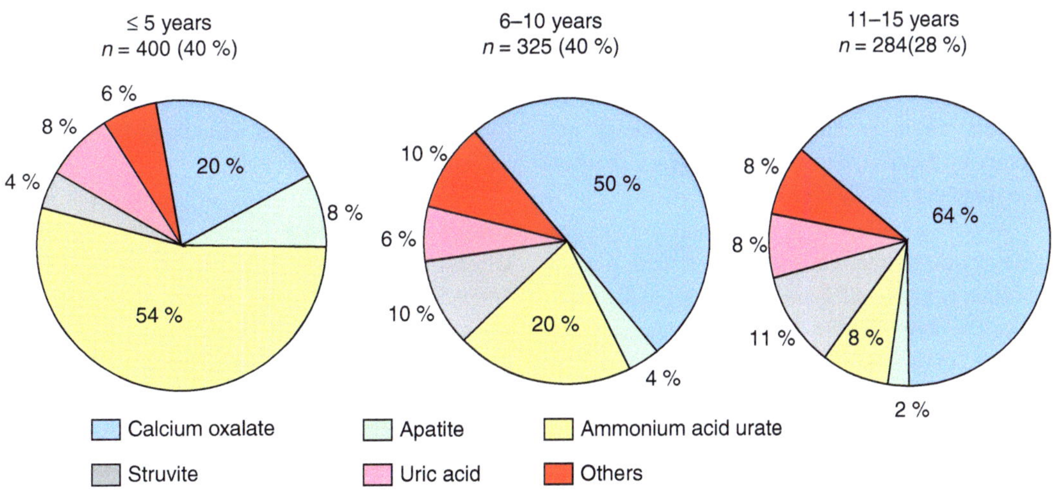

Fig. 30.4 Distribution of pure renal stones in different age groups ($n=1,009$)

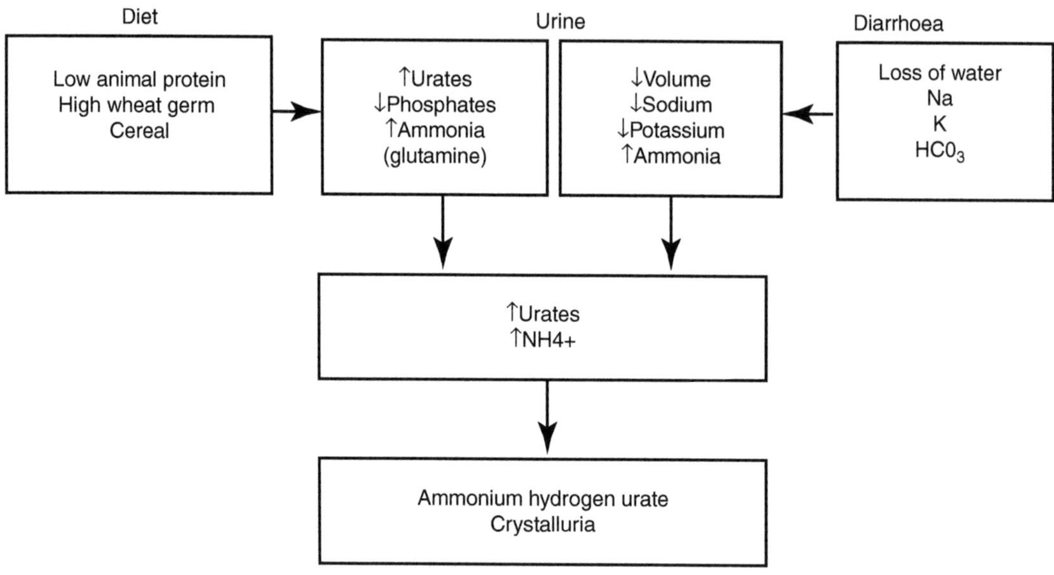

Fig. 30.5 Model of ammonium hydrogen urate stone formation

known risk factors for AHU stone formation (Table 30.2, Fig. 30.5).

High urinary ammonium content is caused by a diet rich in wheat and intracellular acidosis. Low citrate and potassium in the presence of high urate levels leads to AHU stone formation. In contrast, older children without these risk factors form calcium oxalate stones. Separate analysis of the core and surface of the stones showed that stones starting as AHU later grow by addition of calcium oxalate.

30.6.1.3 Role of Diet in Urolithiasis

Diet plays an important role in the pathogenesis and management of pediatric urolithiasis. Stone formers routinely undergo anthropometry and dietary evaluation, and are given dietary protocol to reduce the risk factors.

We use a 7-day food diary and a food frequency questionnaire to obtain information about children's intake of food associated with urolithiasis. These include animal protein, calcium, oxalate, phosphates, purine, sodium, potassium, and refined sugar [17]. Twenty-four-hour fluid intake is assessed by number of glasses consumed. Criteria to analyze fluid intake depends on milliliters per kilogram as recommended.

Anthropometric and dietary analysis. Anthropometric data from 2,372 children with urolithiasis revealed growth deficit and malnutrition in our patient population [15]. The normal Z-score for height and weight, i.e., >−1, was observed in 35 and 24 % of the children, respectively. Of those remaining, 17 % for height and 9 % for weight were severely deficient (Z <−3).

Food frequency questionnaires and dietary recall were analyzed for 2,176 patients and showed low intake of proteins (74 %), potassium (43 %), fiber (48 %), calcium (55 %), and fluids (55 %). High consumption of oxalate in 57 %, sodium in 39 %, purine in 42 %, and refined sugar in 41 % was observed. More than half (60 %) of the population was taking less than the recommended calories [15].

30.6.1.4 Imaging

Ultrasonography

Ultrasound KUB (kidney, ureter, and bladder) is considered as part of the extended physical examination in urology, and the same is true for urolithiasis. It has high sensitivity and specificity for both opaque and non-opaque stones. Stones present as hyperechoic areas in the pelvicalyceal system with negative anechoic areas behind them (posterior

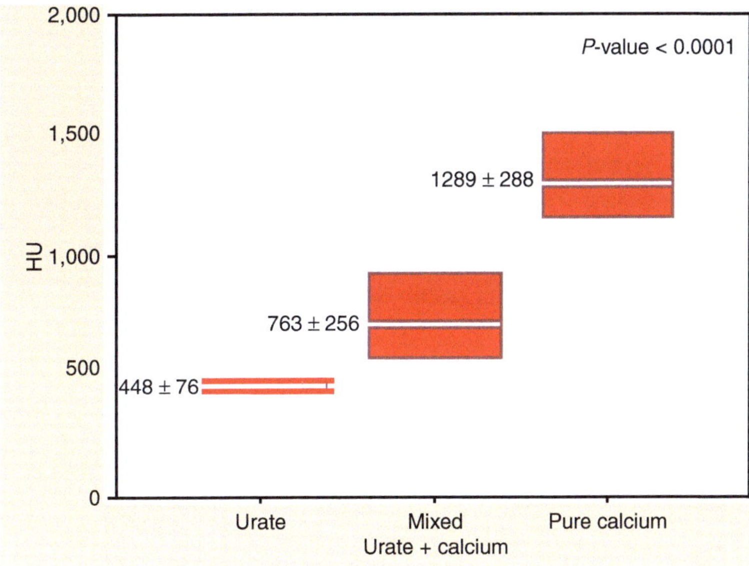

Fig. 30.6 Mean Hounsfield units (HU) in different stone types

acoustic shadowing). Ultrasonography gives an added advantage, in that it can tell us about kidney size and thickness of the cortex, echogenicity of the cortex, hydronephrosis, and any associated hydroureter. Repeat ultrasonograms can be performed for follow-up of the disease.

X-Ray

Plain X-ray KUB was the very first investigation in the evaluation of urolithiasis, although alone it has low sensitivity and specificity. However, this increases to >90 % when sonography and X-ray KUB are combined, and this combination is the only required diagnostic imaging for most of our cases.

IVU

The old time gold standard IVU (intravenous urogram) is now performed in selective cases only with normal renal functions where information regarding the pelvicalyceal system (PCS) is required in greater detail, and where computerized tomography (CT scan) is not available or when CT scan requires general anesthesia. IVU has certain requirements, such as extensive preparation of the bowel, as in children bowel gases obscure key information regarding the stone site and pelvicalyceal anatomy. There is also a risk of allergic reactions and nephropathy. It is also unable to delineate the anatomy of the PCS in renal dysfunction or severe obstruction, and radiation hazards are also a disadvantage.

Non-contrast Computerized Tomography

When any further imaging is required, non-contrast computed tomography has replaced IVU, and it provides extensive details of the stone size, the site, and the anatomy of the PCS. It is the investigation method of choice for patients with ureteric colic, where it identifies ureteric stones, especially mid-ureteric stones, which are almost impossible to detect by USG, X-ray KUB, and IVU together.

Non-contrast CT (NCCT) also provides information about the surrounding tissue, excluding any other pathology, as the cause of acute pain in the surrounding viscera. NCCT can also be helpful in the assessment of stone composition, and can easily differentiate between calcium and non-calcium stones on the basis of attenuation values i.e. Hounsfield units (HU) (Fig. 30.6).

Isotope Scan

An isotope scan, especially using DMSA (dimercaptosuccinic acid – a radioactive tracer), is used to assess the relative function of the kidney.

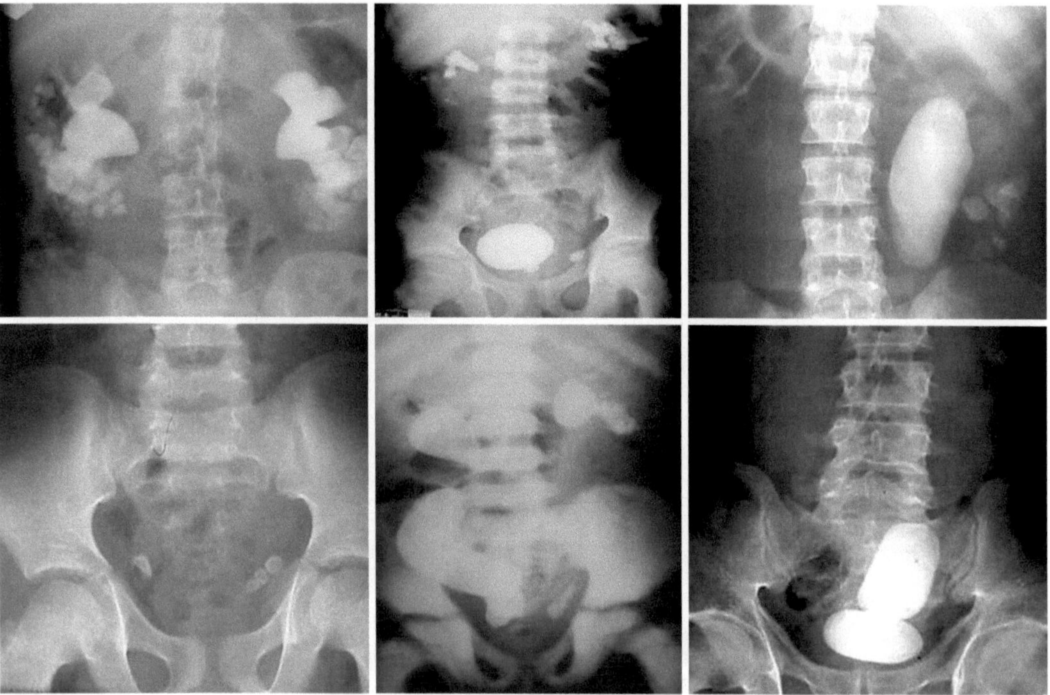

Fig. 30.7 Stone burden: large stones at multiple sites

30.6.2 Management

30.6.2.1 Medical Management

Medical expulsive therapy with alpha blockers is prescribed for ureteric stones and post–ESWL (extracorporeal shock wave lithotripsy). Adequate hydration for the whole 24 h is one of the best measures to prevent kidney stone formation, and therefore we encourage good hydration in our patients on a milliliter per kilogram basis and keep a watch on the urine color to ensure it remains white or light yellow. Two servings of lemon juice daily are recommended to provide a good oral citrate source. Potassium citrate-containing syrup is provided from the hospital for patients with calcium oxalate, cystine, xanthine, and urate stones to maintain adequate urinary alkalinization, and urinary pH is checked with litmus paper. Specific medical therapy is advised on an individual basis.

30.6.2.2 Surgical Management of Urolithiasis in Children

Historically, all patients are managed by open surgery. Advances in technology and invention of pediatric-size endoscopic instruments have created a paradigm shift from open surgical procedures to minimally invasive surgery (MIS) [18]. These include extracorporeal shock wave lithotripsy (ESWL), percutaneous nephrolithotomy (PCNL), retrograde intrarenal surgery (RIRS), ureterorenoscopy (URS) and laparoscopy for renal and ureteric stones, and per urethral and percutaneous cystolithoclast (PUCL/PCCL) for vesical calculi [14]. In developed countries, over 95 % of patients are managed by MIS. Although our experience is similar, we still treat 28 % of patients with open surgery. The main reasons for this, besides anatomical abnormalities, are complex and large stones with atrophic cortices (Fig. 30.7), neglected stones with renal failure, and/or sepsis. Furthermore, many patients come from far-off places where repeat visits are not possible. This compels us to perform the maximum possible clearance in one go with open surgery, with the shortest possible stay in hospital. From 2009 to 2012, 3,434 surgical procedures for stone disease were carried out on 2,861 patients, with a mean age of 6.5 ± 3.5 years (range 2 months to 15 years) (Table 30.3) [19].

Table 30.3 Management of stone disease in the present era (2009–2012)

$n=3,434$		
	No.	%
Open surgery	983	28.6
Pyelolithotomy	735	21.4
Nephrectomy	82	2.4
Ureterolithotomy	10	0.3
Cystolithotomy	64	1.9
Minimally invasive	2,451	71.4
ESWL	568	16.5
PCNL	733	21.3
Lap nephrectomy	25	0.7
URS + laser	529	15.4
PUCL + PCCL	596	17.3

Minimally Invasive Surgery: Our Experience

Extracorporeal Shock Wave Lithotripsy (ESWL)

Since the first clinical report of ESWL in children by Newman et al in 1986, large size stones and even staghorn calculi have been treated with ESWL [11, 20]. Stone-free rates range from 44 to 84 % in different series but these data are difficult to interpret because of discrepancies in the available data with regard to the number of shock waves administered, retreatment rates, stone-free status, and size of residual fragments. ESWL outcome depends on type of lithotripter, operator skills, ESWL protocol used, stone characteristics including location, size, multiplicity, and composition [21].

Our initial experience with ESWL published in 2003, was very satisfactory and showed a stone-free rate of 84 %, with a mean 1.4 sessions given to a stone size ranging from 1.5 to 2.5 cm [11].

In a recent audit of our pediatric renal stones treated with ESWL, we analyzed clearance with renal units treated with ESWL in different stone positions and stone load. In the single stone group of 158 renal units with mean size of 10±2.5 mm, 121 renal units (76 %) cleared in a single session, and 21 units cleared in the second session, giving an overall clearance rate of 89 % in a mean of 1.14 sessions.

In the second group of 58 units comprising multiple stones having a mean size of 17 ± 5.3 mm, 46 % (27 units) cleared in a single session, 32 %(19 units) cleared in the second session, and 7 % (4 units) cleared in the third session, giving an overall clearance rate of 86 % in a mean of 1.54 sessions. These results showed an increase in mean ESWL sessions with an increase in stone burden.

The relationship between stone location and clearance showed that the best clearance rates following a single session of ESWL were found for the upper calyx (87 %) and pelvis (84 %), and the poorest for the lower calyx (67 %). The mean numbers of sessions required for clearance in the upper calyx, pelvis, and middle calyx were 1.1, 1.2, and 1.3, respectively, as compared to the figure for the lower calyx of 1.5.

In a small study of 58 renal units, where we assessed the relationship between the stone densities i.e. hounsefield unit (HU on NCCT) and ESWL, the outcome showed that a lower HU is associated with good clearance for the same size of stone.

ESWL in the pediatric population is carried out under general anesthesia to minimize pain and stone mobility. To avoid repeated anesthesia and to allay the concern of renal damage in the developing kidney and hypertension, we limit our patient population for ESWL to only those cases where complete clearance is expected in a single session. We therefore recommend a maximum stone size of 1.5 cm for a renal stone and, as the lower calyceal anatomy hinders clearance of a stone, a size of 1 cm for lower calyceal stones being managed by ESWL.

Percutaneous Nephrolithotomy (PCNL)

Fernström and Johansson (1976) reported the first case of PCNL carried out in an adult [22]. Its safety and efficacy in the adult population is well established. Parenchymal damage, radiation exposure in children with its effect on the growth of the child, bleeding, and risk of sepsis were serious considerations in the pediatric age group. Woodside and associates in 1985 were the first to present PCNL in the pediatric population with adult instruments [23]; we also initially started off with adult sized instruments.

Miniaturization of the PCNL instruments have facilitated its use in all age group. We usually use a nephroscope of 15, 18, and 20 Fr for PCNL. We have successfully performed more than 1,600

PCNL in children with a mean age of 7.4 ± 3.41 years, 35 % of whom were up to 5 years of age and 10 % were less than 2 years of age.

Although instruments as small as 11 Fr "Mini-Perc" have been reported to be used [24], they go on to the other side of the spectrum and are only for selected cases. Minimal tract dilatation decreases blood loss, allows for increased maneuverability of the instruments, and leads to shorter hospital stays. However, use of these pediatric nephroscopes has to be individualized on the basis of stone location and burden to balance the benefits of small scopes against the concerns of impaired visualization, limitation with the size of grasping forceps, lower irrigation fluid flow, and prolonged operative time.

Our indications for PCNL are stone sizes of 1.5 cm or more with favorable anatomy, previous open surgery on the respective side, failed ESWL, or stones where more than one session of ESWL is expected. All the patients should undergo the proposed evaluation mentioned earlier. Active or untreated UTIs, sepsis, and bleeding diathesis are the few contraindications which should be mentioned. Spinal deformity such as scoliosis and kyphosis should be elucidated prior to surgery.

PCNL is carried out under general anesthesia, and operative considerations include negative urine culture, prophylactic antibiotics, proper draping, isotonic irrigation fluid at body temperature to avoid hypothermia and hyponatremia, and short operative time. The patient is placed in a lithotomy position first for the placement of a ureteric catheter, and then turned prone, taking care of the pressure points and ventilation.

The puncture site is chosen on the basis of the stone location, bulk, and pelvicalyceal anatomy. We prefer subcostal posteriosuperior calyceal punctures when suitable, as this gives access to the majority of the calyces with little torque on the kidney, and also allows access to the pelviureteric junction and lower calyces in the case of stone migration.

In certain situations, the supracostal approach also has be utilized with marginal risks of hydropneumothorax, which can also be avoided in experienced hands.

Table 30.4 Route, calyceal access, and tracts in PCNL

Route	
Subcostal	68 %
Supracostal	32 %
Calyceal access	
Superior	65 %
Inferior	33 %
Middle	7 %
Tracts	
Single tract	95 %
Two tracts	5 %

The procedure involves puncturing of the collecting system through the fornix, along the direction of the infundibulum, to avoid blood vessels adjacent to the infundibulum under ultrasonography or fluoro guidance using C-arm. We occasionally make multiple tracts to clear stones in inaccessible calyces or blind calyces (Table 30.4).

At our center we use an ultrasonic burr and pneumatic lithoclast for stone fragmentation, both being cost effective and reusable (Fig. 30.8). They are used either alone or in combination, depending on the size and hardness of the stone. The holmium:YAG laser is only occasionally used, with deflecting flexible nephroscope, where the stone is found at an acute angle or in calyceal diverticulum with narrow infundibulum. Electrohydraulic Lithoclast (EHL) is known to be very traumatic and therefore has not been used at our centre. We ensure complete stone clearance by checking both fluoroscopically and endoscopically (Fig. 30.9).

Tubeless PCNL has been performed in cases with no significant bleeding, pelvicalyceal breach, and residual fragments. However, we prefer to place a 10–16 Fr nephrostomy tube postoperatively in the majority of our cases for safety reasons.

The variety of stones managed at our center with PCNL range from single pelvic or calyceal stones to partial or complete staghorn stones.

For the purpose of evaluating the results of our PCNL, we divide our stone burden into simple (81 %) and complex (19 %) stones. Simple stones (mean stone burden 2.7 ± 1.5 cm^2) were single stones in the pelvis or calyx or pelvic stones with a single calyceal stone. Complex stones (mean stone burden

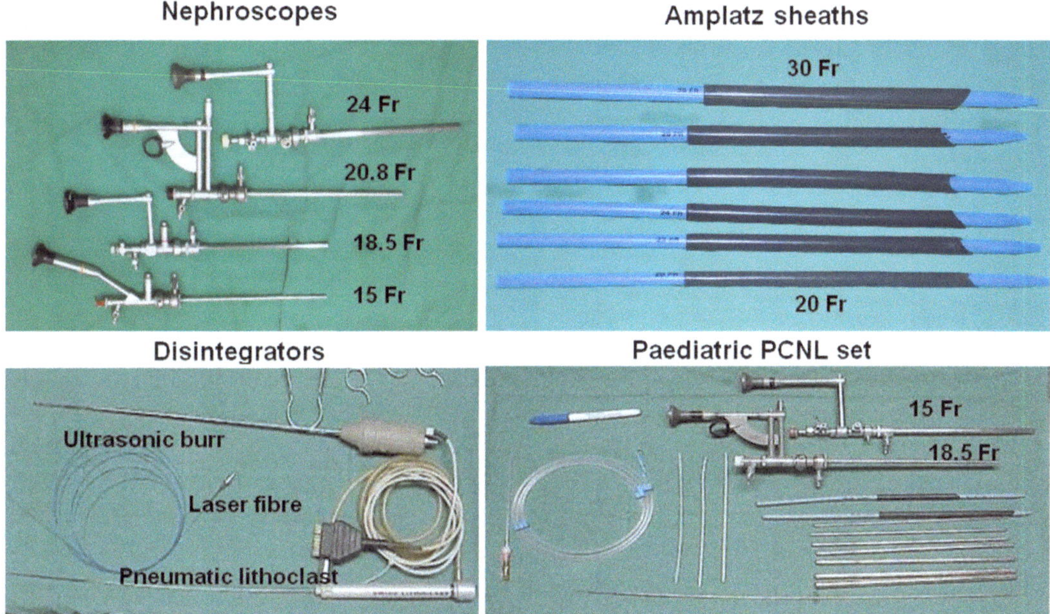

Fig. 30.8 Instruments used for PCNL in children

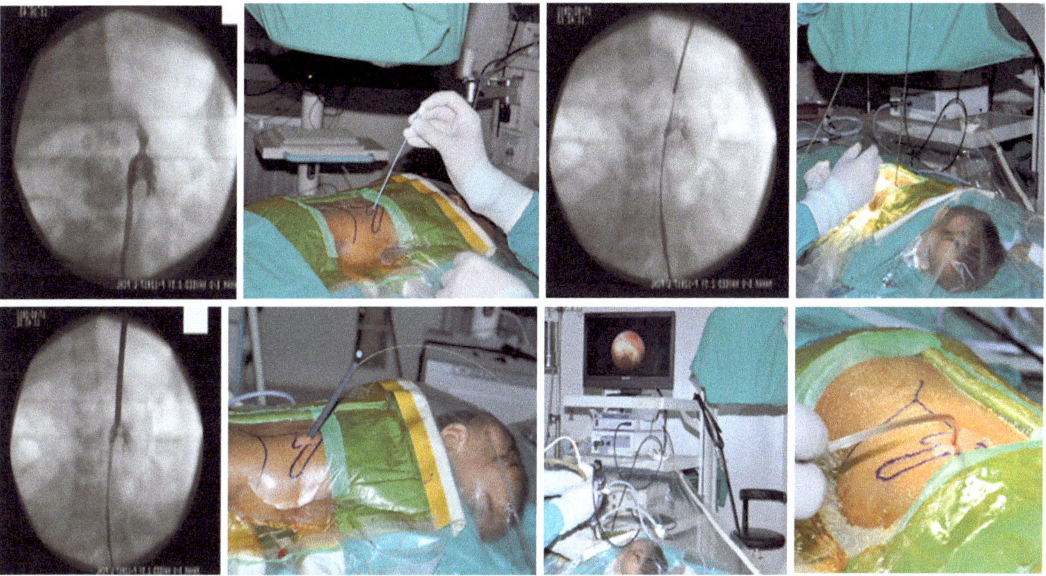

Fig. 30.9 PCNL in progress

5.0±5.8 cm²) were staghorn, partial staghorn, or stones in the pelvis with two or more calyces. The success rate of PCNL as monotherapy is higher in simple stones (89 %) than in complex stones (71.5 %). Those with residual stones required retreatment with Re-PCNL, ESWL, or URS, and stone clearance increased to 95 % in simple stones and 86 % in complex stones.

Preoperatively, patients' mean hemoglobin was 11.1 gm/dl. Of our patients, 14 % required blood transfusion, more in complex stone cases, where more manipulation was carried out.

Our mean operative time was 64.9 min for simple and 92 min for complex stones. Our mean hospital stay was 4.1±3 days. Our patients tend to overstay in hospital as they come from far-off areas, where follow-up facilities are not available.

Conversion to open surgeries (2.6 %) occurred in the early phase of our learning curve. Post-operative complications include hydrothorax in 2 % and urosepsis in 1.6 %, while intraperitoneal and perirenal collections are seen in 1.5 % of cases.

The post-operative effects on renal functions have been evaluated by measuring creatinine levels in all cases and by DMSA scans in selected cases. We did not find any significant deterioration in renal function post-operatively.

To conclude, PCNL is a safe and effective method of renal stone management in all age groups, with acceptable complication rates.

Ureterorenoscopy (URS) and Retrograde Intrarenal Surgery (RIRS)

Ureterorenoscopy and retrograde intrarenal surgery have become the standard urological techniques [14, 18, 25]. They have various diagnostic and therapeutic indications, and their main use is in the management of urolithiasis. The first ureteroscopy was performed in 1912 by Hugh Hampton Young. The first URS in children was performed by Ritchy and colleagues in 1988. With the development of fiber optics, miniaturization of the instruments took place, and thereby semi-rigid and flexible ureteroscopes were developed.

Ureterorenoscopy with a holmium YAG laser is the mainstay of treatment of ureteric stones at our institute. Semi-rigid ureterorenoscopes of size 4.5/6, 6/7.5, and 8/9.8 Fr are used depending on the age and anatomy of the patient and size of the stone, considering the therapeutic requirements. The semi-rigid ureteroscopes are more durable, can access the whole ureter even as far as the PCS, and have better visibility, faster irrigation flow, and larger working channels. In contrast, banding may be difficult and, with large psoas muscles, access to the upper ureter may be limited in comparison to flexible ureteroscopes, which we use infrequently because they are fragile and expensive. The deflectable tip of the flexible scopes is more suitable for retrograde intrarenal surgery.

After complete workup we perform URS under general anesthesia in the lithotomy position with antibiotic prophylaxis and negative urine culture. First a cystoscopy is performed, and a safety guide/glide wire is placed in the ureter under fluoroscopic guidance. Usually no ureteric (VUJ) dilatation is needed, but, in cases where we cannot negotiate the smallest of the scopes (4/6.5 Fr), we use plastic dilators over a guide wire to dilate the ureteric orifice or place a DJ stent for 2–3 weeks, which relieves obstruction and dilates the ureter for the subsequent session of stone fragmentation. Balloon dilatation is not used at our center, being controversial in children and very expensive. Isotonic saline is used at body temperature as an irrigation fluid, and may be used for hydrodilatation of VUJ with caution, taking care to prevent any stone fragment migration and extravasation.

We do not use ureteral access sheaths, which are used with flexible URS to aid in repeated entry into the ureter. The smallest diameter available is 9 Fr, which is too big for our patients.

EHL is too traumatic and cannot be used with small size URS. The pneumatic lithoclast is cost effective, but can only be used with minimum 7 Fr scopes. We use a pneumatic lithoclast in older children with large or hard stones.

Our mainstay of stone disintegration and fragmentation has been the holmium YAG laser, which has revolutionized pediatric ureteric stone management because of its safety and effectiveness in fragmentation of all stone compositions in all age groups, including infants. Its safety is ensured, as most of the laser energy is absorbed by the irrigation fluid, and thus does not damage the ureteric mucosa if the laser fiber is in line with the ureter and not in close proximity to the ureteric wall (0.5–1.0 mm). It produces a photothermal and photomechanical effect, resulting in vaporization of the stone. Typically, 200- to 400-μm fibers are utilized during ureteroscopy. The energy is mostly absorbed by the irrigating solution and the incident angle is kept constant.

We have used the Ho:YAG laser in our patients with a mean age of 6.8±3.5 years, 40 % being less than 5 years of age. Our mean stone size was 8 mm (4–20 mm). The majority (80 %) is in the distal ureter with a stone free rate of 82 % in a single session and 98 % in two sessions. The complications with URS and stone disintegration include extravasation in 2.5 %, UTI in 5 %, and hematuria in 10 %.

30.7 Stones with Renal Failure

About 15–20 % of our pediatric stone patients present with renal dysfunction. There are two major groups of patients presenting with this:

First group: calculus oligo – anuric with two good kidneys or a solitary good/normal functioning kidney, which becomes acutely blocked with bilateral renal and/or mostly ureteric stones. Usually these children are younger with a mean age of 4.3±2.9 years.

Second group: chronic calculus renal failure group, who have been harboring stones for a long period; these stones have slowly and gradually affected/damaged the kidney permanently or irreversibly because of associated chronic obstruction leading to ischemic cortical atrophy, with infection on top of this. Most of these children are in renal dysfunction for extended periods, affecting their body metabolism and growth. Many present with extremes of disease with osteodystrophy, anemia, and severe malnutrition. These children are older than those with calculus oligo/anuria, with mean ages of 6.9±3.4 years.

The majority (89 %) of these patients are from poor socioeconomic backgrounds, 66 % coming from rural areas, and live far away from our health facility, with a mean travel distance of 160±45 km. They therefore present late with advanced uremia, sepsis, fever, tachypnea, and respiratory distress because of fluid overload and or severe acidosis and hyperkalemia.

The initial management in many of these patients requires resuscitation, ventilatory support, and multidisciplinary intensive care management, with immediate imaging, peritoneal or hemodialysis.

Management of the calculus anuria group after evaluation is by placement of the JJ stent under general anesthesia within a few hours of their presentation. There are 24-h services for anesthesia, pediatric nephrology, and urology. This is considered to be the best form of management for these patients, as JJ placement results in relief of obstruction and urine formation. Those who cannot have a JJ stent, and have some plevicalyceal dilatation, are treated by placement of percutaneous nephrostomy.

After evaluation, the chronic calculus renal failure group undergoes immediate management with temporary angio access with double lumen catheter, hemodialysis, and some with peritoneal dialysis. In the calculus anuria group, 90 % of patients had complete recovery of renal function, compared to 54 % in the chronic calculus renal failure group, whereas there was partial recovery in 7 % of the first group and 17 % in the chronic calculus renal failure group. In the chronic calculus renal failure group, no recovery of renal function is observed in 21 %, of which 14 % are on hemodialysis, and 7 % underwent renal transplantation.

References

1. Shattock JG (1905) A pre- historic or pre- dynastic Egyptian calculus. Trans Pathol Soc Lond 61:275
2. Desnos E (1914) The history of urology. Murphy LJT (trans and ed). Paris, Doinlet Fits, pt.1
3. Dimopoulos C, Gialas A, Likourinas M, Androutsos G, Kostakopoulos A (1980) Hippocrates: founder and pioneer of urology. Br J Urol 52(2):73–74
4. Baştuğ F, Düşünsel R (2012) Pediatric urolithiasis: causative factors, diagnosis and medical management. Nat Rev Urol 9(3):138–146
5. Sarica K (2006) Pediatric urolithiasis: etiology, specific pathogenesis and medical treatment. Urol Res 34(2):96–101
6. Bakane BC, Nagtilak SB, Patil B (1999) Urolithiasis: a tribal scenario. Indian J Pediatr 66(6):863–865
7. McCarrison R (1931) A lecture on the causation of stone in India. Br Med J 1(3675):1009
8. Sharma AP, Filler G (2010) Epidemiology of pediatric urolithiasis. Indian J Urol 26(4):516–522
9. Romero V, Akpinar H, Assimos DG (2010) Kidney stones: a global picture of prevalence, incidence, and associated risk factors. Rev Urol 12(2–3):e86
10. Rizvi SAH, Naqvi SAA, Hussain Z, Hashmi A, Hussain M, Zafar MN, Sultan S, Mehdi H (2002) Pediatric urolithiasis: developing nation perspectives. J Urol 168(4):1522–1525

11. Rizvi SAH, Naqvi SAA, Hussain Z, Hashmi A, Hussain M, Zafar MN, Sultan S, Mehdi H (2003) Management of pediatric urolithiasis in Pakistan: experience with 1,440 children. J Urol 169(2):634–637
12. Rhodes C, Churchill D, Hulton SA (2005) Antenatal diagnosis of fetal renal calculus. Ultrasound Obstet Gynecol 25(5):517–518
13. Tannous RJ, Solhaug MJ, Bogdan D, Abuhamad AZ (2000) Prenatal diagnosis of fetal nephrolithiasis. Ultrasound Obstet Gynecol 15(4):331–332
14. Gnessin E, Chertin L, Chertin B (2012) Current management of paediatric urolithiasis. Pediatr Surg Int 28(7):659–665
15. Rizvi SA, Sultan S, Zafar MN, Ahmed B, Faiq SM, Hossain KZ, Naqvi SA (2007) Evaluation of children with urolithiasis. Indian J Urol 23(4):420–427
16. Kovacevic L, Wolfe-Christensen C, Edwards L, Sadaps M, Lakshmanan Y (2012) From hypercalciuria to hypocitraturia—a shifting trend in pediatric urolithiasis? J Urol 188(4):1623–1627
17. Hamill PVV, Drizd TA, Johnson CL, Reed RB, Roche AF, Moore WM (1979) Physical growth: National Center for Health Statistics percentiles. Am J Clin Nutr 32(3):607–629
18. Raju GA, Norris RD, Ost MC (2010) Endoscopic stone management in children. Curr Opin Urol 20(4):309–312
19. Rizvi SA, Sultan S, Ijaz H, Mirza ZN, Ahmed B, Saulat S, Naqvi SA (2010) Open surgical management of pediatric urolithiasis: a developing country perspective. Indian J Urol 26(4):573
20. Lottmann HB, Traxer O, Archambaud F, Mercier-Pageyral B (2001) Monotherapy extracorporeal shock wave lithotripsy for the treatment of staghorn calculi in children. J Urol 165(6):2324–2327
21. Jeong U, Lee S, Kang J, Han DH, Park KH, Baek M (2013) Factors affecting the outcome of extracorporeal shock wave lithotripsy for unilateral urinary stones in children: a 17-year single-institute experience. Korean J Urol 54(7):460–466
22. Fernström I, Johansson B (1976) Percutaneous pyelolithotomy. A new extraction technique. Scand J Urol Nephrol 10(3):257–259
23. Woodside JR, Stevens GF, Stark GL, Borden TA, Ball WS (1985) Percutaneous stone removal in children. J Urol 134(6):1166–1167
24. Jackman SV, Hedican SP, Peters CA, Docimo SG (1998) Percutaneous nephrolithotomy in infants and preschool age children: experience with a new technique. Urology 52(4):697–701
25. Wang AJ, Preminger GM (2011) Modern applications of ureteroscopy for intrarenal stone disease. Curr Opin Urol 21(2):141–144

Renal Transplantation

31

Matteo Ravaioli, Annalisa Amaduzzi, Flavia Neri, and Antonio Daniele Pinna

31.1 Introduction

The first kidney transplantation was performed on 1954, and the graft was successfully transplanted from one healthy twin to his brother who was dying of renal disease, at the Brigham Hospital in Boston. The operation was successful, renal function was restored in the recipient, and the donor suffered no ill effects [1]. Since that date, the procedure improved in the surgical and medical fields, and in particular, the immunosuppressant protocol including CNI (cyclosporine and tacrolimus) and steroids reduced drastically the risk of graft loss due to acute rejection.

The organ shortage encourages specific pediatric allocation policies to minimize the waiting time for deceased donors and to achieve better survival for children with ESRD (end-stage renal disease) (www.optn.org). Renal transplantation is the treatment of choice for young patients affected by ESRD. The 5-year patient survival rate for transplant (94–97 %) exceeds dialysis (75–87 %) [2]. The living kidney donation is the optimal source of organ with optimal recipient outcome and with a possibility to favor preemptive kidney transplantation (before starting dialysis), which avoids the complications related to the dialysis [3]. The future prospective for pediatric kidney transplantation includes therefore living donation, preemptive transplantation, and effective immunosuppression with lower side effects.

31.2 Indication to Kidney Transplant

Incidence of ESRD in children is variable in the different age groups. The registry from the European Society of Pediatric Nephrologists reported the highest incidence in adolescence (8/pmarp), lowest in mild childhood (4.6/pmarp), and intermediate (6.7/pmarp) in children younger than 5 years of age [4]. Causes of ESRD in children are different compared to adults. According to the report of 2010 from the NAPRTCS (North American Pediatric Renal Trials and Collaborative Studies), although the etiology of ESRD varies by the ethnicity and age group, the most common primary diagnosis is renal hypoplasia/dysplasia/aplasia (15.8 %) followed by obstructive uropathy (15.3 %) and FSGS (focal segmental glomerulosclerosis) (11.7 %) which becomes the main cause of ESRD in black patients and increases in frequency with older age [5].

ESRD is a major burden for children as it significantly reduces survival among the young population as well as in the adults. According to a study published on *NEJM* in 2004, the long-term survival

M. Ravaioli, PhD (✉) • A. Amaduzzi, MD
F. Neri, MD • A.D. Pinna, PhD
Department of General Surgery and Transplantation, S. Orsola-Malpighi University Hospital, Via Massarenti 9, 40138 Bologna, Italy
e-mail: matteo.ravaioli@aosp.bo.it; antoniodaniele.pinna@asop.bo.it

M. Lima, G. Manzoni (eds.), *Pediatric Urology: Contemporary Strategies from Fetal Life to Adolescence*, DOI 10.1007/978-88-470-5693-0_31, © Springer-Verlag Italia 2015

rate among children requiring renal-replacement therapy was 79% at 10 years and 66% at 20 years [6]. For pediatric patients, the advantages of renal transplantation over staying on dialysis are considerable not only in terms of improved physical growth and psychological development but also for the overall survival benefit which in some cases can reach 20 years [7]. The importance of early renal transplantation for children caused the adoption of the strategy of preemptive renal transplantation, a revised allocation policy to convey organs from younger donors preferentially to children, and finally the promotion of programs of living donors.

The European registry (ESPN/ERA –EDTA) reported 900 kidney transplantations performed in children in 2008, which accounted for 4.4 % of all the renal transplantation procedures. The median percentage of preemptive and living donor transplantation was, respectively, 17 and 43 % [8]. This tendency to adopt renal transplantation as initial renal replacement therapy for children is witnessed by the OPTN (Organ Procurement and Transplantation Network) annual report; the number of preemptive kidney transplantations in children increased from 23.8 % in the years 2000–2002 to 28.7 % in the years 2010–2012. While the adoption of preemptive transplantation has spread, the diffusion of LDKT (living-donor kidney transplantation) has not followed with the same pace. From the same report, it appears that while the number of total kidney transplantation in children has slightly increased from 2000 to 2012, the percentage of LDKT has dropped from 57.8 % in the years 2000–2002 to 38.5 % around the year 2005 and has remained stable since then. Although the LDKT in children has declined, the percentage of unrelated living donors has increased with respect to the related ones, probably as a reflection of a greater participation to programs of living-donor exchanges. The recipients of less than 6 years underwent the highest percentage of LDKT (45 %) [9].

31.3 Allocation

Since the year 2000, effort has been aimed to give relative priority to children [10], and since 2005, the OPTN implemented a new policy for pediatric kidney allocation (SHARE 35 policy). According to this policy, children had higher priority for younger donors [11] and this leads to increased number of PKT (pediatric kidney transplantation) from deceased donors [12]. The median waiting time for children was reduced from 11.2 months in 1998 to 6.8 months in 2009 [13] as well as the mortality on waiting list; thanks to this new allocation improvement.

Similar allocation systems have been developed in European countries in order to reduce the time in waiting list and the mortality for the pediatric population with ESRD. A recent survey was published concerning the allocation policies adopted in Europe and the associated rates of PKT. The results showed that from the adoption of the new allocation strategies, organs from younger deceased donors were allocated more preferentially to children, and, as a consequence, the rate of PKT increased and a lower proportion of LDKT (living-donor kidney transplantation) was observed. However, a great variability on distribution of donor sources and access to KT was observed among the various countries, due to the economic disparities and the differences in health-care priorities [8].

31.4 Outcome of Kidney Transplant

Kidney transplantation in children has reached nowadays good results in terms of patient survival. According to the latest NAPRTCS report, the survival rate has improved from 90 % at 3 years in the time period 1987–1995 to 96 % in the years 1996–2007; the improvement is even more significant when considering DDKT (deceased-donor kidney transplantation). When considering the age group, the highest patient survival is observed in children 6–11 years old and the lowest for children under 5 years of age for both DDKT and LDKT [5].

The most common causes of death in children after KT are infections (28.5 %), cardiopulmonary diseases (14.7 %), cancer/malignancies (11.3 %), and complications related to dialysis (3.1 %) [14].

When the program of PKT started in the late 1980s, the graft survival was inferior compared to adults. However, it improved significantly to results comparable to adults in 2000 and has remained stable since then. When considering the age groups, the children under 5 years have the lowest 1-year graft survival for deceased donors (89.9 %) but the highest long-term (10 years) graft survival for both deceased (63.9 %) and living donors (80.6 %) [13].

An accurate estimate of long-term outcome of KT is calculated as half-life of the graft which is the time point at which 50 % of the grafts are still functioning; from the OPTN report, the half-life of PKT has increased in the last decades for both deceased (DD) and living donors (LD) (respectively, from 8 to 12 years for DD and from 12.5 to 15.3 years for LD) [9, 14].

The most common cause of graft loss was chronic rejection (41 %), followed by acute rejection which occurs in 14 % of DD and 9 % of LD at 1 year after KT: its incidence increases with time from KT, always more frequent among DD than LD [9–14]. The incidence of vascular thrombosis as cause of graft loss has decreased to 7 % in the more recent years (2000–2007).

31.5 Immunosuppression

From 2000, the field of PKT has seen the advent of tacrolimus as the cornerstone of the immunosuppressive therapy in children as well as in adults since its superiority over cyclosporine in increasing the graft survival was proved in several studies [15]. The use of cyclosporine and azathioprine has decreased consensually to the adoption of tacrolimus and mycophenolate [9]. Administration of steroids to children exerts growth-suppressive effects, and therefore, new immunosuppressive protocols have been developed in the recent years in order to avoid or minimize the use of steroids in post-transplantation immunosuppression. A large randomized multicentric European study was recently conducted on the effects of induction with IL-2 receptor antibody and post-transplant rapid withdrawal of steroids in pediatric recipients. This study showed that steroid tapering was feasible without significant increased risk of rejection and with considerable advantages for metabolic profile and developmental pattern in pediatric recipients [16]. These results supported the use of induction therapy which has therefore been adopted more extensively in the recent years.

Although the latest report by OPTN showed an increased use of T-cell-depleting agents which have been adopted by 56.2 % of the recipients in 2012, their superiority over IL-2 receptor antibodies on preventing rejection or in increasing graft survival has not been shown to be significant in children undergoing kidney transplantation [9, 17].

31.6 Surgical Aspect of KT and Complications

Although surgical and immunosuppressive refinements occurred in the recent years, the renal transplant in pediatric patients remains a challenging procedure because of surgical issues and anesthetic problems related to vascular and hemodynamic changes after the graft revascularization.

In most of the pediatric renal transplant programs, the kidney graft is placed in the standard extraperitoneal iliac fossa as in adult-to-adult transplant when the recipient's weight is over 20 Kg (Figs. 31.1, 31.2, and 31.3); intra-abdominal placement with vascular anastomoses to the infrarenal aorta and IVC is commonly preferred in small children less than 20 Kg (Figs. 31.4, and 31.5). Transplantation in small children is also performed even in younger than 1 year recipients; nevertheless, in the most of the cases, surgeons try to wait for the recipient's weight to reach 10–12 kg and the linked enlargement of blood vessel, supporting the recipient with growth hormone and maximizing the nutrition, to avoid some of the risks of vascular thrombosis.

31.6.1 Transplant Surgery

An oblique Gibson incision from below the thoracic cage to the pubis is performed on the right side to facilitate access to the IVC; the external

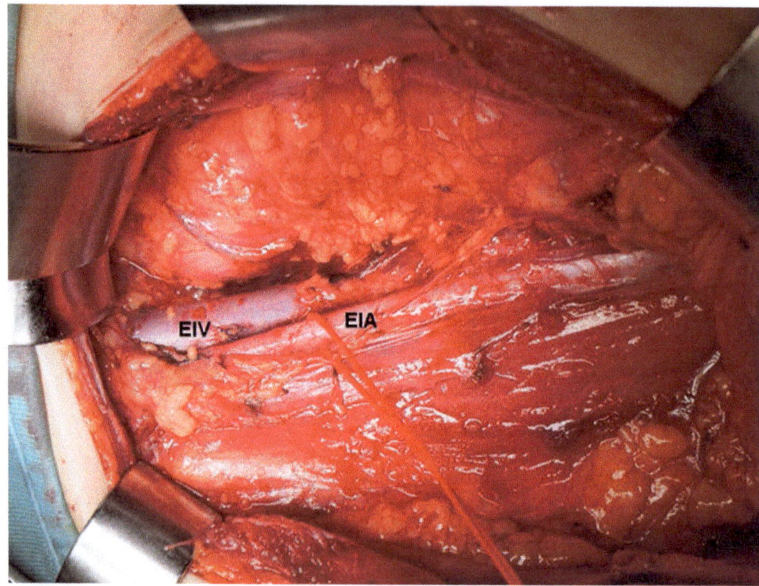

Fig. 31.1 Retroperitoneal approach – Mobilization of the external iliac vessels (artery encircled on vessel loop); *EIV* external iliac vein, *EIA* external iliac artery

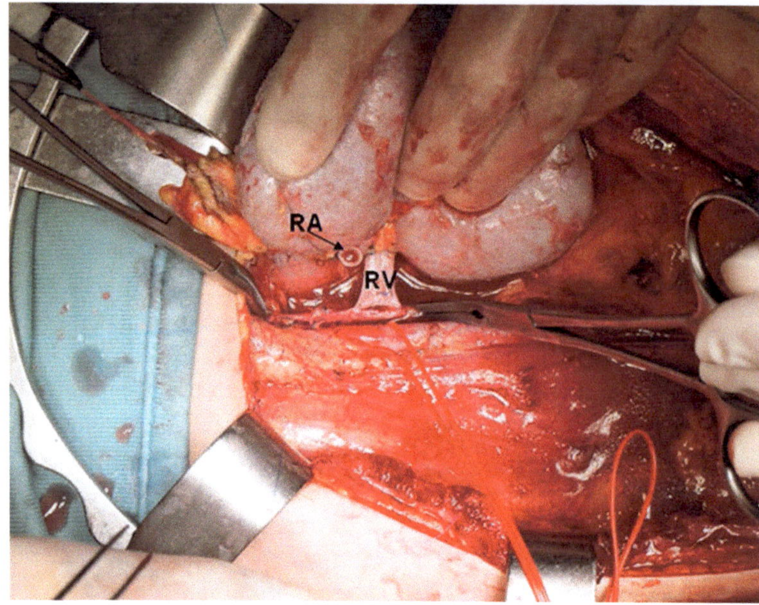

Fig. 31.2 Retroperitoneal approach – Venous anastomosis: renal vein (*RV*) end-to-side to the external iliac vein, *RA* renal artery

oblique, internal oblique, and transversus abdominis muscles are incised, the inferior epigastric vessels legated and divided. An appropriate retroperitoneal room is created sweeping medially the peritoneum. The common and external iliac vessels and the distal end of the aorta and IVC are exposed (Fig. 31.1). The sites for vascular reconstruction are chosen by placing the graft into the iliac fossa to determine the best fit to avoid vessel traction or kinking. Anastomoses to the aorta or IVC can be performed also through an extraperitoneal access in small children. Renal vein and artery anastomoses are performed end to side using a running 6/0 or 7/0 polypropylene suture (Fig. 31.2). Urinary tract reconstruction is carried out by extravesical Lich-Gregoir ureteroneocystostomy with

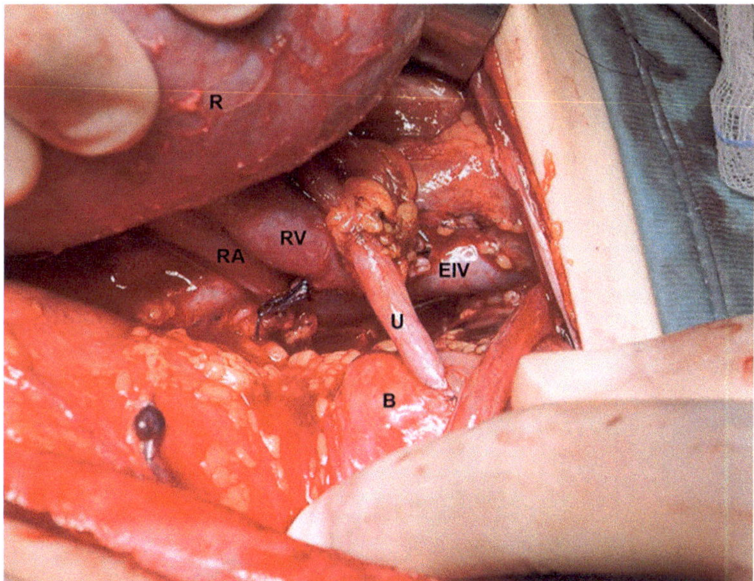

Fig. 31.3 Retroperitoneal approach – *R* renal graft, *RV* renal vein, *RA* renal artery, *EIV* external iliac vein, *U* ureter, *B* bladder

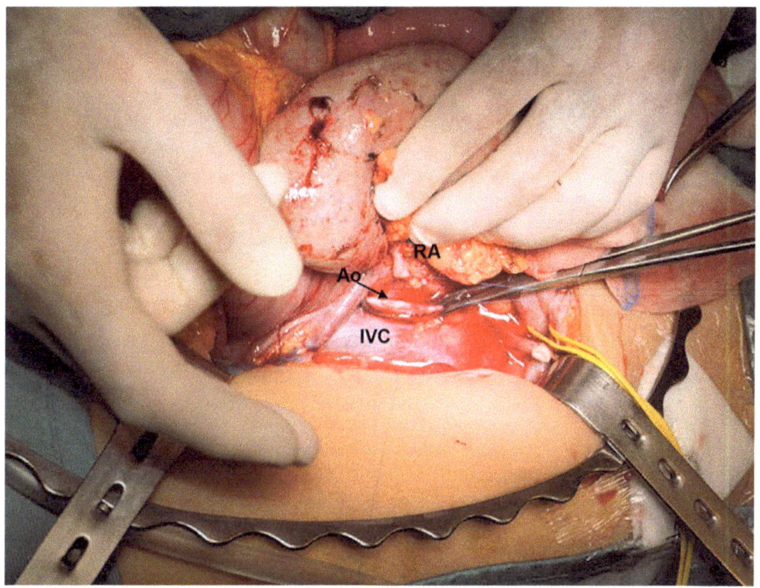

Fig. 31.4 Intraperitoneal approach – Arterial anastomosis: renal artery end-to-side to the aorta, *RA* renal artery, *Ao* aorta, *IVC* inferior vena cava

placement of an internal double-J stent. Antireflux techniques are also used by some surgeons (Fig. 31.3).

Pediatric patient with complex urologic issues may require pretransplant and peritransplant procedures. If the transplant surgeon is not a urologist, good planning among the surgical team is necessary. The percentage of patients with lower urinary tract dysfunction undergoing kidney transplantation ranges from 2 to 6 % [18].

For a long time, patients with end-stage renal disease caused by lower urinary tract dysfunction were considered poor candidates for transplantation because of an increased risk of renal failure attributed to the complications of poor urinary drainage also after kidney transplantation [19].

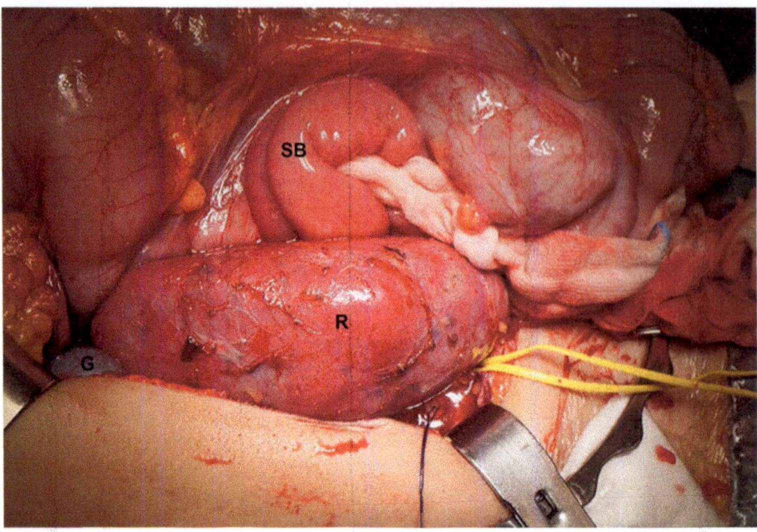

Fig. 31.5 Intraperitoneal approach – *R* renal graft, *SB* small bowel, *G* gall bladder

The growing number of children with end-stage renal disease and severe lower urinary tract abnormalities, together with improvements in the overall results of kidney transplantation programs, has forced to offer kidney transplantations to this group of patients. A urinary reservoir with a good capacity, compliance, and emptying for the transplanted kidney should be planned before transplant or performed at the time of transplant surgery. The main procedures in these patients are bladder augmentation and incontinent ileal conduit diversion; auxiliary urinary stoma (Mitrofanoff) is also created, and voiding is maintained by intermittent catheterization.

There is no full agreement concerning the timing of bladder augmentation and creation of an ileal conduit. Some Authors advocate the fashioning of the ileal conduit simultaneously through the same incision of transplant to avoid adhesions and also to permit a better graft arrangement to avoid kinking of the ureter during creation of the anastomosis to the ileal conduit. In such situations, the kidney has also been placed upside-down, with the ureter going straight up to the extraperitoneal part of the ileal conduit [20].

Most authors perform bladder augmentation before transplantation [21], but some reports indicate that bladder augmentation is safe even at the time of transplantation as well [22]. These patients have higher percentage of urinary tract infections (up to 90 %) compared to the general population of kidney recipients. There is no statistical difference in the rate of occurrence of urinary tract infection between ileal conduits and bladder reconstructions [23]; some authors postulate that urinary tract infection may trigger acute rejections, especially in early postoperative period, and therefore, they recommend early and aggressive treatment of urinary tract infections [24]. On the other hand, the intensive treatment of infection without symptoms may induce resistant bacterial growth; therefore, other authors suggest to use a constant prophylaxis with nitrofurantoin without changing management in cases of positive bacterial cultures without clinical symptoms.

In all patients with augmented bladder, ureter anastomosis to the native bladder is widely recommended. Anastomosis to the bowel segment is also feasible; however, when possible, it should be done to the native bladder. This may be impossible when malformation in a patient with myelomeningocele causes displacement of the bladder, making it difficult to find the native bladder wall. Satisfying results are achieved by routine regular drainage of augmented bladders, preventing symptomatic urinary infections, and by reservoir irrigation with a saline solution to remove enteric secretions that can accumulate and become a source of obstruction and infection. In conclusion, kidney transplantation in children with lower urinary tract dysfunction and end-stage renal failure gives excellent medium-term results, despite nonstandard urinary drainage into an augmented bladder or ileal conduit [20].

31.6.2 Intraperitoneal vs. Extraperitoneal Kidney Transplantation

In smaller children and infants, anastomosis to larger vessels is necessary. Infants weighing 10 kg or less generally undergo a midline laparotomy with vascular anastomosis at the level of the vena cava and the aorta (Fig. 31.4). For children between 10 and 30 kg, there are some variable approaches (retroperitoneal vs. intraperitoneal or common iliac vessels vs. vena cava and aorta) according to surgeon preference. Extraperitoneally allografting with vascular anastomosis to the aorta and the vena cava has been demonstrated to be feasible and preferable by some authors [25] in recipients less than 15 Kg in weight because of the advantages of rapid oral feeding and absence of postoperative intestinal adhesions. For young children with previous intra-abdominal procedures or vascular access issues, the thrombosis of the major intra-abdominal vessels must be carefully evaluated in order to select an appropriately sized donor organ that can be accommodated to small collateral vessels in the abdomen [26]. An adult-sized graft occupies now almost the entire right side of the abdomen; abdominal closure may result difficult in small children, but this is accomplished with the interposition of a biologic biodegradable prosthesis if necessary [27] (Fig. 31.5).

A graft ultrasound Doppler is advised in the early post-transplant hours to detect compartmental syndrome, early vascular or ureteral complications, or perinephric fluid collections that can benefice of an early treatment to save the graft as well as representing a baseline study for subsequent investigation.

31.6.3 Kidney Graft from Donor ≤5 Years of Age

Kidneys from donors ≤5 years of age represent a controversial issue, because of presumed higher rates of technical complications (such as vascular thrombosis and ureteral leak) and suboptimal results were historically not considered as suitable for transplant. Improved transplant technique and better immunosuppression regimens resulted in a better outcome. In order to maximize the donor pool, some centers accept now as kidney donors also infants even less than 5 k of weight, for single or en bloc kidney transplant. According to the data from NAPRTCS 2010, among deceased donor source transplants, only 1.4 % comes from donors less than 24 months old, while 21.2 % comes from donors between 2 and 12 years of age. A recent report promotes the increased use of those donors due to the improved outcome shown [28–30].

The Eurotransplant International Foundation reported that of a total of 501 kidneys from deceased donors ≤5 year from 2000 to 2010, 98 % was allocated as single or en bloc grafts.

The en bloc renal transplant from small pediatric donors represents surgical strategies to facilitate early transplantation among children, even if it is still quite uncommon and underutilized in the pediatric population. The donor kidneys are retrieved en bloc with aorta, vena cava, and bilateral ureters in continuity with donor urinary bladder. The en bloc allografts are commonly placed retroperitoneally in the right iliac fossa. The distal end of the allograft aorta is commonly anastomosed to the common iliac artery end-to-side or to internal iliac artery end-to-end. The venous anastomosis of the allograft vena cava is performed end-to-side to the recipient vena cava or to the external iliac vein end-to-side [31].

The extravesical ureteroneocystostomy is the standard technique for the anastomosis of the graft ureter. The anastomosis of donor bladder patch including both the meatus and the dome of the recipient bladder appears to be at high risk for leak due to vascular insufficiency of the patch [32]; antireflux techniques are also used by some surgeons to reduce the risks of reflux and infections.

Despite surgical improvements, the incidence of technical complication is still high, and it represents an important cause of graft loss. The NAPRTCS data show that graft thrombosis accounts for 9.8 % of all graft loss in pediatric kidney transplant patients [14]. Some authors consider at too high risk the combination of an infant donor and a very small pediatric recipient, and they therefore prefer the use of recipients weighing 15–30 kg in case of infant donor [32]. These kidneys show excellent renal reserve and long-term survival; these grafts adapt to the growing child by increasing glomerular filtration rate over time differently from what happens in the adult patient [33].

The recent data on this strategy showed that the en bloc transplant was safe and feasible. The higher risk of vascular thrombosis was reduced by the growing technical expertise associate to the prophylactic administration of aspirin [31, 34]. Regardless of surgical improvements, the observation of glomerulomegaly on biopsy and a high glomerular filtration rate in many recipients raise potential concern for progressive renal injury from hyperfiltration, which will need to be closely monitored in a longer follow-up [31].

31.6.4 Nephrectomy

Nephrectomy of native kidneys may be required before or during transplant surgery. Indications for nephrectomy are represented by nephrotic syndrome which is also an independent risk factor for clotting, uncontrolled hypertension, or infected kidney or kidney affected by disease leading to polyuria that can put at risk for hypovolemia, hemoconcentration, and clotting in the early postoperative period.

31.6.5 Intraoperative Management

The intraoperative fluid management is crucial especially in small children who receive adult kidney graft. A central venous catheter is generally inserted for monitoring central venous pressures (CVP); of paramount importance is to maintain a mean arterial pressure above 70 mmHg and a CVP as high as 12 mmHg either at the time of anastomoses to ensure adequate perfusion of adult graft which contain a volume of 150–250 ml of blood (about 10 % of a small child's total circulating volume) or in the postoperative period to supply the large urine output and presumably minimize clotting. Colloid and crystalloids are infused; dopamine (2–3 μg/kg/min) and mannitol (1 g/kg) can be administered to optimize renal perfusion and stimulate prompt diuresis; red blood transfusion is quite a common procedure to avoid anemia due to dilution [35]. Occasionally, calcium channel antagonists such as verapamil or papaverine are injected into or simply onto the arterial anastomosis to overcome arterial spasm. Fluid management in the early postoperative period is balanced on the urine volume; some centers supply one to one for urine output less than 200 ml/h and 0.8–1 for greater volume of urine until the young recipient reaches an adequate oral fluid intake.

31.6.6 Graft Dysfunction and Causes

Several complications, surgical and medical, may occur in the transplanted kidney in the different phases of the postoperative period.

Technical complications are represented by arterial or venous thrombosis or stenosis, ureteral leak, stenosis or reflux, and fluid collection (hematoma, sieroma, lymphoceles). Graft thrombosis is a common cause of graft loss in children; it is likely to be related to the disparity between vascular diameters of the donor and recipient and to vascular compromise at the time of surgery. Vascular complications are most severe and frequent in children; they occur from 4 to 18 % according to different experiences. Some studies report better outcome when the vascular anastomosis was performed into the IVC and aorta [36, 37]; other authors use them only if technically necessary [38]. The incidence of ureteric complications (leakage or stenosis) is variable between 7 and 12 %.

31.6.7 Living-Donor Nephrectomy

Most authors suggest that the best option for pediatric patient is first, living-donor transplantation [39]; second, adult-sized deceased donor [40]; and the last one, pediatric donor preferably

>6 years of age [41]. Living-donor nephrectomy is nowadays considered a safe procedure for the donor, subjected to a mortality rate inferior to the 0.03 %. Different surgical techniques to harvest a kidney from living donors have been described. The conventional methods of donor nephrectomy have been challenged by potentially less invasive surgical procedures using laparoscopic techniques or minimally invasive approach in order to limit the donor pain, scarring, morbidity in favor of a short hospital stay, and a fast return to work.

Operating a healthy person who has not received direct therapeutic benefit exposes the surgeon to unusual challenges; the principle of "*primum non nocere*" became extremely important. The entire process of donation from the selection of the donor to the choice of the surgical procedure is ruled by the principle of not to damage the donor and leave the "better kidney" with him.

In the classic transperitoneal approach, the kidney is harvested through a midline or left/right subcostal incision, whereby the peritoneum is opened. In the lumbar approach, the incision is performed underneath the 12th rib (in the most of cases, rib resection is not necessary) or above it; the procedure is completely extraperitoneal, and care must be taken not to open the pleural space. Since 1995 when the first laparoscopic donor nephrectomy has been performed by Ratner [42], the laparoscopic approach has found a worldwide expansion. Developments have included not only better instruments but also new operative techniques such as introduction of hand-assisted [43] laparoscopic approaches [44] and then hand-assisted retroperitoneal approaches [45]. Overcome some concerns over the safety of laparoscopic procedures, it is now considered a feasible and safe procedure for donor and recipient [46].

A Cochrane review published in 2011 comparing open to laparoscopic procedures (different approaches) [47] concluded that laparoscopic donor nephrectomy is associated with reduced analgesia use, shorter hospital stay, and faster return to normal physical functioning. The number of complication and the incidence of perioperative events requiring further intervention are equivalent in the two approaches. Open nephrectomy is associated with shorter operating time when compared to the laparoscopic one; kidneys obtained laparoscopically were exposed to longer warm ischemia period with no associated short-term consequence.

Recipient outcome (DGF rate, decreasing in serum creatinine, and short-term outcome) has been demonstrated to be equivalent with laparoscopic or open nephrectomy.

Hand-assisted technique has been introduced to increase safety and to facilitate the operation. The incision for extracting the kidney is used to insert a hand in the operative field, maintaining the pneumoperitoneum. The tactile feedback makes it easier to learn the procedure, limits the risks connected to the learning curve, permits a rapid extraction of the kidney, and reduces the operating time and its costs [48, 49].

The retroperitoneoscopic procedure combines the advantages of the retroperitoneal approach (reduced risk of visceral injuries, bowel obstruction, and postoperative adhesions) to the better outcome offered by laparoscopic surgery (less pain, better cosmetic result, faster return to work). The technique has found fairly wide acceptance in the urological community; the results of this are so far encouraging, though the smaller operative field is a potential disadvantage [50].

Concluding, an open minimally invasive or laparoscopic approach is now considered the best option for living-donor nephrectomy. The choice between minimally invasive and laparoscopic, and between the different laparoscopic techniques, should be based on the local expertise of the surgeons [51].

References

1. Morris PJ (2004) Transplantation – a medical miracle of the 20th century. N Engl J Med 351(26):2678–2680
2. Horslen S, Barr ML, Christensen LL, Ettenger R, Magee JC (2007) Pediatric transplantation in the United States, 1996–2005. Am J Transplant 7:1339–1358
3. Butani L, Perez RV (2011) Effect of pre-transplant dialysis modality and duration on long-term outcomes of children receiving renal transplants. Transplantation 91(4):447–451
4. Van Stralen KJ, Tizard EJ, Verrina E, Schaefer F, Jager KJ, European Society for Paediatric Nephrology/ European Renal Association-European Dialysis and

Transplant Association (ESPN/ERA-EDTA) registry study group (2010) Demographics of pediatric renal replacement therapy in Europe: 2007 annual report of the ESPN/ERA-EDTA registry. Pediatr Nephrol 25(7): 1379–1382
5. Smith JM, Martz K, Blydt-Hansen TD (2013) Pediatric kidney transplant practice patterns and outcome benchmarks, 1987–2010: a report of the North American Pediatric Renal Trials and Collaborative Studies. Pediatr Transplant 17(2):149–157
6. McDonald SP, Craig JC, Australian and New Zealand Paediatric Nephrology Association (2014) Long-term survival of children with end-stage renal disease. N Engl J Med 350(26):2654–2662
7. Gillen DL, Stehman-Breen CO, Smith JM et al (2008) Survival advantage of pediatric recipients of a first kidney transplant among children awaiting kidney transplantation. Am J Transplant 8:2600–2606
8. Harambat J, van Stralen KJ, Schaefer F, Grenda R, Jankauskiene A, Kostic M, Macher MA, Maxwell H, Puretic Z, Raes A, Rubik J, Sørensen SS, Toots U, Topaloglu R, Tönshoff B, Verrina E, Jager KJ (2013) Disparities in policies, practices and rates of pediatric kidney transplantation in Europe. Am J Transplant 13(8):2066–2074
9. Matas AJ, Smith JM, Skeans MA, Thompson B, Gustafson SK, Schnitzler MA, Stewart DE, Cherikh WS, Wainright JL, Snyder JJ, Israni AK, Kasiske BL (2014) OPTN/SRTR 2012 annual data report: kidney. Am J Transplant 14(Suppl 1):11–44
10. Gritsch HA, Veale JL, Leichtman AB et al (2008) Should pediatric patients wait for HLA-DR–matched renal transplants? Am J Transplant 8:2056–2061
11. Abraham EC, Wilson AC, Goebel J (2009) Current kidney allocation rules and their impact on a pediatric transplant center. Am J Transplant 9:404–408
12. Mage JC, Krishnan SM, Benfield MR et al (2010) Pediatric transplantation in the United States, 1997–2006. Am J Transplant 8(part 2):935–945
13. http://srtr.transplant.hrsa.gov/annual_reports/2010
14. North American Pediatric Renal Trials and Collaborative Studies (2010) NAPRTCS annual transplant report. Available online at: https://web.emmes.com/study/ped/annlrept/annlrept.html
15. Webster A, Woodroffe RC, Taylor RS, Chapman JR, Craig JC (2005) Tacrolimus versus cyclosporine as primary immunosuppression for kidney transplant recipients. Cochrane Database Syst Rev 19;(4)
16. Grenda R, Watson A, Trompeter R, Tönshoff B, Jaray J, Fitzpatrick M, Murer L, Vondrak K, Maxwell H, van Damme-Lombaerts R, Loirat C, Mor E, Cochat P, Milford DV, Brown M, Webb NJ (2010) A randomized trial to assess the impact of early steroid withdrawal on growth in pediatric renal transplantation: the TWIST study. Am J Transplant 10(4):828–836
17. Sampaio MS, Poommipanit N, Kuo HT, Reddy PN, Cho YW, Shah T, Bunnapradist S (2010) Induction therapy in pediatric kidney transplant recipients discharged with a triple drug immunosuppressive regimen. Pediatr Transplant 14(6):770–778
18. Mendiz Abal S, Estornell F, Zamora I et al (2005) Renal transplantation in children with severe bladder dysfunction. J Urol 173:226–229
19. Lawrenson R, Wyndaele JJ, Vlachonikolis I et al (2001) Renal failure in patients with neurogenic lower urinary tract dysfunction. Neuroepidemiology 20:138–143
20. Broniszczak D, Ismail H, Nachulewicz P, Szymczak M, Drewniak T, Markiewicz-Kijewska M, Kowalski A, Jobs K, Smirska E, Rubik J, Skobejko-Włodarska L, Gastoł P, Mikołajczyk A, Kalicinski P (2010) Kidney transplantation in children with bladder augmentation or ileal conduit diversion. Eur J Pediatr Surg 20(1):5–10
21. Nahas WC, Mazzucchi E, Arap MA et al (2003) How to deal with children with end-stage renal disease and severe bladder dysfunction. Transplant Proc 35: 849–850
22. Luke PP, Herz DB, Bellinger MF et al (2003) Long-term results of pediatric renal transplantation into a dysfunctional lower urinary tract. Transplantation 76:1578–1582
23. Hatch DA, Koyle MA, Baskin LS et al (2001) Kidney transplantation in children with urinary diversion or bladder augmentation. J Urol 165:2265–2268
24. Crowe A, Cairns HS, Wood S et al (1998) Renal transplantation following renal failure due to urological disorders. Nephrol Dial Transplant 13:2065–2069
25. ElSheemy MS et al (2014) Surgical complications and graft function following live donor extraperitoneal renal transplantation in children 20Kg or less. J Pediatr Urol. doi:10.1016/j.jpurol.2013.12.013
26. Shapiro R, Sarwal MM (2010) Pediatric kidney transplantation. Pediatr Clin N Am 57(2):393–400
27. Karpelowsky JS, Thomas G, Shun A (2009) Definitive abdominal wall closure using a porcine intestinal submucosa biodegradable membrane in pediatric transplantation. Pediatr Transplant 13:285–289
28. El-Sabrout R, Buch K (2005) Outcome of renal transplants from pediatric donors <5 yr of age. Clin Transpl 19:316
29. Mohanka R, Bsau A, Shapiro R, Kayler LK (2008) Single versus en bloc kidney transplantation from pediatric donors less than or equal to 15 kg. Transplantation 86:264
30. Foss A, Gunther A, Line PD et al (2008) Long-term clinical outcome of paediatric kidneys transplanted to adults. Nephrol Dial Transplant 23:726
31. Butani L, Troppmann C, Perez R (2013) Outcomes of children receiving en bloc renal transplant from small pediatric donors. Ped Transplant 17:55–58
32. Zhao WY, Zhang L, Zhu YH, Chen Y, Zhu FY, Shen Q, Xu H, Zeng L (2014) En bloc kidneys transplanted from infant donors less than 5 kg into pediatric recipients. Transplantation 97(5):555–8
33. Gallinat A, Sotiropoulos GC, Witzke O, Treckmann JW, Molmenti EP, Paul A, Vester U (2013) Kidney grafts from donors ≤ 5 yr of age: single kidney transplantation for pediatric recipients or en bloc transplantation for adults? Pediatr Transplant 17(2): 179–184

34. Lau KK, Berg GM, Schjoneman YG, Perez RV, Butani L (2010) Pediatric en bloc kidney transplantation into pediatric recipients. Pediatr Transplant 14:100–104
35. Salvatierra O Jr, Singh T, Shifrin R et al (1998) Successful transplantation of adult-sized kidneys into infants requires maintenance of high aortic blood flow. Transplantation 66:819–823
36. Becker T, Neipp M, Reichart B, Pape L et al (2006) Pediatric kidney transplantation in small children-a single centre experience. Transpl Int 19:197–202
37. Adam J, Gudemann C, Tonshoff B, Mehls O, Wiesel M (2001) Renal transplantation in small children in small children-a comparison between surgical procedures. Eur Urol 40:552–556
38. Mickelson JJ, MacNeily AE, Leblanc J, White C, Gourlay WA (2006) Renal transplantation in children 15Kg or less: the British Columbia Children's Hospital experience. J Urol 176:1797–1800
39. Humar A, Remucal M, Matas A, Cook ME, Matas AJ, Najarian JS (1998) Kidney transplantation in children younger than 1 year using cyclosporine immunosuppression. Ann Surg 228:421–428
40. Neipp M, Ofner G, Luck R et al (2002) Kidney transplantation in children weighing less than 15 kg: donor considerations and technical considerations. Transplantation 73:409–416
41. Mcenery PT, Stablein DM, Arbus G, Tejani A (1992) Renal transplantation in children: a report of the North American Pediatric Renal Transplant Cooperative Study. N Engl J Med 326:1727–1732
42. Ratner LE, Ciseck LJ, Moore RG et al (1995) Laparoscopic live donor nephrectomy. Transplantation 60:1047–1049
43. Wolf JS Jr, Tchetgen MB, Merion RM (1998) Hand-assisted laparoscopic live donor nephrectomy. Urology 52:885–887
44. Gill IS, Rassweiler JJ (1999) Retroperitoneoscopic renal surgery: our approach. Urology 54:734–738
45. Wadstrom J, Lindstrom P (2002) Hand-assisted retroperitoneoscopic living donor nephrectomy; initial 10 cases. Transplantation 73:1839–1840
46. Matas AJ, Bartlett ST, Leichtman AB, Delmonico FL (2003) Morbidity and mortality after living kidney donation, 1999–2001: survey of United States transplant centers. Am J Transplant 3:830–834
47. Wilson CH, Sanni A, Rix DA, Soomro NA (2011) Laparoscopic versus open nephrectomy for live kidney donors. Cochrane Database Syst Rev 9;(11)
48. Slakey DP, Wood JC, Hender D, Thomas R, Cheng S (1999) Laparoscopic living donor nephrectomy: advantages of the hand assisted method. Transplantation 68:581–583
49. Lindstrom P, Haggman M, Wadstrom J (2002) Hand assisted laparoscopic surgery (HALS) for live donor nephrectomy is more time- and cost-effective than standard laparoscopic nephrectomy. Surg Endosc 16:422–425
50. Gill IS, Uzzo RG, Hobart MG et al (2000) Laparoscopic retroperitoneal live donor right nephrectomy for purpose of allotransplantation and autotransplantation. J Urol 164:1500–1504
51. Abramowicz D, Cochat P, Claas FH et al (2014) European renal best practice guide on kidney donor and recipient evaluation and perioperative care. Nephrol Dial Transplant 9; doi: 10.1093/ndt/gft218 http://ndt.oxfordjournals.org/ at Oxford Journals

Index

M. Lima, G. Manzoni (eds.), *Pediatric Urology: Contemporary Strategies from Fetal Life to Adolescence*,
DOI 10.1007/978-88-470-5693-0, © Springer-Verlag Italia 2015

P

Q

R

S

W

Y

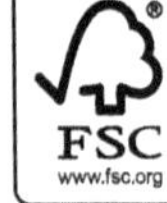

MIX
Papier aus verantwortungsvollen Quellen
Paper from responsible sources
FSC® C105338

If you have any concerns about our products,
you can contact us on
ProductSafety@springernature.com

In case Publisher is established outside the EU,
the EU authorized representative is:
Springer Nature Customer Service Center GmbH
Europaplatz 3, 69115 Heidelberg, Germany

Printed by Libri Plureos GmbH
in Hamburg, Germany